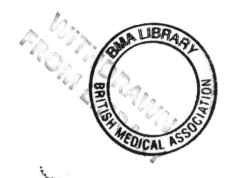

A Companion to Specialist Surgical Practice

Series Editors

O. James Garden
Simon Paterson-Brown

HEPATOBILIARY AND PANCREATIC SURGERY

SIXTH EDITION

Edited by

Rowan W. Parks

MBBCh BAO MD FRCSI FRCS(Ed)

Professor of Surgical Sciences, Clinical Surgery, The University of Edinburgh;
Honorary Consultant HPB Surgeon, Royal Infirmary of Edinburgh, Edinburgh, UK

For additional online content visit ExpertConsult.com

ELSEVIER Edinburgh   London   New York   Oxford   Philadelphia   St Louis   Sydney   2019

ELSEVIER

First edition 1997
Second edition 2001
Third edition 2005
Fourth edition 2009
Fifth edition 2014
Sixth edition 2019

Notice

Practitioners and researchers must always rely on their own experience and knowledge in evaluating and using any information, methods, compounds or experiments described herein. Because of rapid advances in the medical sciences, in particular, independent verification of diagnoses and drug dosages should be made. To the fullest extent of the law, no responsibility is assumed by Elsevier, authors, editors or contributors for any injury and/or damage to persons or property as a matter of products liability, negligence or otherwise, or from any use or operation of any methods, products, instructions, or ideas contained in the material herein.

ISBN: 978-0-7020-7250-5

Printed in China
Last digit is the print number: 9   8   7   6   5   4   3   2

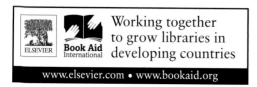

Working together
to grow libraries in
developing countries

www.elsevier.com • www.bookaid.org

Content Strategist: Laurence Hunter
Content Development Specialist: Lynn Watt
Project Manager: Umarani Natarajan
Design: Miles Hitchen
Illustration Manager: Nichole Beard
Illustrator: MPS North America LLC

Contents

Contents

Series Editors' preface

The *Companion to Specialist Surgical Practice* series has now come of age. This Sixth Edition takes the series to a different level since it was first published in 1997. The intention from the outset was to ensure that we could support the educational needs of those in the later years of specialist surgical training and of consultant surgeons in independent practice who wished for contemporary, evidence-based information on the subspecialist areas relevant to their general surgical practice. Although there still seems to be a role for larger reference surgical textbooks, and having contributed to many of these, we appreciate that it is difficult for them to keep pace with changing surgical practice.

This Sixth Edition continues to keep abreast of the increasing specialisation in general surgery. The rise of minimal access surgery and therapy, and the desire of some subspecialities, such as breast and vascular surgery, to separate away from 'general surgery' may have proved challenging in some countries. However, they also underline the importance for all surgeons of being aware of current developments in their surgical field. This series as a consequence continues to place emphasis on the need for surgeons to deliver a high-quality emergency surgical practice. The importance of evidence-based practice remains throughout, and authors have provided recommendations and highlighted key resources within each chapter. The ebook version of the textbook has also enabled improved access to the reference abstracts and links to video content relevant to many of the chapters.

We have recognised in this Sixth Edition that new blood is required to maintain the vitality of content. We are indebted to the volume editors, and contributors, who have stood down since the last edition and welcome the new leadership on several volumes. The contents have been comprehensively updated by our contributors and editorial team. We remain grateful for the support and encouragement of Laurence Hunter and Lynn Watt at Elsevier. We trust that our original vision of delivering an up-to-date affordable text has been met and that readers, whether in training or independent practice, will find this Sixth Edition an invaluable resource.

O. James Garden, CBE, BSc, MBChB, MD, FRCS (Glas), FRCS(Ed), FRCP(Ed), FRACS(Hon), FRCSC (Hon), FACS(Hon), FCSHK(Hon), FRCSI(Hon), FRCS(Engl)(Hon), FRSE
Regius Professor of Clinical Surgery, Clinical Surgery, The University of Edinburgh and Honorary Consultant Surgeon, Royal Infirmary of Edinburgh, Edinburgh, UK

Simon Paterson-Brown, MBBS, MPhil, MS, FRCS(Ed), FRCS(Engl), FCSHK, FFST(RCSEd)
Honorary Clinical Senior Lecturer, Clinical Surgery, The University of Edinburgh and Consultant General and Upper Gastrointestinal Surgeon, Royal Infirmary of Edinburgh, Edinburgh, UK

Editors' preface

The Sixth Edition of *Hepatobiliary and Pancreatic Surgery* builds on the strong foundation provided by my colleague Professor James Garden, who edited the previous five editions and kindly invited me to join him as co-editor for the Fifth Edition. Over the past 20 years, this volume and, indeed, the entire *Companion to Specialist Surgical Practice* series, has become well established with a remarkable reputation. It is a privilege to be able to build on this legacy.

Each new edition brings the opportunity to update and refresh the content and format of the book. For this Sixth Edition, half of the chapters have been delivered by new contributors and, in particular, there is a new section on liver transplantation and an entirely new chapter on pancreas and islet transplantation.

The aim has been to secure further leading international experts to ensure contemporary, evidence-based content on the various aspects of benign and malignant liver, biliary and pancreatic disease. All chapters have been brought up to date with new content highlighting current guidelines and practice, with high-quality images, figures and video content to enhance the resources available to the reader.

Acknowledgements

I am indebted to the input of all previous editions' contributors and, as in selected areas some of the core content has been retained. I would especially like to acknowledge Steven Strasberg, Jean-Francois Gigot, Rene Adam, Graham Poston, Geoffrey Haydon, John Isaac, John Buckels, Simon Olliff, Richard Schlinkert, Leslie Nathanson, Murat Akyol and Jacob Izbicki. I am grateful to colleagues at Elsevier, particularly Laurence Hunter and Lynn Watt, for their guidance and encouragement during this project and for trying to keep progress on schedule. I would also wish to acknowledge the tremendous support and tolerance of my wife, Janet, and my children, Matthew, Amy, Naomi and Thomas, in allowing me to deliver this volume.

Rowan W. Parks
Edinburgh

Evidence-based practice in surgery

Critical appraisal for developing evidence-based practice can be obtained from a number of sources, the most reliable being randomised controlled clinical trials, systematic literature reviews, meta-analyses and observational studies. For practical purposes three grades of evidence can be used, analogous to the levels of 'proof' required in a court of law:

1. **Beyond all reasonable doubt.** Such evidence is likely to have arisen from high-quality randomised controlled trials, systematic reviews or high-quality synthesised evidence such as decision analysis, cost-effectiveness analysis or large observational datasets. The studies need to be directly applicable to the population of concern and have clear results. The grade is analogous to burden of proof within a criminal court and may be thought of as corresponding to the usual standard of 'proof' within the medical literature (i.e. $P < 0.05$).

2. **On the balance of probabilities.** In many cases a high-quality review of literature may fail to reach firm conclusions due to conflicting or inconclusive results, trials of poor methodological quality or the lack of evidence in the population to which the guidelines apply. In such cases it may still be possible to make a statement as to the best treatment on the 'balance of probabilities'. This is analogous to the decision in a civil court where all the available evidence will be weighed up and the verdict will depend upon the balance of probabilities.

3. **Not proven.** Insufficient evidence upon which to base a decision, or contradictory evidence.

Depending on the information available, three grades of recommendation can be used:

a. Strong recommendation, which should be followed unless there are compelling reasons to act otherwise.

b. A recommendation based on evidence of effectiveness, but where there may be other factors to take into account in decision-making, for example the user of the guidelines may be expected to take into account patient preferences, local facilities, local audit results or available resources.

c. A recommendation made where there is no adequate evidence as to the most effective practice, although there may be reasons for making a recommendation in order to minimise cost or reduce the chance of error through a locally agreed protocol.

✔✔ Evidence where a conclusion can be reached **'beyond all reasonable doubt'** and therefore where a **strong recommendation** can be given. This will normally be based on evidence levels:
- Ia. Meta-analysis of randomised controlled trials
- Ib. Evidence from at least one randomised controlled trial
- IIa. Evidence from at least one controlled study without randomisation
- IIb. Evidence from at least one other type of quasi-experimental study.

✔ Evidence where a conclusion might be reached **'on the balance of probabilities'** and where there may be other factors involved which influence the recommendation given. This will normally be based on less conclusive evidence than that represented by the double tick icons:
- III. Evidence from non-experimental descriptive studies, such as comparative studies and case–control studies
- IV. Evidence from expert committee reports or opinions or clinical experience of respected authorities, or both.

Evidence that is associated with either a **strong recommendation** or **expert opinion** is highlighted in the text in panels such as those shown above, and is distinguished by either a double or single tick icon, respectively. The references associated with double-tick evidence are listed as Key References at the end of each chapter, along with a short summary of the paper's conclusions where applicable. The full reference list for each chapter is available in the ebook.

The reader is referred to Chapter 1, 'Evaluation of surgical evidence' in the volume *Core Topics in General and Emergency Surgery* of this series, for a more detailed description of this topic.

Contributors

Ian J. Beckingham, DM, FRCS
Department of Surgery, Queens Medical Centre,
Nottingham, UK

Adam Brooks, MBA, MBChB, FRCS
Consultant HPB Surgeon and Director, East
Midlands Major Trauma Centre, Nottingham
University Hospital NHS Trust, Nottingham, UK

Olivier R.C. Busch, MD, PhD
Gastrointestinal Surgeon, Department
of Surgery, Academic Medical Center, Amsterdam,
The Netherlands

C. Ross Carter, MD, FRCS
West of Scotland Pancreatic Unit, Glasgow Royal
Infirmary, Glasgow, UK

**John Casey, PhD, MBChB, PhD, FRCS(Glasg),
FRCS(Ed), FRCS(Gen Surg), FRCP Edin**
Consultant Surgeon/Hon Senior Lecturer,
Lead Clinician for Transplantation in Scotland,
Lead Clinician for National Islet Transplant
Programme, Chair NHSBT UK Pancreas
Advisory Group, Transplant Unit, Royal Infirmary
of Edinburgh, Edinburgh, UK

Steve M.M. de Castro, PhD, MD
Department of Surgery, OLVG, Amsterdam,
The Netherlands

**Kevin C. Conlon, MBMCh, FRCSI, FRCSEd,
FRCSGlas, FACS, MBA, MA, FTCD**
Professor and Academic Head, Department
of Surgery, Trinity College Dublin; Consultant
Hepatobiliary Surgeon, Department of HPB
Surgery, St Vincent's University Hospital,
Dublin, Ireland

Saxon Connor, MBChB, FRACS
HPB Surgeon, Department of Surgery,
Christchurch Hospital, Christchurch,
New Zealand

Otto M. van Delden, MD, PhD
Department of Radiology, Academic Medical Centre,
Amsterdam, The Netherlands

Cornelis H.C. Dejong, MD, PhD, FRCSED, FEBS
Professor of HPB Surgery, Department of Surgery,
European Surgical Centre Aachen-Maastricht
(ESCAM), Maastricht University Medical Centre,
Maastricht, The Netherlands; Universitätsklinikum
Aachen, Aachen, Germany

Euan J. Dickson, MBChB, MD, FRCS
Consultant Surgeon, West of Scotland Pancreatic
Unit, Glasgow Royal Infirmary, Glasgow, UK

Mary E. Dillhoff, MD, MS
Assistant Professor of Surgery, Department of
Surgery, The Ohio State University Wexner Medical
Center, Columbus, OH, USA

Marcel den Dulk, MD, PhD, FRCS
Consultant HPB and Pediatric Surgeon, Department
of Surgery, European Surgical Centre Aachen-
Maastricht (ESCAM), Maastricht University Medical
Centre, Maastricht, The Netherlands;
Universitätsklinikum Aachen, Aachen, Germany

Olivier Farges, MD, PhD
Department of Surgery, Hôpital Beaujon,
Assistance Publique-Hôpitaux de Paris, University
Paris, Clichy, France

**Stephen W. Fenwick, BMedSci, BMBS,
MD, FRCS**
Consultant Hepatobiliary Surgeon, Department of
Hepatobiliary Surgery, Aintree University Hospital,
Liverpool, UK

Steven Gallinger, MD, MSc, FRCSC
Professor of Surgery, Division of General Surgery
Toronto General Hospital, University Health Network,
University of Toronto, Toronto, Canada

**O. James Garden, CBE, BSc, MBChB, MD
FRCS(Glas), FRCS(Ed), FRCP(Ed), FRACS(Hon),
FRCSC(Hon), FACS(Hon), FCSHK(Hon),
FRCSI(Hon), FRCSEng(Hon), FRSE**
Regius Professor of Clinical Surgery, Clinical
Surgery, The University of Edinburgh and Honorary
Consultant Surgeon, Royal Infirmary of Edinburgh,
Edinburgh, UK

Contributors

William R. Jarnagin, MD
Chief, Hepatopancreatobiliary Service, Benno C. Schmidt Professor of Surgical Oncology, Memorial Sloan-Kettering Cancer Center; Professor of Surgery, Weill Cornell Medical College, New York, NY, USA

Geoffrey W. Krampitz, MD, PhD
General Surgery Resident, Department of Surgery, Stanford University School of Medicine, Stanford, CA, USA

Russell C. Langan, MD
Memorial Sloan Kettering Cancer Center, Surgery, Surgical Oncology, New York, NY, USA

Chetana Lim, MD, PhD
HPB and Liver Transplantation, Henri Mondor Hospital, Creteil, France

Shishir K. Maithel, MD, FACS
Associate Professor of Surgery, Division of Surgical Oncology, Department of Surgery, Emory University, Winship Cancer Institute, Atlanta, GA, USA

Colin J. McKay, MBChB, MD, FRCS
Consultant Pancreatic Surgeon, West of Scotland Pancreatic Unit, Glasgow Royal Infirmary, Glasgow, UK

Carol-anne Moulton, MEd, PhD, FRACS
Associate Professor, Department of Surgery, University of Toronto, Canada

Alex P. Navarro, MBBS, BMedSci(Hons), FRCS, PhD
Consultant HPB and Major Trauma Surgeon, Queens Medical Centre, Nottingham University Hospitals NHS Trust, Nottingham, UK

Stephen O'Neill, MSc, PhD
Surgical Registrar, HPB and Transplant Surgery, Royal Infirmary of Edinburgh, Edinburgh, UK

Gabriel C. Oniscu, MD, FRCS
Consultant Transplant Surgeon, Transplant Unit, Royal Infirmary of Edinburgh; Honorary Clinical Senior Lecturer, Clinical Surgery, University of Edinburgh, Edinburgh, UK

Timothy M. Pawlik, MD, MPH, PhD
Professor and Chair, The Urban Meyer III and Shelley Meyer Chair for Cancer Research; Department of Surgery, The Ohio State University Wexner Medical Center, Columbus, OH, USA

Amir A. Rahnemai-Azar, MD
Surgical Oncology Fellow, Department of Surgery, Division of Surgical Oncology, University of Wisconsin Hospital, Madison, WI, USA

Shaheel M. Sahebally, MB, MRCS
Department of Hepatobiliary Surgery, St Vincent's University Hospital, Dublin, Ireland

Carl Schmidt, MD
Associate Professor of Surgery, Department of Surgery, The Ohio State University Wexner Medical Center, Columbus, OH, USA

Ajith K. Siriwardena, MD, FRCS
Professor of Hepatobiliary Surgery, Regional Hepato-Pancreato-Biliary Unit, Manchester Royal Infirmary, Manchester, UK

Benjamin M. Stutchfield, BSc(Hons), MBChB, MSc, MRCS(Ed), PhD
Clinical Lecturer and Honorary Surgical Registrar, University of Edinburgh, Edinburgh, UK

Andrew Sutherland, MBChB, BSc(Hons), DPhil, FRCSEd
Consultant Surgeon, Transplant Surgery, Royal Infirmary of Edinburgh, Edinburgh, UK

Benjamin N.J. Thomson, MBBS, DMedSc, FACS, FRACS
Clinical Associate Professor, The University of Melbourne; HPB Surgeon & Head of General Surgical Specialties, The Royal Melbourne Hospital, Parkville, Victoria, Australia

Brendan Visser, MD
Associate Professor of Surgery, Hepatobiliary and Pancreatic Surgery, Stanford University School of Medicine, Stanford, CA, USA

Stephen J. Wigmore, BSc(Hons), MBBS, MD, FRCSEd, FRCS(Gen Surg), FRCPEd
Professor of Transplantation Surgery, Clinical Surgery, The University of Edinburgh; Honorary Consultant Surgeon, Royal Infirmary of Edinburgh, Edinburgh, UK

Vincent S. Yip, MBChB, MD, FRCS
Consultant in HPB Surgery, Department of Surgery, Royal Liverpool and Broadgreen University Hospital, Liverpool, UK

Nathan Zilbert, MD, MEd, FRCSC
Hepato-Pancreato-Biliary Surgery Fellow, Department of Surgery, University of Toronto, Toronto, Ontario Canada

1

Liver function and failure

Benjamin M. Stutchfield
Stephen J. Wigmore

Overview of liver functions and evolution

The liver is the largest solid organ in the human body. It has a unique structure with a dual blood supply, being approximately one-third from the hepatic artery and two-thirds from the portal venous system. Within the liver substance blood flows through sinusoids between plates of hepatocytes to drain into central veins, which in turn join the hepatic veins draining into the vena cava. The liver is a major site of protein synthesis exporting plasma proteins to maintain oncotic pressure and coagulation factors. Acute phase proteins that act as antiproteases, opsonins and metal ion carriers are synthesised by the liver in response to injury or infection. Numerous immune cells populate the liver and the resident tissue macrophages, the Kupffer cells, form an important component of the innate immune system. Nutrients are extracted from portal blood by the liver and processed, and the liver acts as an important reservoir for glycogen. Waste products are either modified in the liver for excretion by the kidneys or are excreted into bile. Many drugs are taken up by the liver and metabolised, giving either active metabolites or inactive metabolites for excretion. In humans, as in many vertebrates, the liver's capacity for metabolism and clearance far exceeds what is required for day-to-day life. It is possible that this ability offers a significant advantage in terms of survival from poisoning, starvation or trauma.

Symptoms of liver failure: acute and chronic

In the acute setting, liver failure can present with a number of symptoms, but it is important to note that not all of these may be present at the same time. Typically, a patient with acute liver failure after surgery, transplantation or due to acute poisoning will be confused or mentally slow as a result of encephalopathy, which may progress to loss of consciousness and a need to protect the airway by intubation and mechanical ventilation. Patients are often not immediately jaundiced, but jaundice may develop over the course of several days. Patients may be hypoglycaemic and the requirement for intravenous infusion of dextrose is a sinister development and an indicator of severe acute liver failure. Coagulopathy may develop, with evidence of bruising or bleeding from line sites or surgical scars. Severe acute liver failure can be assessed using the King's College Hospital criteria, which were designed to predict mortality in paracetamol- and non-paracetamol-dependent acute liver failure.[1] Later, this scoring system was adopted in the UK to determine criteria indicating likely benefit from liver transplantation. In the surgical patient, the development of acute liver failure is usually more gradual and less dramatic; a useful scoring system for liver dysfunction in the acute setting has been reported by Schindl et al.[2] (see Box 1.1).

Box 1.1 • Definition of postoperative hepatic dysfunction based on results from blood tests and clinical observation

Total bilirubin (micromol/L)
<20 (0 points)
21–60 (1 point)
>60 (2 points)

Prothrombin time (seconds above normal)
<4 (0 points)
4–6 (1 point)
>6 (2 points)

Serum lactate (mmol/L)
≤1.5 (0 points)
1.6–3.5 (1 point)
>3.5 (2 points)

Encephalopathy grade (West haven Criteria)
None (0 points)
1 and 2 (1 point)
3 and 4 (2 points)

Severity of hepatic dysfunction
None = 0 points; mild = (1–2) points; moderate = (3–4) points; severe (>4) points

Adapted from Schindl MJ, Redhead DN, Fearon KC, et al. The value of residual liver volume as a predictor of hepatic dysfunction and infection after major liver resection. Gut 2005;54:289–96. With permission from the BMJ Publishing Group Ltd.

Common causes of acute liver failure: hepatic insufficiency following liver resection

Liver resection is the only treatment with the potential to cure patients with cancers that have originated in the liver itself (primary liver cancer) or that have originated elsewhere and have subsequently spread to the liver (metastatic liver cancer). Equally, it is a preferred therapy in patients with benign liver tumours that have the potential of malignant transformation (uncertain benign primary liver tumours). Resection of up to 70% of the liver is feasible, because the liver has a remarkable capacity to regenerate. Within 6–8 weeks following 60–70% hepatectomy, the liver has regained nearly its original size and weight.

The most common cause of liver metastases is from primary colorectal cancer, and it is estimated that in the West there is a yearly incidence of 300 new cases of colorectal liver metastases per million population. The current estimate is that this should lead to approximately 100–150 patients per million eligible for liver resection for this indication. To this should be added the patients with primary benign and malignant liver tumours, and hence about 150–200 liver resections should probably be performed per million population each year.

Ever since the first liver resection by Langenbuch in 1887, this procedure has remained a major undertaking and even in the recent past, liver resection was still a dangerous surgical procedure with a high mortality of 20–30% in the 1970s. This was mainly due to excessive intraoperative bleeding but, over the subsequent decades, the procedure has become increasingly safe due to improvements in surgical and anaesthetic techniques. At present, mortality rates are reported to be well below 5%. Currently, the single most important cause of lethal outcome following hepatic resection is liver failure. For this reason, many researchers and clinicians have attempted to design methods to identify patients at risk of liver failure (and hence mortality) following liver surgery. However, the development of such a method has been hampered by several factors, as outlined below.

The critical point determining lethal outcome following liver resection has been a failure of the residual liver to function properly. Focus in this research area has been to determine a single liver function test that identifies patients with impaired liver function. This has proven exceedingly difficult, and such a test is not available for a number of reasons.

First, as outlined above, the liver has a remarkable capacity to regenerate very rapidly, which emphasises that there is tremendous overcapacity of several liver functions. In this context, it is known that it is entirely safe to resect 50% of an otherwise healthy liver, because the residual half liver will simply take over all vital liver functions such as clearing bacteria, urea synthesis and synthesis of crucial proteins. It has been estimated that a crucial liver function, such as urea synthesis, has an overcapacity of 300%, which implies that a static preoperative liver function test will be unable to assess this particular function. An alternative and innovative strategy would be to give a challenge to the liver and measure the ability of the liver to respond or cope – a dynamic test.

✔✔ The critical minimum residual liver volume for healthy liver parenchyma has been estimated to be approximately 25% after resection.[2]

The second crucial problem has been that there is only a poor correlation between volume and function. However, it is still unclear why some patients with smaller hepatic remnants do not develop liver failure whilst some with greater residual volumes do. These observations suggest, however, that peri- and intraoperative events superimposed on the innate hepatic capacity to withstand injury play a role. Hepatic insufficiency in this situation may arise either if not enough liver volume is left after partial hepatectomy or if the residual volume does not function properly. A functional limitation may arise, for example, in patients who have received chemotherapy in order to reduce the number and size of metastases prior to surgical treatment by liver resection. One of the factors contributing to defective defence may be preoperative fasting,[3] but equally, prior chemotherapy and pre-existent steatosis may play a role.

A third important aspect is that during liver surgery, deliberate hypotension and temporary hepatic blood inflow occlusion (the so-called Pringle manoeuvre) are used by many surgeons to reduce blood loss during hepatic surgery (15 minutes ischaemia, 5 minutes reperfusion [15/5 Pringle]). Other surgeons do not use this manoeuvre, assuming that it causes oxidative stress and ischaemia/reperfusion (I/R) injury.[4,5] There is little doubt that this procedure does cause oxidative stress and I/R injury; however, the consequence of this is variable. In a situation where defence mechanisms against oxidative stress are deficient, it may adversely affect liver function. In this situation, hepatic steatosis may constitute an additional predisposing factor to damage by I/R.

✔✔ Ischaemia/reperfusion is the basis of ischaemic preconditioning, a process in which temporary clamping and release of the liver blood flow has been shown to be beneficial in terms of increasing resistance to subsequent injury.[6]

In this situation it is assumed that defence mechanisms against oxidative stress are adequate and are indeed enhanced by short-term I/R injury.[7]

The above three factors explain why it has been exceedingly difficult to design a proper liver function test that reliably singles out those patients at risk of liver failure following liver resection. The term 'liver function' is a rather crude denominator for a range of functions that includes ammonia detoxification, urea synthesis, protein synthesis and breakdown, bile synthesis and secretion, gluconeogenesis and detoxification of drugs, bacteria and bacterial toxins.

Chronic liver failure

The clinical signs of chronic liver failure are often insidious and can also be related to the type of disease. Cirrhosis is associated with a failure of hepatic function and the consequences of increased hepatic vascular resistance. Metabolic impairment is manifest by jaundice, coagulopathy, impaired ammonia clearance and encephalopathy, hypoalbuminaemia and oedema. The presence of increased vascular resistance is associated with the development of splenomegaly, ascites and gastro-oesophageal or abdominal wall varices. The slow progression of many chronic liver diseases, over years, implies a gradual, almost incremental, loss of liver cell mass or function. There are many causes of liver failure, including hepatitis B and C virus, autoimmune diseases such as primary biliary cirrhosis, primary sclerosing cholangitis and autoimmune hepatitis, alcoholic liver disease, Wilson's disease, α_1-antitrypsin deficiency and others. All are associated with chronic or repeated cell injury and attempts at repair. The fibrosis and scarring associated with this regeneration and repair lead to the clinical condition termed cirrhosis, with a typically small shrunken irregular liver and an increased risk of cancer.

The Child–Pugh score for chronic liver disease[8] has served as a useful means of categorising patients based on the severity of their liver disease. It employs five clinical measures of liver disease and each measure is scored 1–3, with 3 indicating the most severe derangement (Table 1.1). In the setting of liver transplantation, the Model for End-stage Liver Disease (MELD) or MELD-Na (MELD including sodium) score or in the United Kingdom UKELD score has replaced Child–Pugh scoring in the assessment of severity of liver disease.

Table 1.1 • Child–Pugh score for chronic liver disease

Measure	1 point	2 points	3 points	Units
Bilirubin (total)	<34 (<2)	34–50 (2,3)	>50 (>3)	µmol/L (mg/dL)
Serum albumin	>35	28–35	<28	g/L
INR	<1.7	1.71–2.20	>2.20	No unit
Ascites	None	Suppressed with medication	Refractory	No unit
Hepatic encephalopathy	None	Grade I–II (or suppressed with medication)	Grade III–IV (or refractory)	No unit

Child-Pugh A = 5–6 points; Child-Pugh B = 7–9 points; Child-Pugh C =10–15 points. 1 year survival: A = 100%; B = 80%; C = 45%.

Metabolic liver function

The liver plays a central role in fat, carbohydrate and protein metabolism, as well as in acid–base homeostasis. In the context of liver failure, disturbances of fat metabolism are probably not crucially important. With respect to carbohydrate metabolism, it is well known that the liver plays a central role in the conversion of lactate to glucose. Part of this lactate is formed due to anaerobic metabolism of, amongst others, glucose in skeletal muscle. This metabolic route of glucose to lactate (muscle) and then back to glucose (liver) is very important for glycaemic homeostasis and is called the Cori cycle. Liver failure will be manifested by lactic acidosis and hypoglycaemia.

Next to its role in carbohydrate metabolism, the liver plays a central function in nitrogen homeostasis. Hepatic synthesis and breakdown of proteins and amino acids, and detoxification and clearance of the nitrogenous waste products from other organs are of central importance. For example, the gut uses the amino acid glutamine as a fuel for enterocytes, which results in the production of waste end-products of intestinal metabolism, such as ammonia. This ammonia is then transported via the portal vein to the liver, where it is detoxified with the formation of urea.

Why do patients die from liver failure?

The failing liver can trigger a range of events resulting in multi-organ failure, sepsis and death. When three or more organs are involved, the chance of death approaches 80%.[9] Bacterial infection and hepatic encephalopathy are the leading causes of death in this group who experience progressive systemic failure.

Risk of bacterial infection is increased considerably following partial hepatectomy.[2] Immune function is compromised as the liver's phagocytic and synthetic capacity is impaired by its reduced size. The shear force generated by increased portal venous blood flow per unit area, as well as ischaemic injury at the time of surgery, can further impair immune capacity.[10] Management of sepsis in these patients necessitates intensive care multi-organ support and broad-spectrum antibiotics subsequently guided by culture results.

Hepatic encephalopathy is a reversible neuro-psychiatric syndrome, with multifactorial cause. It is characterised by cerebral oedema, raised intracranial pressure, with risk of brain herniation and death.[11] A range of factors may contribute to this phenomenon, including rising concentration of ammonia, glutamine and lactate. Ammonia has a range of effects on brain function, affecting neurotransmission as well as impairing mitochondrial function and key cellular transport systems. There is a direct correlation between arterial ammonia concentration and the presence of brain herniation.[12] Brain glutamine concentration is elevated in acute liver failure, which may influence the development of hepatic encephalopathy through toxic metabolites, modulation of hepatic blood flow or by amplifying the toxic effects of ammonia.[13] Lactate can result in significant swelling of astrocytes in culture[14] and raised brain lactate concentration is seen in a wide range of experimental models of acute liver failure.

Therapeutic approaches in hepatic encephalopathy aim to address these areas with strategies to lower ammonia levels, protect systems by inducing mild hypothermia, reduce blood–brain ammonia transfer, decrease brain lactate synthesis and reduce inflammation. However, in the face of overwhelming liver failure, attempts to modulate these mechanisms of hepatic encephalopathy have been shown at best to prolong life by hours to a few days. In some selected patients, this may provide a 'bridge to liver transplantation'; however, patients undergoing surgery for metastatic disease are ineligible for transplantation and therefore their only hope lies in the intrinsic ability of the liver to regenerate.

Assessment of the liver

Measuring liver volume

Advances in imaging techniques have permitted the development of in vivo imaging of the liver. Three-dimensional models of the liver can be constructed from computed tomography (CT) or other cross-sectional imaging modalities, such as magnetic resonance imaging (MRI). The volume of the liver can then be calculated based on known separation of image slices combined with planar mapping of cross-sectional areas. In addition, such three-dimensional computer models can be simulated to map the effects of surgery by performing virtual hepatic resection, and studies have demonstrated that there is a good correlation between computer modelling and actual resection weight of surgical liver specimens (**Figs 1.1–1.3**).[2,15] Some centres use 3D printers to create a replica of the patient's liver. This enables the relationship between the tumour and the vascular/biliary anatomy of the liver to be better understood, aiding complex liver resections.[16]

Blood tests of liver function

As part of many blood chemistry analyses, it is possible to request liver function tests. These tests

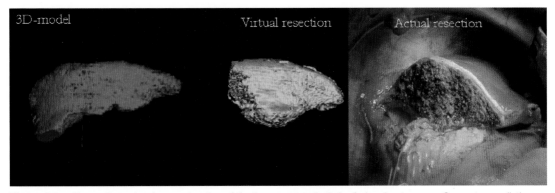

Figure 1.1 • Three-dimensional reconstruction of the liver preoperatively (red) showing tumours. Computer prediction of residual liver volume based on virtual hepatectomy of 3-D model (yellow) and actual photograph of resection showing residual liver segments.
Reproduced from Schindl MJ, Redhead DN, Fearon KC, et al. The value of residual liver volume as a predictor of hepatic dysfunction and infection after major liver resection. Gut 2005;54:289–96. With permission from the BMJ Publishing Group Ltd.

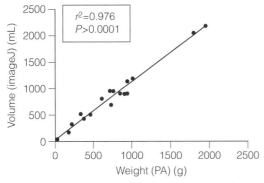

$r^2 = 0.976$
$P > 0.0001$

Figure 1.2 • Correlation between volume of resection calculated with ImageJ and actual measured weights of the resection specimens ($n = 15$, Pearson's test).
Reproduced with permission from Dello SA, van Dam RM, Slangen JJ, et al. Liver volumetry plug and play: do it yourself with ImageJ. World J Surg 2007;31(**11**):2215–21.

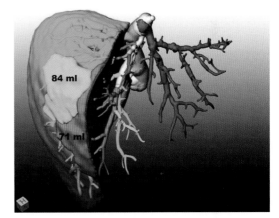

Figure 1.3 • Mapping the territory of the right hepatic lobe drained by the middle hepatic vein. The numbers represent the volumes of the territories at risk if segment 5 and 8 tributaries of the middle hepatic vein were not reconstructed in a potential right lobe living-donor liver transplant.
Reproduced with permission of MeVis imaging technologies, Bremen, Germany. Kindly provided by H. Lang and A. Radtke, Plainz, Germany.

refer to the transaminases, alkaline phosphatase, γ-glutamyl transferase and bilirubin. They are not truly measures of function but do give an indication of processes going on within the liver. Aspartate aminotransferase and alanine aminotransferase are hepatocyte enzymes that are released in conditions in which hepatocytes are damaged or killed, such as ischaemic injury, hepatitis, severe sepsis and in response to cancer. Liver-specific alkaline phosphatase is expressed predominantly in the biliary epithelium and is elevated in conditions such as cholangitis or biliary obstruction. γ-Glutamyl transferase is expressed by both hepatocytes and biliary epithelium, and can also be induced by high alcohol consumption.

Biochemical markers of true liver function vary depending on whether acute or chronic liver failure or injury is being considered (Table 1.2).

Table 1.2 • Blood tests useful to assess function in acute and chronic liver injury

	Acute	**Chronic**
Albumin	–	+++
Prothrombin time	+++	+++
Bilirubin	+	+++
Lactate	++	–
Glucose requirement	++	–
Ammonia	+	+

Tests of liver function measuring substance clearance

The ability to accurately predict postoperative outcome based on preoperative liver function would be a valuable addition to preoperative assessment. The tests currently in common use include the indocyanine green (ICG) clearance test, hepatobiliary scintigraphy with radioisotope clearance, lidocaine clearance test, the aminopyrine breath test and the galactose elimination test. These tests aim to provide an indicator of dynamic liver function, in that they can provide real-time assessment of liver function in response to a challenge. However, none of these tests challenge the liver to demonstrate its full functional capacity. Serum bilirubin and clotting factors provide a static indirect estimation of liver metabolism and synthetic function, but are influenced by a range of other factors that limit their relevance and suitability to predict postoperative outcome. The most commonly used test for liver function prior to liver resections is the ICG clearance test.

Indocyanine green (ICG)

ICG is a compound that is used widely to measure liver function. It is rapidly cleared from blood, specifically by hepatocytes, and is excreted into bile without enterohepatic circulation. Hepatocytes are highly effective at clearing ICG such that hepatic blood flow is the limiting factor in patients with otherwise normal liver parenchyma. In more severe liver disease both hepatic blood flow and hepatocyte function may be compromised, so impairing the clearance of ICG. ICG clearance can be measured as 'disappearance' from the blood or can also be measured as accumulation in bile. Liver dysfunction is suggested by a slower rate of clearance from the blood and is usually expressed as percentage retention at 5 or 15 minutes after injection. Continuous measurement of ICG clearance can also be performed, offering potentially improved accuracy, by measurement of the area under the clearance curve (**Fig. 1.4**). In some centres ICG clearance is routinely performed during preoperative work-up, with cut-off values set for which patients are 'safe' to proceed to resection. However, there is no evidence to suggest that outcomes are improved in centres that use this test compared to centres that do not. In chronic liver disease, the discriminative ability of ICG clearance is greatest in those with intermediate to severe liver failure. Addition of this test to the MELD score can improve prognostic accuracy for patients with intermediate to severe liver dysfunction.[17] However, given the relationship with hepatic blood flow, caution should be exercised when interpreting ICG clearance in the context of abnormally high cardiac output.

Hepatobiliary scintigraphy and SPECT

Using a radiolabelled tracer that is eliminated exclusively by the liver, such as [99mTc]mebrofenin (technetium is a gamma-emitting radioisotope), blood clearance and hepatic uptake can be measured using a gamma camera to provide an indication of hepatic function (**Fig. 1.5**). Hepatobiliary scintigraphy may improve predictive value compared to future liver remnant volume, especially in patients with uncertain quality of liver parenchyma.[18] Combining nuclear medicine techniques with CT (SPECT: single-photon emission computed tomography) enables the generation of a 3D image of liver function which can be related to liver volume. Using this technique, segmental liver function and liver functional volume can be calculated.

De Graaf et al. demonstrated in 2010 that by combining CT with [99mTc]mebrofenin SPECT, the function of the proposed future liver remnant can be accurately obtained.[19] This group, based at the Amsterdam Medical Centre, subsequently demonstrated that routine implementation of this technique for patients requiring major liver resection significantly reduced postoperative liver failure and failure-related mortality.[20] The authors reported that a better understanding of preoperative liver function improved patient selection and led to an increased use of portal vein embolisation to optimise the future liver remnant.

> ✔✔ Combining CT with nuclear medicine techniques enables regional liver function to be calculated and can be used to assess preoperative function.[19,20]

Lidocaine (MEG-X)

Lidocaine, also known as monoethylglycinexylidide (MEG-X), is a local anaesthetic that is taken up by the liver and undergoes biotransformation by a cytochrome P450 enzyme, CYP1A2. The rate of disappearance of lidocaine from plasma correlates with liver function; however, measurement of lidocaine is more complex than that of ICG.

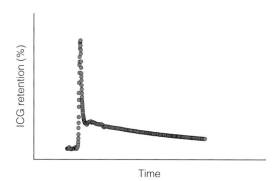

Figure 1.4 • Typical ICG clearance curve for a subject with healthy liver function.

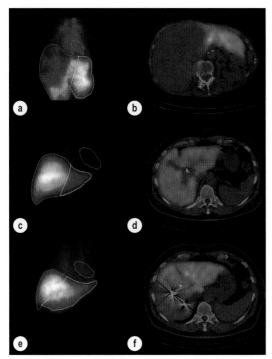

Figure 1.5 • Hepatobiliary scintigraphy before major liver surgery in a patient with a large hepatocellular carcinoma of the right liver **(a, b)** and a patient with a Klatskin type IIIa tumour before **(c, d)** and 3 weeks after portal vein embolisation **(e, f)**. Panels A and B show a large afunctional right-sided hepatic mass with sufficient future liver remnant function in segments 2–3. Panels C and D show relatively small liver segments 2–3 with insufficient future liver remnant function ($1\%/min/m^2$). Volume and function of segments 2–3 increased significantly after PVE (panels E and F) with sufficient future liver remnant function ($2.7\%/min/m^2$) for safe resection (extended right hemihepatectomy).
Images courtesy of R. Bennink, Amsterdam Medical Centre, Netherlands.

Aminopyrine breath test

The aminopyrine breath test was the first breath test proposed for the assessment of liver function in patients with liver disease. The test uses $^{13}C_2$-aminopyrine, which is a stable, non-radioactive, isotopically labelled compound eliminated almost exclusively by the liver. Following oral intake, the compound is taken up by the gut and then transported to the liver, where it is metabolised by microsomal cytochrome P450 function. This metabolism liberates $13CO_2$, which can be measured non-invasively in exhaled air. This test is not readily available at the bedside and requires fairly sophisticated apparatus to measure stable isotopic enrichment in the exhaled air. Induction of microsomal metabolism by various drugs may constitute a problem.

Urea synthesis

Recently, the feasibility of measuring urea synthesis using stable isotopes and relating this to liver volume in patients undergoing liver resection was explored.[21] As liver failure is almost always accompanied by hyperammonaemia, it was hypothesised that this is related to a presumed failure of hepatic urea synthesis. Using stable isotopically ^{13}C-labelled urea, urea synthesis was measured before and after major hepatic resection, and liver volumes before and after resection were determined using CT.

> ✅✅ Major hepatic resection did not affect total body ureagenesis, because the synthesis of urea per gram of residual liver increased 2.6-fold.[21] Therefore, it is unlikely that urea synthesis is a limiting factor in the initial aetiology of liver failure and this test is not likely to contribute to predicting liver failure following liver resection.

Glutathione synthesis

Unfortunately, most of the above tests focus on very specific functions or pathways. None of them assesses the main hepatic protection system against many diverse forms of stress and intoxications: the intracellular content and synthesis of glutathione (GSH). It is generally accepted that GSH plays a key role in the protection of the liver against many forms of stress, ischaemia and toxic compounds such as paracetamol. Unfortunately, there is currently no adequate test to assess hepatic GSH synthesis and metabolism in vivo in humans, even though such a test would be of great clinical importance. We have previously explored the feasibility of measuring GSH synthesis in vivo during liver surgery in humans using stable isotopically labelled $^{2}H_2$-glycine, a component of GSH (γ-glutamyl-cysteinyl-glycine), but this approach was not suitable, because part of the deuterium label of glycine was lost (unpublished data). Future research will have to focus on designing a test that is both dynamic and focuses on the GSH system, making it possible to determine liver function correlated to liver volume, and assess an individual's risk of developing liver failure following hepatic resection.

Measuring liver blood flow

Blood flow in the splanchnic area, particularly the gut and liver, can be measured in a number of ways. These can basically be either invasive (i.e. intraoperative) or non-invasive. During open abdominal surgery, blood flow can be measured in the portal vein and hepatic artery. Portal vein blood flow measurements provide predominantly information on the flow across the intestines. By summing up the blood flow in the hepatic artery and portal vein, total hepatic blood flow can be calculated. Theoretically, this could also be achieved by measuring hepatic venous outflow, but this is impractical in humans because of the short common outflow tract of the three hepatic veins. Non-invasive MRI-based techniques are being developed that may offer improved accuracy of measurement of liver blood flow and provide the potential for repeat measurements.[22] The ratio of portal vein to hepatic artery blood flow changes with increasing resistance of the liver and may indicate the development of fibrosis or cirrhosis. Methodology for assessing the importance of blood flow as a predictor of liver parenchymal condition has not been fully evaluated, but may provide a means of determining regenerative capacity and safety of surgery in some patients.

Such measurements of hepatic and portal arterial blood flow can be obtained using 6–8 mm and 12–14 mm handle ultrasonic flow probes (Transonic Systems, Kimal PLC, Uxbridge, UK). Essentially, the vessels have to be dissected free for this flow measurement and the three-quarters circular probe is applied to the vessel. These probes are believed to provide the most accurate technique for assessing flow in relatively small vessels. However, there is considerable variability in measurement related to Doppler ultrasound signal strength and coupling with the vessel wall. Also, there are likely to be changes in diameter of the artery, in particular related to its handling during surgery. However, the advantage is that repeated measurements can be obtained and the surgeon can operate this application without help from a radiologist. Furthermore, post-resection blood flow measurements can be taken before closure of the abdomen, typically 1–2 hours after the first measurement. This gives an impression of blood flow across the residual liver following major resection.

During liver surgery, organ blood flow can also be measured by means of colour Doppler ultrasound scanning (e.g. Aloka Prosound SSD 5000; Aloka Co. Ltd, Tokyo, Japan). A 5-MHz probe is used to trace the vessels and calculate the cross-sectional area. Then, time-averaged mean velocities of the bloodstream are measured at the point where the cross-sectional area of the portal vein and hepatic artery have been measured. For accurate velocity measurements, care must be taken to keep the angle between the ultrasonic beam direction and blood flow direction below 60°. If an accessory hepatic artery is present, flow in both arteries should obviously be measured.[23,24] In our experience, this method gives roughly the same values as the ultrasonic flow measurement described above. Theoretically, it is possible to perform such flow measurements preoperatively or postoperatively using a percutaneous approach, although the measurement in the hepatic artery requires a skilled ultrasonographer.

In recent years, technical improvements in hardware and software applications for MRI have made it possible to measure blood flow in the portal vein and hepatic artery non-invasively. By linking this method of flow measurement to hepatic volumetry, blood flow per volume unit of liver can be calculated.[25,26] It has been suggested that MRI may provide a more accurate and reliable assessment of portal vein and hepatic artery blood flow than ultrasonography, particularly given the wide interobserver variability seen with the latter technique.[22] Although limited to the preoperative period, MRI flow studies may provide complementary information to intraoperative ultrasonography.

A further technique that is emerging is the use of near-infrared spectroscopy. This technique measures absorption of near-infrared wavelength light and from this can be calculated tissue oxygenation, since haemoglobin oxygenation status alters absorption of this wavelength light. This technique is more useful for estimating tissue oxygenation and perfusion at a sinusoidal level, but could potentially be combined with other measures to estimate liver blood flow.[27]

Effect of major liver resection on hepatic blood flow

Direct measurement of hepatic artery and portal vein blood flow before and after liver resection reveals interesting results. When expressed as absolute values, portal blood flow does not change significantly whereas hepatic artery blood flow generally falls. Typically, portal vein flow is approximately 840 mL/min and post-resection 805 mL/min, whereas hepatic artery flow pre-resection is approximately 450 mL/min and post-resection 270 mL/min. When these flows are expressed in relation to the preoperative and residual postoperative liver volume, it can be seen that the portal blood flow increases from a mean of 0.55 ml/min per gram of liver to 1.09 ml/min per gram of liver, and the hepatic artery flow remains relatively constant (**Fig. 1.6**).

In experimental research, pressure measurements can also be obtained using radial artery invasive monitoring to estimate hepatic artery pressure and direct portal vein pressure measurement, using a small needle coupled to a pressure transducer similar to that used for measuring central venous pressure. The combination of flow and pressure measurement then allows calculation of hepatic sinusoidal resistance (**Fig. 1.6**).

Assessment of innate immunity

The liver forms an important part of the innate immune system by producing acute-phase proteins and other opsonins, proteins that bind to bacteria facilitating their phagocytosis. In addition, 85% of

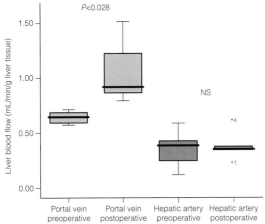

$P<0.028$

NS

*4

*1

Liver blood flow (mL/min/g liver tissue)

Portal vein preoperative | Portal vein postoperative | Hepatic artery preoperative | Hepatic artery postoperative

Figure 1.6 • Directly measured blood flow intraoperatively in six patients during major hepatic resection. Measurements were taken from the main portal vein and the main hepatic artery simultaneously using multichannel Transonics ultrasound flow probes. During the liver resection one branch of each of the portal vein and hepatic artery is ligated. The post-resection blood flow measurement has been taken just before closure of the abdomen, typically 1–2 hours after the first measurement. Results are expressed per gram of liver tissue.

as antiproteases. Liver failure or liver surgery may be associated with a reduction in synthesis of some of these acute-phase proteins (mannan-binding lectin, haptoglobin, α-fetuin and fibronectin), whereas the concentrations of others may be increased despite a reduction in functional liver tissue (C-reactive protein, liver fatty acid-binding protein; unpublished data). The exact significance of these changes is unclear but may contribute to a global impairment in innate immunity in the injured liver.

Liver regeneration

The liver is unique in that it is the only organ in the adult that is capable of regenerating or renewing itself to restore the ratio between pre-injury liver volume and body weight. Knowledge of the capacity for the liver to regenerate is presumed to be ancient and is the basis for the punishment meted out by Zeus to Prometheus, who according to Greek mythology was chained to a rock and had his liver eaten daily by an eagle, only for it to regenerate overnight. This continued for several years until the eagle was finally killed by Hercules, who also released Prometheus. While the speed of liver regeneration is exaggerated in this myth, it is true that it is an extremely rapid process. In the context of surgery, liver regeneration happens very rapidly, with most of the cell division required for regeneration occurring within 72 hours of injury in mice. Full liver function and volume are usually restored within 6–12 weeks in humans. In chronic injury or in the presence of fibrosis, liver regeneration can be chaotic with repeated insults causing scarring, and nodular regeneration with disordered architecture leading to cirrhosis.

Molecular signals for hepatic regeneration

At a cellular level, liver regeneration depends on the coexistence of three key factors: changes in the microenvironment of the liver cell supporting growth, the ability of differentiated hepatocytes to proliferate and inhibition of processes, linking injury to programmed cell death.

Stimuli for liver regeneration stimulate transcription factors that turn on a variety of genes expressing growth factors. Although not direct growth factors, the hormones insulin and adrenaline potentiate the effects of growth factors on hepatocyte regeneration. All elements of the liver are required to regenerate; however, the coordination of these processes is complex. Removal of the stimulus for regeneration by growth to pre-injury capacity and transforming growth factor-β act as brakes that slow regeneration of liver elements (**Fig. 1.7**). Barriers to hepatic regeneration include cirrhosis and fibrosis and ongoing liver injury such as might occur with biliary obstruction or sepsis.

the reticuloendothelial system is located in the liver (Kupffer cells) and clearly surgical resection will involve a reduction of this cell mass.

It is not unreasonable to expect that major liver resection might result in some impairment of innate immunity. Our group has previously demonstrated that major liver resection is associated with increased frequency of infection as well as increased likelihood of objective evidence of liver function impairment.[2]

In a separate study, our group has also shown that major liver resection is associated with a temporary defect in the ability of the reticuloendothelial system to clear albumin microspheres that were used as a surrogate for bacteria.

> ✔ Loss of approximately 50% of liver volume, such as might occur during a right hepatectomy, is associated with impairment of reticuloendothelial cell clearance equivalent to that of non-surgical patients with Child C chronic liver disease.[28]

The liver also synthesises and exports many acute-phase proteins involved in innate immunity or homeostasis. C-reactive protein, for example, binds to phosphoryl choline moieties of encapsulated bacteria and acts as an opsonin, promoting phagocytosis. Mannan-binding lectin, complement fragments and α_1-acid glycoprotein (orosomucoid) can also act as opsonins. Transferrin and caeruloplasmin are important in the binding and carriage of free metal ions and α_1-antitrypsin and α_1-antichymotrypsin act

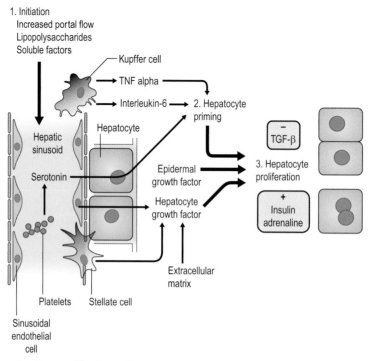

1. Initiation
Increased portal flow
Lipopolysaccharides
Soluble factors

Kupffer cell

TNF alpha

Interleukin-6 → 2. Hepatocyte priming

Hepatocyte

Hepatic sinusoid

− TGF-β

Serotonin

Epidermal growth factor

3. Hepatocyte proliferation

Hepatocyte growth factor

+ Insulin adrenaline

Extracellular matrix

Platelets   Stellate cell

Sinusoidal endothelial cell

Figure 1.7 • Schematic of some of the factors known to regulate liver regeneration.

Cell populations involved in liver regeneration

Histology of normal liver regeneration following resection or acute injury shows the presence of high mitotic rates in mature hepatocytes. Normally, these cells are mitotically quiescent but can move into S phase extremely rapidly. For example, following 70% hepatectomy in rat, approximately 30–40% of hepatocytes are seen to be undergoing mitosis within 48 hours of surgery and the liver will regain its normal size within 10 days. The situation is more complex in chronically injured liver (e.g. cirrhotic liver); here, the hepatocytes are less able to undergo mitosis and are frequently in cell cycle arrest. Furthermore, the accumulation of excess scar tissue deposited in cirrhosis contributes to the inability of the liver to respond to injury and regenerate effectively. In this setting a second population of cells becomes activated and may contribute to parenchymal regeneration. These intrahepatic cells are located in the canal of Hering (the most distal branch of the biliary tree); termed hepatic progenitor cells (HPCs), they are bipotential and are capable of giving rise to both biliary and hepatocyte populations under the influence of macrophage-derived factors.[29] This response is seen in chronic or severe injury and sometimes appears as a ductular reaction. It is also worth noting that there is an increasing recognition that intrahepatic stem cells are a likely source of a

significant proportion of liver cancers. The role of circulating extrahepatic cells in liver regeneration has received interest recently and the potential bone marrow origin of hepatocytes has been suggested. However, if this phenomenon occurs at all, it is extremely rare. The bone marrow does, however, supply macrophages and myofibroblasts that are involved in the liver's scarring response to injury. The relationship between bone marrow-derived cells and the response to injury is complex, with different macrophage subtypes shown to either promote fibrosis or repair. However, administration of bone marrow-derived macrophages to the fibrotic liver via the portal vein has been shown to reduce fibrosis and improve markers of regeneration in preclinical models.[30] The use of bone marrow populations to stimulate liver regeneration in both animal models and clinical studies is likely to be an area of future development (see later).

Consequences of surgery

Unfortunately, at present it is unclear what the key mechanisms of liver failure are, and why the liver usually regenerates but sometimes progresses into liver failure. It is believed that ischaemia/reperfusion (I/R) injury plays an important role in the sequence of events leading to liver failure. Hepatic resections are major surgical procedures, often leading to significant blood loss. In order to reduce blood loss, central venous pressure is reduced during liver surgery and hepatobiliary surgeons frequently occlude hepatic blood inflow temporarily (Pringle manoeuvre). Obviously, all these factors may contribute to an I/R injury in the liver. A key component of I/R injury is the generation of oxygen free radicals. The latter can induce ischaemic necrosis and caspase-dependent apoptosis, and may contribute to failure of vital metabolic synthetic pathways. However, it remains to be investigated which one of these plays a key role during liver failure. In this context, it has been proposed that the balance between hepatocyte regeneration and apoptosis can be tipped towards either side by hepatic defence mechanisms against oxygen free radical damage. Also, oxygen free radicals play a role in determining whether apoptosis or ischaemic necrosis occurs in the liver. Apparently, the equilibrium between oxygen free radicals and their scavengers plays a pivotal role in determining whether regeneration or decay occurs. Glutathione (GSH) is the principal oxygen free radical scavenger in the liver and the principal defence mechanism against I/R damage. Hepatic GSH levels decrease following I/R damage, inflammation and nutritional deprivation. It seems conceivable that a reduction in liver volume following surgery contributes to insufficient hepatic free radical scavenging capacity as a consequence of reduced GSH synthesis. I/R injury may aggravate this situation.

Small-for-size syndrome

The original descriptions of small-for-size syndrome described a condition arising in split liver transplantation characterised by the development of ascites, portal hypertension and liver dysfunction in an otherwise healthy transplanted portion of liver. The underlying cause for this syndrome is believed to relate to blood flow and the failure of a small liver volume to cope with often very high blood flows in patients with previous chronic liver disease undergoing transplantation. The validity of this hypothesis was supported by the observation that partial diversion of portal blood flow into the graft using a portocaval shunt could limit or prevent the development of small-for-size syndrome. Subsequently, other manoeuvres have

also been effected, such as ligation or embolisation of the splenic artery, which works in the same way by reducing portal vein flow.

In patients undergoing even very major liver resection it is rare to develop small-for-size syndrome. Some patients do, however, develop ascites, jaundice and chronic liver dysfunction, and it is more likely that this syndrome is more dependent on a failure to regenerate than on excessive blood flow.

Hepatic steatosis

Fat infiltration of the liver is an increasing problem with increased prevalence of obesity and the metabolic syndrome (obesity and type 2 diabetes). Macroscopically the liver may appear enlarged, pale or yellow-coloured with rounded edges. Microscopically the liver can have microsteatosis (small fat droplets within every hepatocyte) or macrosteatosis (regional infiltration of hepatocytes with large fat droplets) (see **Fig. 1.8**).

Assessment of steatosis

Assessment of hepatic steatosis is notoriously difficult. Experienced surgeons can estimate liver fat by judging the size, rounded or sharp edges of the liver and its appearance. Even using colour as an estimate is prone to error, as can be seen in **Fig. 1.9**.

The gold standard for hepatic fat assessment is histology. Trucut or wedge biopsies can be assessed by a pathologist and a reliable estimate of the percentage fat content produced. In addition, useful information including the distribution – macrosteatosis or microsteatosis – and the presence of fibrosis or

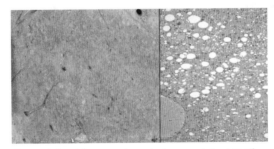

Figure 1.8 • Macroscopic and microscopic images of steatotic liver.

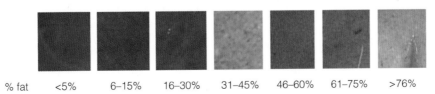

| % fat | <5% | 6–15% | 16–30% | 31–45% | 46–60% | 61–75% | >76% |

Figure 1.9 • Physical appearance of livers with varying fat content confirmed by histology to demonstrate the poor correlation between colour and objective measurement of fat content.

inflammation can be provided. New MRI techniques are, however, challenging the accuracy of pathological assessment of steatosis and offer the potential advantage of being non-invasive.[31]

Chemotherapy-induced liver changes

Increased usage of neoadjuvant chemotherapy, particularly oxaliplatin and irinotecan, has resulted in liver changes. These range from a soft, fragile pale liver to steatosis, steatohepatitis and sinusoidal dilatation. Surgery should be deferred until 6 weeks after chemotherapy and studies, although conflicting, suggest that tolerance of major liver resection may be reduced and complications more frequent in individuals who have received chemotherapy. A study by Mehta et al. showed that oxaliplatin-based chemotherapy was associated with increased blood loss and prolonged hospital stay.[32]

Portal vein embolisation

Morbidity and mortality after hepatectomy have constituted a limitation on the number of patients eligible for resection, and currently only 8% of patients with colorectal liver metastases are candidates for curative hepatic resection. Liver function is correlated with liver volume, and consequently hepatic insufficiency in this situation may arise because not enough functional liver volume is left after surgical removal of part of the liver. As noted above, removal of part of the liver induces the residual liver regenerating to the point where the preoperative liver weight to body weight ratio is regained. This notion led to the belief that if it were possible to increase preoperatively the volume of the future residual liver, it would be possible to perform more extensive liver resections and more patients would be eligible for hepatic resection. It has long been recognised that interruption of one part of the liver portal blood flow usually leads to hypertrophy of normally vascularised liver. This has been observed in patients with Klatskin tumours, which have a tendency to invade the portal vein, causing ipsilateral atrophy and contralateral hypertrophy. This concept has subsequently been harnessed by manoeuvres such as portal vein embolisation (PVE). Embolising the right portal vein prior to surgical resection leads to hypertrophy of the left liver lobe and facilitates the subsequent safe extensive resection of the right liver (extended right hepatectomy) 6 weeks later (**Fig. 1.10**). This phenomenon has been harnessed to maximise the residual functional liver volume of patients who are predicted to have a small remnant liver volume.

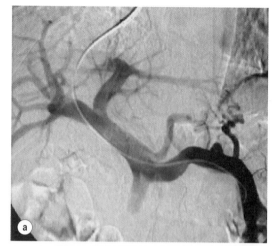
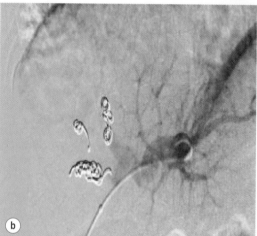

Figure 1.10 • Portal venograms showing the main left and right branches prior to embolisation **(a)** and after embolisation of the right portal vein **(b)**.

This approach is fully based on the concept that, in the normal liver, volume is correlated to function and hence liver failure occurs when residual liver volume is too small. A completely different and novel approach would be to improve liver function per volume unit of liver. Recent evidence from studies using mebrofenin suggests that functional improvement of the future liver remnant following PVE may precede changes in liver volume.[33] This important observation suggests that surgery earlier after PVE may be possible. Limitations to PVE-induced hypertrophy include pre-existing hepatic fibrosis or cirrhosis and technical or anatomical inability to completely obstruct a major portal vein branch.

Technique

The most common technique of PVE is to puncture a branch of the vein using a percutaneous approach.

A venogram is obtained to demonstrate all of the relevant branches and then the branch to be embolised is cannulated and coils and embolic material delivered to obstruct portal flow. A check angiogram can be performed to demonstrate success of the technique. Usually either a left or right main branch is occluded. To obtain hypertrophy of segments 2 and 3 in large right-sided tumours, it is not sufficient to embolise just the right portal vein and it is recommended that the branches supplying segment 4 should also be embolised. Patients usually tolerate PVE remarkably well, presumably because of the dual blood supply of the liver, and complications are uncommon. Significant hypertrophy can be achieved, as can be seen in **Fig. 1.11**.

Associating liver partition and portal vein ligation for staged hepatectomy (ALPPS procedure)

This technique, first described in 2011, aims to enable surgery with curative intent in patients who would otherwise be unsuitable for liver resection due to insufficient future liver remnant volume and in whom PVE is not possible or did not achieve sufficient hypertrophy.[34] The technique involves two distinct stages. The first stage involves division of the liver along the line of proposed resection (between segment 2/3 and segment 4) and ligation of the portal blood supply to liver segments 4–8. Segments 4–8 retain both arterial blood supply and biliary drainage, so enabling these de-portalised liver segments to provide auxiliary support to the future liver remnant (segments 2/3) while they undergo a process of hypertrophy and hyperplasia. Tumours within segments 2/3 can also be removed at this stage. On completion of the first stage, the future liver remnant enlarges rapidly over several weeks. When the future liver remnant (segment 2/3) has enlarged sufficiently (1–2 weeks) the right side (segments 4–8 + 1) is then removed. Early attempts were plagued by complications, including bleeding and liver failure with high mortality rates. However, there are patients who may benefit from this approach. It has become clear that identifying the most appropriate candidates, ensuring sufficient enlargement and function of the future liver remnant and further refinement of the technique are crucial to successful outcomes.

Supporting the failing liver

N-Acetyl cysteine

Glutathione depletion is a major problem in patients with paracetamol (acetaminophen) toxicity. N-acetyl cysteine has been used for many years as a treatment for early paracetamol poisoning. It is thought to act by replenishing glutathione stores and by providing alternative thiol groups to which damaging reactive oxygen species can bind. The realisation that reactive oxygen species can be generated by conditions other than paracetamol poisoning such as sepsis and ischaemia/reperfusion has led to N-acetyl cysteine being used in a more general way to support patients with early evidence of liver dysfunction or failure.

Nutritional support in liver failure

The role of nutritional support in acute liver failure is uncertain, largely because of a lack of evidence in the literature. Enteral nutrition is known to preserve gut barrier function and thus might be considered to be beneficial in the context of liver failure. In addition, the provision of energy might be considered beneficial in the context of glycogen storage failure, and to fuel the regeneration of liver tissue and recover function. The limited ability of the failing liver to handle nitrogen and synthesise urea (potentially exacerbating encephalopathy) would argue against excessive provision of proteins unless these were in a form where they did not contribute to the circulating ammonia load.

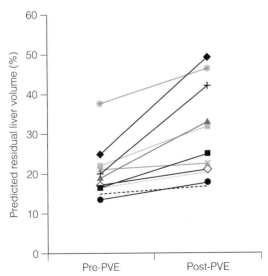

Figure 1.11 • Calculated residual liver volumes before and after portal vein embolisation (PVE) in patients scheduled to undergo major liver resection.

Extracorporeal liver support

For the vast majority of patients who take toxic doses of paracetamol, suffer alcohol-induced liver injury or develop liver dysfunction following liver resection, the regenerative capacity of the liver is sufficient to prevent irretrievable liver failure and death. However, when this regenerative capacity is overwhelmed treatment strategies to temporarily or permanently replace the failing liver are required. The ability to provide short-term extracorporeal liver support, either during the wait for transplantation or to facilitate liver regeneration and avoid transplantation, is an attractive option. A range of devices have been developed, either focusing on the detoxification functions of liver (artificial liver support) or also incorporating bioreactors intended to perform synthetic liver functions (bioartificial liver support). Assessment of efficacy has been hampered by the limited number of randomised controlled trials and small sample size, but a recent meta-analysis does suggest overall survival benefit in acute liver failure.[35]

Artificial liver support

Artificial systems include the MARS (Molecular Adsorbent Recirculating System) device, Prometheus and the BioLogic-DT (now called the Liver Dialysis Device, currently being redesigned). The greatest experience has been with the MARS device, which deploys an albumin dialysis circuit to remove both water-soluble and protein-bound toxins.[36] Thus, a low Fischer ratio can be corrected by recirculating albumin dialysis.[37] Because the system preferentially removes AAAs, compared with BCAAs, the Fischer ratio significantly increases, predominantly by the removal of AAAs in a small series of patients.[37–40] MARS has been shown to be useful in fulminant hepatic failure, by attenuating the increase in intracranial pressure, which plays a major role in this situation.[33] There may also be an effect on survival and improvement of degree of hepatic encephalopathy in patients with acute or chronic liver failure.[39,41] Equally, the system has been tested on artificial neuronal networks showing a normalisation of abnormal signals if the medium (plasma derived from rats with liver failure) was pretreated with MARS. The role of MARS in a more chronic situation of mild hepatic encephalopathy, when correction of an abnormal Fischer ratio would likely be more important if this were a major pathogenetic factor, is still largely unknown and deserves further study.[42] It has been suggested that the role of MARS and bioartificial liver support systems should be limited to carefully designed clinical trials.[43] It is currently uncertain how hepatic excretory assistance devices, such as MARS, compare with bioartificial liver assistance devices, which in addition to their excretory functions aim to provide biosynthetic capacity.[39]

Bioartificial liver systems

Bioartificial systems incorporate a bioreactor containing either human hepatoblastoma cell lines (e.g. the HepatAssist device) or porcine hepatocytes (e.g. the ELAD – Extracorporeal Liver Assist Device), through which the patient's blood is perfused. An additional filter component may be included to aid detoxification and improve bioreactor survival.

One of the major problems with these systems is what type of cells to use, and a variety of different approaches have been taken. Animal hepatocytes perform many of the same functions as human hepatocytes, although some of the proteins produced are obviously different. Human immortalised cell lines are an attractive proposition and some of the more differentiated cell lines can replicate many of the normal hepatocyte functions. Regardless, the true functionality of these cells in the clinical setting is uncertain. The design of bioartificial liver systems is challenging and the large surface area of hepatocytes needed to be effective is difficult. Engineering scaffolds of membranes or tubules has been the most popular approach. In normal liver, hepatocytes are polarised and have an epithelial surface. However, it is still to be determined how to recreate this polarity and its absolute importance has yet to be defined. Hepatocytes proliferate and function better in association with non-parenchymal cells; however, the creation of co-cultures in reactors produces its own problems. Cells must maintain viability or be able to be replenished to provide liver support over a prolonged period of time. In addition, very sick patients require a short time period to set up the support system, and the reactor must be easy to use by critical care nurses, safe from contamination and not overly expensive. For all of these reasons, bioartificial liver systems remain a tantalising prospect that has yet to break through into routine clinical practice.

Liver transplantation

Irreversible acute or chronic liver failure is amenable to treatment by liver transplantation. It is extremely uncommon for patients who have undergone liver resection to subsequently require or proceed to liver transplantation. The most obvious reason for this is that many patients who undergo liver resection do so for metastatic or primary liver cancer and transplantation would be contraindicated because of the risk of immunosuppression and aggressive recrudescence of the tumour. A number of patients with bile duct injury have progressed to transplantation, usually in a chronic setting following the development of biliary stricture, cholangitis and secondary biliary cirrhosis. Similarly, a number of patients who have undergone a 'cancer resection' for what turned out to be a benign biliary stricture, perhaps due to primary sclerosing cholangitis, fail to regenerate their livers and may progress to transplantation.

Cell therapy for liver failure: general principles

A number of key principles have operated as key drivers for the development of cell therapies for clinical treatment of liver failure. Firstly, it is recognised that the injured liver usually provides a rich environment stimulating tissue regeneration and the liver can normally 'heal' itself. Secondly, in animal models there is evidence that stem cells or non-parenchymal cells can support regeneration of hepatocytes. Thirdly, it is recognised that the difference between liver failure and compensated liver function in terms of cellular functional equivalents is probably very small. Finally, it would be preferable to support the liver by techniques that were within the body rather than using extracorporeal devices. This desire has stimulated research into therapeutic application of cell or stem cell transplantation.

The dual goals of stem cell therapy in the context of acute liver failure or injury are to promote rapid recovery of hepatocyte function and to allow regeneration of liver tissue without excessive scarring. Direct administration of hepatocytes or stem cell-derived hepatocytes to the injured liver has been met with little success in preclinical studies. However, bone marrow-derived cells to support endogenous processes may support the regenerating liver, enabling effective regeneration.[44]

Haemopoetic stem cell therapy for liver disease in humans

There are several reports in the scientific literature of bone marrow (BM) stem cell therapy in patients with advanced liver disease. It was first reported that BM stem cells could increase the liver's ability to regenerate in patients who were undergoing hepatic resection for various liver cancers sited in the right lobe. Here the patients underwent embolisation of the right branch of the portal vein prior to surgery to stimulate compensatory hypertrophy of the left lobe. Autologous CD133-positive BM stem cells were injected into the blood vessels that supply the left liver lobe shortly after the surgery and accelerated regeneration of the non-embolised section of the liver was seen compared with control patients.[45] The second report used BM stem cells in patients with liver cirrhosis.[46] CD34-positive stem cells were isolated from the patients' own blood following granulocyte colony-stimulating factor (GCSF)-induced haematopoietic stem cell mobilisation and were re-injected into the blood supply to the liver – preliminary results appeared to show improvement in liver function in three out of five of the patients. In the third study, patients with liver cirrhosis had mononuclear cells isolated from their own BM during general anaesthesia.[47] These cells were re-injected into the patient's bloodstream and again the patient's liver function appeared to improve. Although these studies are very encouraging, they are preliminary, of small numbers and non-randomised. Furthermore, in none of these studies were the cells marked to enable identification either by radiological tracking or in subsequent biopsies of the liver tissue. Therefore, a number of important questions are unanswered. It is not certain that these cells definitely settled in the liver over a period of time, whether some of the cells engrafted other organs in the body and by what mechanisms the cells were having their positive effects within the recipients' livers.

Future developments

The ability to exert greater control in modulating liver volume and function in the surgical patient would be a major advantage. Preoperative functional enhancement might expand the group of patients who would be amenable to surgery, while postoperative intervention might be useful in liver resection, transplantation and acute liver failure as a means of rescuing a failing liver. The potential to use autologous stem cells derived from bone marrow to stimulate liver regeneration is enormous if its positive effects are seen in larger randomised studies.

Key points

- Conventional measures of liver function are poor and take no account of liver volume.
- Liver resection leaving a residual liver volume of <25% is associated with a high risk of liver dysfunction and infection.
- In patients with chronic liver disease, smaller resections can be dangerous.
- The combination of liver dysfunction and sepsis can be fatal.
- Preoperative portal vein embolisation and newer regenerative strategies may improve the safety of liver surgery.

Key references

2. Schindl MJ, Redhead DN, Fearon KC, et al. The value of residual liver volume as a predictor of hepatic dysfunction and infection after major liver resection. Gut 2005;54:289–96. PMID: 15647196.

   The first paper providing strong evidence of an association between residual liver volume and clinical infection.

6. Clavien PA, Yadav S, Sindram D, et al. Protective effects of ischemic preconditioning for liver resection performed under inflow occlusion in humans. Ann Surg 2000;232:155–62. PMID: 10903590.

   The first randomised clinical trial demonstrating benefit in clinical markers from ischaemic preconditioning of the liver in patients undergoing liver resection.

21. van de Poll MC, Wigmore SJ, Redhead DN, et al. Effect of major liver resection on hepatic ureagenesis in humans. Am J Physiol Gastrointest Liver Physiol 2007;293:G956–62. PMID: 17717046.

   Clinical experimental study demonstrating the relationship between liver volume and urea synthesis in patients undergoing varying degrees of liver resection.

2

Hepatic, biliary and pancreatic anatomy

Vincent S. Yip
Stephen W. Fenwick

This chapter will provide a basic anatomical foundation for performing liver, biliary and pancreatic surgery. Anatomical features that are clinically unimportant have been omitted. It is self-evident that surgeons operating in this area must have a full working knowledge of the anatomy of the liver, biliary system and pancreas. Furthermore, with ongoing advances in modern imaging techniques, surgeons must be able to translate their understanding of anatomy from the screen to the patient. Surgeons must also be aware that whilst there is a normal or *prevailing pattern* of anatomy, variations, which are termed *anomalies*, are frequent.

Liver

Overview of hepatic anatomy and terminology

The most significant advances in the understanding of the surgical anatomy of the liver were made by the late French surgeon and anatomist Claude Couinaud, during his studies with vasculo-biliary casts of the liver during the 1950s.[1] This work demonstrated that the liver appeared to consist of eight distinct functional segments, with each segment having its own dual vascular inflow, biliary drainage and lymphatic drainage (**Fig. 2.1**). Although more recent studies have questioned the validity of some aspects of this system, it remains the most relevant for the hepatic surgeon. It is clearly important to have uniformity and clarity of anatomical nomenclature pertaining to liver

resectional surgery. Previously this was somewhat chaotic, with multiple terms being used for the same structure or operation, or some individual terms being used for more than one structure or operation. As a result, a terminology committee was formed by the International Hepato-Pancreato-Biliary Association (IHPBA), and the proposed system, which is primarily based on hepatic artery and bile duct ramifications, will be used throughout this chapter.[2]

Divisions of the liver based on the hepatic artery

The proper hepatic artery arises as a branch of the common hepatic artery. The primary (first-order) division of the proper hepatic artery is into the right and left hepatic arteries (**Fig. 2.2**). These branches supply arterial inflow to the right and left hemilivers (**Fig. 2.3**). The plane between the two distinct zones of vascular supply is called a watershed. The border or watershed of the first-order division is called the *midplane of the liver*. It intersects the gallbladder fossa and the fossa for the inferior vena cava (IVC) (**Fig. 2.4**). The right hemiliver usually has a larger volume than the left hemiliver (60:40), although this is variable.

The second-order divisions (Figs 2.2 and 2.4) of the hepatic artery supply four distinct zones of the liver. Each is referred to as a *section*. The right liver is divided into two sections, the *right anterior section* and the *right posterior section*. These sections are supplied by the right anterior sectional hepatic artery and the right posterior sectional hepatic artery (Fig. 2.2). The plane between these sections is the *right intersectional plane*, which does not have

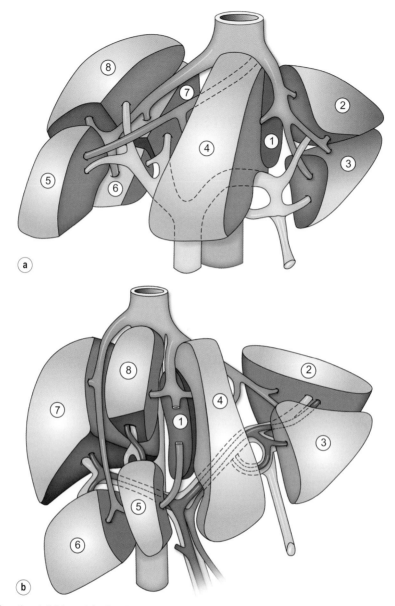

Figure 2.1 • Functional division of the liver into eight segments as described by Coinaud: **(a)** as observed in the anatomical position in the patient; **(b)** as observed ex vivo.
Adapted from Poston GJ, D'Angelica M, editors. Surgical management of hepatobiliary and pancreatic disorders. 2nd ed. 2010. Informa Healthcare, Taylor and Francis Group. Chapter 1, Figure 1.7.

any surface markings to indicate its position. The left liver is also divided into two sections, the *left medial section* and the *left lateral section* (Fig. 2.4), which are supplied by the left medial sectional hepatic artery and the left lateral sectional hepatic artery (Fig. 2.2). The plane between these sections is referred to as the left intersectional plane, which is marked on the surface of the liver by the umbilical fissure and the line of attachment of the falciform ligament. The third-order divisions of the hepatic

artery divide the right and left hemilivers into *segments* (Sg) 2–8 (Figs 2.2 and **2.5**). Each of the segments has its own feeding segmental artery. The left lateral section is divided into Sg2 and Sg3. The ramification of vessels within the left medial section does not permit subdivision of this section into segments, each with its own arterial blood supply. Therefore, the left medial section and Sg4 are synonymous. However, Sg4 is arbitrarily divided into superior (4a) and inferior (4b) parts

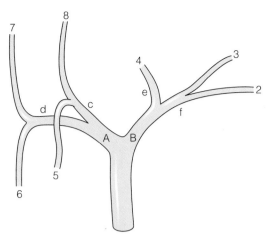

Figure 2.2 • Ramification of the hepatic artery in the liver. The prevailing pattern is shown. The first-order division of the proper hepatic artery is into the right **(A)** and left **(B)** hepatic arteries, which supply right and left hemilivers (see Fig. 2.3), respectively. The second-order division of the hepatic arteries supplies the four sections (see Fig. 2.4). The third-order division supplies the segments (see Fig. 2.5). The caudate lobe is supplied by branches from **(a)** and **(b)**. Bile duct anatomy and nomenclature is similar to that of the hepatic artery. © Washington University in St Louis.

without an exact anatomical plane of separation. The right anterior section is divided into two segments, Sg5 and Sg8. The right posterior section is divided into Sg6 and Sg7. The planes between segments are referred to as intersegmental planes. The ramifications of the bile ducts are identical to that described for the arteries, as are the zones of the liver drained by the respective ducts.

Segment 1 (caudate lobe) is a distinct portion of the liver, separate from the right and left hemilivers (**Fig. 2.6**). It is appropriately referred to as a lobe since it is demarcated by visible fissures. It consists of three parts: the bulbous left part (Spiegelian lobe), which wraps around the left side of the vena cava and is readily visible through the lesser omentum; the paracaval portion, which lies anterior to the vena cava; and the caudate process, on the right. The caudate process merges indistinctly with the right hemiliver. The caudate lobe is situated posterior to the hilum and the portal veins. Lying anterior and superior to the paracaval portion are the hepatic veins, which limit the upper extent of the caudate lobe[1,3] (Fig. 2.6). The caudate lobe receives vascular supply from both right and left hepatic arteries and portal veins. Caudate bile ducts drain into both right and left hepatic ducts.[1] The caudate lobe is drained by several short caudate veins that enter the IVC directly from the caudate lobe. Their number and size are variable, and they must be ligated when mobilising the caudate lobe from the vena cava. Commonly, these veins enter the IVC on either side of the midplane of the vessel, an anatomical feature that allows the creation of a tunnel behind the liver on the surface of the IVC without encountering the caudate veins. A 'hanging manoeuvre' can be performed by lifting up on a tape placed through this tunnel (see below).

Resectional terminology

The terminology of hepatic resections is based upon the terminology of hepatic anatomy. Resection of one side of the liver is called a hepatectomy or hemihepatectomy (Fig. 2.3). Resection of the right side of the liver is a right hepatectomy or

Anatomical term	Couinaud segments referred to	Term for surgical resection	Diagram (pertinent area is shaded)
Right hemiliver or Right liver	Sg5–8 (+/–Sg1)	Right hepatectomy or Right hemihepatectomy (stipulate +/– segment 1)	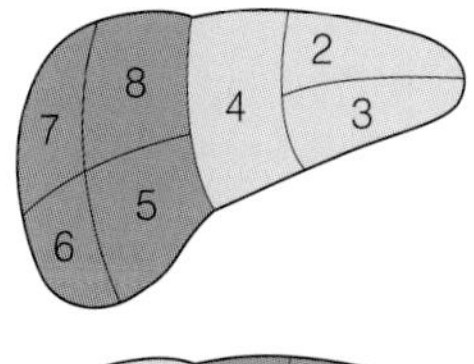
Left hemiliver or Left liver	Sg2–4 (+/–Sg1)	Left hepatectomy or Left hemihepatectomy (stipulate +/– segment 1)	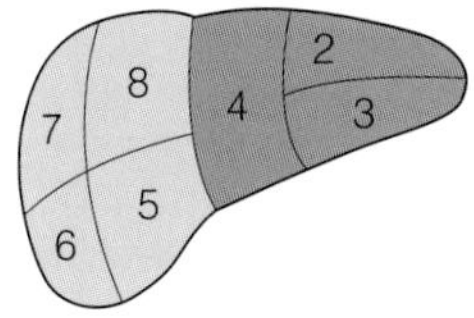

Border or watershed: The border or watershed of the first-order division which separates the two hemilivers is a plane which intersects the gallbladder fossa and the fossa for the IVC and is called the midplane of the liver.

Figure 2.3 • Nomenclature for first-order division anatomy (hemilivers or livers) and resections. © Washington University in St Louis.

Second-order division
(second-order division based on bile ducts and hepatic artery)

Anatomical term	Couinaud segments referred to	Term for surgical resection	Diagram (pertinent area is shaded)
Right anterior section	Sg 5,8	Add (-ectomy) to any of the anatomical terms as in Right anterior sectionectomy	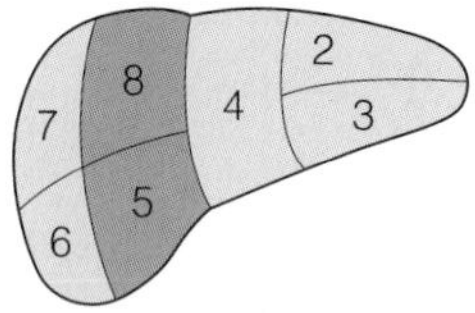
Right posterior section	Sg 6,7	Right posterior sectionectomy	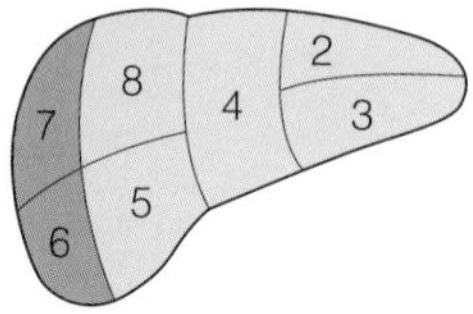
Left medial section	Sg 4	Left medial sectionectomy or Resection segment 4 (also see third order) or Segmentectomy 4 (also see third order)	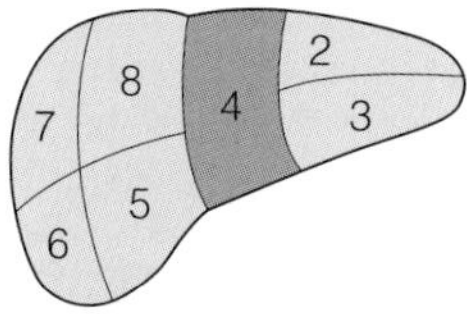
Left lateral section	Sg 2,3	Left lateral sectionectomy or Bisegmentectomy 2,3 (also see third order)	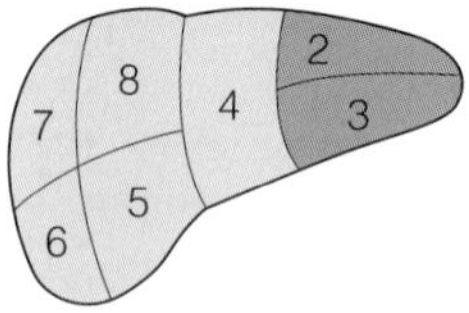

Other sectional liver resections

	Sg 4–8 (+/–Sg1)	Right trisectionectomy (preferred term) or Extended right hepatectomy or Extended right hemihepatectomy (stipulate +/– segment 1)	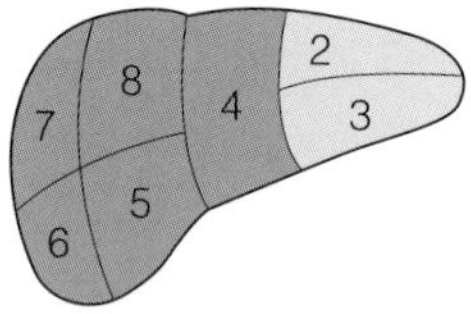
	Sg 2,3,4,5,8 (+/–Sg1)	Left trisectionectomy (preferred term) or Extended left hepatectomy or Extended left hemihepatectomy (stipulate +/– segment 1)	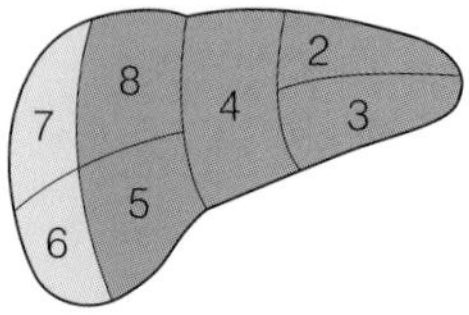

Border or watershed: The borders or watersheds of the sections are planes referred to as the right and left intersectional planes. The left intersectional plane passes through the umbilical fissure and the attachment of the falciform ligament. There is no surface marking of the right intersectional plane.

Figure 2.4 • Nomenclature for second-order division anatomy (sections) and resections including extended resections. © Washington University in St Louis.

Third-order division

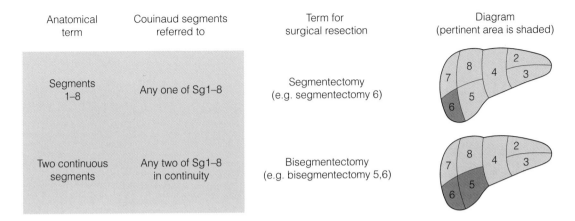

Anatomical term	Couinaud segments referred to	Term for surgical resection	Diagram (pertinent area is shaded)
Segments 1–8	Any one of Sg1–8	Segmentectomy (e.g. segmentectomy 6)	
Two continuous segments	Any two of Sg1–8 in continuity	Bisegmentectomy (e.g. bisegmentectomy 5,6)	

Border or watershed: The borders or watersheds of the segments are planes referred to as intersegmental planes.

Figure 2.5 • Nomenclature for third-order division anatomy (segments) and resections. © Washington University in St Louis.

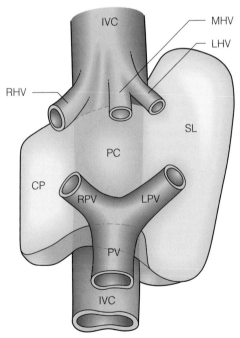

Figure 2.6 • Schematic representation of the anatomy of the caudate lobe. The caudate lobe consists of three parts: the caudate process (*CP*), on the right, the paracaval portion anterior to the vena cava (*PC*) and the bulbous left part (Spiegelian lobe, *SL*). *IVC*, inferior vena cava; *PV*, portal vein; *RHV*, *MHV*, *LHV*, right hepatic, middle hepatic and left hepatic vein, respectively. © Washington University in St Louis.

hemihepatectomy and resection of the left side of the liver is a left hemihepatectomy or hepatectomy. Resection of a liver section is referred to as a sectionectomy (Fig. 2.4). Resection of the liver to the left side of the umbilical fissure is a left lateral sectionectomy. The other sectionectomies are named accordingly, e.g. right anterior sectionectomy. Resection of the right hemiliver plus Sg4 is referred to as a right trisectionectomy (Fig. 2.4). Similarly, resection of the left hemiliver plus the right anterior section is referred to as a left trisectionectomy.

Resection of one of the numbered segments is referred to as a segmentectomy (Fig. 2.5).

Surgical anatomy for liver resections

Hepatic arteries and liver resections

In the prevailing anatomical pattern, the coeliac artery terminates to divide into left gastric, splenic and common hepatic arteries. The common hepatic artery runs for 2–3 cm anteriorly and to the right to ramify into gastroduodenal and proper hepatic arteries. The proper hepatic artery enters the hepatoduodenal ligament and normally runs for 2–3 cm along the left side of the common bile duct and terminates by dividing into the right and left hepatic arteries, the right immediately passing behind the common hepatic duct. The four sectional arteries arise from the right and left arteries 1–2 cm from the liver (**Fig. 2.7**). While this is the commonest pattern,

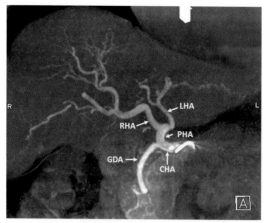

Figure 2.7 • Cone beam computed tomography image of conventional hepatic arterial anatomy. (*CHA*, common hepatic artery; *PHA*, proper hepatic artery; *GDA*, gastroduodenal artery; *LHA*, left hepatic artery; *RHA*, right hepatic artery.)

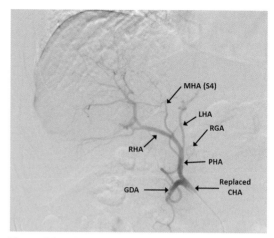

Figure 2.8 • Superior mesenteric arteriogram showing replaced common hepatic artery. *CHA*, common hepatic artery; *PHA*, proper hepatic artery; *GDA*, gastroduodenal artery; *RHA*, *LHA*, *MHA*, right hepatic, middle hepatic and left hepatic artery, respectively; *RGA*, Right gastric artery.

variations from this pattern are also very common. Thus it is imperative that the surgeon does not make assumptions regarding hepatic arteries based on size or position, but instead on complete dissection, trial clamping and intraoperative imaging. 'Replaced' and 'aberrant' arteries are surgically important anomalies. 'Replaced' means that the artery supplying a particular volume of liver is in an unusual location and also that it is the sole supply to that volume of liver. 'Aberrant' means the structure is in an unusual location. While the definition of 'aberrant' does not state whether the structure provides sole supply, it is usually considered to be synonymous with 'replaced' in respect to these arteries. 'Accessory' refers to an artery that is additional, i.e. is present in addition to the normal structure and as a result is *not* the sole supply to a volume. Consequently, ligation of an accessory artery does not result in ischaemia.

In about 25% of individuals, part or all of the liver is supplied by a replaced (or aberrant) artery. The *replaced right hepatic artery* arises from the superior mesenteric artery. It runs from left to right behind the lower end of the common bile duct to emerge and course on its right posterior border. It may supply a segment, section or the entire right hemiliver. Rarely, this artery supplies the entire liver and then it is called a *replaced hepatic artery* (**Fig. 2.8**). The *replaced left hepatic artery* arises from the left gastric artery and courses in the lesser omentum in conjunction with vagal branches to the liver (hepatic nerve). As with the right artery, it may supply a segment, section (usually the left lateral section), hemiliver or very rarely the whole liver. Sometimes left hepatic arteries arising from the left gastric artery are actually accessory rather than replaced and exist in conjunction with normally situated left hepatic

arteries. Knowledge of these particular arterial variations is of importance not only in hepatobiliary surgery, including transplantation, but also in gastric surgery and pancreatic surgery. Transection of the left gastric artery at its origin during gastrectomy may cause ischaemic necrosis of the left hemiliver if a replaced left artery is present. The same may occur on the right side as a result of injury to a replaced right artery. Also, and of particular importance, these vessels must be preserved and perfused during donor hepatectomy for transplantation.

Replaced arteries may confer an advantage during surgery. For instance, when a replaced left artery supplies the left lateral section, it is possible to resect the entire proper hepatic artery when performing a right trisectionectomy for hilar cholangiocarcinoma. The replaced right artery is sometimes invaded by pancreatic head tumours and is in danger of injury during pancreatico-duodenectomy. This is only a brief description of replaced arteries and there are many variations of replaced arteries, especially on the right, depending on the relationship of the artery to the pancreatic head and neck, the bile duct and the portal vein.[4]

In performing hepatectomies by the standard technique of isolating individual structures instead of pedicles it is critical to correctly identify the particular artery(ies) supplying the volume of liver to be resected. One important anatomical point is that an artery located to the right side of the bile duct always supplies the right side of the liver, but arteries found on the left side of the bile duct may supply either side of the liver. Therefore, when using the individual vessel ligation method it is important to be aware of the position of the common hepatic duct. A trial occlusion of an artery with an atraumatic clamp should always be performed in order to be sure that there is a good pulse to the future remnant liver.

Bile ducts and liver resections

Prevailing pattern and important variations of bile ducts draining the right hemiliver

Normally only a short portion of the right hepatic duct, approximately 1 cm, is in an extrahepatic position. The prevailing pattern of bile duct drainage from the right liver is shown in **Fig. 2.9(a)**. The segmental ducts from Sg6 and Sg7 (called *B6, B7*) unite to form the *right posterior sectional bile duct* and the segmental ducts from Sg5 and Sg8 (*B5, B8*) unite to form the *right anterior sectional bile duct* (Fig. 2.9a). The sectional ducts unite to form the *right hepatic duct*, which unites with the left hepatic duct at the *confluence* to form the common hepatic duct.

There are two important sets of biliary anomalies on the right side of the liver. The first involves insertion of a right sectional duct into the left bile duct. This is a common anomaly. The right posterior sectional duct inserts into the left hepatic duct in 20% of individuals (Fig. 2.9b) and the right anterior bile duct does so in 6% (Fig. 2.9c). In these situations there is no right hepatic duct. A right sectional bile duct inserting into the left hepatic duct is in danger of injury during left hepatectomy if the left duct is divided at its termination. Therefore, when performing left hepatectomy, the left hepatic duct should be divided close to the umbilical fissure to avoid injury to a right sectional duct.

The second important anomaly is insertion of a right bile duct into the biliary tree at a lower level than the prevailing site of confluence. Low union may affect the right hepatic duct, a sectional right duct, a segmental duct or a subsegmental duct. A right bile duct unites with the common hepatic duct below the prevailing site of confluence in about 2%

of individuals. Sometimes the duct unites with the cystic duct and then with the common hepatic duct. The latter anomaly places the aberrant duct at great risk of injury during laparoscopic cholecystectomy.

Very rarely the right hepatic duct terminates in the gallbladder. This may be congenital or acquired. In the latter case a gallstone has effaced a cystic duct which united with the right hepatic duct, giving the appearance that it joins the gallbladder. An extremely rare anomaly is the absent common hepatic duct. In these cases the right and left hepatic duct enters the gallbladder and the duct emerging from the gallbladder runs downward to join with the duodenum.[5] In the presence of these anomalies, which would be extremely difficult to detect, a complete cholecystectomy will result in ductal injury. These ducts should not be confused with ducts of Luschka (see below).

The right *posterior* sectional duct normally hooks over the origin of the right *anterior* sectional portal vein ('Hjortsjo's crook'),[6] where it is in danger of being injured if the right anterior sectional pedicle is clamped too close to its origin (**Fig. 2.10**).

Prevailing pattern and important variations of bile ducts draining the left hemiliver

The prevailing pattern of bile duct drainage from the left liver is shown in **Fig. 2.11a**. It is present in only 30% of individuals, i.e. variations (anomalies) are present in the majority of individuals. In the prevailing pattern, the segmental ducts from Sg2 and Sg3 (**B2, B3**) unite to form the *left lateral sectional bile duct*. This duct passes behind the umbilical portion of the portal vein and unites with the duct from Sg 4 (**B4**; also called the left medial sectional duct since section and segment are synonymous for this volume of liver). The site of union of these ducts to form the left hepatic duct lies about one-third of the distance between the umbilical fissure and the midplane of the liver. The left hepatic duct continues

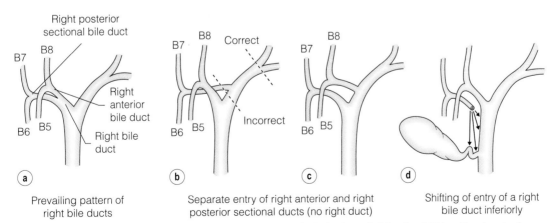

(a) Prevailing pattern of right bile ducts

(b) Separate entry of right anterior and right posterior sectional ducts (no right duct)

(d) Shifting of entry of a right bile duct inferiorly

Figure 2.9 • Prevailing pattern **(a)** and important variations **(b–d)** of bile ducts draining the right hemiliver (see text).
© Washington University in St Louis.

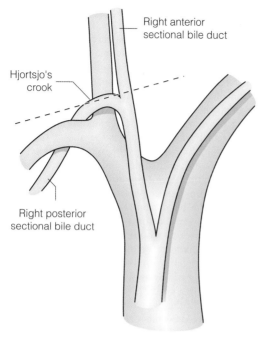

Right anterior
sectional bile duct

Hjortsjo's
crook

Right posterior
sectional bile duct

Figure 2.10 • Hjortsjo's crook. Note that the right posterior sectional bile duct (RPSBD) crosses the origin of the right anterior sectional portal vein.
© Washington University in St Louis.

from this point for 2–3 cm along the base of Sg4 to its confluence with the right hepatic duct. Note that it is in an extrahepatic position and that it has a much longer extrahepatic course than the right bile duct. The extrahepatic position of the left hepatic duct is a key anatomical feature, which makes this section of duct the prime site for high biliary–enteric anastomoses.

The main anomalies of the left ductal system involve variations in site of insertion of B4 (Fig. 2.11b), multiple ducts coming from B4 (Fig. 2.11c) and primary union of B3 and B4 with subsequent union of B2 (Fig. 2.11d). B4 may join the left lateral sectional duct to the left or right of its point of union in the prevailing pattern (Fig. 2.11b); in the former case the insertion of B4 is at the umbilical fissure and in the latter the insertion may occur at any place to the right of the prevailing location up to the point where the left hepatic duct normally unites with the right hepatic duct. In the latter instance, which according to Couinaud is present in 8% of individuals, there is no left hepatic duct. Instead there is a confluence of three ducts, the left lateral sectional duct, B4 and the right hepatic duct, to form the common hepatic duct. These variations are important in split liver transplantation and in diagnosis and repair of biliary injuries.

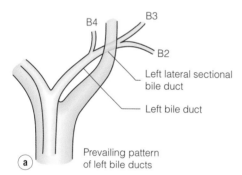

B4   B3

B2

Left lateral sectional
bile duct

Left bile duct

Prevailing pattern
of left bile ducts

(a)

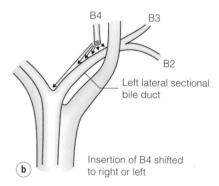

B4   B3

B2

Left lateral sectional
bile duct

Insertion of B4 shifted
to right or left

(b)

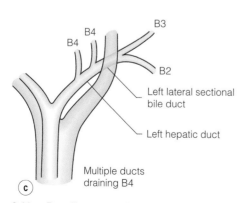

B3

B4
B4

B2

Left lateral sectional
bile duct

Left hepatic duct

Multiple ducts
draining B4

(c)

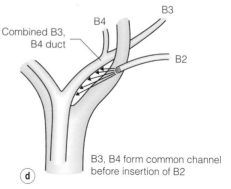

B3

B4

Combined B3,
B4 duct

B2

B3, B4 form common channel
before insertion of B2

(d)

Figure 2.11 • Prevailing pattern **(a)** and important variations **(b–d)** of bile ducts draining the left hemiliver.
© Washington University in St Louis.

The bile duct to Sg3 has been used to perform biliary bypass and can be isolated by following the superior surface of the ligamentum teres down to isolate the portal pedicle to Sg3. The technique is less commonly used now that internal endoscopic bypass has been developed.

Prevailing pattern of bile ducts draining the caudate lobe (Sg1)

Normally, two to three caudate ducts enter the biliary tree. Their orifices are usually located posteriorly on the left duct, right duct or right posterior sectional duct.

Portal veins and liver resections

On the right side of the liver the portal vein divisions correspond to those of the hepatic artery and bile duct, and they supply the same hepatic volumes. Therefore, there is a right portal vein that supplies the entire right hemiliver (**Fig. 2.12**). It divides into two sectional and four segmental veins, as do the arteries and bile ducts. On the left side of the liver, however, the left portal vein is quite unusual because of the fact that its structure was adapted to function in utero as a conduit between the umbilical vein and the ductus venosus, whilst postnatally the direction of flow is reversed. The left portal vein consists of a *horizontal or transverse portion*, which is located under Sg4, and a *vertical part or umbilical portion*,

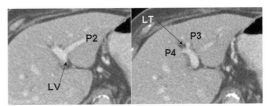

Figure 2.13 • Ramification of the left portal vein as seen on computed tomography. Note the branches to segments 2–4 and the ligamentum teres (*LT*). The arrow pointing to the ligamentum venosum (*LV*) and the groove between the left lateral section and the caudate lobe. This is also the site of origin of the ligamentum venosum, where the transverse portion of the left portal vein becomes the umbilical portion of the vein, proving conclusively that the branch to Sg2 is not part of a terminal division of the transverse portion of the vein as might be concluded from case studies (also see reference 7).
© Washington University in St Louis.

which is situated in the umbilical fissure (**Fig. 2.13**). Unlike the right portal vein, neither portion of the left portal vein actually enters the liver, but rather they lie directly on its surface. Often the umbilical portion is hidden by a bridge of tissue passing between left medial and lateral sections. This bridge of liver tissue may be as thick as 2 cm or be only a fibrous band. The junction of the transverse and umbilical portions of the left portal vein is marked by the attachment of a stout cord – the ligamentum venosum. This structure, the remnant of the fetal ductus venosus, runs in the groove between the left lateral section and the caudate lobe and attaches to the left hepatic vein/IVC junction.

Ramification of the left portal vein

The transverse portion of the left portal vein sends only a few small branches to Sg4. Large branches from the portal vein to the left liver arise exclusively beyond the attachment of the ligamentum venosum, i.e. from the umbilical part of the vein.[7] These branches come off both sides of the vein – those arising from the right side pass into Sg4 and those from the left supply Sg2 and Sg3. There is usually only one branch to Sg2 and Sg3, but often there is more than one branch to Sg4. The left portal vein terminates in the ligamentum teres at the free edge of the left liver. Note that the umbilical portion of the portal vein has a unique pattern of ramification. The pattern is similar to an air-conditioning duct that sends branches at right-angles from both of its sides to supply rooms (segments), tapering as it does so, finally to end blindly (in the ligamentum teres). Other vascular and biliary structures normally ramify by dividing into two other structures at their termination and not by sending out branches along their length.

Although the divisions of the portal vein are unusual, for the embryonic reasons described above,

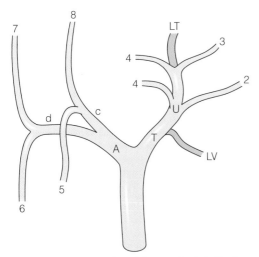

Figure 2.12 • Ramification of the portal vein in the liver. The portal vein divides into right (*A*) and left (*T*) branches. The branches in the right liver correspond to those of the hepatic artery and bile duct (Fig. 2.2). The branching pattern on the left is unique. The left portal vein has transverse (*T*) and umbilical portions (*U*). The transition point between the two parts is marked by the attachment of the ligamentum venosum (*LV*). All major branches come off the umbilical portion (see text). The vein ends blindly in the ligamentum teres (*LT*).
© Washington University in St Louis.

it is uncommon to have variations from this pattern. Probably the most common variation is absence of the right portal vein. In these cases the right posterior and right anterior sectional portal veins originate independently from the main portal vein. Under these circumstances the anterior sectional vein is usually quite high in the porta hepatis and may not be obvious. An unsuspecting surgeon may divide the posterior sectional vein thinking that it is the right portal vein and become confused when the anterior sectional vein is subsequently revealed during hepatic transection.

The portal vein branches to Sg4 may be isolated in the umbilical fissure on the right side of the umbilical portion of the left portal vein. The veins here are associated with the bile ducts and the arteries passing to Sg4, i.e. they enter sheaths as they go into the liver substance. Isolation in this location may provide extra margin when resecting a tumour in Sg4 that impinges upon the umbilical fissure. Normally the branches to Sg4 are isolated after dividing the parenchyma of the liver of Sg4 close to the umbilical fissure, an approach that is used to avoid injury to the umbilical portion of the left portal vein. Injury to this vein could, of course, deprive Sg2 and Sg3 of portal vein supply as well as Sg4. For instance, if this occurs when performing a right trisectionectomy, the only portion of the liver to be retained would be devascularised of portal vein flow. However, isolation of these structures within the umbilical fissure does provide an extra margin of clearance on tumours and can be done safely if care is taken to ascertain the position of the portal vein. Likewise, it is possible to isolate the portal vein branches going into Sg2 and Sg3 in the umbilical fissure and to extend a margin when resecting a tumour in the left lateral section. For the same reasons given above, caution must be taken when doing this in order not to injure the umbilical portion of the portal vein. In order to access the portal vein in this location it is usually necessary to divide the bridge of liver tissue, between the left medial and lateral sections. This is done by passing a blunt instrument behind the bridge before dividing it, usually with cautery. Note that arteries and bile ducts passing to the left lateral section are in danger of being injured as one isolates the most posterior–superior portion of the bridge. To facilitate passage of an instrument behind the bridge, the peritoneum at the base of the bridge may be opened in a preliminary step. The instrument being passed behind the bridge should never be forced.

Hepatic veins and liver resection (Fig. 2.14)

There are normally three large hepatic veins. These run in the midplane of the liver (middle hepatic vein), the right intersectional plane (right hepatic vein) and the left intersectional plane (left hepatic vein). The

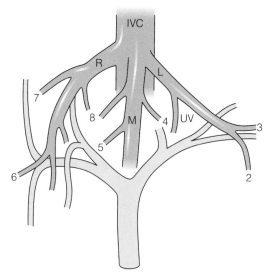

Figure 2.14 • Hepatic veins. There are normally three hepatic veins: right (R), middle (M) and left (L). Note the segments drained. The umbilical vein (UV) normally drains part of Sg4 into the left hepatic vein. The latter is proof that the terminal portion of the left vein lies in the intersectional plane of the left liver. IVC, inferior vena cava. © Washington University in St Louis.

left hepatic vein actually begins in the plane between Sg2 and Sg3 and travels in that plane for most of its length. It becomes quite a large vein even in that location. It leaves the plane between Sg2 and Sg3 and enters the left intersectional plane about 1 cm from where it terminates by uniting with the middle hepatic vein to form a common channel that enters the IVC. It receives the umbilical vein from Sg4 in its short course in the left intersectional plane. Note that this is the same plane in which the umbilical portion of the left portal vein lies. It is important not to confuse the 'umbilical portion of the left portal vein' with the 'umbilical vein'. The latter is a tributary of the left hepatic vein that normally drains the most leftward part of Sg4.[8,9] The left and middle hepatic veins usually fuse at a distance of about 1–2 cm from the IVC, so that when viewed from within the IVC there are only two hepatic vein openings. Rarely, hepatic veins join the IVC above the diaphragm.

In about 10% of individuals there is more than one large right hepatic vein. In these people, in addition to the right superior hepatic vein (normally called the right hepatic vein), which enters the IVC just below the level of the diaphragm, there is a right inferior hepatic vein that enters the IVC 5–6 cm below this level. If this inferior hepatic vein is present, resections of Sg7 and Sg8 may be performed, including resection of the right superior vein, without compromising the venous drainage of Sg5 and Sg6.

The caudate lobe is drained by its own veins – several short veins that enter the IVC directly from the caudate lobe. When performing a classical right hepatectomy, caudate veins are divided in the preliminary stage of the dissection. As dissection moves up the anterior surface of the vena cava to isolate the right hepatic vein, one encounters a bridge of tissue lateral to the IVC referred to as the hepato-caval ligament.[10] It connects the posterior portion of the right liver to the caudate lobe behind the IVC. This bridge of tissue usually consists of fibrous tissue, but occasionally is a bridge of liver parenchyma. It limits exposure of the right side of the IVC at a point just below the right hepatic vein and must be divided in order to isolate the right vein extrahepatically. This must be done with care as the ligament may contain a large vein and forceful dissection of the ligament may also result in injury to the right lateral side of the IVC. Isolation of the right hepatic vein is also aided by clearing the areolar tissue between the right and middle hepatic veins down to the level of the IVC when exposing these veins from above.

Another approach to right hepatectomy is to leave division of the caudate and right hepatic veins until after the liver is transected. In this case an instrument may be passed up along the anterior surface of the vena cava from below to emerge between the right and middle hepatic veins. Once an umbilical tape is passed, the liver may be hung to facilitate transection ('hanging manoeuvre').[11]

The left and middle veins can also be isolated prior to division of the liver. There are several ways to achieve this anatomically. One method is to divide all the caudate veins as well as the right hepatic vein. This exposes the entire anterior surface of the retrohepatic vena cava and leaves the liver attached to the vena cava only by the middle and left hepatic veins, which are then easily isolated. This is suitable when performing a right hepatectomy or extended right hepatectomy, especially when the caudate lobe is also to be resected. The advantage of having control of these veins during operations on the right liver is that total vascular occlusion is possible without occlusion of the IVC and haemodynamically the effect is not much different from occlusion of the main portal pedicle alone (Pringle manoeuvre).

In performing a left hepatectomy the right hepatic vein is conserved and a different anatomical approach to isolation of the left and middle hepatic veins is required. They may be isolated from the left side by dividing the ligamentum venosum, where it attaches to the left hepatic vein, then dividing the peritoneum at the superior tip of the caudate lobe and gently passing an instrument on the anterior surface of the vena cava to emerge between the middle and right veins and/or between the left and middle veins. Again, care needs to be applied when

performing this manoeuvre in order to avoid injury to the structures.

Isolation of the vena cava above and below the hepatic veins is also a technique that should be in the armamentarium of every surgeon performing major hepatic resection. It is not usually necessary when performing standard liver resections but surgeons should be familiar with the anatomical technique of doing so. Isolation of the vena cava superior to the hepatic veins is done by dividing the left triangular ligament and the lesser omentum, being careful to first look for a replaced left hepatic artery. The peritoneum on the superior border of the caudate lobe is then divided and a finger is passed behind the vena cava to come out just inferior to the crus of the diaphragm. The crus of the diaphragm makes an easily identified column on the right side. This column passes across the right side of the vena cava and dissection of the space inferior to this column and behind the vena cava facilitates passage of the finger from the left side to the right side in the space behind the vena cava. Isolation of the vena cava below the liver is more straightforward but one should be aware of the position of the adrenal vein and in some cases it is necessary to isolate the adrenal vein if bleeding is persisting after occlusion of the vena cava above and below the liver.

Finally, the surgeon should be aware that during transection of the liver large veins will be encountered in certain planes of transection. For instance, in its passage along the midplane the middle hepatic vein usually receives two large tributaries, one from Sg5 inferiorly and the other from Sg8 superiorly. Both are routinely encountered in performing right hepatectomy. The venous drainage of the right side of the liver is highly variable and additional large veins, including one from Sg6, may also enter the middle hepatic vein.

Liver capsule, attachments and the plate system

The liver is encased in a thin fibrous capsule, called Glisson's capsule, which covers the entire organ except for a large bare area posteriorly where the organ is in contact with the IVC and with the diaphragm to the right of the IVC. The bare area stretches superiorly to include the termination of the three hepatic veins and ends in a point, which is also where the attachment of the falciform ligament ends. The limit of the bare area, where the peritoneum passes between the body wall and the liver, is called the coronary ligament. It is one of three structures that connect the liver to the abdominal wall 'dorsally', the other two being the right and left triangular ligaments. The liver also has another bare area, best thought of as a bare crease, where the hepatoduodenal ligament and the lesser omentum attach on the 'ventral' surface. It is through this crease that the portal structures enter the liver at the hilum. The other ligamentous structures of interest to surgeons are the ligamentum teres, falciform ligament and the ligamentum venosum. The ligamentum teres (teres = 'round') is the obliterated left umbilical vein and runs in the free edge of the falciform ligament from the umbilicus to the termination of the umbilical portion of the left portal vein. The falciform (falciform = 'scythe shaped') is the filmy fold that runs between the anterior abdominal wall above the umbilicus and attaches to the anterior surface of the liver between the left medial and left lateral sections.

There are four fibrous plates on the surface of the liver (hilar, cystic, umbilical and arantian) (**Fig 2.15**). These fibrous plates are condensations of Glisson's capsule. The hilar plate is the most important plate in liver surgery. Incising the junction between the base of Sg4 and the hilar plate is referred to as 'lowering the hilar plate' and is an important step in the surgical exposure of the extrahepatic bile ducts, particularly the left hepatic duct.

The sheath of the right portal pedicle extends off the hilar plate like a sleeve into the liver surrounding the portal structures, i.e. portal vein, hepatic artery and bile duct. The combined structure is referred to as a 'portal pedicle'. As the right portal pedicle enters the liver it divides into a right anterior and right posterior portal pedicle supplying the respective sections, and then segmental pedicles supplying the four segments. On the left side, only the segmental structures are sheathed. There is no sheathed main portal pedicle because the main portal vein, proper hepatic artery and common hepatic duct are not close enough to the liver to be enclosed in a sheath.

The cystic plate is the ovoid fibrous sheet on which the gallbladder lies (Fig. 2.15). When a cholecystectomy is performed, this plate is normally left behind. In its posterior extent the cystic plate narrows to become a stout cord that attaches to the anterior surface of the sheath of the right portal pedicle. The latter is a point of anatomical importance for the surgeon wishing to expose the anterior surface of the right portal pedicle, since this cord must be divided to do so.[12] With severe chronic inflammation the cystic plate may become shortened and thickened so that the distance between the top of the cystic plate and the right portal pedicle is likewise much shorter than usual. This places the structures in the right pedicle in danger during cholecystectomy when dissection is performed 'top down' as a primary strategy. The other plates are the umbilical and arantian, which underlie the umbilical portion of the left portal vein and the ligamentum venosum, respectively (Fig. 2.15). The other sheaths carry segmental bilovascular pedicles of the left liver and caudate lobe.

In performing a right hepatectomy there are two methods of managing the right-sided portal vessels and bile ducts. The first is to isolate the hepatic artery, portal vein and bile duct individually and either control them or ligate them extrahepatically, and the second is to isolate the entire portal pedicle and staple the pedicle. Isolation of the right portal pedicle can be performed by making hepatotomies above the right

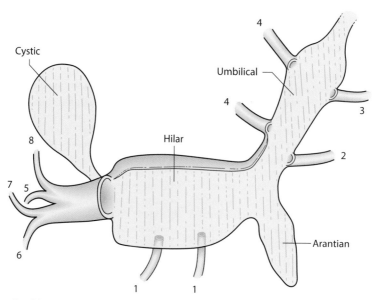

Figure 2.15 • The plate/sheath system of the liver.
Adapted from Strasberg SM, Linehan DC, Hawkins WG. Isolation of right main and right sectional portal pedicles for liver resection without hepatotomy or inflow occlusion. J Am Coll Surg 2008;206:390–6. With permission of the Journal of the American College of Surgeons.

portal pedicle in Sg4 and in the gallbladder fossa after removing the gallbladder. A finger is passed through the hepatotomy to isolate the right portal pedicle. This technique usually requires inflow occlusion. It can also be done without inflow occlusion by lowering the hilar plate and coming around the right portal pedicle directly on its surface (**Fig. 2.16**).[13] It is advisable to divide caudate veins in the area below the vena caval ligament before performing pedicle isolation, since haemorrhage from these veins can be considerable if they are injured during isolation of the right portal pedicle.

Liver volume and regeneration

The normal adult human liver is approximately 2% of total body mass. This represents a relative surplus of functioning liver tissue. A key factor that must be considered when planning a liver resection is the likely volume of the future remnant liver. For patients with healthy liver parenchyma, this can be as low as 30% of original hepatic volume. Resecting beyond this risks the development of post hepatectomy liver failure. When a proposed liver resection risks leaving a small future remnant, or where there is concern regarding the quality of the liver parenchyma, it is possible to induce relative regeneration in the future remnant liver, largely through hyperplasia. This is most often achieved by means of partial vascular occlusion to the part of the liver resected, commonly through ligation or embolisation of the respective branch of the portal vein. This principle can be adapted to enable a two-stage procedure, which is usually indicated when a patient requires a right hemihepatectomy along with multiple resections from the left hemiliver. The first stage involves the clearance of all disease from the left hemiliver and ligation of the right portal vein. The patient is then given 4–6 weeks during which the left hemiliver regenerates, following which a right hepatectomy can be safely performed. A more recent evolution of the principle of the two-stage resection is the ALPPS procedure (Associating Liver Partition and Portal vein ligation for Staged hepatectomy). This involves the addition of a parenchymal separation of the future remnant liver during the first-stage operation.[14] The ALPPS procedure is controversial, as although it produces rapid hypertrophy of the future liver remnant permitting the second-stage resection to be performed within one week, early reports have been associated with increased morbidity and mortality.

Gallbladder and extrahepatic bile ducts

Gallbladder

The gallbladder lies on the cystic plate. The edge of the gallbladder forms one side of the hepatocystic triangle. The other two sides are the right side of the common hepatic duct and the liver. Eponyms covering this anatomy (Calot, Moosman, etc.) are confusing and should be abandoned. The hepatocystic triangle contains the cystic artery and cystic node and a portion of the right hepatic artery, as well as fat and fibrous tissue. Clearance of this

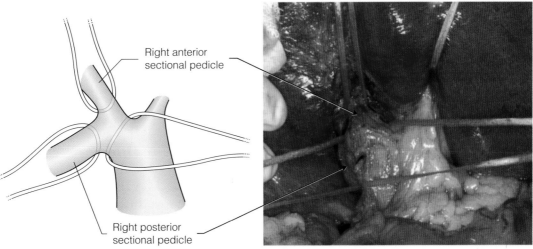

Right anterior
sectional pedicle

Right posterior
sectional pedicle

Figure 2.16 • Isolation of right portal pedicle and sectional pedicles by the technique of dissection on the surface of pedicles. No inflow occlusion or separate hepatotomies are used (see reference 13). The umbilical tape in the upper right of the photograph is around the bridge of liver tissue over the umbilical fissure.
Reproduced from Strasberg SM, Linehan DC, Hawkins WG. Isolation of right main and right sectional portal pedicles for liver resection without hepatotomy or inflow occlusion. J Am Coll Surg 2008;206:390–6. With permission of the Journal of the American College of Surgeons.

triangle along with isolation of the cystic duct and elevation of the base of the gallbladder off the lower portion of the cystic plate gives the 'critical view of safety' that has been described for identification of the cystic structures during laparoscopic cholecystectomy[15] (**Fig. 2.17**). A large number of curiosities of the gallbladder, e.g. the phrygian cap, have been described. The following are anomalies of importance to the biliary surgeon.

Agenesis of the gallbladder

Agenesis occurs in approximately 1 in 8000 patients. It can be difficult to recognise but when it is suspected, axial imaging may confirm. If doubt remains, laparoscopy is definitive.

Double gallbladder

This is also a very rare anomaly but can be the cause of persistent symptoms after cholecystectomy. The gallbladder may also be bifid which typically does not cause symptoms, or have an hourglass constriction which may cause symptoms due to obstruction of the upper segment.

Cystic duct

This structure is normally 1–2 cm in length and 2–3 mm in diameter. It joins the common hepatic duct at an acute angle to form the common bile duct. The cystic duct normally joins the common hepatic duct approximately 4 cm above the duodenum. However, the cystic duct may enter at any level from the biliary confluence down to the ampulla. The cystic duct may also join directly into the right hepatic duct, either when the right duct is in its normal position or in an aberrant location.

There are three patterns of confluence of the cystic duct and common hepatic duct (**Fig. 2.18**). In 20% of patients there is a parallel union and the surgeon approaching the common hepatic duct by dissecting the cystic duct is at risk of injuring the side of the former structure (Fig. 2.18). When making a choledochotomy in this situation, the incision should be started on the lateral side of the midplane of the bile duct in order to avoid entering a septum between the two fused ducts. When performing cholecystectomy, the cystic duct should be occluded in such a way that there is a visible section of cystic duct between the clip and the common bile duct.

Although a gallbladder with two cystic ducts has been described, the author has not seen convincing proof that this anomaly actually exists. If it does, it must be an anomaly of extreme rarity.

Cystic artery

The cystic artery is about 1 mm in diameter and normally arises from the right hepatic artery in the hepatocystic triangle (**Fig. 2.19a**). Typically the cystic artery runs for 1–2 cm to meet the gallbladder superior to the insertion of the cystic duct. The artery ramifies into an anterior and posterior branch at the point of contact with the gallbladder and these branches continue to divide on their respective surfaces. Sometimes the cystic artery divides into branches

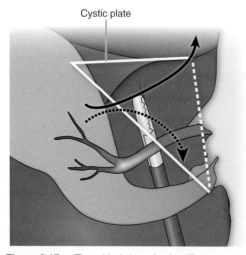

Cystic plate

Figure 2.17 • The critical view of safety. The hepatocystic triangle has been dissected free of fat and fibrous tissue. Gallbladder, right side of the common hepatic duct (not displayed) and the liver form the border of the hepatocystic triangle. The cystic artery is within the hepatocystic triangle, and is branched into anterior and posterior branches. The arrows (solid and dotted) indicate the direction of dissection during cholecystectomy. The dotted arrow indicates leaving areolar tissue on the cystic plate; whereas the solid arrow indicates leaving the areolar tissue with the gallbladder during dissection.

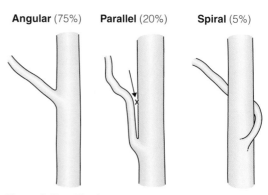

Angular (75%)   **Parallel** (20%)   **Spiral** (5%)

Figure 2.18 • The three types of cystic duct/common hepatic duct confluence. The parallel union confluence is shown in the middle. Dissection of this type of cystic duct (*arrow*) may lead to injury to the side of the common hepatic duct during laparoscopic cholecystectomy. This is often a cautery injury.
Adapted from Warrren KW, McDonald WM, Kune GA. Bile duct strictures: new concepts in the management of an old problem. In: Irvine WT, editor. Modern trends in surgery. London: Butterworth; 1966. With permission from Elsevier.

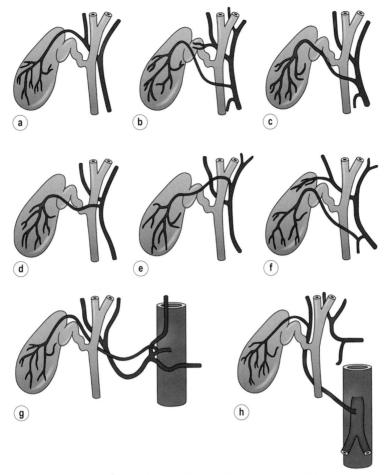

Figure 2.19 • The eight common anatomical variations of the cystic artery to the gallbladder.
(Adapted from Poston GJ, Blumgart LH, editors. Surgical management of hepatobiliary and pancreatic disorders. 2nd ed. 2010. Ch. 2, p. 10. Boca Raton: CRC Press.)

before the gallbladder is reached. In this situation, the anterior branch may be mistaken as the cystic artery proper and the posterior branch will not be discovered until later in the dissection, when it may be divided inadvertently. The artery may ramify into several branches before reaching the gallbladder, giving the impression that there is no cystic artery. The anterior and posterior branches may arise independently from the right hepatic artery, giving rise to two distinct cystic arteries. It is important to bear in mind other anatomical variations which are of significance during cholecystectomy including (Fig. 2.19):

1. A cystic artery that arises from the hepatic artery proper and runs anterior to the common hepatic duct (Fig. 2.19c).
2. A cystic artery that arises from the right hepatic artery on the left side of the common hepatic duct (Fig. 2.19d) or from the left hepatic artery (Fig. 2.19e) and runs anterior to the common

hepatic duct, while the right hepatic artery runs behind it. Such cystic arteries tend to tether the gallbladder and make dissection of the hepatocystic triangle more difficult.
3. A cystic artery that arises from the gastroduodenal artery (GDA) (Fig. 2.19f) or an aberrant right hepatic artery coming off the superior mesenteric artery (SMA) (Fig. 2.19h). In this case the cystic artery and not the cystic duct tends to be in the free edge of the fold leading from the hepatoduodenal ligament to the gallbladder. This should be suspected whenever the 'cystic duct' looks smaller than the 'cystic artery'.

Multiple small cystic veins drain into intrahepatic portal vein branches by passing into the liver around or through the cystic plate. Sometimes there are cystic veins in the hepatocystic triangle that run parallel to the cystic artery and enter the main portal vein.

The **cystic plate** has been described above. Small bile ducts may penetrate the cystic plate to enter the gallbladder. These 'ducts of Luschka' are very small, usually submillimetre accessory ducts. However, when divided during cholecystectomy, postoperative bilomas may occur if they are not visualised and occluded. Bilomas and haemorrhage may also be caused by penetration of the cystic plate during dissection. In about 10% of patients there is a large peripheral bile duct immediately deep to the plate, disruption of which will cause copious bile drainage. The origin of the middle hepatic vein is also in this location, and if it is injured massive haemorrhage may ensue. There is areolar tissue between the muscularis of the gallbladder and the cystic plate. At the top of the gallbladder the layer is very thin. This areolar layer thickens if retrograde dissection from the top of the gallbladder in a medial direction is performed. If areolar tissue is left on the cystic plate, the surgeon will arrive on the posterior surface of the cystic artery and cystic duct (Fig. 2.17, *dotted arrow*). Conversely, if dissection is performed on the cystic plate leaving the areolar tissue on the gallbladder, the surgeon will arrive at the right portal pedicle (Fig. 2.17, *solid arrow*). If this is not anticipated, structures in the right portal pedicle may be injured. This dissection method is significantly more challenging in the presence of an inflamed gallbladder or Mirizzi syndrome, when the areolar tissue between the gallbladder and cystic plate is fused together.

Extrahepatic bile ducts

The common hepatic duct (CHD) is a structure formed by union of the right and left hepatic ducts. The union normally occurs at the right extremity of the base of Sg4, anterior and superior to the portal vein bifurcation. The CHD travels in the right edge of the hepatoduodenal ligament for 2–3 cm, where it joins the cystic duct to form the common bile duct (CBD). The latter has a supraduodenal course of 3–4 cm and then passes behind the duodenum to run in or occasionally behind the pancreas to enter the second portion of the duodenum. Details of its lower section and relation to the pancreatic duct are described in the final section of this chapter. The external diameter of the common bile duct varies from 5 to 13 mm when distended to physiological pressures. However, the duct diameter at surgery, i.e. in fasting patients with low duct pressures, may be as small as 3 mm. Radiologically, the internal duct diameter is measured on fasting patients. Under these conditions the upper limit is normally 8 mm. Size should never be used as a sole criterion for identifying a bile duct. Caution is required in situations where a structure seems larger than expected. Although the cystic duct may be enlarged due to passage of stones, the surgeon should take extra precaution before dividing a 'cystic duct' that is greater than 2 mm in diameter because the common bile duct can be 3 mm in diameter and aberrant ducts may be smaller.

Anomalies of extrahepatic bile ducts

As already noted, there are biliary anomalies of the right and left ductal systems that can affect the outcome of hepatic surgery. The same is true for biliary surgery. The most important clinical anomaly is low insertion of right hepatic ducts referred to above. Because of its low location, it may be mistaken as the cystic duct and be injured during cholecystectomy. This is even more likely to occur when the cystic duct unites with an aberrant duct as opposed to joining the common hepatic duct. Left hepatic ducts can also join the common hepatic duct at a low level. They are less prone to injury since dissection during cholecystectomy is on the right side of the biliary tree.

Extrahepatic arteries

The course of these arteries has been described above. Anomalies of the hepatic artery are important in gallbladder surgery. Normally the right hepatic artery passes posterior to the bile duct (80%) (Fig. 2.19a) and gives off the cystic artery in the hepatocystic triangle. However, in 20% of cases the right hepatic artery runs anterior to the bile duct (Fig. 2.19b–f). The right hepatic artery may lie very close to the gallbladder and chronic inflammation can draw the right hepatic artery directly on to the gallbladder, where it lies in an inverse U-loop and is prone to injury. In the 'classical injury' in laparoscopic cholecystectomy when the common bile duct is mistaken for the cystic duct, an associated right hepatic artery injury is very common.

Blood supply of bile ducts

Many studies, dating back to the 19th century, have examined the blood supply of the extrahepatic bile ducts in cadaveric specimens. A key observation made by Rappaport is that the bile ducts are supplied by the hepatic artery only,[16] unlike the liver, which has a dual blood supply from the hepatic artery and the portal vein. The arterial blood supply can be thought of as having three anatomical elements. The first consists of afferent vessels from the hepatic artery and its branches (**Fig. 2.20a**). The second element is longitudinal arteries that run parallel to the long axis of the bile duct and that receive blood from the afferent vessels (**Fig. 2.20b**). The third element is an arterial plexus encasing the bile ducts that receives blood from the marginal arteries (**Fig. 2.20c**). Tiny branches of the plexus pierce the bile duct wall to supply the capillaries of the bile duct.

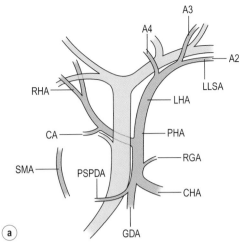

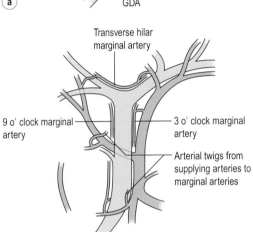

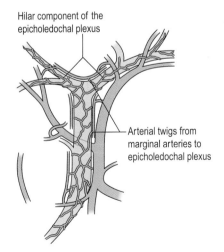

Figure 2.20 • **(a)** The supplying arteries. All arteries shown can all give branches to the marginal arteries or in some cases directly supply the epicholedochal plexus. (*A2*, *A3*, *A4*, arteries to Sg2, 3 and 4; *CA*, cystic artery; *CHA*, common hepatic artery; *GDA*, gastroduodenal artery; *LHA*, left hepatic artery; *LLSA*, left lateral sectional artery; *PHA*, proper hepatic artery; *PSPDA*, posterior superior pancreaticoduodenal artery, the most important and constant artery; *RHA*, right hepatic artery). Replaced arteries arising from the superior mesenteric artery may also supply the bile ducts. **(b)** Marginal arteries. Marginal arteries are disposed at 3 and 9 o'clock (and occasionally at 12 o'clock) on the common bile duct/common hepatic duct. The hilar marginal artery runs across the top of the confluence of the right and left hepatic ducts. **(c)** Epicholedochal plexus. The epicholedochal plexus is supplied by the marginal arteries. Adapted from Strasberg SM, Helton WS. An analytical review of vasculobiliary injury in laparoscopic and open cholecystectomy. HPB 2011;13(1):1–14. With permission from John Wiley & Sons.

The afferent vessels are branches of the hepatic arteries and less commonly of the superior mesenteric artery or other upper abdominal arteries. The most constant and important artery supplying the bile duct is the posterior superior pancreaticoduodenal artery, usually the first branch of the GDA. Arterial branches pass to the duct as the artery winds around the lower end of the duct. These branches supply much of the retroduodenal and intrapancreatic bile duct, but also ascend the bile duct to supply the supraduodenal bile duct. The lowest portion of the duct near the ampulla is also supplied by the anterior superior pancreatic artery from the inferior pancreatico-duodenal artery. Other vessels that commonly send afferents to the supraduodenal duct are the proper hepatic artery, cystic artery and artery to Sg4. Furthermore, body wall collaterals such as phrenic arteries can at times supply the bile ducts (as well as the liver) since bile duct infarction is much more common when there is occlusion of the common hepatic artery after a transplant than it is in an in situ liver. The notion that the extrahepatic bile duct is supplied by arteries that join it only at the bottom and top of its course is incorrect. Supplying arteries from the cystic artery, right and left hepatic arteries and proper hepatic artery may also supply it.

The afferent vessels usually supply the longitudinal or 'marginal' arteries that run parallel to the long axis of the bile ducts (also called 'marginal anastomotic loop').[17] These vessels are disposed at 3 and 9 or, less commonly, at 12 o'clock on the common bile duct/common hepatic duct, or run across the top of the confluence and the right and left bile ducts. This 'hilar marginal artery' has been called the 'caudate arcade' or 'communicating arcade'. This artery is of great importance in maintaining blood supply to the liver when one hepatic artery (right or left) is occluded.[18]

The third element of this system is the 'epicholedochal plexus', a fine arterial plexus that lies on and surrounds the entire common bile duct and the left and right bile ducts. The latter is the hilar component of the epicholedochal plexus. The vessels of the plexus tend to run along the long axis of the ducts so that on the common duct many of the vessels are vertical while those around the confluence and the right and left ducts are disposed horizontally. In the portion of the biliary tree that lies adjacent to the hilar plate or which has entered the fibrous sheaths, the epicholedochal plexus lies between the sheath and the wall of the bile duct. Dissection in this plane has the potential to devascularise bile ducts.[19]

Transection of the bile duct may result in ischaemia of the duct. For instance, if the duct is transected at the level of the duodenum, ischaemia of a portion of the bile duct above this level may occur since blood flow originating from the superior pancreatico-duodenal artery and passing up along the marginal artery is cut off. Similarly, in a high transection at the level of the confluence, the lower cut end of the duct may become ischaemic. This problem is thought to be an important contributory cause to the frequent failure of choledocho-choledochotomy as a form of biliary reconstruction. To avoid this problem, the bile duct is trimmed back to within 1 cm of the confluence and a hepatico-jejunostomy is fashioned.

Pancreas

Embryological development of the pancreas

The thickening of the endoderm on the dorsal side of the gut tube opposite the hepatic bulge marks the development of the dorsal pancreas. The bulging of the dorsal pancreas into the mesenchyme becomes paired with the growth of the ventral foregut endoderm, which becomes the ventral pancreas. During the clockwise rotation of the gut tube, the ventral and dorsal buds come together and subsequently fuse. Pancreatic progenitor cells undergo further differentiation and commit to the major pancreatic lineages depending on either endocrine or exocrine pathways. Acinar cells are produced and proliferate around the epithelial tip, whilst islets of Langerhans are derived at a later stage, and continue to develop beyond the first week of the postnatal period.

Anatomical structure and functions of the pancreas

The pancreas is a retroperitoneal organ lying obliquely across the upper abdomen so that the tail is superior to the head. It is approximately 22 cm in length. The head of the pancreas is discoid in shape and terminates inferiorly and medially in the hook-like uncinate process. The neck, body and tail are shaped like a flattened cylinder, sometimes somewhat triangular in cross-section with a flat anterior and pointed posterior surface. These divisions of the organ are somewhat arbitrary, but the neck of the pancreas sits anterior to the superior mesenteric and portal vein. Normally the consistency of the gland is soft.

The pancreas has two key functions, which are endo- and exo-crine functions. For the exocrine function, pancreatic juice is secreted from acinar cells to intralobular ducts, which in turn drain into the main pancreatic duct and then to the duodenum. The enzyme produced from the acinar cell is secreted as an inactive form, called zymogen, which is then cleaved and activated by enteropeptidase upon reaching the duodenum (**Fig. 2.21**).

The endocrine function of the pancreas is contributed by four types of pancreatic islet cells, namely α-(alpha-)cells (secreting glucagon), β-(beta-)cells (insulin), δ-(delta-)cells (somatostatin) and γ-(gamma-)cells (pancreatic polypeptide). Insulin acts to decrease blood glucose level, whereas glucagon balances it out. These hormones are secreted by the islet cells directly into the bloodstream, and function independently from the exocrine role of the pancreas.

Pancreatic ducts

The prevailing anatomical pattern of the pancreatic duct is the result of union of the ventral main duct (Wirsung) with the dorsal accessory duct (Santorini), along with partial regression of the dorsal duct in the head. The 'genu' of the duct (genu = knee) is the bend in the duct where the ventral duct joins the dorsal duct. In the prevailing pattern, both ducts communicate with the duodenum, the dorsal duct entering at the minor papilla approximately 2 cm above and 5 mm anterior to the major papilla. Other ductal patterns are possible that involve various degrees of dominance or regression of portions of the ducts in the head of the pancreas. For instance,

the ducts may not unite, resulting in separate drainage from the ventral and dorsal pancreas (pancreas divisum), the dorsal duct may lose its connection to the duodenum; or the dorsal duct in the head may lose its connection to the rest of the ductal system and drain only a small section of the head into the duodenum. Alternatively, the ventral duct may regress and the dorsal duct drain more or all of the pancreas through the minor ampulla. The uncinate process is served by its own duct, which joins the main pancreatic duct 1–2 cm from its entry into the duodenum.

The pancreatic duct (and pancreas) are often referred to as proximal (head) and distal (tail). These may be confusing terms – as may the terms proximal and distal bile duct. The bile duct nearest to the ampulla is commonly referred to as 'distal', but the pancreatic duct in this region as 'proximal'. An alternative is to refer to the pancreatic portion or lower bile duct and the upper extrahepatic or hilar bile duct. For the pancreas, the duct may be referred to as the 'pancreatic head duct', 'pancreatic body duct', etc.

The ventral duct usually joins the common bile duct to form a common channel several millimetres from the ampulla of Vater, usually within the wall of the duodenum. The bile duct traverses the duodenal wall obliquely and the pancreatic duct at a right-angle. Each duct and the common channel have their own sphincters. The common channel may

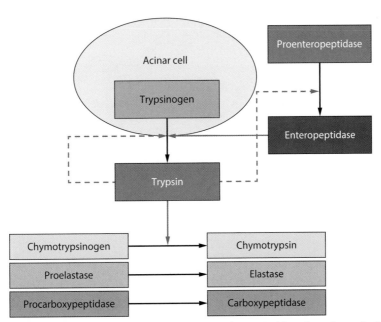

Figure 2.21 • Pancreatic zymogen activation cascade. Trypsinogen is secreted from the acinar cells. Upon reaching the duodenum, trypsinogen is cleaved and activated by enteropeptidase to become trypsin, which then activates chymotrypsinogen, proelastase, procarboxypeptidase. The formation of trypsin also allows the cleavage of more trypsinogen and the precursor of enteropeptidase.

be longer or absent, with both ducts entering the duodenum separately, the pancreatic duct more inferiorly. In performing a sphincteroplasty, it is advisable to open the common opening superiorly (10–12 o'clock position in the mobilised duodenum) to avoid the orifice of the pancreatic duct (4 o'clock). The ampulla is normally at the midpoint of the second part of the duodenum. It is rarely higher but can be as low as the midpoint of the third part of the duodenum. When the dorsal duct has its own communication with the duodenum, it is found at the 'minor papilla', about 2 cm proximal and 1 cm anterior to the major papilla.

Blood supply of the pancreas

The arterial supply of the pancreas consists of two vascular systems, one supplying the head and uncinate, and the other the body and tail. The neck is a watershed area between these two vascular systems.[20] The head and uncinate process are supplied by the pancreatico-duodenal arcade, which consists of two to several loops of vessels that arise from the superior pancreatico-duodenal (branch of the GDA) and inferior pancreatico-duodenal (branch of the SMA) arteries. The arcades run on the anterior and posterior surface of the pancreas next to the duodenum, the anterior arcade lying somewhat closer to the duodenum. The second system arises from the splenic artery, which gives rise to three arteries into the dorsal surface of the gland (**Fig. 2.22**). The dorsal pancreatic artery is the most medial of the three and the most important. It anastomoses with the pancreatico-duodenal arcade in the neck of the pancreas. It is the most aberrant artery in the upper abdomen and may arise from vessels that are routinely occluded during pancreatico-duodenectomy, which may account in part for fistula formation after this procedure.

This unique arterial arcade between the inferior pancreatico-duodenal and the GDA at the head of the pancreas provides an additional surgical option in achieving resectability for pancreatic body tumours encasing the coeliac axis in these rare circumstances. By resecting the coeliac axis the liver will then rely on the backflow arterial supply from the GDA to the hepatic artery proper, and that GDA will also provide the only arterial supply to the stomach via the gastroepiploic artery, since the left gastric and splenic arteries will have been sacrificed during the coeliac axis resection. This procedure is known as the 'Appleby' procedure, which was first described by Lyon Appleby in 1953.[21]

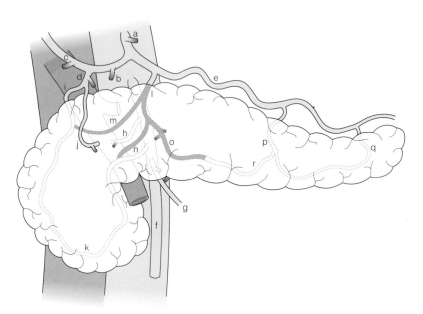

Figure 2.22 • Arterial blood supply to the pancreas. The dorsal pancreatic artery is shown shaded. Alternative origins of the artery are shown as black stumps. Key: *a*, coeliac artery; *b*, common hepatic artery; *c*, right hepatic artery; *d*, gastroduodenal artery; *e*, splenic artery; *f*, superior mesenteric artery; *g*, middle colic artery; *h*, right hepatic artery (aberrant); *i*, superior pancreatico-duodenal artery; *j*, right gastroepiploic artery; *k*, inferior pancreatico-duodenal artery; *l*, dorsal pancreatic artery (DPA); *m*, right anastomotic branch of DPA to superior part of pancreatico-duodenal arcade; *o*, left anastomotic branch of DPA becomes transverse pancreatic artery; *p*, pancreatica magna artery; *q*, caudal pancreatic artery; *r*, transverse pancreatic artery.
© Washington University in St Louis.

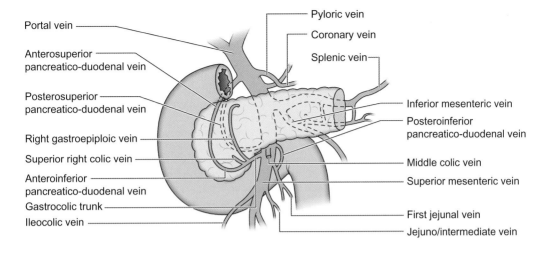

Portal vein

Anterosuperior pancreatico-duodenal vein

Posterosuperior pancreatico-duodenal vein

Right gastroepiploic vein

Superior right colic vein

Anteroinferior pancreatico-duodenal vein

Gastrocolic trunk

Ileocolic vein

Pyloric vein

Coronary vein

Splenic vein

Inferior mesenteric vein

Posteroinferior pancreatico-duodenal vein

Middle colic vein

Superior mesenteric vein

First jejunal vein

Jejuno/intermediate vein

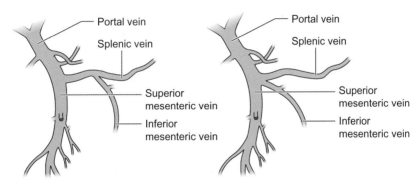

Portal vein

Splenic vein

Superior mesenteric vein

Inferior mesenteric vein

Portal vein

Splenic vein

Superior mesenteric vein

Inferior mesenteric vein

Figure 2.23 • Venous drainage of the pancreas. Variations in the relation of the portal, splenic, superior mesenteric and inferior mesenteric veins are shown at the bottom.
Adapted from Vickers SM, Arnoletti JP, Brunicardi FC, Andersen DK. Pancreas anatomy and physiology. In: Mulholland MW, Lillemoe KD, Doherty GM, editors. Greenfield's surgery: scientific principles and practice. 4th edition. Philadelphia: Lippincott Williams & Wilkins; 2006. Copyright © 2006 Lippincott Williams & Wilkins.

Venous drainage generally follows the arterial supply (**Fig. 2.23**). The veins of the body and tail of the pancreas drain into the splenic vein, which lies partly embedded in the posterior surface of the gland. These veins are short and fragile. The right gastroepiploic and anteroinferior pancreatico-duodenal veins provide drainage for the head and uncinate process. These two tributaries form the gastrocolic trunk, which in turn drains into the superior mesenteric vein (SMV) on the right lateral side, and then to the portal vein (PV) above the porto-splenic confluence. The gastrocolic trunk is a key tributary that is ligated during pancreatico-duodenectomy. A nearly constant posterosuperior pancreatico-duodenal vein enters the right lateral side of the portal vein at the level of the duodenum. During the isolation of all venous tributaries prior to performing a SMV/PV resection, it is important to be mindful of the insertion of the coronary vein, which provides drainage for the left gastric vein immediately above the porto-splenic confluence. The inferior mesenteric vein (IMV) normally drains into the splenic vein. However, the IMV can occasionally drain directly to the SMV, and can be damaged during surgical dissection.

Lymphatics of the pancreas

For surgical purposes, the lymphatic drainage of the pancreas is best considered with respect to resection of the pancreatic head and resection of the pancreatic body and tail. Nomenclature for nodal stations is currently based on the classification of the Japanese Pancreas Society as recommended by the International Study Group on Pancreatic Surgery (ISGPS).[22]

There is a ring of nodes around the pancreas that drain the adjacent sections of the gland and are denoted by various lymph node stations (Ln), depending on their location.[23] The lymphatics of the head and uncinate process drain into lymph nodes in the pancreatico-duodenal groove anteriorly (Ln17) and posteriorly (Ln13), and infrapyloric nodes inferiorly (Ln6). These in turn drain into nodes adjacent to the common bile duct (Ln12) and hepatic artery superiorly (Ln8), and into nodes along the SMA (Ln14), coeliac axis (Ln9) and aorta (axial nodes). Understanding these lymph node stations is important as current practice is a standard lymphadenectomy for pancreatico-duodenectomy, which does not include coeliac (Ln9), splenic (Ln11) and left gastric (Ln7) nodes.

The lymphatics of the body and tail are shown in **Fig. 2.24**. These are lymph nodes around the splenic hilum (Ln10), splenic artery (Ln11) and inferior border of body/tail of pancreas (Ln18). Resection of Ln9 is only indicated in tumours involving the body of the pancreas.

Anatomical relations and ligaments of the pancreas

The pancreas is a deeply seated organ that, unlike the liver and most of the biliary tree, is not obvious when opening the abdomen. The anatomical relations of the pancreas are very important in pancreatic surgery. The structures emphasised in the following section are those that are commonly invaded by tumours.

The pancreas lies in the pararenal space anterior to the anterior renal fascia and behind the peritoneum. Posteriorly, the pancreas is related, from right to left, to the right kidney and perinephric fat, IVC and right gonadal vein, aorta, left renal vein (slightly inferior), retropancreatic fat, left adrenal gland and the superior pole of the left kidney. All of the former structures lie in the perirenal space and behind the anterior renal fascia. In the case of oncological resections, the plane of dissection should be behind the anterior renal fascia in order to

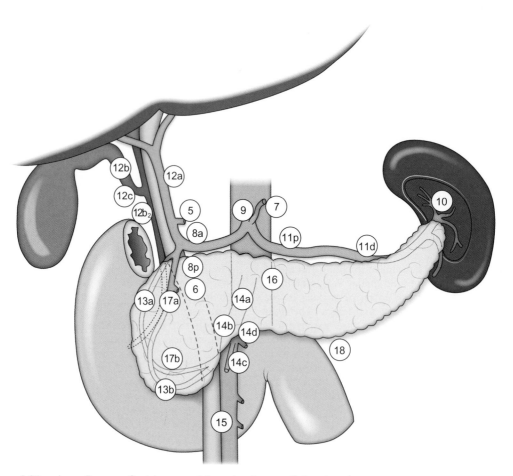

Figure 2.24 • Japan Pancreas Society nomenclature of peripancreatic lymph nodes.
Adapted from Japan Pancreas Society. Classification of pancreatic carcinoma. 2nd English edition. Tokyo: Kanehara & Co. Ltd; 2003.

maximise the chance of obtaining negative margins as described for the radical antegrade modular pancreatosplenectomy (RAMPS) procedure.[24]

The SMV and portal vein are posterior relations to the neck of the pancreas, and *splenic vein* to the body and tail. The SMA is a posterior relation of the junction of the neck and body of the gland lying posterior and medial to the SMV. The SMA and SMV are both related to the uncinate process and give branches into and receive tributaries from the uncinate process, respectively. Often the uncinate veins enter a large tributary of the SMV, the first jejunal vein, which also abuts the uncinate process. These short arteries and veins are of importance surgically as they are divided when the head of the pancreas is resected. The *coeliac artery* rises vertically superior to the SMA close to the superior edge of the pancreas, where it gives off the common hepatic artery and the *splenic artery*. The former runs anteriorly and to the left in approximation to the superior border of the pancreas. At the point where the artery passes in front of the portal vein, it divides into the *gastroduodenal artery*, which passes anterior to the neck of the pancreas, sometimes buried within it. It terminates in the right gastroepiploic artery that rises in a fold of tissue toward the pylorus, a fold that also contains the right gastroepiploic vein and subpyloric nodes. The splenic artery snakes along the superior border of the pancreas to leave it 2–3 cm from the termination of the pancreas.

The head of the pancreas is wrapped in the first three parts of the duodenum and the tail ends in relation to the splenic hilum. There is variability in the proximity of the tail of the pancreas to the spleen. In some cases the pancreas terminates 2 cm from the splenic substance and in others it abuts it. The anterior surface of the body and tail of the pancreas is covered by peritoneum, which is the posterior wall of the lesser sac, and then by the posterior wall of the stomach anterior to this. The transverse mesocolon is related to the inferior border of the pancreas, and the right and left extremities of the transverse colon are related to the head and tail of the gland. The inferior mesenteric vein is related to the inferior border of the neck of the pancreas and may pass behind it to enter the splenic vein or turn medially to enter the SMV.

The pancreas is normally accessed surgically by entering the lesser sac either by division of the greater omentum below the gastroepiploic arcade or by releasing the greater omentum from its attachment to the transverse colon. When the lesser sac is entered, the anterior surface of the neck, body and tail are often visible, but may be obscured by congenital filmy adhesions to the posterior wall of the stomach. To expose the head of the pancreas it is necessary to mobilise the right side of the transverse colon and hepatic flexure inferiorly and to divide the right gastroepiploic vein. The latter crosses the inferior border of the pancreas to join with the middle colic vein to form the gastrocolic trunk, which then enters the SMV. For complete exposure, e.g. for a Frey procedure, the right gastroepiploic artery is also divided and it and the subpyloric nodes are swept upwards off the pancreas. To access the SMV at the inferior border of the pancreas the peritoneum at the inferior border of the neck is divided and the dissection is carried inferiorly and laterally to open a groove between the uncinate process and the mesentery. Division of the right gastroepiploic vein at the inferior border of the pancreas greatly facilitates this manoeuvre. Normally no veins enter the SMV or PV from the posterior surface of the neck of the pancreas. Consequently the neck of the pancreas can be separated from the anterior surface of the SMV/PV in this avascular plane. The peritoneum at the inferior border of the neck, body and tail of the pancreas is avascular, and there are few vascular connections between the back of the body and tail of the pancreas and retroperitoneal tissues. As a result the pancreas may be readily dissected free from the retroperitoneum. The splenic vein is partly embedded in the back of the pancreas from the point that it reaches the gland on the left to about 1 cm from its termination at its confluence with the SMV.

Innervation of the pancreas

The pancreas is a highly innervated visceral organ. Pancreatic nerves are sensitive to both chemical and mechanical stimuli. These nerves transmit nociceptive and visceral afferent signals to the coeliac plexus, which is the largest of the three plexuses of the sympathetic system. Normally, the preganglionic efferent fibres exit the spinal cord to form the sympathetic chain. Instead of synapsing at the sympathetic chain, the greater, lesser and least splanchnic nerves pass through the sympathetic chain to form the coeliac ganglia, and provide the major preganglionic contribution to the coeliac plexus. The parasympathetic supply of the pancreas is provided by the left and right vagal trunks, which do not connect at the coeliac ganglia. This coeliac plexus most commonly consolidates around the origin of the coeliac axis and SMA.[25]

An understanding of this pancreatic innervation has led to the development of various non-surgical and surgical techniques for treating pain in chronic pancreatitis. These include the coeliac plexus block most commonly performed under endoscopic guidance[26] and selective pancreatic denervation by splanchnicectomy and ganglionectomy.[27,28]

Key points

- A prevailing pattern of hepatic, biliary and pancreatic anatomy exists but variations (anomalies) are frequent.
- All HPB operations should be conducted with the strong suspicion that an anatomical anomaly may be present.

⊕ Full references available at **http://expertconsult.inkling.com**

Key references

2. Terminology Committee of the IHPBA. The Brisbane 2000 Terminology of Liver Anatomy and Resections. HPB 2000;2:333–9.

   The Scientific Committee of the IHPBA created a Terminology Committee to deal with the confusion in nomenclature of hepatic anatomy and liver resections. The resulting terminology is presented in this paper. This use of agreed anatomical and surgical terms permits a meaningful and consistent approach to liver resection terminology in all clinical and academic writing.

14. Schnitzbauer AA, Lang SA, Goessmann H, et al. Right portal vein ligation combined with in situ splitting induces rapid left lateral liver lobe hypertrophy enabling 2-staged extended right hepatic resection in small-for-size settings. Ann Surg 2012;255:405–14. PMID: 22330038.

    First report of a novel two-stage hepatic resection performing surgical exploration, portal vein ligation, and in-situ splitting, resulting in marked and rapid hypertrophy of functional liver tissue enabling curative resection of marginally resectable liver tumours or metastases.

15. Strasberg SM, Brunt LM. Rationale and use of the critical view of safety in laparoscopic cholecystectomy. J Am Coll Surg 2010;211:132–8. PMID: 20610259.

    This paper describes the use of the critical view of safety (CVS) method of identification of the cystic duct and cystic artery during laparoscopic cholecystectomy, in order to minimise the risk of common bile duct injury.

22. Tol JA, Gouma DJ, Bassi C, et al. Definition of a standard lymphadenectomy in surgery for pancreatic ductal adenocarcinoma: a consensus statement by the International Study Group on Pancreatic Surgery (ISGPS). Surgery 2014;156(3):591–600. PMID: 25061003.

    This paper describes the lymph node stations surrounding the pancreas, and provides the definitions required for standard lymphadenectomy in surgery for ductal adenocarcinoma located in different parts of the pancreas.

3

Staging and assessment of hepatobiliary malignancies

Steve M.M. de Castro
Otto M. van Delden
Olivier R.C. Busch

Introduction

Tumour staging including assessment of potential metastases in patients with HPB malignancy is of the utmost importance. Patient selection should ideally identify those who might benefit from surgery and those who will not. Palliation for the majority of patients with unresectable or metastatic disease can be undertaken using minimally invasive techniques (i.e. endoscopic or percutaneous biliary stenting, radio- and/or chemotherapy). Technological advances have changed the approach to evaluate patients with suspected HPB malignancies. Modern state-of-the-art imaging now allows physicians to focus on two key questions in patients with suspected HPB tumours. Is there really a malignant tumour present (diagnosis)? If so, can it be removed with an R0 resection (staging)?

This chapter focuses on the diagnostic work-up of patients with the most common HPB malignancies and discusses the staging and assessment, mainly focusing on resectability.

Colorectal liver metastases

Imaging of colorectal liver metastases (CRLM) is important in patient assessment for several reasons. Firstly, to detect all the liver metastases present with their exact location within the liver, in order to maximise the chance of achieving complete clearance of disease at surgery. Secondly, to characterise any benign liver lesions that may be present, so as to avoid unnecessary surgical procedures. Thirdly,

to provide anatomical information necessary to perform a complete and safe resection or ablative procedure.

Transabdominal ultrasound

Ultrasound has a diagnostic sensitivity of only 36–61% for detecting lesions measuring 1–2 cm even when performed by experienced radiologists.[1] It is very useful in guiding fine-needle aspiration (FNA) to confirm unresectability by cytopathology. However, FNA has a risk of seeding metastases in up to 10% of patients and is associated with a risk of false-negative results, which does not justify its use in patients suitable for potentially curative therapy.[2]

A meta-analysis of the performance of ultrasound for CRLM found a pooled sensitivity of 63% (95% CI 56–70%; five studies) with a specificity of 97.6% (95% CI 95.6–99.5%; four studies).[3]

Ultrasound can be very useful as a problem-solving tool when computed tomography (CT) or magnetic resonance imaging (MRI) is uncertain. Targeted ultrasound of a suspicious lesion can often discriminate between a benign (e.g. cyst) or malignant lesion.

Computed tomography and magnetic resonance imaging

Nowadays, cross-sectional imaging CT and MRI are the most commonly used modalities for staging and follow-up of patients with colorectal cancer. Current multidetector CT scanners allow for multiplanar reformatting with the same resolution as the original axial images. This improves detection and characterisation of small lesions.[3] Multiplanar reformatting also enables the demonstration of hepatic arterial, venous and portal anatomy, which is necessary for preoperative planning.[4] CT allows for accurate volumetric assessment of tumour size and volume, and future liver remnant volume.[5]

A multiphase contrast-enhanced CT should be performed to stage CRLM. The study should include unenhanced, arterial, portal-venous and delayed phases. CRLM may show an enhancing rim in the arterial phase and are hypodense when compared to liver parenchyma on portal-venous phase imaging (**Fig. 3.1**). A slice thickness of 3 mm or less is recommended for axial viewing.

A meta-analysis on the performance of CT found a pooled sensitivity of 74.8% (95% CI 71.2–78.3; 12 studies) and specificity of 95.6% (95% CI 93.4–97.8; seven studies).[3]

MRI of the liver may involve numerous sequences. The standard MRI protocol includes T2-weighted, unenhanced T1-weighted and dynamic contrast-enhanced T1-weighted sequences, as well as diffusion-weighted imaging (DWI) sequences. T2-weighted and DWI images are used for the detection and characterisation of lesions (e.g. hemangioma, liver cyst).[6,7]

A meta-analysis on the performance of MRI found a pooled sensitivity of 81.1% (95% CI 76.0–86.1; five studies) and specificity of 97.2% (95% CI 94.5–99.9; two studies).[3] On individual lesion analysis, MRI appeared to show higher sensitivities across individual studies compared to CT. Pooled data showed comparable results, with MRI having a combined sensitivity of 88% and accuracy of 87%, compared to CT with a sensitivity of 74% and accuracy of 78%.

Subgroup analyses of these studies showed that MRI has better sensitivity at picking up smaller lesions (<1 cm) compared to CT and positron emission tomography (PET-CT).[8] The majority of lesions missed by CT were metastases <1 cm in diameter. This meta-analysis concluded that MRI was the preferred first-line modality for liver evaluation. It has high overall sensitivity and specificity and can accurately depict lesions smaller than 10 mm. MRI also provides excellent anatomical detail.

Positron emission tomography

Fluorine-18-2-fluoro-2-deoxy-D-glucose positron emission tomography (FDG-PET) is a well-established non-invasive functional scanning method where a labelled glucose molecule is injected intravenously. The principle of FDG-PET is that malignant cells have a higher glucose uptake than regular cells. The scanner performs a rapid non-invasive interrogation of glycolytic activity throughout the whole body in a single imaging session. Besides being used for the detection of primary malignant tumours, it can also be used to detect regional and distant metastases, to differentiate benign from malignant disease or recurrent cancer from treatment-related scarring, and to evaluate response to therapy.

With PET-CT combination it is possible to produce fusion images with high-resolution anatomical localisation of the CT together with functional data of the FDG-PET. This combination of scanning characteristics is becoming more widely available (**Fig. 3.2**).

Kinkel et al.[9] performed a meta-analysis and concluded that, at equivalent specificity, PET-CT is more sensitive than US, CT and MRI for the detection of hepatic metastases from gastrointestinal cancers. Bipat et al.[10] also performed a meta-analysis

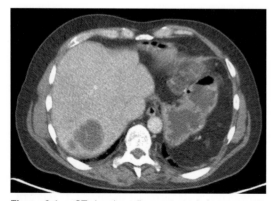

Figure 3.1 • CT showing a liver metastasis in segment 7 with a small adjacent satellite lesion.

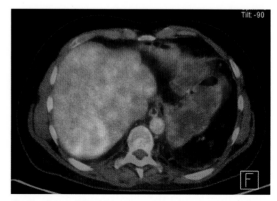

Figure 3.2 • PET-CT in the same patient showing two distinct colorectal liver metastases.

and concluded that PET-CT is the most sensitive diagnostic tool for the detection of CRLM on a per patient basis, but not on a per lesion basis. The authors suggest that in patients requiring further work-up, FDG-PET can be used as a second-line modality because both sensitivity and specificity were fairly high and FDG-PET plays a crucial role in detecting extrahepatic disease.

Mainenti et al.[11] found that PET-CT showed a trend to perform better than the other modalities. The pooled estimate of a meta-analysis for PET-CT was 93.8% (95% CI 90.0–97.7; six studies) and specificity per patient was 98.7% (95% CI 97.2–100; six studies).[3]

A recent trial in patients with potentially resectable CRLM found that the use of PET-CT compared to CT alone did not result in frequent change in surgical management, raising questions about the value of PET-CT in this setting.[12]

Diagnostic laparoscopy and laparoscopic ultrasound

Diagnostic laparoscopy is used to detect small peritoneal metastases or subcapsular liver metastases, which can be missed on cross-sectional imaging. The addition of laparoscopic ultrasound (LUS) may increase the detection of small intrahepatic metastases. There are not many prospective studies on patients with CRLM and most retrospective series also include patients with other liver tumours (i.e. hepatocellular carcinoma or metastases from non-colorectal gastrointestinal malignancies).

Recent prospective studies have reported a limited benefit of LUS, documenting that an unnecessary laparotomy can be prevented in 10%[13] to 13%[14] of patients with CRLM, which is considerably lower than earlier reports of 12–33%.[15–17]

One reason for the lower yield is that the indications for resection of CLRM have changed towards a more aggressive approach including resection of multiple lesions and bilobar disease. Furthermore, the use of local ablative techniques such as radiofrequency ablation (RFA) and microwave ablation (MWA) in combination with resection, and downsizing with chemotherapy have extended the possibilities for surgical treatment even further. Currently the only absolute restrictions for curative resection include unresectable extrahepatic dissemination and limited function of the future liver remnant (FLR). The general consensus is that 20–30% of healthy normal functioning liver should be left in situ. Liver function may be a better predictor of liver failure than volumetry.[18] The varying definition of unresectability has a linear correlation with the yield of laparoscopy. In addition, improved

cross-sectional imaging techniques in recent years have resulted in a decreased yield of diagnostic laparoscopy.

Several centres favour the selective use of laparoscopy. Jarnagin et al.[14] have described a clinical risk score (CRS) that predicts survival after hepatic resection and may be suitable in identifying high-risk patients most likely to benefit from laparoscopy. In a study of 103 patients, occult unresectable disease was found in 12% of patients with a low score versus 42% of patients with a high score.[14,19] Similarly, in a series of 200 patients, a detection rate of only 6% was reported in patients with the lowest CRS, whereas this was 75% for the highest CRS scores.[15] Another study demonstrated a yield of 50% in a selected group of patients, while in the group of 49 patients selected for direct surgical exploration 46 patients (94%) were eventually resected.[16]

Staging and assessment of resectability

The optimal selection of patients for hepatic resection is evolving, and the criteria for resectability differ among individual liver surgeons. A consensus statement in 2005 defined resectability as absence of non-treatable extrahepatic disease, fitness for surgery, ability to leave 30% of residual liver parenchyma in healthy livers and disease in no more than six segments.[20] Modern multidisciplinary consensus defines resectable CRLM simply as tumours that can be resected completely, leaving an adequate liver remnant.[21] Before surgical exploration, most surgeons would require that there was no radiographic evidence of involvement of the hepatic artery, major bile ducts, main portal vein, or coeliac/para-aortic lymph nodes, and a predicted hepatic remnant with adequate function.[22] Some centres with extensive expertise do perform resections directly adjacent to major vascular structures with margins less than 10 mm, even laparoscopically, but a margin of 10 mm is still recommended by many authors.[23–25] This may be different in the era of preoperative chemotherapy where a 1-mm margin has been described as the minimum. If a limited number of lung lesions are also present, liver resection is generally performed first, followed by resection of the lung. There is no reason to refrain from liver resection in a patient with advanced age who has good general (cardio/pulmonary) fitness. Risk scoring systems (such as the CRS[26] and others[27–29]) to predict which patients with CRLM are most likely to benefit from resection are of uncertain clinical utility, particularly since most patients undergo different neoadjuvant chemotherapy regimens. Some studies have shown that the risk scoring system needs refinement[30,31] and that the outcome in patients treated by neoadjuvant chemotherapy was not predicted by the traditional clinical scoring system, but rather by response to chemotherapy as evaluated by CT and PET-CT.[32]

> ✓✓ MRI and CT are both well suited to be used as a first-line modality for evaluating patients with CRLM; both provide anatomic details and have a high detection rate, especially MRI for lesions smaller than 10 mm. FDG-PET is valuable in the detection of extrahepatic disease but with little added benefit according to a multicentre trial.[12]

Hepatocellular carcinoma

> ✓ The diagnosis of hepatocellular carcinoma (HCC) is challenging as it has a variable appearance on imaging and because lesion detection is difficult against the inhomogeneous background of liver cirrhosis with dysplastic and regenerating nodules mimicking HCC.

Transabdominal ultrasound

Transabdominal ultrasound is recommended by the European Association for Study of the Liver (EASL), the American Association for Study of Liver Disease (AASLC) and the Asian Pacific Association for the Study of Liver Disease (APASL) as a surveillance tool for patients at high risk of developing HCC. Meta-regression analysis has demonstrated a significantly higher sensitivity for early HCC with US every 6 months than with annual surveillance.[33]

Computed tomography and magnetic resonance imaging

Multiphase contrast-enhanced CT or MRI should be performed when evaluating HCC. The hallmark of HCC on CT and MRI is enhancement on arterial phase imaging (**Fig. 3.3**) and washout of contrast-agent on delayed phase imaging (**Fig. 3.4**).[34] This feature in particular enables differentiation from dysplastic nodules, regenerative nodules or intrahepatic cholangiocarcinoma, the latter showing delayed enhancement.[35]

HCC arising in a non-cirrhotic liver is often larger, due to its long asymptomatic course and late presentation.[36] This contrasts with the multifocal tumours more commonly found in patients with chronic liver disease who are often in surveillance

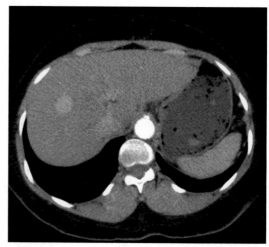

Figure 3.3 • CT of patient with hepatocellular carcinoma in the liver showing arterial enhancement of the lesion.

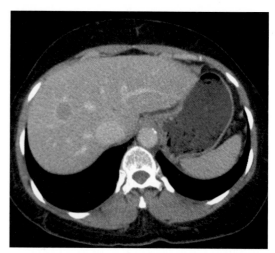

Figure 3.4 • CT of same patient with hepatocellular carcinoma in the liver showing venous washout of the lesion with enhancing rim.

programmes. CT features of HCC which help in differentiating it from other causes of a focal liver mass include a mosaic appearance with fibrous septa separating areas of variable attenuation, representing internal regions of haemorrhage, necrosis, fatty degeneration and fibrosis. The fibrous capsule has a low attenuation on unenhanced images and enhances on the portal venous phase.

A number of benign lesions, including haemangiomas, focal confluent fibrosis, peliosis, benign regenerative nodules and pseudo-lesions like transient hepatic attenuation difference, can mimic small HCC lesions on CT.[37]

On MRI, HCC can have a variable appearance on unenhanced T1-weighted images and typically show an increased signal on T2-weighted and

DWI images.[38] Following gadolinium administration, HCC demonstrates characteristic early enhancement on arterial phase imaging[39] and washout on delayed images, resulting in a hypointense lesion compared to the surrounding parenchyma.[40]

Diagnostic laparoscopy and laparoscopic ultrasound

Laparoscopic evaluation can avoid exploratory laparotomy in 45–63% of patients with unresectable disease.[41,42] The procedure has been reported as accurate in assessing the presence of advanced intrahepatic disease and the quality of the liver remnant, but less sensitive in determining the extent of local invasion, especially in large (>10 cm) tumours. Another study clearly showed the value of laparoscopic ultrasonography in detecting small HCCs; 134 new nodules were visualised by this technique in 64 of 186 (34%) patients in whom 28 nodules (in 23 patients) were histologically diagnosed as HCC.[43] Of these 23 patients, 18 had been diagnosed as having a solitary HCC before laparoscopy. Similarly, new lesions of histologically proven HCC were found in 22% of patients.[44] Even when preoperative staging included a CT, laparoscopic ultrasonography was superior in detecting additional tumours.[45] Ultrasonography confirmed all 201 tumours seen on CT and detected 21 additional tumours (9.5%) in 11 patients (20%).

Staging and assessment of resectability

Tumour staging to select a treatment regimen is complicated by the fact that many of the staging systems (including the TNM staging system of the American Joint Committee on Cancer [AJCC], Table 3.1) are based on surgical findings, while surgery is applicable to only about 5% in this group of patients. Others recommend the Barcelona Clinic Liver Cancer (BCLC) staging system.[47] The Barcelona algorithm does not address the value of resection for some subgroups of patients with HCC who may potentially benefit from this approach, including some patients defined as being 'early stage' (with a single tumour >2 cm in size or multiple nodules) and 'intermediate stage' (patients who have multiple tumours but a good performance status). The Milano/Mazzaferro criteria for liver transplantation of HCC (i.e. solitary tumour ≤5 cm or up to three tumours all ≤3 cm) are widely accepted.[48] However, according to the Barcelona algorithm, only selected patients with three nodules ≤3 cm (those without 'associated diseases') should undergo liver transplantation.[47] The American Hepato-Pancreato-Biliary Association (AHPBA)/ American Joint Commission on Cancer (AJCC) Consensus Conference on HCC in 2002 concluded that no single staging system could be used to accurately stage patients across the spectrum of HCC.[48,49]

Table 3.1 • TNM staging for hepatocellular cancer

Primary tumour (T)	
TX	Primary tumour cannot be assessed
T0	No evidence of primary tumour
T1	Solitary tumour without vascular invasion
T2	Solitary tumour with vascular invasion or multiple tumours none more than 5 cm
T3a	Multiple tumours more than 5 cm
T3b	Single tumour or multiple tumours of any size involving a major branch of the portal vein or hepatic vein
T4	Tumour(s) with direct invasion of adjacent organs other than the gallbladder or with perforation of visceral peritoneum
Regional lymph nodes (N)	
NX	Regional lymph nodes cannot be assessed
N0	No regional lymph node metastasis
N1	Regional lymph node metastasis
Distant metastasis (M)	
M0	No distant metastasis
M1	Distant metastasis
Fibrosis score (F)*	
F0	Fibrosis score 0–4 (none to moderate fibrosis)
F1	Fibrosis score 5–6 (severe fibrosis or cirrhosis)

(Continued)

Table 3.1 • TNM staging for hepatocellular cancer—cont'd

Anatomic stage/prognostic groups				5-year survival after resection,[†] n = 13 772[46]
Stage I	T1	N0	M0	70
Stage II	T2	N0	M0	58
Stage IIIA	T3a	N0	M0	41
Stage IIIB	T3b	N0	M0	
Stage IIIC	T4	N0	M0	
Stage IVA	Any T	N1	M0	25
Stage IVB	Any T	Any N	M1	15

Note: cTNM is the clinical classification, pTNM is the pathological classification.

[*]The fibrosis score as defined by Ishak is recommended because of its prognostic value in overall survival. This scoring system uses a 0–6 scale.

[†]Data from AJCC 6th edition

Used with the permission of the American Joint Committee on Cancer (AJCC), Chicago, Illinois. The original source for this material is the AJCC Cancer Staging Manual, 7th edition (2010), published by Springer New York, Inc.

The ideal patient for resection has a solitary HCC confined to the liver that shows no radiographic evidence of invasion of the hepatic vasculature, no evidence of portal hypertension and well-preserved hepatic function. According to the current TNM/UICC staging system for HCC (Table 3.1), most consider stage IIIB, IIIC, IVA or IVB disease to be incurable by resection. However, hepatic resection for stage IIIB, IIIC and IVA disease may be considered in some centres of excellence as clinical benefits and long-term survival can be achieved in a selected minority of patients.

Assessment of hepatic reserve is paramount to selection for resection. Postoperative mortality is twice as high in cirrhotic as in non-cirrhotic patients unless proper patient selection is applied. For patients with cirrhosis, surgical resection can safely be performed in those with Child–Pugh grade A disease. Indications for therapies such as liver transplantation, radiofrequency ablation (RFA), transarterial chemoembolisation (TACE) are discussed elsewhere.

✔✔ Surveillance US at 6 months is recommended as a screening tool in cirrhotic patients, while CT and MRI are most useful to confirm the diagnosis and stage HCC. Laparoscopic staging may be useful in these patients as they have a high risk of being unresectable. Laparoscopy may also allow guided biopsy of the future liver remnant in patients with cirrhosis.

Pancreatic and periampullary carcinoma

Most pancreatic tumours are located in the head of the pancreas (60–65%), while 20% are present in the body and 10% in the tail region. Unfortunately only a minority (5–20%) of pancreatic tumours are resectable. Tumours in the pancreatic head often present earlier due to compression of the common bile duct causing obstructive jaundice. Therefore, these tumours are often smaller at the time of presentation and more likely to be resectable. These smaller tumours (<2 cm) without liver metastases have better 5-year survival.[50]

The goal of imaging for pancreatic tumours is twofold. The first is to accurately identify tumours with local invasion or distant metastases to tailor the treatment strategy, and the second is to accurately image the anatomical variations prior to resection.

Transabdominal ultrasound

This is usually the first screening examination of the abdomen in patients with obstructive jaundice. It is a useful diagnostic modality with a high sensitivity (>90%) for detecting bile duct obstruction, and a reasonable sensitivity for determining the level of obstruction (e.g. intrahepatic, proximal or distal) and identifying the presence of gallstone disease.[51] Transabdominal ultrasound is widely available but highly operator-dependent and often limited by the inability to adequately visualise the pancreas due to bowel gas interference. The goal of ultrasound is therefore to primarily establish a differential diagnosis among the various causes of obstructive jaundice and identify liver metastases. Ultrasound is highly sensitive in detecting gallbladder stones (>90%),[52] but this sensitivity drops to 50–75% for the detection of bile duct stones.[53] On ultrasound, a pancreatic tumour appears as a hypoechoic (poorly reflective) mass. A tell-tale sign suggestive of malignant obstruction is the combined presence of a dilated common bile duct (CBD) and pancreatic duct (double duct sign). Ultrasound is able to detect most pancreatic masses of at least 3 cm as was shown in a meta-analysis of 14 studies.[54] Pancreatic tumours (irrespective of size) yielded a sensitivity of 76% and a specificity of 75%. However, these results were from studies performed in centres with significant experience in the diagnostic work-up of patients with pancreatic cancer. Doppler ultrasound can show vascular involvement of portal and mesenteric veins and arteries.

Additionally, transabdominal ultrasound has a reasonable sensitivity for detecting liver metastases and a high sensitivity for detecting ascites. FNA can be accurately performed using ultrasound guidance. Sensitivity for liver lesions depends on the size of the lesion and is >90% for lesions >2 cm in diameter, 60% for lesions in the range 1–2 cm and 20% for lesions <1 cm.[1]

Computed tomography and magnetic resonance imaging

Computed tomography is the most widely used imaging modality for pancreatic disease and for staging pancreatic tumours. Multidetector CT enables evaluation of the vascular and ductal structures, and mapping of the anatomy and anatomical variations. The most important goal of CT, besides the detection of tumours, is the assessment of resectability.

Tumour conspicuity depends heavily on CT scanning phases. Currently, a combination of pancreatic and portal phase CT is the optimal technique for pancreatic lesions. The best oral contrast is water. The optimal CT section thickness is 2 mm.

The arterial phase optimally demonstrates the arterial vessels (superior mesenteric artery, coeliac artery and hepatic artery) and their relation to the pancreatic tumour (**Fig. 3.5**). The portal venous phase demonstrates the portal and superior mesenteric

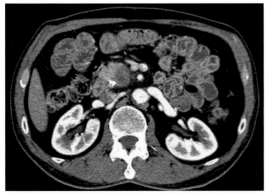

Figure 3.5 • CT of patient with pancreatic head mass with no vascular involvement.

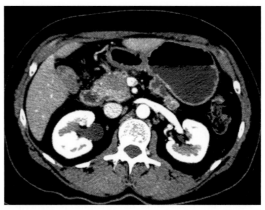

Figure 3.6 • CT of patient with pancreatic head mass with portal contact of approximately 90°.

veins and the confluence area at the pancreatic neck (**Fig. 3.6**). The parenchymal phase is between these two phases and a pancreatic adenocarcinoma will appear hypovascular compared to the rest of the parenchyma.

The double duct sign appears when both the CBD and the pancreatic duct are dilated. Smooth dilatation is more suggestive of pancreatitis, whereas irregular or beaded dilatation is more suggestive of malignancy. Tumours that extend beyond the contours of the pancreas with infiltration of the peripancreatic fat show blurring of the normal dark peripancreatic fat. The sensitivity and specificity of CT for detection of a pancreatic head mass is 91% and 85% respectively, versus 84% and 82% for MRI in a pooled meta-analysis.[54] It is important that radiologists and clinicians use a uniform definition of 'pancreatic mass' since it has been shown that this will improve inter-observer agreement.[55]

CT has been reported to have a positive predictive value of 100%, negative predictive value of 56% and overall accuracy of 70% for unresectable pancreatic carcinoma.[56] This ability to predict unresectability preoperatively is superior to the ability to predict resectability, particularly because the detection of small liver and peritoneal metastases is limited. Specific clinical and imaging characteristics to indicate the absence of a malignancy lack sufficient discriminatory value.[57]

Endoscopic retrograde cholangiopancreatography

Endoscopic retrograde cholangiopancreatography (ERCP) has been performed as an initial diagnostic investigation in patients with obstructive jaundice for many years. However, the advent of improved non-invasive diagnostic modalities such as CT, MRI and endoscopic ultrasound (EUS) has led to less frequent use of invasive ERCP as a diagnostic procedure itself. ERCP is associated with a morbidity rate of 5–10% and a mortality rate of 0.1–1%. The most common complications include pancreatitis (5–10%), bleeding (1–2%) and perforation (<0.3%).[58] A recent randomised clinical trial showed that early surgery without preoperative biliary drainage did not increase the risk of postoperative complications, and the complications associated with the drainage itself were fairly high.[59]

Magnetic resonance cholangiopancreaticography (MRCP) closely mimics the imaging capacity of ERCP but is non-invasive. The advantage of MRCP is that cross-sectional imaging information regarding the tumour and its relation to surrounding structures is also obtained during the same examination. In addition, distant metastases can be detected with MRI. The results of MRCP in visualisation of the biliary system are similar to ERCP in clinical studies, with a sensitivity of 71–93% versus 81–86% and specificity of 92–94% versus 82–100%, respectively. When comparing ERCP with EUS; the sensitivity was 75–89% versus 85–89% and specificity of 65–92% versus 80–96%, respectively.[60] There are no known direct comparisons between ERCP and CT. If ERCP is performed, it is possible to perform brush cytology, bile aspiration cytology and even intraductal biopsies. These examinations are highly sensitive but lack specificity.

The detection rate of malignancy was not significantly different for brush cytology compared to bile cytology (sensitivity of 33–100% and specificity of 6–50%, respectively) and also not significantly different for FNA cytology compared to brush cytology (25–91% and 8–56%, respectively). Forceps biopsy compared to brush cytology was also not significantly different (43–81% and 18–53%, respectively).[60] Other new modalities such as intraductal cholangiopancreaticoscopy and intraductal endosonography have yet to be proven in larger series.

Endoscopic ultrasound (EUS)

Endoscopic ultrasound (EUS) allows a sonographic transducer to be placed in close proximity to the pancreas. In doing so, interference from overlying bowel gas is eliminated and higher frequencies can be used, resulting in markedly improved resolution. EUS was considered superior to the other imaging modalities prior to the recent refinements made in CT,[61] because most CT studies dated from the period 1994 to 2000. EUS was considered more sensitive in one systematic review describing nine studies of EUS compared to CT for diagnostic effectiveness.[62] The most valuable role of EUS in these studies was detecting relatively small tumours (<2 cm). The

pooled sensitivity was 85% with a specificity of 94%, but heterogeneity was an issue in this pooled analysis. FNA can be performed when differentiating between malignancy and pancreatitis, with a lower risk of causing peritoneal carcinomatosis than with transabdominal aspiration. A study in 62 patients with pancreatic cancer which compared EUS, CT and MRI with the gold standard of surgery found that a sequential approach consisting of helical CT as an initial test and EUS as a confirmatory technique when in doubt seemed to be the most reliable and cost effective strategy.[63] Thus EUS is not mandatory in the work-up of patients with pancreatic cancer. In those cases with potentially resectable tumours, an EUS-guided (fine-needle aspiration) biopsy has a pooled sensitivity for malignant cytology of 85% (95% CI 0.84–0.86) and a pooled specificity of 98% (95% CI 0.97–0.99).[64] The major limitations of this technology are operator dependence and a limited field of visualisation for the detection of distant metastases. This modality should be used on a selective basis (e.g. to obtain preoperative tissue biopsy for patients scheduled for neoadjuvant therapy) and in centres with experience.

Positron emission tomography

Preliminary reports indicate that FDG-PET may provide additional information regarding the M status of a patient and can change the therapeutic option in up to 16% of patients.[65] A meta-analysis of PET in patients with a positive, negative and inconclusive CT found a sensitivity and specificity of 92% and 68%, respectively, after a positive CT, 73% and 86%, respectively, after a negative CT and 100% and 68%, respectively, after an inconclusive CT.[66] Its usefulness will vary depending upon the pretest probability of the patient and the results of CT. FDG-PET is most often used for response evaluation in neoadjuvant chemoradiotherapy trials.

Diagnostic laparoscopy and laparoscopic ultrasound

Despite best efforts, there are still the unexpected occasions when the intraoperative findings are contrary to those reported by the preoperative investigations, especially with regard to resectability. These patients consequently still undergo an unnecessary laparotomy, along with its accompanying risks, albeit small, of postoperative morbidity and mortality. The quality of life becomes further diminished in a patient population whose survival is already limited. The detection of small liver and peritoneal metastases (**Fig. 3.7**) is an important motivation for performing diagnostic

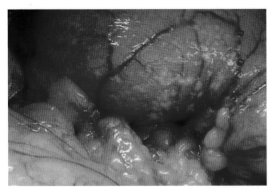

Figure 3.7 • Peritoneal metastases on the first part of the duodenum found during laparotomy in a patient with a periampullary carcinoma.

or staging laparoscopy, since this might avoid unnecessary, open exploration. CT has excellent accuracy in predicting unresectability; however, sensitivity for assessment of resectability remains much lower. This is due to its inability to detect very small liver lesions (<1 cm) or peritoneal deposits.

Despite the logical rationale behind its use, laparoscopy continues to provoke considerable debate. Advocates have reported that laparoscopy can identify occult metastases, which were not detected by a preceding CT, in 30% of patients.[67] Consequently, the resection rates after laparoscopy have been reported to be 75–92%.[68] Because of these results, some centres strongly recommend the use of diagnostic laparoscopy as a routine procedure but to some extent this may reflect the quality of prelaparoscopy imaging as well.

Critics argue that routine laparoscopy is therefore not cost-effective. With the newer generations of CT scanners, the incidence of missed hepatic or peritoneal metastases is less than 20%. The implication is that performing routine laparoscopy adds unnecessary surgical time and expense to the remaining 80% of patients with resectable disease or, if locally unresectable, precludes them from surgical palliation, which is considered superior.[69,70]

The yield of additional laparoscopic staging is influenced greatly by the quality of the prelaparoscopic staging process. Incorrect staging with poor quality CT, for example, results in an overestimation in the yield of diagnostic laparoscopy and laparoscopic ultrasonography. While the most important objective in laparoscopy is to prevent an unnecessary laparotomy, a number of patients will benefit from a subsequent laparotomy for palliation (e.g. bypass procedure for gastrointestinal obstruction), although these may also be done laparoscopically. The limited detection rate for unresectable metastatic disease and the likely absence of a large gain after switching from surgical to endoscopic palliation, prompted many centres not

to routinely perform laparoscopy in patients with periampullary carcinoma.[70] In a study assessing 233 patients with upper gastrointestinal malignancy, of whom 114 patients had a periampullary tumour, laparotomy was avoided initially in 17 patients (15%) but five of these patients subsequently required laparotomy for duodenal obstruction.[61] This reduced the overall efficacy of laparoscopy in preventing unnecessary laparotomies from 15% to 11%. In a more recent study of 297 patients, the laparoscopic yield decreased to only 13% (39 patients), probably due to improved radiological staging techniques.[70] This, combined with an increasingly critical view of resectability and palliation, has resulted in a decreased benefit of laparoscopic staging making it unsuitable for routine use. Staging laparoscopy done in the same setting, especially when done by surgeons who can perform laparoscopic bypass surgery, may be more useful.

> ✓ Diagnostic laparoscopy is advised to identify true locally advanced disease when chemoradiation is considered to 'downstage' the tumour, thus minimising the number of patients with undetected metastases on preoperative imaging.

Staging and assessment of resectability

Staging is according to the TNM-atlas, 7th edition, 2009 (Tables 3.2–3.4). Most clinicians agree that a tumour is considered incurable if there are distant metastases (liver, lung, lymph nodes outside the (radical) lymph node dissection area as defined by Pedrazzoli)[74] or if there is local invasion into arterial structures such as the superior mesenteric artery, coeliac trunk or common hepatic artery (Table 3.5). Arterial resections with reconstruction have been described in small retrospective studies, with almost no survival benefit, but increased mortality and morbidity, ranging from 21% to 40% and 2% to 35%, respectively, and should therefore be abandoned as a useful treatment.[75]

Criteria to assess vascular ingrowth on CT include tumour involvement of any of the major pancreatic vessels (coeliac artery, hepatic artery, superior mesenteric artery, superior mesenteric vein, or portal vein) that exceeds half of the circumference of the vessels (**Fig. 3.8**). This is especially specific for the involved arteries. Contour deformity, obliteration and thrombosis of the veins is also highly suspicious of vascular involvement.[76] Additional radiological features that suggest vascular invasion include perivascular cuffing, described as increased attenuation of the normal perivascular fat, and the

Table 3.2 • TNM staging system for exocrine and endocrine tumours of the pancreas

Primary tumour (T)	
TX	Primary tumour cannot be assessed
T0	No evidence of primary tumour
Tis	Carcinoma in situ*
T1	Tumour limited to the pancreas, 2 cm or less in greatest dimension
T2	Tumour limited to the pancreas, more than 2 cm in greatest dimension
T3	Tumour extends beyond the pancreas but without involvement of the coeliac axis or the superior mesenteric artery
T4	Tumour involves the coeliac axis or the superior mesenteric artery (unresectable primary tumour)
Regional lymph nodes (N)	
NX	Regional lymph nodes cannot be assessed
N0	No regional lymph node metastasis
N1	Regional lymph node metastasis
Distant metastasis (M)	
M0	No distant metastasis
M1	Distant metastasis

Anatomic stage/prognostic groups				5-year survival after resection,[†] $n = 21\,512$[71]
Stage 0	Tis	N0	M0	
Stage IA	T1	N0	M0	31
Stage IB	T2	N0	M0	27
Stage IIA	T3	N0	M0	16
Stage IIB	T1	N1	M0	8
	T2	N1	M0	
	T3	N1	M0	
Stage III	T4	Any N	M0	7
Stage IV	Any T	Any N	M1	3

Note: cTNM is the clinical classification, pTNM is the pathological classification.

*This includes lesions classified as PanIn III classification.

[†]Data from AJCC 6th edition.

Used with the permission of the American Joint Committee on Cancer (AJCC), Chicago, Illinois. The original source for this material is the AJCC Cancer Staging Manual, 7th edition (2010), published by Springer New York, Inc.

Table 3.3 • TNM staging for ampullary carcinoma

Primary tumour (T)	
TX	Primary tumour cannot be assessed
T0	No evidence of primary tumour
Tis	Carcinoma in situ
T1	Tumour limited to the ampulla of Vater or sphincter of Oddi
T2	Tumour invades duodenal wall
T3	Tumour invades pancreas
T4	Tumour invades peripancreatic soft tissues or other adjacent organs or structures other than pancreas
Regional lymph nodes (N)	
NX	Regional lymph nodes cannot be assessed
N0	No regional lymph node metastasis
N1	Regional lymph node metastasis
Distant metastasis (M)	
M0	No distant metastasis
M1	Distant metastasis

Table 3.3 • TNM staging for hepatocellular cancer—cont'd

Anatomic stage/prognostic groups				5-year survival after resection,[†] $n = 1301$[72]
Stage 0	Tis	N0	M0	
Stage IA	T1	N0	M0	60
Stage IB	T2	N0	M0	57
Stage IIA	T3	N0	M0	30
Stage IIB	T1	N1	M0	22
	T2	N1	M0	
	T3	N1	M0	
Stage III	T4	Any N	M0	27
Stage IV	Any T	Any N	M1	0

Note: cTNM is the clinical classification, pTNM is the pathological classification.
[†]Data from AJCC 6th edition
Used with the permission of the American Joint Committee on Cancer (AJCC), Chicago, Illinois. The original source for this material is the AJCC Cancer Staging Manual, 7th edition (2010), published by Springer New York, Inc.

Table 3.4 • TNM staging system for distal cholangiocarcinoma

Primary tumour (T)	
TX	Primary tumour cannot be assessed
T0	No evidence of primary tumour
Tis	Carcinoma in situ
T1	Tumour confined to the bile duct histologically
T2	Tumour invades beyond the wall of the bile duct
T3	Tumour invades the gallbladder, pancreas, duodenum, or other adjacent organs without involvement of the coeliac axis, or the superior mesenteric artery
T4	Tumour involves the coeliac axis, or the superior mesenteric artery
Regional lymph nodes (N)	
NX	Regional lymph nodes cannot be assessed
N0	No regional lymph node metastasis
N1	Regional lymph node metastasis
Distant metastasis (M)	
M0	No distant metastasis
M1	Distant metastasis

Anatomic stage/prognostic groups				5-year survival after resection,[†] $n = 779$[73]
Stage 0	Tis	N0	M0	
Stage IA	T1	N0	M0	60
Stage IB	T2	N0	M0	
Stage IIA	T3	N0	M0	39
Stage IIB	T1	N1	M0	
	T2	N1	M0	
	T3	N1	M0	
Stage III	T4	Any N	M0	34
Stage IV	Any T	Any N	M1	10

Note: cTNM is the clinical classification, pTNM is the pathological classification.
[†] Data from AJCC Cancer Staging Manual, 6th edition.
Used with the permission of the American Joint Committee on Cancer (AJCC), Chicago, Illinois. The original source for this material is the AJCC Cancer Staging Manual, 7th edition (2010), published by Springer New York, Inc.

Table 3.5 • Resectability of pancreatic tumours

Resectable	Borderline	Unresectable
No tumour abutment with vessel	>90° tumour abutment with PV or SMV >5-mm length of PV or SMV contact	>180° tumour abutment with PV or SMV PV/SMV constriction or thrombus or Teardrop deformation of SMV Any ingrowth in SMA
No distant metastasis		Distant metastasis

PV, portal vein; SMA, superior mesenteric artery; SMV, superior mesenteric vein.

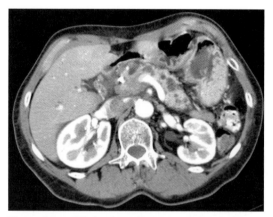

Figure 3.8 • CT of patient with pancreatic head mass with portal contact of more than 180°.

presence of dilated collateral veins. The 'teardrop' sign, which describes the deformity of the otherwise round shape of the superior mesenteric vein, suggests venous invasion. Nevertheless, there is much debate over the exact definition of vascular involvement in relation to resectability.

Successful resection of (a part of) the superior mesenteric vein or portal vein has been described and could be advantageous, provided that a R0 resection can be achieved. In a review by Ramacciato et al.,[77] 12 series are described with a total of 399 patients; the morbidity ranges from 16.7% to 54% and mortality from 0 to 7.7%, with a median survival of 13–22 months and a 5-year survival of 9–18%. Muller et al. also described 110 patients following resection of venous invasion with a morbidity of 41.8% and mortality of 3.6%.[78] The survival was not increased by the addition of a venous resection with bypass, because earlier local recurrence and/or distant metastases arose in this group of patients

compared with patients who had no invasion of the vein. Glanemann et al. reported a morbidity of 21–42% and mortality of 0–5.9% when pooling a series of 1967 patients reported in the literature.[79] The 5-year survival in this study ranged from 7% to 20%. The systematic review of Siriwardena found no survival benefit nor disadvantage due to complications from resection of venous structures with invasion.[75]

Size is the only characteristic of a pancreatic tumour that can be determined preoperatively. A review by Garcea et al.[80] used the size measured at histopathology. In these studies the cut-off value varied, but most studies suggested 2 cm. In these combined studies, the median survival of patients with tumours <2 cm was 35.5 months versus 14 months for larger tumours. Although the studies varied in quality, this meta-analysis concluded that size (< or >2 cm), is an (independent) prognostic factor for median survival (OR = 2.52, 95% CI 1.95–3, P <0.001). One relatively small study used size of the tumour on preoperative imaging and found that prognosis correlated with the size determined on CT.[81]

✔✔ Staging and assessment of patients with pancreatic or periampullary tumours is important because distant metastases and extensive arterial ingrowth preclude a resection with curative intent. A pancreas protocol CT is the most important factor in the staging and assessment of pancreatic cancer for the local extent as well as the presence of distant metastases.

✔ There is still some controversy concerning the maximal degree of vascular ingrowth and resectability. It is clear that extensive arterial involvement precludes a curative resection. Patients with borderline tumours with limited vascular involvement might benefit from vascular resection and should undergo explorative laparotomy.

Proximal bile duct tumours

Patients with proximal bile duct tumours generally present with jaundice. Patients with jaundice and a hilar stricture will either have a benign biliary stricture or a malignancy that has obstructed the hepatic confluence.[82,83] The differential diagnosis includes benign biliary strictures (postoperative bile duct injury, primary sclerosing cholangitis (PSC), HIV cholangiopathy, Mirizzi syndrome) or other malignancies such as gallbladder cancer or lymphoma. Diagnosis of a hilar cholangiocarcinoma can be challenging, particularly in patients with PSC who may have multiple stenoses and mass lesions without significant intrahepatic biliary dilation.

Transabdominal ultrasound

Abdominal ultrasound is often the first diagnostic study when jaundice occurs to confirm biliary ductal dilatation, identify the level of obstruction and exclude gallstones.[84] Duplex ultrasound has also been useful to assess vascular involvement in patients with proximal biliary tumours.[85]

Computed tomography and magnetic resonance imaging

Computed tomography is used to establish the presence of a tumour, its location as well as local spread, vascular ingrowth and distant metastases. Magnetic resonance (MR) cholangiography is comparable to endoscopic retrograde cholangiopancreatography (ERCP) in the detection of biliary malignancy. An advantage offered by MR cholangiography is that it can identify the luminal involvement and thus provide more accurate staging of the tumour without cannulation of the bile ducts and risk of infection. It allows visualisation of both the obstructed and non-obstructed ducts, and gives important information such as the extent of tumour within the biliary tree and in periductal tissue, vascular and nodal involvement, lobar atrophy, invasion of adjacent liver parenchyma and distant metastases.[86] If imaging studies demonstrate a focal stenotic lesion of the bile duct in the absence of previous biliary tract surgery, an assumptive diagnosis of hilar cholangiocarcinoma is made until proven otherwise.[83]

Endoscopic retrograde cholangiopancreatography

ERCP and percutaneous transhepatic cholangiography (PTC) allow for tissue sampling for pathology and collection of bile for cytology. The value of cytology has recently been stressed;[87] however, histological confirmation is not mandatory before surgical exploration. In patients that require biliary drainage preoperatively, it is unclear whether PTC is preferable over ERCP, but this is being studied in the randomised controlled multicentre DRAINAGE trial.[88]

Positron emission tomography

PET has been shown to have a high sensitivity for diagnosing biliary malignancy. The limitation of the method is that patients with an inflammatory process of the biliary tree (i.e. PSC) can have false-positive findings. In a prospective study by Kim et al.,[89] PET proved significantly more accurate in identifying distant metastases compared with CT (58% vs 0%). Other studies have confirmed the usefulness of PET for detecting metastases not found by other imaging,[90] ultimately influencing clinical management in up to 25% of patients.[91] The sensitivity of FDG-PET for detecting primary intrahepatic cholangiocarcinoma has been estimated at 78%.[91] However, Petrowsky et al.[92] found PET-CT to be more sensitive (93% vs 55%) and specific (80% vs 33%) in detecting intrahepatic versus extrahepatic cholangiocarcinoma.[81] Another limitation reported by Kluge et al., despite a sensitivity of 92% in detecting hilar cholangiocarcinoma, was that the rate of detection of extrahepatic tumours was dependent on the shape of the tumour.[93]

Diagnostic laparoscopy and laparoscopic ultrasound

Information on the additional value of diagnostic laparoscopy for malignant proximal bile duct obstruction is limited. In a pilot study from our institution, advanced disease was diagnosed in 19 of 47 patients (40%) by laparoscopy.[94] A recent meta-analysis found that the pooled analyses of the data suggested that one in four patients with potentially resectable hilar cholangiocarcinoma benefited from diagnostic laparoscopy.[95] However, given the considerable heterogeneity, a trend to lower yield in more recent studies and further improvement of preoperative imaging over time, the routine use of diagnostic laparoscopy is now being questioned. Another study found that tumour size ≥4.5 cm, bilateral portal vein involvement and suspected lymph node or extrahepatic metastases on imaging were independent factors associated with unresectability at diagnostic laparoscopy.[96] A proposed risk score using these variables appeared promising to improve the yield of diagnostic laparoscopy. A more recent study of 110 consecutive patients in our institution confirmed these findings.[97] Laparoscopy revealed histologically proven incurable disease in 44 patients (41%). Of the 65 patients who underwent laparotomy, 35 patients (54%) were unresectable. Although laparotomy was avoided in 41% of cases, laparoscopy was unable to assess resectability correctly in 44% of patients. These findings were similar to results from the Memorial Sloan Kettering Cancer Center involving 100 patients with carcinoma of the extrahepatic biliary tree.[98] Thirty-five patients (35%) were identified as having unresectable disease at laparoscopy. Of the 65 patients who underwent laparotomy, a further

34 tumours (52%) were unresectable, resulting in an overall accuracy of 51%. Finally, in a series of 401 patients with hepatobiliary cancer, the highest yield for laparoscopy was found in patients with biliary cancer, but the study emphasised that the surgeon's preoperative impression of resectability was as important as the laparoscopic staging procedure itself.[13] Recently, a study from our centre found that the yield has decreased to 12% in recent years due to better preoperative imaging.[99] During staging laparoscopy, nodal sampling, for instance of the station 8 hepatic artery lymph node, is also feasible.

Laparoscopic ultrasonography has not been very useful in staging the local tumour spread of proximal bile duct cancer. Patients with unresectable disease most often have locally advanced tumours, but laparoscopic ultrasonography did not contribute to the assessment of resectability in these patients.[98] Furthermore, extensive biliary and vascular involvement can be determined with high accuracy (91%) using external colour Doppler ultrasonography, as well as thin-slice contrast-enhanced multislice CT.[100] The additional value of laparoscopic ultrasonography is therefore too low for it to be performed routinely.

Staging and assessment of resectability

The American Joint Committee on Cancer (AJCC) TNM staging system is most commonly used to stage hilar cholangiocarcinoma (Table 3.6). However, this system is based on pathology criteria

Table 3.6 • TNM staging system for perihilar cholangiocarcinoma

Primary tumour (T)

TX	Primary tumour cannot be assessed
T0	No evidence of primary tumour
Tis	Carcinoma in situ
T1	Tumour confined to the bile duct, with extension up to the muscle layer or fibrous tissue
T2a	Tumour invades beyond the wall of the bile duct to surrounding adipose tissue
T2b	Tumour invades adjacent hepatic parenchyma
T3	Tumour invades unilateral branches of the portal vein or hepatic artery
T4	Tumour invades main portal vein or its branches bilaterally; or the common hepatic artery; or the second-order biliary radicals bilaterally; or unilateral second-order biliary radicals with contralateral portal vein or hepatic artery involvement

Regional lymph nodes (N)

NX	Regional lymph nodes cannot be assessed
N0	No regional lymph node metastasis
N1	Regional lymph node metastasis (including nodes along the cystic duct, common bile duct, hepatic artery, and portal vein)
N2	Metastasis to periaortic, pericaval, superior mesenteric artery and/or coeliac artery lymph nodes

Distant metastasis (M)

M0	No distant metastasis
M1	Distant metastasis

Anatomic stage/prognostic groups

Stage 0	Tis	N0	M0
Stage I	T1	N0	M0
Stage II	T2a-b	N0	M0
Stage IIIA	T3	N0	M0
Stage IIIB	T1-3	N1	M0
Stage IVA	T4	N0-1	M0
Stage IVB	Any T	N2	M0
	Any T	Any N	M1

Note: cTNM is the clinical classification, pTNM is the pathological classification.
Used with the permission of the American Joint Committee on Cancer (AJCC), Chicago, Illinois. The original source for this material is the AJCC Cancer Staging Manual, 7th edition (2010), published by Springer New York, Inc.

The preoperative clinical T-staging system (Table 3.7) as proposed by Jarnagin and Blumgart[101,102] defines both the radial and longitudinal extension of hilar cholangiocarcinoma, which are critical factors in the determination of resectability. This Memorial Sloan-Kettering Cancer Center (MSKCC) staging system incorporates three factors based on preoperative imaging studies: (1) location and extent of ductal involvement; (2) presence or absence of portal vein invasion; and (3) presence or absence of hepatic lobar atrophy. Criteria for unresectability include locally advanced tumour extending to secondary biliary radicles (that is, sectional bile ducts [right anterior, right posterior, left lateral and left medial]) bilaterally, to unilateral sectional bile ducts with contralateral portal vein branch involvement, encasement or occlusion of the main portal vein proximal to its bifurcation, atrophy of one hepatic lobe with contralateral portal vein involvement, or atrophy of one hepatic lobe with contralateral tumour extension to sectional bile ducts. A recently designed new system of staging incorporates the size of the tumour, extent of the disease in the biliary system, involvement of the hepatic artery and portal vein, evidence of lymphadenopathy, distant metastases and the putative future liver remnant (Table 3.8).[103]

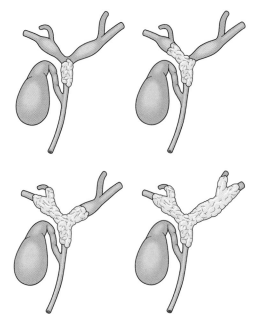

Figure 3.9 • Classification of Klatskin tumours according to Bismuth–Corlette, type I, II, IIIa and IV. Type I and II tumours are limited to the confluence of the right and left hepatic duct. In type III tumours, the segmental branches of the right or left hepatic duct are involved (type IIIa or IIIb, respectively). In type IV tumours, the tumour extends into the segmental branches of both right and left hepatic duct.

and does not provide information on the potential for resectability. Therefore, other staging systems have been used to predict resectability and to assess the extent of resection. The Bismuth–Corlette classification (**Fig. 3.9**) stratifies patients based on extent of biliary involvement by tumour. In brief, type I: tumours below the confluence of the left and right hepatic duct; type II: tumours reaching the confluence; type IIIa and IIIb: tumours occluding the common hepatic duct and either the right or the left hepatic duct, respectively; and type IV: tumours involving the confluence and both the right and left hepatic ducts.

✔✔ Staging and assessment of proximal bile duct tumours is difficult and usually requires a combination of investigations including US, CT and MRI. More invasive tests should only be performed if necessary in order to avoid procedure-related complications and delay of surgery. Preoperative biopsy and brush cytology are not always reliable and should not delay surgical exploration.

✔✔ The older staging and classification systems were of limited use in guiding preoperative decision-making. This led to the development of new modified clinical staging systems which have overcome these limitations and can aid with preoperative decision-making.

Table 3.7 • Jarnagin–Blumgart clinical T-staging system[101]

	Biliary involvement	**PV involvement**	**Lobar atrophy**
T1	Hilus ± unilateral sectional bile ducts	No	No
T2	Hilus ± unilateral sectional bile ducts	+ Ipsilateral	± Ipsilateral
T3	Hilus + bilateral sectional bile ducts	Yes/No	Yes/No
	Hilus + unilateral sectional bile ducts	+ contralateral	Yes/No
	Hilus + unilateral bile ducts	Yes/No	+ Contralateral
	Hilus ± unilateral sectional bile ducts	Bilateral	Yes/No

Sectional bile ducts = right anterior, right posterior, left medial, left lateral. PV, portal vein.

Table 3.8 • Classification system proposed by DeOliveira et al.[103]

Bile duct (B)[†]		
B1		Common bile duct
B2		Hepatic duct confluence
B3	R	Right hepatic duct
B3	L	Left hepatic duct
B4		Right and left hepatic duct
Tumour size (T)		
T1		<1 cm
T2		1–3 cm
T3		≥3 cm
Tumour form (F)		
Sclerosing		Sclerosing (or periductal)
Mass		Mass-forming (or nodular)
Mixed		Sclerosing and mass-forming
Polypoid		Polypoid (or intraductal)
Involvement (>180°) of the portal vein (PV)		
PV0		No portal involvement
PV1		Main portal vein
PV2		Portal vein bifurcation
PV3	R	Right portal vein
PV3	L	Left portal vein
PV4		Right and left portal veins
Involvement (>180°) of the hepatic artery (HA)		
HA0		No arterial involvement
HA1		Proper hepatic artery
HA2		Hepatic artery bifurcation
HA3	R	Right hepatic artery
HA3	L	Left hepatic artery
HA4		Right and left hepatic artery
Liver remnant volume (V)		
V0		No information on the volume needed (liver resection not foreseen)
V%	Indicate segments	Percentage of the total volume of a putative remnant liver after resection
Underlying liver disease (D)		
		Fibrosis
		Non-alcoholic steatohepatitis
		Primary sclerosing cholangitis
Lymph nodes (N)[‡]		
N0		No lymph node involvement
N1		Hilar and/or hepatic artery lymph node involvement
N2		Periaortic lymph node involvement
Metastases (M)[§]		
M0		No distant metastases
M1		Distant metastases (including liver and peritoneal metastases)

[†]Based on the Bismuth classification.
[‡]Based on the Japanese Society of Biliary Surgery classification.
[§]Based on the TNM classification.

Key points

- CT or MRI are equally accurate and should be performed for staging patients with HCC or CRLM depending on local expertise.
- Although PET-CT may provide additional information in the work-up of patients with CRLM it does not alter the overall resection rate or survival.
- Abdominal ultrasonography is highly accurate in identifying bile duct obstruction and stone disease but is of limited use in detecting and staging pancreatic tumours.
- CT is the investigation of choice for the diagnostic work-up and staging of pancreatic tumours.
- The accuracy of non-invasive cross-sectional imaging with CT, MRI/MRCP and EUS is superior to the more invasive ERCP in diagnosis of malignant bile duct obstruction.
- FDG-PET plays no routine role in patients with a pancreatic mass because it is associated with a high rate of false-negative results.
- EUS is the most accurate technique for detecting smaller tumours (<1 cm) and for differentiating between focal pancreatitis and malignancy.
- Diagnostic laparoscopy and laparoscopic ultrasound have a limited yield in patients with CRLM and pancreatic cancer but are useful in hepatocellular carcinoma. The role of diagnostic laparoscopy in proximal bile duct tumours is uncertain.
- The presence of vascular invasion and hepatocellular function determine the treatment of patients with cancer of the proximal biliary tract.
- Surgery for HPB tumours demands careful multidisciplinary preoperative assessment of risk factors and subsequent selection of patients. This should be done in a multidisciplinary meeting which includes HPB specialists in the field of medical oncology, radiotherapy, gastroenterology, (interventional) radiology and surgery.

🌐 Full references available at **http://expertconsult.inkling.com**

Key references

3. Floriani I, Torri V, Rulli E, et al. Performance of imaging modalities in diagnosis of liver metastases from colorectal cancer: a systematic review and meta-analysis. J Magn Reson Imaging 2010;31(1):19–31. PMID: 20027569.
   This study provides evidence for the use of MRI for the detection of colorectal liver metastases.

10. Bipat S, van Leeuwen MS, Comans EF, et al. Colorectal liver metastases: CT, MR imaging, and PET for diagnosis – meta-analysis. Radiology 2005;237(1):123–31. PMID: 16100087.
    A good quality meta-analysis that compares the most common diagnostic modalities to detect colorectal liver metastases.

12. Moulton CA, Gu CS, Law CH, et al. Effect of PET before liver resection on surgical management for colorectal adenocarcinoma metastases: a randomized clinical trial. JAMA 2014;311(18):1863–9. PMID: 24825641.
    This randomised trial shows that PET-CT compared with CT alone does not result in frequent change in surgical management of patients with colorectal liver metastases.

14. Jarnagin WR, Conlon K, Bodniewicz J, et al. A clinical scoring system predicts the yield of diagnostic laparoscopy in patients with potentially resectable hepatic colorectal metastases. Cancer 2001;91(6):1121–8. PMID: 11267957.
    A clinical tool to identify high-risk patients with colorectal liver metastases most likely to benefit from diagnostic laparoscopy.

29. Nordlinger B, Guiguet M, Vaillant JC, et al. Surgical resection of colorectal carcinoma metastases to the liver: a prognostic scoring system to improve case selection, based on 1568 patients. Association Francaise de Chirurgie Cancer 1996;77(7):1254–62. PMID: 8608500.
    A simple prognostic scoring system to evaluate the chances of cure in patients following resection of colorectal liver metastases.

49. Henderson JM, Sherman M, Tavill A, et al. AHPBA/AJCC consensus conference on staging of hepatocellular carcinoma: consensus statement. HPB (Oxford) 2003;5(4):243–50. PMID: 18332995.
    Excellent consensus statement on the staging of hepatocellular carcinoma.

59. van der Gaag NA, Rauws EA, van Eijck CH, et al. Preoperative biliary drainage for cancer of the head of the pancreas. N Engl J Med 2010;362(2):129–37. PMID: 20071702.
    A randomised trial which shows that routine preoperative biliary drainage in patients undergoing

surgery for cancer of the pancreatic head increases the rate of complications.

69. Van Heek NT, De Castro SM, van Eijck CH, et al. The need for a prophylactic gastrojejunostomy for unresectable periampullary cancer: a prospective randomized multicenter trial with special focus on assessment of quality of life. Ann Surg 2003;238(6):894–902. PMID: 14631226.
A randomised trial showing that a prophylactic gastrojejunostomy significantly decreases the incidence of gastric outlet obstruction without increasing complication rates.

75. Siriwardana HP, Siriwardena AK. Systematic review of outcome of synchronous portal-superior mesenteric vein resection during pancreatectomy for cancer. Br J Surg 2006;93(6):662–73. PMID: 16703621.
The largest collective report to date on portal-superior mesenteric vein resection in pancreatectomy showing that cure is unlikely, even with radical resection.

81. Phoa SS, Tilleman EH, van Delden OM, et al. Value of CT criteria in predicting survival in patients with potentially resectable pancreatic head carcinoma. J Surg Oncol 2005;91(1):33–40. PMID: 15999356.
CT signs of local irresectability and a tumour diameter of >3 cm predict a poor survival after resection.

4

Benign liver lesions

Marcel den Dulk
Cornelis H.C. Dejong

Introduction

Benign liver tumours are common and are frequently found coincidentally. Most benign liver lesions are asymptomatic, although larger lesions can cause non-specific complaints such as vague abdominal pain. Although rare, some of the benign lesions, e.g. large hepatic adenomas, can cause complications such as rupture or bleeding.

Ultrasound, computed tomography (CT) and magnetic resonance imaging (MRI) of the liver are the routine imaging modalities for the liver. Ultrasound is often a good screening investigation and can differentiate a cystic from a solid lesion. CT (with contrast enhancement) and MRI can be used to study the number and size of lesions, and often provide further characterisation of lesions. However, even with these imaging modalities, it may be challenging to differentiate between a benign liver lesion, such as a hepatic adenoma, and a malignancy, such as a well-differentiated hepatocellular carcinoma. Liver biopsies are in general only undertaken if there is doubt about the diagnosis and if results of the biopsy could influence the management strategy.

Asymptomatic lesions are often managed conservatively by observation. Surgical resection can be performed for symptomatic lesions or when there is a risk of malignant transformation. The type of resection is variable, from small, simple, peripheral resections or enucleations, to large resections or even liver transplantation for severe polycystic liver disease.

This chapter will focus on the description of benign liver lesions in the normal liver. These lesions can be classified by their origin, as is shown in Table 4.1.

Hepatocellular liver lesions

Focal nodular hyperplasia (FNH)

General

Focal nodular hyperplasia (FNH) is the second commonest benign solid liver tumour, with a prevalence of approximately 0.2%.[1] It has a higher incidence in females, mainly between 20 and 40 years of age, but also occurs in men and even in children. It is a rare finding in children but is more commonly observed after treatment for childhood cancer, with haematopoietic stem cell transplantation as the most important risk factor. Because of the predominant occurrence in females and the young age at onset, a role for female hormones has been suggested, but a relationship with oral contraceptives has not been clearly demonstrated.[2] In men, the lesions are often smaller and less typical.[3]

Clinical presentation

FNH lesions are often asymptomatic and found during imaging for unrelated reasons.[4] However, a small proportion of patients experience symptoms such as abdominal pain or a palpable mass.[3] In up to 20%, other liver lesions are found, such as

Table 4.1 • Classification of benign liver lesions by their origin

Hepatocellular	Focal nodular hyperplasia
	Hepatocellular adenoma
	Nodular regenerative hyperplasia
	Dysplastic nodules
Cholangiocellular	Bile duct cysts (simple or polycystic)
	Mucinous biliary cystadenoma
	Bile duct adenoma (biliary hamartoma/von Meyenburg complexes)
	Intraductal papillary neoplasm of the bile duct
Mesenchymal	Cavernous haemangioma
	Lipoma
	Angiolipoma
Inflammatory	Hepatic abscess (pyogenic, amoebic)
	Hydatid cysts
Others	Mesenchymal hamartoma
	Focal fatty infiltration
	Hepatic pseudotumours

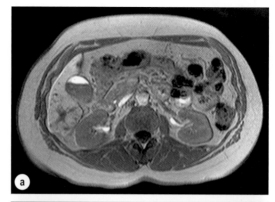

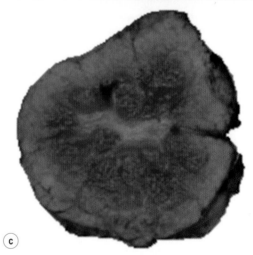

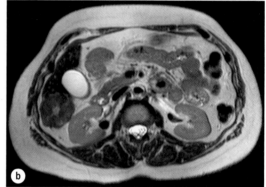

hepatic haemangiomata or adenomas.[3] Although FNH is commonly observed, complications are very rare; there are only a few published cases of spontaneous rupture resulting in intraperitoneal haemorrhage.

Diagnosis

Ultrasound is often the initial imaging investigation when a hepatic lesion is found. There is only a subtle difference in echogenicity between FNH and the surrounding normal liver.[5] Although the accuracy of the diagnosis increases with the use of contrast-enhanced ultrasound and colour Doppler, ultrasound is currently not the modality of choice for characterisation of an FNH.

On CT, FNH is usually homogeneous and isoattenuating to the normal liver before contrast injection. FNH lesions are hypervascular in the arterial phase and typically have a central scar (hypodense).[5] In the portal phase, a typical FNH returns to isoattenuating compared to the normal liver.[5] In the delayed phase, hyperattenuation of the central scar and septae are often seen.

MRI has a higher sensitivity (70%) and specificity (98%) for FNH than ultrasonography or CT.[6] Typically, FNH is iso- or hypointense on T1-weighted images, is slightly hyper- or isointense on T2-weighted images, and has a hyperintense central scar on T2-weighted images (**Fig. 4.1**). A typical FNH

Figure 4.1 • Focal nodular hyperplasia caudal in the right liver lobe (segment 6). On MRI T1-weighted images **(a)** late phase after Primovist, FNH may be iso- to hypointense on T1, with a hypointense central scar. On the T2-weighted images **(b)** the FNH is mainly slightly hyper- to isointense, with a hyperintense scar. A cross-sectional image of the resection specimen of the same patient is seen in **(c)**, showing the central scar.

demonstrates intense homogeneous enhancement during the arterial phase of gadolinium-enhanced imaging and enhancement of the central scar during later phases.[6]

Pathology

FNH is typically a lobulated lesion composed of nodules surrounded by fibrous septa originating from a central scar in an otherwise normal liver (Fig. 4.1).[6] On histological analysis, a classic FNH shows nodular hyperplastic parenchyma. The hepatic plates may be moderately thickened (two or three cells in thickness) with normal-appearing hepatocytes. The central scar contains fibrous connective tissue, cholangiolar proliferation with surrounding inflammatory infiltrates and malformed vessels of varying calibre, including tortuous arteries with thickened walls, capillaries but no portal veins. Approximately 50% of lesions show some degree of fatty infiltration, compared to the surrounding liver. In less than 20% of FNH lesions, the liver shows signs of steatosis.[6]

The development of FNH is thought to be caused by an injury to the portal tract resulting in the formation and enlargement of arterial to venous shunts.[7] This in turn causes hyperperfusion in local arteries resulting in oxidative stress that triggers a response from hepatic stellate cells to produce the typical central scar.[7]

Management

In general, the diagnosis can be made on MRI or CT, and routine biopsy is not indicated.[7] However, when imaging is not typical or if there is doubt about the diagnosis, e.g. with a differential diagnosis of hepatic adenoma or hepatocellular adenocarcinoma, a biopsy can be considered. FNH is currently not considered premalignant.[5]

In asymptomatic patients with typical features of FNH on imaging, no further treatment or follow-up is required. However, further evaluation is recommended for symptomatic lesions when the diagnosis cannot be firmly established. The current American College of Gastroenterology guidelines recommend follow-up with an annual ultrasound for 2–3 years in women diagnosed with FNH who wish to continue using oral contraceptives. In individuals with a firm diagnosis of FNH who are not using oral contraceptives, follow-up imaging is not required.[7]

> ✅ The diagnosis of FNH can be made on MRI or CT, and routine biopsy is not indicated. However, when imaging is not typical or if there is doubt about the diagnosis, e.g. with a differential diagnosis of hepatic adenoma or hepatocellular adenocarcinoma, biopsy can be an option. FNH is not a precursor of malignancy. In asymptomatic patients with typical features of FNH on imaging, no further treatment or follow-up is required. However, further evaluation is recommended for symptomatic lesions in which the diagnosis cannot be firmly established.

Hepatocellular adenoma

General

Hepatocellular adenomas (HCA) are rare benign hepatic neoplasms in otherwise normal livers with a prevalence of around 0.04% on abdominal imaging.[1] HCAs are predominantly found in women of child-bearing age (2nd to 4th decade) with a history of oral contraceptive use; they occur less frequently in men.[8,9] The association between oral contraceptive usage and HCA is strong and the risk for a HCA increases if an oral contraceptive with high hormonal potency is used, and if it is used for over 20 months. Long-term users of oral contraceptives have an estimated annual incidence of HCA of 3–4 per 100 000.[8] More recently, an increase in incidence in men has been reported, probably related to the increase in obesity, which is reported as another risk factor for developing HCA. In addition, anabolic steroid usage by body builders and metabolic disorders such as diabetes mellitus or glycogen storage disease type I are associated with HCAs. HCAs in men are generally smaller but have a higher risk of developing into a malignancy.

In the majority of patients, only one HCA is found, but in a minority of patients more than 10 lesions have been described (also referred to as liver adenomatosis).

Clinical presentation

Small HCAs are often asymptomatic and found on abdominal imaging being undertaken for other purposes, during abdominal surgery or at autopsy. Some patients present with abdominal discomfort, fullness or (right upper quadrant) pain due to an abdominal mass. It is not uncommon that the initial symptoms of a HCA are acute onset of abdominal pain and hypovolaemic shock due to intraperitoneal rupture. In a series of patients who underwent resection, bleeding was reported in up to 25%.[10,11] The risk of rupture is related to the size of the adenoma.[11] Exophytic lesions (protruding from the liver) have a higher chance of bleeding compared to intrahepatic or subcapsular lesions (67% vs 11% and 19%, respectively, $P < 0.001$).[12] Lesions in segments II and III are also at higher risk of bleeding compared to lesions in the right liver (35% vs 19%, $P = 0.049$).

Diagnosis

HCAs are often detected first by ultrasound during investigation of right upper quadrant discomfort. The high lipid content of adenomas may contribute to the hyperechoic appearance of these lesions.[13] The ultrasound appearance is often heterogeneic due to haemorrhage, necrosis and fat content. Colour Doppler ultrasound can be used to differentiate HCA from FNH. However, the diagnosis of adenoma is not usually made definitely at ultrasonography, and subsequent CT or other imaging modalities are often required to confirm the diagnosis.[13]

Multiphasic helical CT allows more accurate detection and characterisation of focal hepatic lesions. The degree of attenuation of the adenoma relative to the background liver depends on the composition of the tumour and liver.[13] CT may demonstrate a hypoattenuating mass due to the presence of intratumoural fat, or the lesion may be nearly isoattenuating relative to normal liver on unenhanced, portal venous-phase and delayed-phase images (most of the adenomas; Fig. 4.2). Alternatively, the lesion may be hyperattenuating in all phases of both contrast enhanced and unenhanced images in fatty livers.[13] Due to the presence of large subcapsular feeding vessels, peripheral enhancement may be seen on contrast-enhanced CT, with a centripetal pattern of enhancement. Small HCAs may enhance rapidly and are often hyperattenuating relative to the liver. The enhancement usually does not persist in adenomas due to arteriovenous shunting. Larger HCAs may be more heterogeneous than smaller lesions, and their CT appearance is less specific.[13]

On MRI, HCAs are usually heterogeneous in appearance. They are typically bright on T1-weighted MRI, and predominantly hyperintense relative to liver on T2-weighted images (Fig.4.2).[13] Almost one-third of adenomas have a peripheral rim corresponding to a fibrous capsule (Fig. 4.2). If there is still doubt about the diagnosis, a positron emission tomography (PET)-CT scan with 18 F-fluoromethylcholine be considered as this imaging modality has recently been shown to differentiate between HCA and FNH with a sensitivity of 100% and a specificity of 97%.[14] Alternatively, a biopsy can be considered in very selected cases when there is persistent doubt about the diagnosis.[15]

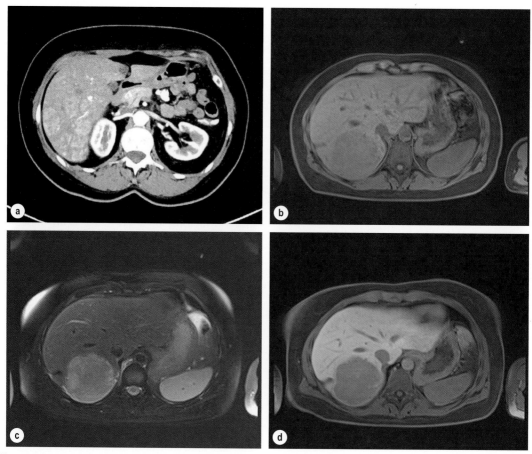

Figure 4.2 • A patient with adenomatosis of the liver **(a)** and another patient with a hepatocellular adenoma posteriorly in the right liver lobe (segment 7; **b**, **c** and **d**). **(a)** shows CT appearance of multiple heterogenous hyperdense lesions during the arterial phase. On MRI, the signal of the adenoma depends both on the fat composition of the liver and the adenoma. This adenoma is isointense on the T1-weighted images **(c)**, is heterogeneous hyperintense on T2-weighted images **(d)**, and there is no substantial uptake or retention after administration of Primovist (hepatocellular-specific contrast agent).

Pathology

HCAs are typically nodular lesions with a size ranging from microscopic to lesions as large as 20 cm.[9] They are relatively uniform, although areas of congestion, necrosis, haemorrhage, or fibrosis can be observed. Often large subcapsular vessels are seen as well as intratumoural fat. On microscopic examination, HCA is defined as a tumoural monoclonal proliferation of well-differentiated, usually bland-looking hepatocytes arranged in sheets and cords that are usually one, or at most two, cells in width.[9]

More recently, molecular classification has revealed four major subtypes of HCA (the Bordeaux classification): HNF1A (coding for hepatocyte nuclear factor 1a) inactivating mutations (30–40%), inflammatory adenomas (40–50%), β-catenin-mutated HCAs (β-HCA; 10–15%) and unclassified HCAs (10%).[16] Inflammatory HCAs can also be β-catenin activated (10%). It is important to differentiate between these subclasses, as β-catenin mutations appear to be associated with a higher risk of malignant transformation.[16]

Management

HCAs have a risk of spontaneous rupture and malignant transformation. The risk of rupture is related to the size of the adenoma.[11] In a group of 124 patients, 25% of HCAs ruptured, but no rupture was observed in lesions <5 cm.[11] Recent hormonal treatment was also a risk factor for haemorrhage.[11] Mortality after spontaneous rupture is approximately 5–10%.

Stoot et al. performed a systematic review and studied 1635 HCAs.[17] They concluded that only 4.2% of patients with a HCA had malignant transformation, and malignant transformation in lesions <5 cm was a very rare finding. The risk of malignant transformation is much higher in men, and in some studies it is reported to be as high as 47%.[18]

There is no guideline for the treatment of HCAs, although there are general agreements. In men, all lesions should be considered for surgical resection independent of size, given the high risk of malignant transformation, while taking into account comorbidity and location of the lesion. Resection should also be considered in patients with HCAs due to a metabolic disorder.[15] In women, lesions <5 cm can be observed with sequential imaging after cessation of oral contraceptive treatment.[19] In larger tumours, treatment strategies vary. Some clinicians have proposed non-surgical management if hormone therapy is stopped and patients are followed up with serial radiological examinations. The time period of waiting is still under debate, however recent studies indicate that a waiting period of longer than 6 months could be justified.[20,21] Others have advocated resection of adenomas because of the risk of haemorrhage and malignancy.[7] Alternatively, elective transarterial embolisation could be a valid approach in women.

Hepatic arterial embolisation can be effective for controlling bleeding in patients who present with acute haemorrhage.[22] If the lesion is atypical, resection could be considered, but if there is no suspicion of a malignancy it is best to wait for resorption of the haematoma before further therapy.[22] HCAs tend to grow during pregnancy.[15] Pregnancy should not be discouraged in the presence of a small HCA; however, close sonographic surveillance is recommended.[15]

Orthotopic liver transplantation has been performed for HCAs. However, liver transplantation should be reserved for exceptional cases, such as for hepatic adenomatosis in patients with a metabolic liver disease (e.g. glycogen storage disease) or in patients with hepatic adenomatosis and (a suspicion of) malignant transformation.

More recently, the subtypes of the Bordeaux classification of HCA have been studied related to their risk of complications. Some groups report that percutaneous core needle biopsy is of limited value because the therapeutic strategy is based primarily on patient sex and tumour size.[23] Others report a different therapeutic approach based on subtype. Thomeer et al. concluded that there was no evidence to support the use of subtype classification in the stratification and management of individual patients related to risk of bleeding.[15] Size still remains the most important feature to predict those at risk of bleeding during follow-up. However, malignant transformation does seem to be related to differences in subtypes. β-catenin-mutated HCAs trigger a potent mitogenic signalling pathway that is prominent in HCC.[15] Cases of inflammatory HCAs can also show activation of the β-catenin pathway with a risk of developing malignancy.[9] Therefore, β-catenin-mutated and inflammatory HCAs are prone to malignant degeneration, and particularly if >5 cm.[15] In these circumstances, invasive treatment should be considered.

✔ There is currently no guideline for the treatment of HCAs, although there are some general agreements. In men, all lesions should be considered for surgical resection independent of size, given the high risk of malignant transformation, while taking into account comorbidity and location of the lesion. Resection should also be considered in patients with HCAs due to a metabolic disorder. In women, lesions <5 cm can be observed with sequential imaging after cessation of oral contraceptive treatment. In larger tumours, treatment strategies vary. Some advocate non-surgical management in which hormone therapy is stopped and patients are followed up with serial radiologic examinations. The waiting period should be at least 6 months, although recent publications have shown that a longer period is necessary. Others resect larger adenomas because of the risk of haemorrhage and malignancy. More recently, it was found that the HCA subtype with a β-catenin-mutation is more prone to malignant transformation, and in these patients invasive treatment should be considered. For patients with acute haemorrhage from a HCA, hepatic arterial embolisation can be effective for controlling bleeding, after which either resection or observation (with or without biopsy) could be considered.

Nodular regenerative hyperplasia

Nodular regenerative hyperplasia (NRH) is the transformation of normal hepatic parenchyma into small regenerative nodules, also known as micronodular transformation.[7] This condition should not be confused with regeneration nodules found in cirrhotic patients, which are different entities. NRH nodules are thought to be related to altered blood flow; obstructive portal venopathy causes ischaemia, which in turn leads to hyperplasia of hepatic acini with adequate blood flow in order to compensate for atrophied hepatocytes.[24] In a retrospective study of autopsies, NRH was found in 2.1–2.6% of cases, all middle-aged to elderly adults with a female to male ratio of 2:1,[25] although this was not confirmed in all studies. NRH has been associated with immunological and haematological disorders, cardiac and pulmonary disorders, several drugs and toxins, neoplasia and organ transplantation.[24] It has been suggested by some that NRH is a premalignant condition, although others think that NRH is a condition secondary to HCC or its treatment.

NRH is often discovered incidentally. The majority of patients are asymptomatic, although some patients have signs of portal hypertension.[7] The nodules have variable echogenicity on ultrasonography and are often hypodense on CT without significant enhancement. Unfortunately, even MRI is not very helpful to distinguish the lesions as they are often small and difficult to characterise.[7] Therefore, histological examination is necessary to make the diagnosis of NRH. A correct diagnosis is often difficult using percutaneous needle biopsy, and in these cases laparoscopically guided liver biopsy or wedge biopsy for diagnosis may be considered.[7]

The management depends on the presenting symptoms, but should at least focus on treating the underlying condition.[7,24] If there is portal hypertension, treatment options include medication or sometimes portosystemic shunt procedures, but it may also be necessary to treat complications such as ascites or oesophageal varices. Liver failure is a rare complication for which liver transplantation may be the only solution.[24]

Cholangiocellular liver lesions

Simple cysts of the liver

General

Hepatic cysts are relatively common, and seen in approximately 6% of ultrasound procedures.[1] The incidence increases with age, with more than half of patients over 60 years of age having one or more simple cysts.[26] These non-parasitic cysts can occur as single, multiple or diffuse cysts (polycystic liver disease will be discussed separately). Cysts can range from 1 mm to >20 cm (containing several litres of fluid). Some groups report that cysts are more frequent in women with a female to male ratio of approximately 2:1, but others indicate a more even distribution. Symptomatic cysts are reported up to 10 times more commonly in women than in men.[27]

Simple cysts contain clear, bile-like fluid, but have no communication with bile ducts. As bile duct epithelium covers the cyst inner lining, it is hypothesised that simple cysts arise during embryogenesis when intrahepatic ductules fail to connect with intra- or extrahepatic ducts.[26]

Clinical presentation

In the majority of patients the cysts are discovered incidentally.[26] A small fraction of patients, mainly with large cysts, experience symptoms such as abdominal pain, early satiety, nausea and vomiting due to a mass effect.[26] Physical examination may reveal a palpable abdominal mass or hepatomegaly. Complications such as haemorrhage, rupture and biliary obstruction are rare and are more likely in larger cysts.[26]

Diagnosis

The diagnosis of a simple cyst can be made by ultrasound. Ultrasound has a sensitivity and specificity of approximately 90% for diagnosing cysts.[26] CT shows a well-demarcated, water-attenuated, smooth lesion without an internal structure, and no enhancement with contrast (**Fig. 4.3**).[7] MRI T1-weighted sequences show low signal intensity, whereas T2-weighted sequences show extremely high signal intensity, which does not enhance after contrast injection. MRI has a diagnostic accuracy of 97% for cysts. Aspiration of the cyst for diagnosis is not needed or recommended.[7]

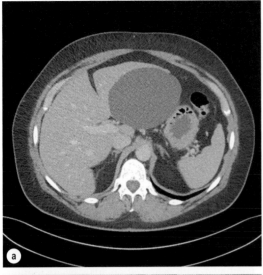
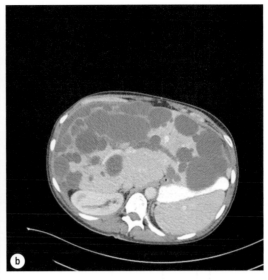
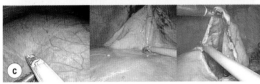

Figure 4.3 • **(a)** CT of a solitary liver cyst in segment 2/3. **(b)** CT of a patient with polycystic liver disease. **(c)** Laparoscopic cyst fenestration.

If intracystic haemorrhage occurs, ultrasound typically shows a hyperechogenic pattern with suggestion of septations or solid portions.[26] In general, when irregularities and nodules in the cystic wall are identified, these should be considered neoplastic.[26] Simple cysts rarely have calcifications and this is more characteristic of hydatid cysts.

Management

Asymptomatic cysts do not require treatment, but symptomatic cysts may require intervention. Percutaneous aspiration does not provide definitive treatment as the cyst typically recurs; however, it may help to clarify if abdominal pain is related to a cyst.

Percutaneous aspiration sclerotherapy is recommended by many as the preferred first treatment.[26,28] Wijnands et al. performed a systematic literature review and reported excellent results with respect to long-term efficacy and safety after aspiration sclerotherapy of hepatic cysts.[28] Recurrence rates of aspiration sclerotherapy range between 20% and 30%. A primary surgical approach should be considered if it is difficult to rule out cystadenoma or malignancy. Surgery may also be indicated if there is biliary communication and infection, when sclerotherapy has been ineffective, and in patients with recurrence.[29]

Surgical deroofing or fenestration of the cystic wall results in excellent reduction of symptoms.[30] Historically, this was done as an open procedure but nowadays a laparoscopic approach can be performed safely with minimal morbidity (Fig. 4.3). Recurrence rates of 10–25% are reported.[30] Excision of a simple cyst is usually not necessary and can result in additional morbidity and mortality as there is often no dissection plane between the cyst and crucial structures in the liver. However, in selected cases a more radical resection with emphasis on preserving functional hepatic parenchyma may be necessary. If histology of the partially removed cyst wall is abnormal or suggestive of a cystadenoma, hepatic resection is indicated.

Polycystic liver disease

General

Polycystic liver disease (PLD) is a condition which is characterised by the development of multiple hepatic cysts.[31] Similar to simple liver cysts, it is a congenital malformation of biliary ducts. Three PLD entities are recognised in adults: (1) Von Meyenburg complexes (biliary hamartoma; hepatic cystic hamartoma) with characteristic small, non-hereditary nodular cystic lesions; (2) isolated polycystic liver disease with innumerable hepatic cysts (autosomal dominant; PCLD), and (3) autosomal dominant polycystic kidney disease (ADPKD) with cysts in both kidneys and in many cases hepatic cysts. The incidence of Von Meyenburg complexes is estimated at 0.7–5.6%, the prevalence of ADPKD 1/400 to 1/1000, and the prevalence of PCLD is 1/100 000 to 1/1 000 000.[31] Von Meyenburg complexes will be addressed later in this chapter. This section will focus on the other two entities.

Variants of three genes have been associated with PCLD and are present in approximately 25% of cases: protein kinase C substrate 80 K-H (PRKCSH), SEC63 homologue (SEC63), and low-density lipoprotein receptor-related protein 5 (LRP5).[32] In ADPKD, variants in two genes are responsible for ADPKD in virtually all cases: polycystic kidney disease 1 (PKD1; 85%) and polycystic kidney disease 2 (PKD2; 15%).[32,33] Studies have shown that in families with PLD, the clinical presentation can be heterogeneous, and that between families there is a considerable phenotypic variability of hepatic cysts.[31]

Clinical presentation

The majority (>80%) of PLD patients are clinically asymptomatic. When symptoms arise, they are associated with the extent of hepatomegaly or due to compression of neighbouring organs. Symptoms include pain, abdominal discomfort, pyrosis, early satiety, weight loss and anorexia. In general, women present with larger-sized liver cysts and are more frequently symptomatic, suggesting that a hormonal component may play a role.

Complications can occur, such as cyst haemorrhage, rupture and infection. These complications appear to occur more frequently in ADPKD compared to PCLD.[31] Rupture and jaundice have only occasionally been described. In advanced stages, portal hypertension, ascites and liver failure can be found.

The main difference between ADPKD and PCLD is the presence of polycystic kidneys. The prognosis of these diseases is different, as the majority of ADPKD patients develop enlarged kidneys and end-stage renal disease. In PCLD patients, a few renal cysts may be present, but this does not result in renal failure.[31]

Imaging is similar to that for simple cysts and typically includes assessment by MRI or CT (Fig. 4.3). However, it should be remembered that in patients who present with multiple liver cysts, imaging of the kidneys should also be performed. Several clinical classifications have been proposed to grade the severity of PLD, e.g. Gigot's classification, Qian's classification and Schnelldorfer's classification. These classifications use factors such as symptoms, number and size of cysts to grade the severity of PLD.[34]

Management

The primary aim of treatment of PCLD and ADPKD is to reduce symptoms.[31] Treatment varies depending on the phenotype of PLD; patients with a few large cysts require a different approach to those with many small cysts.

In asymptomatic patients, no therapy is warranted. Women should be advised to stop oral contraceptives. More recently, treatment with somatostatin analogues has shown a reduction in liver volume after 6 months of therapy, but only a modest improvement in quality of life.[35] Therefore, these drugs should be used only in a trial setting.[7] Analgesics can be administered for symptomatic relief of pain.

In patients with large symptomatic dominant cysts, invasive treatments may be considered. Several studies have shown beneficial effects of invasive treatments, including aspiration sclerotherapy or laparoscopic cyst deroofing.[31] However, it is recognised that a high percentage of patients require further intervention (approximately 50% for PLD).[31] In selected cases, hepatic resection combined with fenestration may be an option.[34] Liver transplantation may be indicated for patients with liver failure.

Cystadenoma

General

Cystadenomas of the liver are rare tumours, accounting for <5% of biliary tumours.[7] They are solitary, usually multilocular, almost always found in women, with a preference for presentation in the fourth decade of life. No association between cystadenomas and oral contraceptive use has been found.[36] Cystadenomas >20 cm in diameter have been reported. In the majority of cases (95%), the content of the cyst is mucin.[7]

Histologically, cystadenomas are multilocular with benign cuboidal to columnar epithelium. In the past it was thought that all lesions had an ovarian-like stroma, but cystadenomas without ovarian-like stroma have been reported in 15% of patients.[36]

Various hypotheses about the origin of the ovarian-like stroma in hepatic cystadenomas exist. One explanation is that during embryological development, when the gonads are located directly under the diaphragm, ectopic ovarian cells migrate to the liver and eventually form the lesion. This would explain the predominance of cystadenomas in segment 4. However, ovarian stroma also resemble embryonic mesenchyma of the embryonic gallbladder and large bile ducts. Another hypothesis is therefore that cystadenomas are remnants of ectopic tissue destined to form the gallbladder.

Cystadenoma is thought to be a precursor of cystadenocarcinoma.[7] Malignancy has been identified in approximately 10% of resections for presumed cystadenoma.[37] In contrast to cystadenomas, hepatic cystadenocarcinomas are found more equally distributed in men and women. Furthermore, cystadenocarcinoma follows a more aggressive course in men (more often in a cystadenoma without ovarian-like stroma). Therefore, a lesion that is considered to be a cystadenoma in a man should always raise the suspicion of a malignancy.

Clinical presentation

Cystadenomas are often found incidentally. Larger cysts can be symptomatic and present with abdominal pain, abdominal fullness, early satiety and weight loss. Laboratory values are usually normal.[37]

Imaging

On ultrasonography, cystadenomas typically have irregular walls and internal septations forming loculi (small spaces or cavities within the main cystic lesion).[7] If a complex cyst is found on ultrasound investigation, cross-sectional imaging with CT and MRI should always be obtained. CT and MRI can help identify heterogeneous septations, irregular papillary growths and thickened cyst walls (**Fig. 4.4**). The cysts are typically hyperintense on T2 weighting, although because of mucinous content they may appear heterogeneous.[7]

It is difficult to differentiate cystadenomas from cystadenocarcinomas preoperatively on imaging. However, the presence of calcifications along with mixed solid and cystic components on imaging is associated with cystadenocarcinoma.[7] Also, a

mural or septal nodule and a nodule diameter >10 mm on conventional ultrasound are suggestive of cystadenocarcinoma. Aspiration or biopsy is not recommended as it has limited sensitivity and there is a risk of disseminating malignancy if there is an underlying cystadenocarcinoma.[7] Besides, it does not alter the management strategy as the recommended treatment for both is resection.

Management

If a cystadenoma is diagnosed, complete tumour excision is the standard treatment, both to obtain a definitive histological diagnosis and to prevent malignant transformation. Recurrence rates are low with either standard hepatic resection or enucleation, but are approximately 60% following aspiration or partial resection.[37] Therefore, if cyst fenestration has been performed for what was thought to be a simple cyst, but the definitive histology confirms a cystadenoma, resection is indicated. After excision of a cystadenoma, long-term outcome is good; however, the prognosis for patients with a cystadenocarcinoma is worse.[37]

Bile duct adenoma

Bile duct adenomas, also referred to as bile duct hamartomas or Von Meyenburg complexes, are benign bile duct malformations. They are composed of dilated intrahepatic bile ductules embedded in fibrous stroma and usually appear as subcapsular or parenchymal nodules <10 mm in diameter. In general, these lesions do not cause clinical symptoms, but they can cause a diagnostic dilemma when liver metastases are suspected. When found during surgery, a biopsy may be necessary to differentiate between a bile duct adenoma and hepatic malignancies, such as cholangiocarcinoma or metastasis. Treatment is usually not required.

Intraductal papillary neoplasm of the bile duct

Intraductal papillary neoplasm of the bile duct (IPNB) is a rare bile duct tumour and is, along with biliary intraepithelial neoplasia, thought to be a precursor lesion of cholangiocarcinoma. It is characterised by papillary growth within the bile duct lumen and is regarded as a biliary counterpart of intraductal papillary mucinous neoplasm (IPMN) of the pancreas.

Patients present with repeated episodes of abdominal pain, jaundice and acute cholangitis, although some patients experience no complaints (mainly in the group of patients with non-mucinous-producing biliary papillomatosis).[38] The most

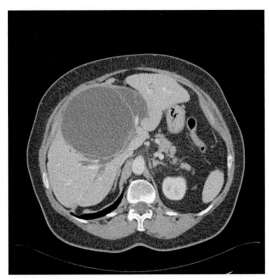

Figure 4.4 • CT showing central cystic liver lesion with a thickened wall and sepatations with secondary biliary duct dilatation. Histology confirmed a cystadenoma.

common radiological findings for IPNB are bile duct dilatation and intraductal masses. The patterns of bile duct dilatation are diffuse duct ectasia, localised duct dilatation and cystic dilatation.[38] Some groups recommend cholangioscopy to confirm the histology and view the extent of the tumour.[39]

All patients with IPNB should be considered for treatment. IPNB (and associated mucin) often cause recurrent cholangitis and obstructive jaundice, even if these tumours are not malignant.[39] Patients without distant metastasis should be considered for surgical resection. Intraoperative frozen section of the resection margin of the bile duct and regional lymph node excision are recommended.[39] Patients treated by curative resection have a good prognosis.[38]

Mesenchymal liver lesions

Haemangiomata

General

Haemangiomata are the commonest benign liver lesions, with an incidence of approximately 3%.[1,40] Liver haemangiomata are more frequently observed in women than in men (ratio 5:1).[2] The mean age at diagnosis is around 50 years.[1] The size of the lesions varies from some millimetres to >20 cm. In a study of more than 45 000 hospital patients undergoing liver ultrasonography, the mean diameter of haemangiomata was 2 cm.[1] Classically, giant haemangiomata were defined as haemangiomata greater than 4–5 cm in diameter.[41] However, in recent years more groups are defining giant haemangiomata as lesions >10 cm.[4] These giant haemangiomata are mainly found in women, and a role for female hormones in progression has been considered, although a strong association with the oral contraceptive pill has not been demonstrated.

In the majority of cases (77%), haemangiomata are solitary lesions, but a minority (1.6%) of patients have >5 haemangiomata.[1] A few cases of familial cavernous liver haemangiomata have been described, with similar lesions in other organs such as cerebral cavernous malformations.

Clinical presentation

Haemangiomata are most frequently found incidentally during abdominal ultrasonography for unrelated reasons.[5] Most haemangiomata are small. Sometimes patients with larger haemangiomata present with non-specific abdominal complaints such as vague abdominal pain, fullness, early satiety, nausea or vomiting. This might be explained by compression of adjacent organs or stretch of Glisson's capsule.

Presentation with spontaneous rupture or bleeding from a haemangioma is rare and in a large retrospective cross-sectional study it was observed mainly in large, peripherally located exophytic growing haemangiomata.[40] Even if symptoms are present, the majority of patients have other explanations for these complaints. In a study by Farges et al. 54% of patients with symptoms had another cause for their symptoms.[42] Furthermore, half of the patients with no other explanation for their complaints were still symptomatic after treatment (resection [n=8], embolisation [n=5] and hepatic artery ligation [n=1]), which questions whether the haemangioma itself was the real cause of the initial complaints.[42] However, some patients do present with pain from haemangiomata; these lesions are often located on the surface of the liver and resection of the haemangioma may result in resolution of symptoms.

A rare presentation in patients with a giant haemangioma is thrombocytopenia and hypofibrinogenaemia caused by consumption of coagulation factors, also known as Kasabach–Merritt syndrome. This is a serious complication and mortality ranges between 10% and 37%.

Diagnosis

As the majority of patients are asymptomatic, haemangiomata are often found by coincidence during imaging studies. The majority of haemangiomata can be diagnosed accurately by imaging alone. On ultrasonography, haemangiomata typically appear as well-defined, lobulated, homogeneous hyperechoic masses, but may also have hypoechoic portions due to haemorrhage, fibrosis or calcification. The diagnostic accuracy of ultrasound is reported to be 70–80%.[5] However, unenhanced ultrasound alone cannot differentiate a small haemangioma from a hepatocellular carcinoma, liver cell adenoma, FNH or solitary metastasis. Contrast enhanced ultrasound has been found to increase accuracy to >90%.

The 2014 American College of Gastroenterology guidelines strongly recommended that an MRI or CT is undertaken to confirm the diagnosis of haemangioma.[7] On CT prior to administration of intravenous contrast, haemangiomata appear as a well-demarcated hypodense mass. After intravenous contrast, haemangiomata classically have peripheral nodular enhancement and progressive centripetal fill-in (**Fig. 4.5**).[7] The best imaging modality for haemangiomata is MRI, with a reported sensitivity and specificity of >90% (Fig. 4.5). It has been suggested that MRI is used when lesions are <3 cm, close to the heart, or close to intrahepatic vessels.[24] Haemangiomata are bright on T2-weighted imaging and on enhanced T1-weighted imaging show a similar pattern as found on enhanced CT with peripheral nodular enhancement.

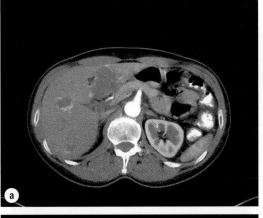

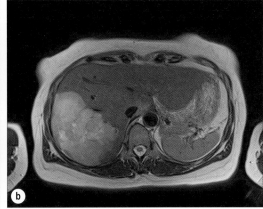

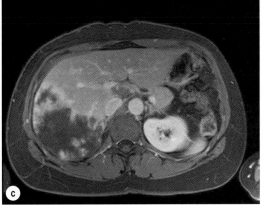

Figure 4.5 • (a) CT after intravenous contrast administration in the arterial phase shows several haemangiomata as nodular, discontinuous, enhancement. In portal and late venous phase there is progressive centripetal filling (not shown on this image). **(b)** T2-weighted MRI of a patient with a giant haemangioma. The haemangioma is seen as a hyperintense lesion. **(c)** Enhanced T1-weighted image (gadolinium enhancement) in the same patient. The lesion does not show uptake of the contrast and a peripheral nodular enhancement pattern is seen.

Single-photon emission CT (SPECT) using technetium-99 m-labelled red blood cells was previously found to be a helpful tool in the diagnosis of larger haemangiomata and those not located near large vessels. However, with improved technology, increased availability and decreased costs of MRI, there is now only a limited role for SPECT.

Pathology

Macroscopically, haemangiomata are well-circumscribed compressible tumours with a dark colour.[5] Microscopically, they are composed of multiple blood vessels lined by a single layer of endothelial cells within a thin, fibrous stroma.[4] Their blood supply is from the hepatic artery.

Needle biopsy is not necessary, and should only be considered in exceptional cases if the findings are atypical. It is debatable whether a needle biopsy of a hypervascular tumour, like a haemangioma, can be safely performed. In a retrospective study of 38 patients with haemangiomata ranging from 1 cm to 13.5 cm in size, no haemorrhage was reported after percutaneous needle biopsy.[43] However, others have reported bleeding after needle biopsy.

Management

Trastek et al. retrospectively studied 36 patients with hepatic haemangiomata >4 cm that were managed conservatively. They found no need for surgery after an observation period of up to 15 years (mean 5.5 years).[44] Furthermore, the majority of haemangiomata remained stable over time.[42] Complications are very rare, and therefore conservative management is in general appropriate.[7]

For larger or symptomatic lesions, the risk of intervention should be weighed against the benefit of resection. Surgical intervention can be considered in patients with a growing lesion that becomes very large (>10 cm) or if the patient begins to report symptoms such as recurrent pain. Follow-up imaging is not required for classical haemangiomata.

If intervention for a haemangioma is performed, complete surgical resection or enucleation of the lesion is the best treatment option.[41] If possible, enucleation of the lesion is preferred rather than hepatic resection, to avoid loss of functional liver tissue, to reduce blood loss and reduce the risk of postoperative complications.[41,45] Surgical intervention for hepatic haemangiomata should not be underestimated as it carries a high risk of major perioperative bleeding.

In a small prospective series, selective transarterial embolisation of haemangioma as the only treatment appeared to improve symptoms, although the size of the lesions did not change.[46] Transarterial embolisation as the only treatment is rarely used. Rupture of a (giant) haemangioma is uncommon (1–4% of cases), but if it does occur initial embolisation of the haemangioma to temporarily control the bleeding before resection should be performed. Others use this strategy for elective resections of giant haemangiomata. More recently, other treatment options such as radio-frequency ablation (RFA) with or without preoperative arterial embolisation have been used successfully.[45] Although very rare, liver transplantation has been performed for technically unresectable, complicated, giant haemangiomata.

✔ Conservative management is appropriate for asymptomatic haemangiomata <4 cm in diameter. For larger or symptomatic lesions, the risk of intervention should be weighed against the benefit of resection. Surgical intervention can be considered in patients with a growing lesion that becomes very large (>10 cm) or if the patient has symptoms such as recurrent pain. Follow-up imaging is not required for classic haemangiomata.

Hepatic lipoma and angiolipoma

Lipomatous tumours, such as hepatic angiomyolipoma or hepatic lipoma, are very rare benign tumours.[5] They are often asymptomatic, although abdominal discomfort could be a presenting symptom. Hepatic angiolipomas may be part of the clinical manifestations of tuberous sclerosis (also called Morbus Bourneville-Pringle, a rare genetic disease that causes benign tumours to grow in different organs including brain, skin, kidney and liver). For atypical cases it may be necessary to perform a biopsy to differentiate them from other hypervascular tumours, including HCC, FNH and haemangiomata.[5] The prognosis of these tumours is favourable, although resection may be necessary due to symptoms.

Inflammatory liver lesions

Pyogenic liver abscess

General

Liver abscess is a rare but potentially lethal condition which in the USA at the end of the last century accounted for approximately 20 per 100 000 hospital admissions.[47] The aetiology has changed over time. Historically, the commonest cause of a liver abscess was acute appendicitis, but in the era of modern surgery and antibiotics, this cause has declined drastically in importance. Other causes for hepatic abscesses include diverticular disease and inflammatory bowel disease (e.g. Crohn's disease). However, biliary causes are now the most frequent known cause of pyogenic liver abscesses. In earlier reports, benign obstruction of the bile duct, commonly due to choledocholithiasis, was the predominant cause of liver abscesses, whereas in more recent publications there is an increase in malignant biliary obstruction as the main aetiological factor.[47] Other rarer, non-gastrointestinal sources of hepatic abscesses include bacterial endocarditis, urinary sepsis, pneumonia, osteomyelitis and intravenous drug abuse. Direct extension into the liver from perforation of an adjacent organ, such as from the gallbladder, colon, stomach or duodenum are other sources of a hepatic abscess.

Clinical presentation

The commonest presenting features are vague non-specific symptoms. Patients present with fever, chills, right upper quadrant pain, jaundice, anorexia and malaise.[47] Almost all patients will have an elevated C-reactive protein (CRP), most will have an elevated white blood cell count, and more than half of patients will have abnormal liver enzymes with cholestatic parameters.

Diagnosis

Ultrasonography generally demonstrates a fluid-filled cavity. It can provide information on the number of lesions, the diameter and anatomical location, as well as information on the presence of bile duct dilatation. CT can be helpful to further evaluate the liver for the number of abscesses and to provide anatomical information required to make treatment decisions (**Fig. 4.6**). Gas in the abscess is only observed in approximately 20% of cases. An MRI or MRCP should be considered if a biliary cause of a hepatic abscess is suspected, such as in patients with distended bile ducts or obstructive liver function tests.

Management

Hope et al. studied 107 patients with hepatic pyogenic abscesses managed in a single centre and found that abscesses <3 cm could be treated successfully with antibiotics only.[48] For abscesses >3 cm that were unilocular, a combination of antibiotics and percutaneous drainage was successful in 83%, whereas for complex multiloculated abscesses >3 cm this regimen was only successful in 33% of patients. Given the non-

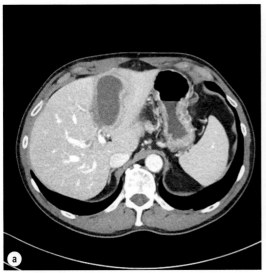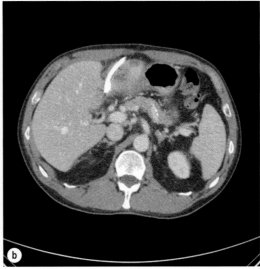

Figure 4.6 • CT in the portal-venous phase after intravenous contrast enhancement. **(a)** shows a hypodense lesion measuring 10 x 8.2 x 4.6 cm in the left lobe of the liver with a thick wall with contrast enhancement suggestive of a liver abscess, probably originating from diverticular disease. **(b)** shows CT after percutaneous drainage of the abscess with the drain located in the abscess **(b)**.

significant difference in mortality in this last group between patients drained percutaneously and those operated, the authors suggested that this last group of abscesses should be treated by surgery. In our opinion, all hepatic abscesses that are not caused by a malignancy should be first treated with antibiotics and (multiple) percutaneous (catheter) drainage (Fig. 4.6). If this fails, an operation can be considered, e.g. video-assisted abscess debridement, laparoscopic drainage, or resection in exceptional cases.

Recently, a meta-analysis comparing percutaneous needle aspiration with catheter drainage concluded that both techniques are safe methods to manage liver abscesses.[49] However, percutaneous catheter drainage was more effective as it facilitated a higher success rate and reduced the time required to achieve clinical relief. It is recommended that drained pus is sent for analysis to determine the responsible micro-organisms and to ensure appropriate antibiotics are administered. Virtually all micro-organisms have been cultured, although enteric organisms are most commonly identified (*Escherichia coli* and *Klebsiella pneumonia*).

In addition to treating the hepatic abscess, the underlying cause should also be treated. Although mortality has dropped drastically with current treatment regimens, mortality for patients with liver abscesses is still relatively high, with mortality rates of approximately 7–10%. For those admitted to the intensive care unit, mortality rates of up to 28% have been reported.[50]

Amoebic liver abscess

General

Amoebic liver abscesses caused by *Entamoeba histolytica* account for 10% of liver abscesses and are predominantly found in areas were *E. histolytica* is endemic, such as in tropical areas.[51] In Mexico 8.4% of the population have serum antibodies against *E. histolytica*. Only 10% of patients experience symptoms, mainly of amoebic colitis. Liver abscesses are the commonest extraintestinal manifestation of this infection. They are found in 1% of clinically infected patients, and primarily affect men between the ages of 18 and 50 years.[52]

E. histolytica trophozoites normally remain confined to the bowel lumen. However, some virulent trophozoites can migrate through the mucosa of the bowel and reach the liver through the portal system. There they can provoke enzymatic focal necrosis of hepatocytes and multiple micro-abscesses that eventually coalesce to form a single lesion. The central cavity contains a homogeneous thick liquid, with typically reddish-brown and yellow colour similar to 'anchovy paste'.[53] This material is almost always sterile, except when a secondary infection has occurred, and this allows differential diagnosis from a pyogenic abscess. The amoebae can be found at the edge of the lesion, but are rarely detected in the pus or within the abscess cavity itself.[53]

Clinical presentation

Right upper quadrant pain, fever and hepatomegaly are the predominant symptoms of hepatic amoebiasis, which can occur without any symptom of intestinal amoebiasis.[52,53] Patients with an amoebic abscess are usually more acutely ill than patients with a pyogenic abscess, have high fever and abdominal pain in the right upper quadrant. They are also younger and are usually from high-prevalence areas or recent travellers to such areas. Amoebic abscesses are more often found in individuals with suppressed cell-mediated immunity. Jaundice is an unusual symptom and is found in patients with multiple lesions or very large abscesses, and is associated with adverse prognosis.[53]

Both ultrasound and CT are sensitive in the detection of amoebic liver abscesses. In many patients, it is difficult to differentiate amoebic abscesses from pyogenic abscesses, but epidemiologic and clinical information in conjunction with positive amoebic titres may suggest the diagnosis. The lesion is typically oval or round and located near the liver capsule. On contrast-enhanced CT, amoebic abscesses usually appear as rounded well-defined lesions, with an enhancing wall 3–15 mm in thickness, and a peripheral zone of oedema around the abscess that is somewhat characteristic. The central abscess cavity may contain multiple septa or fluid-debris levels.

The diagnosis can be confirmed by demonstrating *E. histolytica* trophozoites in aspirated pus, or more frequently from the necrotic material obtained by needle biopsy of the edge of the lesion. However, the amoeba will be found in only a small percentage of cases.[53] In contrast, serum antibodies to *Entamoeba* species are present in >90% of cases.[52] False-negative serology tests may be obtained early in the infection (first 7–10 days), but repeated tests usually will come back positive.[51]

Management

Most amoebic liver abscesses can be treated with metronidazole treatment alone.[51,52] The role of therapeutic aspiration remains controversial. It is reasonable to reserve aspiration for individuals in whom the diagnosis is uncertain, when there is no response to metronidazole, in individuals with large left lobe abscesses (because of the risk of rupture into the pericardium), and in severely ill patients.[52] Individuals with an amoebic liver abscess should also be treated to eliminate intestinal colonisation by *E. histolytica*.[51,52]

Hydatid cysts

General

Echinococcosis or hydatid disease is a parasitic illness caused by the tapeworm *Echinococcus*. The liver is the most commonly infected organ.[54] Hepatic echinococcosis is (if not treated on time)

a life-threatening disease caused by *Echinococcus granulosus* or *Echinococcus multilocularis*, respectively causing a cystic and alveolar form.[55] Infection with *E. granulosus* is more common whereas *E. multilocularis* infection is more serious.[54]

E. granulosus has a worldwide distribution, with the highest prevalence found in Mediterranean countries, Russia, China, North and East Africa, South America and Australia.[55] The parasite life cycle involves dogs (or coyotes, dingoes and red foxes) as definitive hosts and ungulates (sheep, pigs, goats and horses) as intermediate hosts. Humans can accidentally become 'aberrant' intermediate hosts, after ingestion of *Echinococcus* eggs excreted by infected carnivores. The eggs grow inside the host organs (mainly the liver) and form a cyst (hydatid cyst). Hydatid cysts are round in shape and are usually filled with a clear fluid. The inner part of the cyst features a germinating membrane while the outer part features a laminated layer.[54] In time, the parasite cysts expand and cause a granulomatous inflammatory reaction which leads to the cyst becoming walled off by fibrous tissue.[54,55] Maturing cysts may develop daughter cysts (cyst in a cyst) and septations.[5,55] Peripheral calcifications are common in both viable and non-viable cysts.[5]

E. multilocularis is endemic in the northern hemisphere, including North America, Asia and some European countries (mainly France, Switzerland, Austria and Germany).[55] However, due to migration of refugees, the disease is increasingly found in non-endemic areas. The definitive hosts are wild carnivores (such as the red fox) and domestic cats and dogs, intermediate hosts are small rodents, whereas humans are aberrant hosts who ingest embryonated eggs.[55] Echinococcal larvae form alveolar structures with multiple vesicles of different sizes within the liver.[54] Alveolar echinococcosis may spread locally or metastasise to the brain, bones or lungs via the blood.[54]

Clinical presentation

The majority of patients are asymptomatic, since the cyst grows only slowly in the liver (1–5 mm per year).[54,55] Liver lesions are therefore often found incidentally. The most common presenting symptoms are right upper quadrant discomfort and loss of appetite.[54] Complications from hydatid cysts include cyst leakage or rupture resulting in anaphylaxis, cholangitis due to obstruction of bile ducts by daughter cysts or rupture of a cyst into a biliary duct, or secondary infection of the cysts.[54,55] *E. multilocularis* is initially found in the liver (usually the right lobe), but later in the infection it is possible to find metastasis to lung, brain, bones and local extension of the lesion (in the abdomen, retroperitoneum, or diaphragm).[55] In late-stage disease, patients with alveolar echinococcosis may present with liver failure.

Diagnosis

Ultrasound is a good tool for screening and follow-up. With ultrasound imaging, hydatid sand (scolices in the cyst fluid from ruptured vesiculae which form a white sediment), floating membranes, daughter cysts and vesicles inside the cyst can be identified. CT can identify cyst wall or septal calcifications, internal cystic structures and assess for complications (**Fig. 4.7**). MRI is superior for demonstrating cyst wall defects, biliary communication and neural involvement. Serological diagnosis is useful to confirm a radiological diagnosis and may also be an important tool for follow-up after surgical or pharmacological treatment. However, not all patients with cystic echinococcosis have a detectable immune response as this is dependent on the degree of echinoccal antigen secretion.[55]

Management

The treatment options for cystic echinococcosis include surgery, percutaneous treatments and medical treatment with a benzimidazole (such as albendazole or mebendazole), and should be undertaken in a centre with expertise in this disease.[54,55] The most appropriate treatment option depends on multiple variables such as disease-specific characteristics (cyst number, size, site and presence of cystobiliary communication) and clinical condition of the patient.

Surgery is currently reserved for complicated cysts (biliary fistula), multiseptated cysts, cysts with daughter cysts and large superficial cysts with a high risk of perforation.[54] If feasible, surgical removal of hydatid cysts offers the best chance to completely cure the disease.[55] A benzimidazole is often given to reduce the risk of anaphylaxis and secondary cystic echinococcosis.

Another treatment option is the PAIR method; an acronym which stands for Puncture, Aspiration, Injection, Re-aspiration. With this strategy, the cyst is punctured under ultrasound guidance, the cyst fluid is aspirated, a protoscolicidal agent (e.g. hypertonic saline or ethanol) is injected and the fluid re-aspirated. In selected patients, a success rate of up to 97% has been reported, but this method is less suitable for cysts that have daughter cysts.[54] Furthermore, PAIR should not be used if a cystobiliary communication is present, due to the risk of developing sclerosing cholangitis. To minimise the risk of secondary echinococcosis, concurrent treatment with a benzimidazole is recommended. This is usually given 4 hours before the puncture and continued for a month.[55] An alternative percutaneous method is placement of a broad tube to remove the solid components of the cysts as well as the daughter cysts.[54]

Medical treatment without surgery or PAIR may be used for patients with small cysts (<5 cm) without daughter cysts or septations. Otherwise, this treatment should be restricted to patients that cannot undergo surgical or percutaneous treatment.[54,55] It is reported that complete cure (i.e. cyst disappearance) only occurs in approximately a third of patients treated with a benzimidazole alone.[55]

E. multilocularis cysts are treated with surgery or pharmacotherapy. Surgery is the first choice option in all operable patients.[54,55] Liver transplantation may be an option in patients with advanced liver failure. Albendazole treatment should be given for a prolonged period after surgery (at least 2 years) and patients should be monitored for recurrent disease. For patients not suitable for surgery, the optimal duration of therapy is not clear and a benzimidazole could even be necessary for life.[55]

Other liver lesions

Mesenchymal hamartoma is an uncommon benign liver lesion that mainly occurs in young children (<2 years of age), although cases in adults have been reported. These lesions consist of a mixture of epithelial and mesenchymal structures. If the lesions enlarge, surgical resection is recommended. Transformation to undifferentiated (embryological) sarcoma has rarely been described.

Focal steatosis and fatty sparing (also referred to as focal fatty change of the liver) are a frequent findings on liver imaging and can mimic solid lesions. Regional variations in the degree of fat accumulation in the liver can be related to vascular anomalies, metabolic disorders, use of certain drugs or coexistence of hepatic masses. If the diagnosis is made (with or without biopsy), no further treatment is necessary.

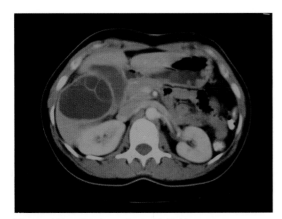

Figure 4.7 • CT of a patient with *Echinococcus granulosus* showing a non-calcified hydatid cyst with daughter cysts.

Inflammatory hepatic pseudotumours are rare hepatic lesions that can mimic malignant lesions. They can occur at all ages. The aetiology is unclear, but an underlying infectious cause has been suggested. Patients can present without any symptoms or with fever, weight loss or upper abdominal pain. A biopsy can be necessary to differentiate the lesion from other tumours. On histological examination myofibroblasts, polyclonal plasma cells and fibrous tissue can be found. The course of the disease is unpredictable. Spontaneous regression has been reported, although recurrence after regression has also been described.[56] Treatment with antibiotics or steroids should be considered.

Key points

- Benign liver lesions are common and often asymptomatic.
- Asymptomatic lesions can usually be managed conservatively.
- Haemangiomata are the commonest benign liver lesion, and can be >10 cm in diameter (giant haemangioma). They are more common in females.
- Haemangiomata are managed conservatively, although for lesions with recurrent pain and very large lesions, resection might be considered.
- Focal nodular hyperplasia (FNH) is the second commonest benign liver tumour, and if the diagnosis is certain neither a resection, nor follow-up of asymptomatic patients is necessary.
- Hepatocellular adenomas are rare hepatic tumours, mainly found in women of child-bearing age and are associated with the use of oral contraceptives.
- The risk of bleeding and malignant transformation increases with hepatocellular adenomas >5 cm in diameter; the risk of malignancy is higher in men.
- Hepatic cysts are common and if asymptomatic need no further treatment.
- Cystadenomas are rare benign cystic tumours of the liver that should be considered for resection.
- Cystadenomas are more frequently found in women, and if found in men carry a higher risk of a malignancy.
- Hepatic liver abscesses should be treated with antibiotics and/or percutaneous drainage.
- Amoebic liver abscesses should be treated initially with metronidazole.
- Hepatic echinococcosis is a parasitic illness, in which humans are an accidental intermediate host. Although the disease is mainly found in endemic areas, it is increasingly found in non-endemic areas due to migration of refugees and should be managed in centres with expertise in the disease.

🌐 Full references available at **http://expertconsult. inkling.com**

Key references

7. Marrero JA, Ahn J, Rajender Reddy K, et al. ACG clinical guideline: the diagnosis and management of focal liver lesions. Am J Gastroenterol 2014;109: 1328–47; quiz 48. PMID: 25135008.

In this guideline of the American College of Gastroenterology the authors provide an evidence-based approach to the diagnosis and management of a focal liver lesion; Clinicians should consider not only malignant liver lesions, but also benign solid and cystic liver lesions such as haemangioma, focal nodular hyperplasia, hepatocellular adenoma and hepatic cysts.

15. Thomeer MG, Broker M, Verheij J, et al. Hepatocellular adenoma: when and how to treat? Update of current evidence. Therap Adv Gastroenterol 2016;9:898–912. PMID: 27803743.

Review that discusses the decision-making processes and associated risk analyses for hepatocellular adenoma based on lesion size and subtype. Hepatocellular adenomas >5 cm present for 6 months after stopping oral contraceptives, lesions with a β-catenin mutation, or lesions in male patients, associated with steroid use, glycogen storage disease, or underlying viral hepatitis should be considered for an intervention.

16. Blanc JF, Frulio N, Chiche L, et al. Hepatocellular adenoma management: call for shared guidelines and multidisciplinary approach. Clin Res Hepatol Gastroenterol 2015;39:180–7. PMID: 25434466.

Describes the molecular subtypes of hepatocellular adenomas and their potential relevance for management. β-catenin-mutated hepatocellular adenomas are associated with a higher risk of malignancy, but also other mutations in the heterogenic group of hepatocellular adenomas are discussed.

17. Stoot JH, Coelen RJ, De Jong MC, et al. Malignant transformation of hepatocellular adenomas into hepatocellular carcinomas: a systematic review including more than 1600 adenoma cases. HPB (Oxford) 2010;12:509–22. PMID: 20887318.

A systematic review of hepatocellular adenomas focusing on malignant transformation. The authors conclude that malignant transformation of hepatocellular adenomas is rare (4.2%) and is mainly observed in lesions >5 cm.

26. Lantinga MA, Gevers TJ, Drenth JP. Evaluation of hepatic cystic lesions. World J Gastroenterol 2013;19:3543–54. PMID: 23801855.

This review article describes the literature and an algorithm to guide clinicians in characterising hepatic cystic lesions. The diagnosis of simple liver cysts is based on typical ultrasound characteristics, whereas serodiagnostic tests and microbubble contrast-enhanced ultrasound are invaluable in differentiating complicated cysts, echinococcosis and cystadenoma/cystadenocarcinoma when ultrasound, CT and MRI show ambiguous findings.

28. Wijnands TF, Gortjes AP, Gevers TJ, et al. Efficacy and safety of aspiration sclerotherapy of simple hepatic cysts: a systematic review. AJR Am J Roentgenol 2017;208:201–7. PMID: 27824501.

A systematic review, in which the efficacy and safety of aspiration sclerotherapy is studied. In the majority of studies a reduction in volume of the cyst and a decrease or disappearance of symptoms was found.

37. Arnaoutakis DJ, Kim Y, Pulitano C, et al. Management of biliary cystic tumors: a multi-institutional analysis of a rare liver tumor. Ann Surg 2015;261:361–7. PMID: 24509187.

Describes a retrospective study of 248 patients with a biliary cystic tumour. Among patients undergoing surgery for biliary cystic tumours, associated malignancy was found in 10% of patients and no preoperative findings reliably predicted underlying biliary cystadenocarcinoma.

41. Hoekstra LT, Bieze M, Erdogan D, et al. Management of giant liver hemangiomas: an update. Expert Rev Gastroenterol Hepatol 2013;7:263–8. PMID: 23445235.

A literature review on giant haemangiomata, defined as >5 cm. In patients with a giant liver haemangioma, observation is justified in the absence of symptoms, whereas surgical resection could be considered in selected patients with abdominal (mechanical) complaints or complications, or when diagnosis remains inconclusive.

49. Cai YL, Xiong XZ, Lu J, et al. Percutaneous needle aspiration versus catheter drainage in the management of liver abscess: a systematic review and meta-analysis. HPB (Oxford) 2015;17:195–201. PMID: 25209740.

A systematic review and meta-analysis on the treatment of liver abscesses. Percutaneous catheter drainage is more effective than percutaneous needle aspiration because it facilitates a higher success rate and reduces the time required to achieve clinical relief.

52. Stanley SL, Jr, Amoebiasis. Lancet 2003;361:1025–34. PMID: 12660071.

Describes epidemiology, diagnosis and treatment of amoebiasis. Amoebic liver abscesses grow inexorably and, at one time, were almost always fatal, but now even large abscesses can be cured by one dose of antibiotic.

54. Mihmanli M, Idiz UO, Kaya C, et al. Current status of diagnosis and treatment of hepatic echinococcosis. World J Hepatol 2016;8:1169–81. PMID: 27729953.

Reviews the diagnosis and treatment of E. granulosus and E. multilocularis infections. The available treatment options for E. granulosus infection include open surgery, percutaneous interventions and pharmacotherapy, whereas E. multilocularis is treated with aggressive surgery as the first-choice treatment, while pharmacotherapy is used as an adjunct to surgery.

5

Primary malignant tumours of the liver

Chetana Lim
Olivier Farges

With the exception of hepatocellular carcinoma (HCC), which is one of the most common malignancies, primary tumours of the liver are relatively rare in adults. HCC arises from hepatocytes and cirrhosis is its main aetiological factor. This tumour remains a subject of considerable interest due to its rising incidence and the development of innovative treatments. Intrahepatic cholangiocarcinoma (ICCA) arises from the peripheral intrahepatic biliary radicles, and other rare primary tumours arise from mesodermal cells and include angiosarcoma, epithelioid haemangioendothelioma and sarcoma.

Hepatocellular carcinoma

HCC accounts for 90% of all primary liver malignancy and its incidence continues to increase. It is the sixth most common neoplasm, accounting for more than 5% of all cancers, and is the second most common cause of cancer-related deaths worldwide. The International Agency for Research on Cancer has estimated in 2012 through its GLOBOCAN series that primary liver cancer caused more than 745 000 deaths worldwide (9.1% of the total).[1]

HCC usually occurs in male patients, and cirrhosis precedes its development in most cases. Due to better medical management of cirrhosis, survival of cirrhotic patients has steadily increased in the last two decades resulting in a greater risk of developing HCC. Cohort studies have reported that in patients with HCC, the death rate due to cancer is 50–60% while hepatic failure and gastrointestinal bleeding are responsible for approximately 30% and 10% of the deaths, respectively. HCC may now be identified at an early stage, particularly through the screening of high-risk patients.

Control of HCC nodules may be achieved successfully by surgical resection and by percutaneous treatment but their precise role will depend on the morphological features of the tumour and the functional status of the non-tumourous liver. Unfortunately tumour recurrence is common due to the persistence of the underlying cirrhosis, which represents a preneoplastic condition. Liver transplantation may seem a logical alternative treatment but has its own limitations, including tumour recurrence, limited availability of grafts and cost. The most exciting areas of progress are the control of hepatitis B virus (HBV) or hepatitis C virus (HCV), prevention of carcinogenesis in patients with chronic liver disease, early radiological screening and the development of medical therapies. In the setting of liver surgery, better liver function assessment and understanding of the segmental liver anatomy with more accurate imaging evaluation are the most important factors that have led to a decrease in postoperative mortality rates. Active follow-up and treatment of recurrence have also contributed to increase the 5-year survival to as much as 70%.[2]

Incidence of HCC

The world age-adjusted incidence of HCC in men is 14.9 per 100 000. Geographical variation related to the prevalence of hepatitis B (HBV) and hepatitis C virus infections are the two main risk factors worldwide, and account for more than three-quarters of all cases (Table 5.1). The incidence may be as high

Table 5.1 • Age and prevalence of HBV and HCV among patients with HCC in different geographical areas

Area	Age (years)	HBV (%)	HCV (%)	Combined (%)
Africa	47	47	18	65
USA	63	16	48	64
South America	55	43	21	64
Western Europe	65	18	44	62
Eastern Europe	60	51	15	66
South-Western Asia	52	42	27	69
Japan	65	15	75	91
China, Korea	52	70	18	88
World		53	25	78

as 99 per 100 000 in Mongolian men. Other high-rate areas include Eastern and South-Eastern Asia (>20 cases per 100 000). By contrast, Northern Europe and South Central Asia are areas with low incidences (<5 cases per 100 000); in these areas, HCV is the main risk factor, together with alcohol abuse, non-alcoholic fatty liver disease and obesity. Southern Europe and North America have intermediate rates.

The rising incidence of HCC was first documented in the USA, where this doubled between the late 1970s and early 1990s, reaching 3 cases per 100 000. The epidemic of HCV infection probably accounted for a large part of this increase. Alternative explanations include ageing of the population, increased detection, improved survival of cirrhotic patients and the epidemic of obesity and type II diabetes.

It has been estimated that HCV began to infect large numbers of young adults in North America and South and Central Europe in the 1960s and 1970s as a result of intravenous drug use. The virus moved into national blood supplies and circulated until a screening test was developed in 1990, after which time rates of new infection decreased dramatically. In Canada, Australia, Japan and various European countries, where HCV infection spread earlier than in the USA, a similar trend was observed, but in some countries the incidence of HCC is now decreasing.

Due to recent advances with the advent of the new direct-acting antivirals, current HCV infection cure rates may reach 90% and this major progress may be associated with several beneficial consequences.[3] Firstly, the incidence of HCV-related HCC will decrease as a result of the eradication of HCV infection and secondly, the evolution of HCV-infected patients progressing to cirrhosis and the need for transplantation will also decrease.[4]

Risk factors for HCC

The main risk factor for HCC is liver cirrhosis. Once present, male gender, age (as a marker of the duration of exposure to a given aetiological agent), stage of cirrhosis and diabetes are additional independent risk factors.

Cirrhosis vs no underlying liver disease

Up to 80–90% of HCC arise in patients with underlying liver disease. The risk of tumour development varies with the type of cirrhosis; the highest risk is reported for chronic viral hepatitis, whereas lower risks are associated with other forms of cirrhosis such as primary biliary cirrhosis.

HCC developing in the absence of cirrhosis is found in 10–20% of patients. The term 'absence of cirrhosis' appears more appropriate than 'normal liver' as these patients frequently have some degree of mild fibrosis, necro-inflammation, steatosis or liver cell dysplasia. HCC in the absence of cirrhosis may be related to some of the same aetiologies as those responsible for HCC in cirrhotic livers such as HBV infection or alcohol abuse. Alternatively, HCC may occur as a result of conditions that infrequently lead to cirrhosis such as α_1-antitrypsin deficiency, haemochromatosis, or in the setting of specific aetiologies that do not result in cirrhosis such as hormonal exposure or glycogenosis.

HBV infection

Chronic HBV infection is the most frequent risk factor for HCC worldwide, and accounts for more than 50% of all cases. It is estimated that 40 million people are currently affected by HBV, particularly in less industrialised countries; HBV infection should, however, begin to decline as a result of increased utilisation of HBV immunisation.

There is evidence that HBV-DNA sequences integrate into the genome of malignant hepatocytes and can be detected in the liver tissue of patients with HCC despite the absence of classical HBV serological markers. HBV-specific protein may also interact with liver genes. HBV is therefore a direct risk factor for HCC and can occur in patients without cirrhosis.

The risk of HBV-associated HCC increases with the severity of the underlying hepatitis, age at infection and duration of infection, as well as level of viral replication. An Asian patient with HBV-related cirrhosis has a 17% cumulative risk of developing HCC over a 5-year period. In the West, this cumulative risk is 10%. This may be explained by the earlier acquisition of HBV in Asia through vertical transmission (rather than horizontal transmission in the West, through sexual or parenteral routes), longer duration of disease, or additional exposure to environmental factors. Ongoing HBV replication or hepatitis Be antigen (HBeAg) infection accelerates the progression to cirrhosis and also to HCC. A study conducted in Taiwanese men reported that the risk of HCC increased 10-fold when HBsAg was present and 60-fold when HBeAg was present. Similarly, HBV-DNA levels greater than 10^4 or 10^6 copies/mL are associated with a 2.3 and 6.1 hazard risk respectively, compared to patients with lower levels of replication.[5] Additional cofactors that increase the risk of HCC are male gender (3–6 times higher risk), age >40 years, concurrent HCV infection (twofold increased risk), HDV co-infection (threefold), heavy alcohol consumption (two- to threefold) and, in endemic regions, aflatoxin ingestion.

HCV infection

The expansion of HCV infection probably accounts for a significant proportion of the increased incidence of HCC observed over the past 10 years. In Western countries, up to 70% of HCC patients have anti-HCV antibodies in their serum and the mean time for developing HCC following HCV infection is approximately 30 years.

In HCV-positive patients with initially compensated viral cirrhosis, HCC is both the most frequent and first complication. The annual incidence of HCC is 0–2% in patients with chronic hepatitis and 1–4% in those with compensated cirrhosis, although rates as high as 7% have been reported in Japan. In patients with cirrhosis, additional independent risk factors increasing the risk of HCC are age >55 years (two- to fourfold), male gender (two- to threefold), diabetes (twofold), alcohol intake greater than 60–80 g/day (two- to fourfold) and HBV co-infection (two- to sixfold). Obesity is also a likely cofactor. In contrast, the viral genotype or viral concentration has no impact on the risk of HCC.

The mechanism of HCV-related HCC is still not very clear. The great majority of patients with HCV-related HCC have cirrhosis, suggesting that it is the presence of cirrhosis that is crucial for the development of this tumour.

> ✅ Because anti-HCV vaccination is not available, prevention of HCV infection and of progression of chronic HCV infection to cirrhosis through antiviral treatment is the only means to reduce the incidence of HCV-related HCC. Sustained virological response in HCV-infected patients is associated with a significantly decreased risk of developing HCC.[6] New direct-acting antivirals have raised several promising perspectives that will likely decrease both the incidence of HCV-related HCC and the requirement for transplantation.

Human immunodeficiency virus (HIV) infection

The incidence of HCC is expected to rise in HIV-positive persons predominantly because of the higher prevalence of associated well-known risk factors: not only co-infection with HCV and HBV, but also alcohol abuse, non-alcoholic steatohepatitis (NASH) and diabetes. HIV-positive patients who are co-infected with HBV or HCV may have more rapidly progressive liver disease, and when they become cirrhotic they are also at increased risk of HCC. The Mortavic study indicated that HCC caused 25% of all liver-related deaths among HIV patients.[7]

Cirrhosis and HCC occur 15–20 years earlier in HIV-HCV co-infected patients than in patients infected by HCV alone. The course of the disease is also considered more aggressive.[8] Screening for HCC should, however, be the same as in HIV-negative patients.

Other viral infections

Infection with the hepatitis delta virus (HDV) is found in patients who are also infected with HBV. Hepatitis A virus (HAV) and hepatitis E virus (HEV) infection cause neither chronic hepatitis nor HCC.

Alcohol

Heavy (>50–70 g/day) and prolonged alcohol ingestion is a classical risk factor for cirrhosis and therefore HCC. Data available from cohort studies of European or US patients with alcohol-related cirrhosis suggest an annual incidence of HCC of 1.7% (as compared with 2.2% and 3.7% in patients from the same geographical area with HBV- or HCV-associated cirrhosis). Alcohol is also a very frequent additional risk factor in patients with HBV or HCV cirrhosis, as well as in those with chronic liver disease associated with the metabolic syndrome.

Non-alcoholic fatty liver disease (NAFLD)

NAFLD has been recognised as being one of the most common causes of liver disease in the USA (and other Western countries). Histological changes in the liver range from simple steatosis to more severe forms of NASH, including cirrhosis. It is closely associated with type II diabetes, central obesity and dyslipidaemia as part of the metabolic syndrome, the prevalence of which has increased as an epidemic. Sixty percent of patients older than 50 years with diabetes and obesity are likely to have NASH with advanced liver fibrosis.[9] Chronic medical conditions such as obesity and diabetes increase the risk of HCC.[10,11]

✔ Obesity and diabetes increase the risk of HCC.

An association between NAFLD and HCC was first identified in 2002 by several studies focusing on HCC patients with chronic liver disease in the absence of HBV/HCV infection or alcohol abuse. In this population, there was a much higher prevalence of obesity, diabetes, hypertriglyceridaemia and pathological features of NAFLD. At the same time, evidence was accumulating linking common features of the metabolic syndrome/NASH with HCC. In particular, obesity increases mortality from liver cancer, far more than for any other cancer. Similarly, diabetes was found to increase the risk of HCC with and without acute or chronic liver disease.

The incidence of HCC among patients with NAFLD increases with male gender, increasing age, sinusoidal iron deposition and severity of underlying liver disease. In surgical series, overt cirrhosis is present in only one-third of patients, while the others have less severe liver damage.[12] In addition, there is also evidence that NAFLD may act synergistically with other risk factors such as chronic HCV or alcoholic consumption to potentiate the development of HCC.

As obesity and the metabolic syndrome are growing epidemics worldwide, the incidence of HCC will undoubtedly increase in the future. Nearly 25% of patients with metabolic syndrome develop cirrhosis. After cirrhosis develops, 4–27% of patients develop HCC.[13] In surgical series, the prevalence of metabolic syndrome-related HCC is approximately 6–10%.[14,15] Compared to HCV, NASH-related HCC as an indication for liver transplantation increased nearly fourfold from 2002 to 2012.[16]

Hereditary haemochromatosis

Hereditary haemochromatosis (HH) is an autosomal recessive disorder associated with homozygosity for the *C282Y* mutation in the haemochromatosis gene and is characterised by excessive gastrointestinal absorption of iron. HH is a long-known risk factor for HCC, and the risk is increasing in patients with cirrhosis. Other risk factors include male gender and diabetes. Several additional risk factors such as HBV infection (4.9-fold), age greater than 55 years

(13.3-fold) and alcohol abuse (2.3-fold) may act synergistically with iron overload to increase the risk of HCC among patients with cirrhosis caused by HH. In a recent meta-analysis including nine studies of 1102 patients with HCC, mainly from European populations, it has been reported that C282Y mutation was associated with an increased risk of HCC (4-fold) in alcoholic liver cirrhosis patients, but not for the viral liver cirrhosis population.[17] Interestingly, pathological conditions other than HH that are associated with iron overload, such as homozygous β-thalassaemia or the so-called African overload syndrome, are also associated with an increased risk of HCC. Similarly, there is also evidence of a link between iron deposits within the liver and HCC in patients with and without cirrhosis.

Cirrhosis of other aetiologies

Primary biliary cirrhosis (PBC) has been considered as a low risk factor for HCC, not only because of its rare incidence but also because it predominantly affects women (with a sex ratio of 9:1). A recent meta-analysis of 12 studies reported that PBC is significantly associated with an increased risk of HCC (18.8-fold) compared to the general population.[18] However, there were several confounding factors in this meta-analysis, such as advanced histological stage of PBC, history of blood transfusion, smoking or drinking habit, which might be associated with increased probability for HCC development in PBC patients or directly associated with PBC development. In contrast, HCC development in patients with secondary biliary cirrhosis is exceptionally rare, if it even exists.

Autoimmune hepatitis has a low risk of HCC development. Potential reasons are the female predominance and the delayed development of cirrhosis through corticosteroid therapy. HCV infection needs to be ruled out as it may induce autoantibodies. Recent data reported that cirrhosis at presentation is an important prognostic risk factor for HCC. In a prospective multicentre cohort study evaluating 193 Japanese patients with autoimmune hepatitis, seven (3.6%) developed HCC during the 8-year period, all of whom had underlying cirrhosis.[19]

Aflatoxin

Aflatoxin B1 has also long been associated with the development of HCC, because areas with a large consumption of this toxin coincide with areas of high incidence of HCC (Asia and sub-Saharan Africa). Aflatoxin is ingested in food as a result of contamination of imperfectly stored staple crops by *Aspergillus flavus*. It is thought to induce HCC through mutation of the tumour suppressor gene *p53*. Although some studies suggest that it is an independent risk factor, others suggest that it could be a co-carcinogen only in patients with HBV infection. HCC in this setting frequently develops in a non-cirrhotic liver.

Metabolic liver diseases and HCC

An increased risk of HCC is recognised in some other forms of metabolic liver diseases such as α_1-antitrypsin deficiency, porphyria cutanea tarda, tyrosinaemia and hypercitrullinaemia. Patients with glycogenosis type IV, hereditary fructose intolerance and Wilson disease may also develop HCC, but with a lower risk. There is evidence that iron and copper overload in haemochromatosis and Wilson disease generate, respectively, oxygen/nitrogen species and unsaturated aldehydes that cause mutations in the *p53* tumour suppressor gene.

Adenoma, contraceptives and androgens

As with adenoma in other locations, hepatocellular adenomas (HCAs) have a risk of malignant transformation and hepatocyte dysplasia is the intermediate step between HCAs and HCC. A recent systematic review estimated the risk to be 4.2%.[20] This risk and the treatment strategy to prevent it may, however, be refined.

HCAs are most classical in women of child-bearing age and are associated with the prolonged use of oral contraceptives and oestrogen treatments. Discontinuation of oral contraceptives does not completely avoid the risk of transformation. Malignancy within HCAs <4cm in this context is exceptional. There is also recent evidence that HCAs may develop in men, frequently in a context of metabolic syndrome. The risk of malignant transformation in men is 50% (10 times higher than in women) and malignancy can occur in HCAs as small as 1cm.[21] Therefore, whereas resection of HCAs >4cm is warranted in women, all HCAs irrespective of size should be resected (or ablated) in men.[22]

The number of HCAs does not appear to increase the risk of malignant transformation and in particular, patients with adenomatosis are not at increased risk.[21,23,24]

Malignant transformation of HCAs has also been linked to the genotype and phenotype of HCAs. It is more prevalent in telangiectatic or atypical HCAs than in steatotic HCAs. Most importantly, the presence of a β-catenin mutation (observed in approximately 10–15% of HCAs) confers a particularly high risk of malignancy.[23]

Malignant transformation of HCAs may also occur within known specific aetiologic contexts, such as with type I glycogenosis, use of anabolic steroids or androgen treatments and Fanconi disease. Recreational anabolic steroid use is also known to potentially result in the development of adenoma, and malignant transformation to HCC has been reported.

Pathology of HCC and of nodular lesions in chronic liver disease

Preneoplastic lesions are morphologically characterised by the appearance of dysplastic lesions in the form of microscopic dysplastic foci and macroscopic dysplastic nodules (DNs).

Dysplastic foci are microscopic lesions composed of dysplastic hepatocytes <1 mm in size, and occur in chronic liver disease, particularly in cirrhosis. DNs are divided into low and high grade depending on the degree of cytological or architectural atypia. DNs are defined as a nodular region <2 cm in diameter with dysplasia but without definite histological criteria of malignancy. Low-grade DNs are approximately 1 cm in diameter, slightly yellowish and have a very low probability of becoming malignant. High-grade DNs are less common with slightly larger nodules (up to 2 cm) and characterised by increased cell density with an irregular thin-trabecular pattern and occasionally unpaired arteries. These are often difficult to differentiate from highly differentiated HCC. They may contain distinct foci of well-differentiated HCC and are therefore considered as precancerous lesions and become malignant in a third of cases. It must, however, be appreciated that lesions <2 cm may also represent HCC.

HCCs can be subdivided according to their gross morphology, degree of differentiation, vascularity, presence of a surrounding capsule and presence of vascular invasion. All of these criteria have practical implications.

On gross morphology, HCCs can be solitary or multinodular, consisting of either a collection of discrete lesions in different segments developing synchronously (multicentric HCC) or as one dominant mass and a number of 'daughter' nodules (intrahepatic metastases) located in the adjacent segments. Diffuse HCCs are relatively rare at presentation and consist of poorly defined, widely infiltrative masses that present particular diagnostic challenges on imaging. A third type is the infiltrating HCC, which typically is less differentiated with ill-defined margins.

Microscopically, HCCs exhibit variable degrees of differentiation that are usually stratified into four different histological grades, known as Edmondson grades 1–4, which correspond to well-differentiated, moderately differentiated, poorly differentiated and undifferentiated types. The degree of differentiation typically decreases as the tumour increases in diameter. Very well-differentiated HCC can resemble normal hepatocytes and the trabecular structure may reproduce a near normal lobar architecture so that histological diagnosis by biopsy or following resection may be difficult. A number of immunomarkers have been described to selectively identify the malignant nature of these HCCs, not only in resected specimens but also in liver biopsies: Glypican 3 (GPC3), Heat Shock Protein 70 (HSP70) and Glutamine Synthetase (GS). Positive staining for any two markers can detect early and well-differentiated HCC in 50–73% of cases, with 100% specificity when the analysis is performed on resected specimens.[25]

Our understanding of the molecular pathogenesis of HCC has significantly advanced with the identification of the major driver genes mutated in HCC over the last decade. TERT promoter mutations are the most frequent mutation (60%) observed in HCC development and progression.[26] The subsequent increase in telomerase expression is a determinant of malignant transformation. The use of these molecular markers, obtained from biopsy or resection specimens, may be useful to determine prognosis, select treatment and assess response to chemotherapy.

Vascularisation is a key parameter in differentiating HCC from regenerating nodules. Progression from macroregenerative nodule to low-grade DN, high-grade DN and frank HCC is characterised by loss of visualisation of portal tracts and development of new non-triadal arterial vessels which become the dominant blood supply in overt HCC lesions. This arterial neoangiogenesis is the landmark of HCC diagnosis and the rationale for chemoembolisation and anti-angiogenic treatment.

Tumour nodules may be surrounded by a distinct fibrous capsule. This capsule, present in 80% of resected HCCs, has a variable thickness, which may not be complete, and is frequently infiltrated by tumour cells. Capsular microscopic invasion by tumour cells is present in almost one-third of tumours <2 cm in diameter, as compared with two-thirds of those with a larger diameter.

HCC has a great tendency to spread locally and to invade blood vessels. The rate of portal invasion is higher in the expansive type, in poorly differentiated HCC and in large tumours. Characteristically, microscopic vascular invasion involves 20% of tumours <2 cm in diameter, 30–60% of cases in nodules 2–5 cm and up to 60–90% in nodules >5 cm in size. The presence of portal invasion is the most important predictive factor associated with recurrence. The tumour thrombus has its own arterial supply, mainly from the site of the original venous invasion. Once HCC invades the portal vein, tumour thrombi grow rapidly in both directions, and in particular towards the main portal vein. As a consequence, tumour fragments spread throughout the liver as the thrombus crosses segmental branches. Once the tumour thrombus

has extended into the main portal vein, there is a high risk of complete thrombosis and increased portal hypertension. This accounts for the frequent presentation with fatal rupture of oesophageal varices, or liver decompensation including ascites (**Fig. 5.1**), jaundice and encephalopathy. Invasion of hepatic veins is possible, although less frequent. The thrombus eventually extends into the suprahepatic vena cava or the right atrium and is associated with a high risk of lung metastases. Rarely, HCC may invade the biliary tract and give rise to jaundice or haemobilia. Mechanisms of HCC-induced biliary obstruction include:

- intraductal tumour extension;
- obstruction by a fragment of necrotic tumour debris;
- haemorrhage of the tumour resulting in haemobilia;
- metastatic lymph node compression of major bile ducts in the porta hepatis.

The rate of invasion of the portal vein, hepatic vein and bile duct at the time of diagnosis is 15%, 5% and 3%, respectively. However, it is estimated that during the natural history of HCC, approximately 1 in 3 patients will develop portal vein thrombosis.

When present, metastases are most frequently found in the lung. Other locations, in decreasing order of frequency, are: adrenal glands, bones, lymph nodes, meninges, pancreas, brain and kidney. Large tumour size, bilobar disease and poor differentiation are risk factors for metastatic disease.

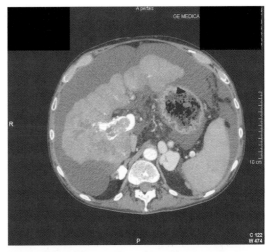

Figure 5.1 • CT scan of a patient with a tumour thrombus originating from an HCC located in the right liver. The thrombus extends in the main portal vein. Ascites is present.

Clinical presentation

HCC rarely occurs before the age of 40 years and reaches a peak at around 70 years of age. The age-adjusted incidence in women is two to four times less than in men and the difference is most pronounced in medium-risk south European populations and premenopausal women. Reasons for this higher rate in men include differences in exposure to risk factors, higher body mass index and higher levels of androgenic hormones.

There are basically three circumstances of diagnosis: (1) incidental finding during routine screening; (2) incidental finding during assessment of patients with deranged liver function tests or of another pathological condition; and (3) presence of liver- or cancer-related symptoms, the severity of which depends on the stage of the tumour and the functional status of the non-tumourous liver. In industrialised countries, a growing number of tumours are discovered incidentally at an asymptomatic stage. As tumours increase in size, they may cause abdominal pain, malaise, weight loss, asthenia, anorexia and fever. These symptoms may be acute as a result of tumour extension or complication.

Spontaneous rupture occurs in 5–15% of patients and is observed particularly in patients with superficial or protruding tumours. The diagnosis should be suspected in patients with known HCC or cirrhosis presenting with acute epigastric pain as well as in Asian or African men who develop an acute abdomen (**Fig. 5.2**). Minor rupture manifests as abdominal pain or haemorrhagic ascites, and hypovolaemic shock is present in only approximately half of patients. Portal vein invasion may manifest as upper gastrointestinal bleeding or acute ascites and invasion of hepatic veins or the inferior vena cava may result in pulmonary embolism or sudden death.

Clinical symptoms resulting from biliary invasion or haemobilia are present in 2% of patients. Possible paraneoplastic syndromes associated with HCC include polyglobulia, hypercalcaemia and hypoglycaemia. Finally, in patients with underlying liver disease, a sudden onset or worsening ascites or liver decompensation may be the first evidence of HCC formation.

Clinical examination may reveal only large or superficial tumours. There may be clinical signs of cirrhosis, in particular ascites, a collateral circulation, umbilical hernia, hepatomegaly and splenomegaly.

Liver function tests and tumour markers

Liver function tests

Liver function test impairment is non-specific and reflects the underlying liver pathology or the presence of a space-occupying lesion. Because most HCCs develop within a cirrhotic liver and since HCCs in normal livers are usually large, normal liver function tests are exceptional. Jaundice is most frequently the result of liver decompensation.

Serum tumour markers
Alpha-fetoprotein

Serum α-fetoprotein (AFP) is the most widely recognised serum marker of HCC. It is secreted during fetal life but the residual levels are very low in the adult (0–20 ng/mL). It may increase in HCC patients and serum levels greater than 400 ng/mL can be considered as diagnostic for HCC, with 95% confidence. Levels may exceed 10 000 ng/mL in 5–10% of patients with HCC. Very high levels usually correlate with poor differentiation, tumour aggressiveness and vascular invasion. However, an AFP >20 ng/mL has a sensitivity of 60% (i.e. a surveillance programme using this cut-off value would miss 40% of tumours). If a value of >200 ng/mL is used, 22% of tumours would be missed. Only 10% of small tumours are associated with raised levels whereas 30% of patients with chronic active hepatitis without an HCC have a moderately increased AFP. This usually correlates with the degree of histological activity and raised levels of transaminase, and it may therefore fluctuate. Tumours other than HCC can also be associated with increased AFP levels but these are rare (non-seminal germinal tumours, hepatoid gastric tumours, neuroendocrine tumours).

Others serum tumour markers

Alternative serum markers for HCC, such as des-γ-carboxy prothrombin (DCP) or prothrombin induced

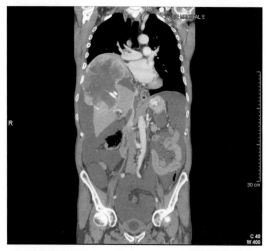

Figure 5.2 • CT of a patient with a ruptured HCC. Note that the rupture is limited at the upper part of the liver. This patient had haemorrhagic ascites.

by vitamin K absence [PIVKA-II (>40 mAU/mL)] and AFP-L3 (>15%) have not come into common practice except in Japan, where they are covered under a national health insurance. A prospective cohort study in at-risk patients comparing the accuracy of AFP and DCP in the early detection of HCC showed that the combination of both markers increased the sensitivity, from 61% and 74% for each marker alone, to 91% for both markers combined.[27]

Morphological studies

The aims of imaging in the context of HCC are to screen high-risk patients, differentiate HCC from other space-occupying lesions and select an appropriate treatment.

Differentiation of HCC from other tumours relies on its vascularisation. The most reliable imaging features of an HCC are the presence of hyperarterialisation of the nodule in the early (arterial) phase and washout during the portal or late phase following injection (the tumour becomes hypovascular compared to the adjacent parenchyma). By definition, the term 'washout' can only be applied to tumours that are hypervascular in the arterial phase (although this may be very transient).

Critical in choosing the most appropriate treatment are the number of lesions, their size and extent, and the presence of daughter nodules, vascular invasion, extrahepatic spread and underlying liver disease.

Assessment may be achieved by ultrasonography (US), contrast-enhanced US, computed tomography (CT), magnetic resonance imaging (MRI), angiography or a combination of these.

> ✅ Imaging aims to:
> * screen patients for the development of HCC and this is best achieved by US;
> * differentiate potential HCC from other tumours and this is best achieved by demonstrating the presence of hypervascularisation during the arterial phase and washout during the portal or late phase.

Ultrasound

Ultrasound (US) is the first-line investigation for screening because of its low cost, high availability and high sensitivity in identifying a focal liver mass. In experienced hands, US may identify 85–95% of lesions measuring 3–5 cm diameter and 60–80% of lesions measuring 1 cm. Differences in accuracy worldwide may be explained by steatosis rates and heterogeneity of the underlying liver disease. Typically, small HCCs are hypoechoic and homogeneous and cannot be differentiated from regenerating or dysplastic nodules. With increasing size, they may become hypo- or hyperechoic but most importantly heterogeneous. A hypoechoic peripheral rim corresponds to the capsule. The infiltrating type is usually very difficult to identify in a grossly heterogeneous cirrhotic liver. Besides echogenicity, the accuracy of US depends on the dimension and location of the tumour, as well as operator experience. A 1-cm diameter tumour can be visualised if it is deeply located, whereas the same lesion located on the surface of the liver can be missed. Similarly, tumours located in the upper liver segments or on the edge of the left lateral segment may be missed. Tumours detected at an advanced stage despite surveillance are frequently located at one of these two sites. Obesity may also prevent accurate assessment of the liver (thickened abdominal wall or steatotic liver). Doppler US may demonstrate a feeding artery and/or draining veins. US is also accurate in identifying vascular or biliary invasion and indirect evidence of cirrhosis such as segmental atrophy, splenomegaly, ascites or collateral veins. Tumour thrombosis is associated with enlargement of the vascular lumen, and an arterial signal may be detected by duplex Doppler.

Computed tomography

Computed tomography (CT) is more accurate than US in identifying HCCs and their lobar or segmental distribution, particularly with the development of helical and multislice spiral scanners. Spiral CT is undertaken without contrast and during arterial (25–50 s), portal (60–65 s) and equilibrium (130–180 s) phases after contrast administration. In addition, it is useful for identifying features of underlying cirrhosis, accurately measuring liver and tumour volumes, and assessing extrahepatic tumour spread. HCCs are usually hypodense and spontaneous hyperdensity is usually associated with iron overload or fatty infiltration, which is seen in 2–20% of patients. Specific features are early uptake of contrast and a mosaic shape pattern. During the portal phase, the density diminishes sharply and results in washout (tumour is hypodense compared to adjacent parenchyma) during the late phase (**Fig. 5.3**). HCCs may show variable vascularity depending on tumour grade and some are poorly vascularised. The capsule, when present, is best seen during the portal or late phase as an enhanced thickening at the periphery (delayed vascular enhancement is characteristic of fibrosis). Vascular invasion of segmental branches may also be identified. Intratumoural arterioportal fistula may occur and present as an early enhancement of portal branches or as a triangular area distal to the tumour with contrast enhancement different from the adjacent parenchyma. Nonetheless, such fistulas are seen frequently in cirrhotic patients without HCC as subcentimetre hypervascular subcapsular lesions.

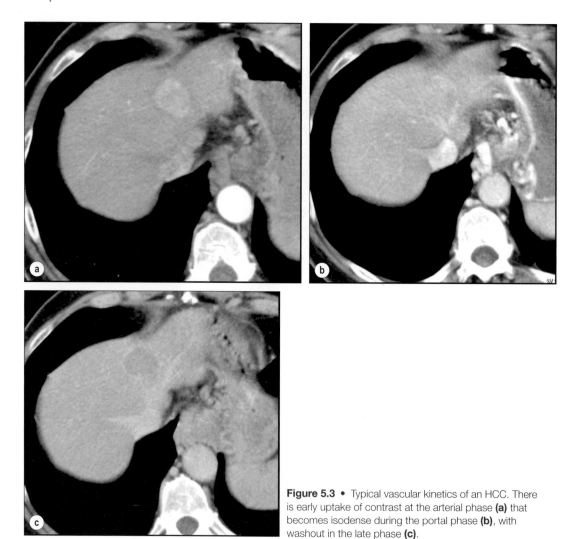

Figure 5.3 • Typical vascular kinetics of an HCC. There is early uptake of contrast at the arterial phase **(a)** that becomes isodense during the portal phase **(b)**, with washout in the late phase **(c)**.

Magnetic resonance imaging

Magnetic resonance imaging (MRI) tends to be more accurate than other imaging techniques in differentiating HCC from other liver tumours, especially those >2 cm. As for CT, the technique of MRI should be accurate with T1- and T2-weighted images and with early, intermediate and late phases following contrast injection of gadolinium. The characteristics of an HCC are the mosaic shape structure and the presence of a capsule. Tumours are hypointense on T1-weighted images and hyperintense on T2-weighted images, but these characteristics are present in only 54% of patients; 16% of HCCs demonstrate hypointensity on both T1 and T2 images. Hyperintensity on T1-weighted images is also possible, and associated with fatty, copper or glycogen infiltration of the tumour. The kinetics of vascular enhancement following injection of contrast is the same as during CT with early uptake and late washout. Recently, liver-specific magnetic resonance contrast medium such as Gd-EOB-DTPA that accumulates in Kupffer cells (due to phagocytosis) or in hepatic cells, has increased the accuracy of MRI, but has not yet come into common practice except in Eastern countries.

Contrast-enhanced ultrasound

Contrast-enhanced US (CEUS) is the most recent technique to assess vascularisation of tumours. A contrast agent (stabilised microbubbles) is administered intravenously via bolus injection followed by saline flush. Enhancement patterns are typically described during the arterial (10–20 s post injection), portal venous (30–80 s) and late (120–360 s) phase. Whereas US microbubbles are confined to the vascular spaces, contrast agents for CT and MRI are rapidly cleared from the blood into the extracellular space. The sensitivity of CEUS to detect arterial enhancement is greater than that of CT or MRI because of the continuous monitoring of the images. Washout is slower for well-differentiated than for poorly differentiated tumours. However, it is subject to the same limitations as other US modes: if the baseline scan is unsatisfactory, the CEUS study will also be unsatisfactory. The advent of the second-generation US contrast agent Sonazoid, approved exclusively in Japan in 2007, has made Sonazoid-CEUS more effective for screening and staging than CEUS using other vascular agents such as SonoVue. Sonazoid contrast agent is taken up by Kupffer cells in the postvascular phase or Kupffer phase (starting 10 min post injection) and provides extremely stable Kupffer images suitable for repeated scanning from 10 to about 120 minutes after injection (**Fig. 5.4**).[28]

Other imaging

Angiography

Although the diagnostic usefulness of angiography has been considerably reduced, it is still widely used as part of arterial chemoembolisation. Arteriography shows early vascular uptake (blush) and, if used, Lipiodol injection is retained selectively for a prolonged period by the tumour. On subsequent CT, the retained radiodense Lipiodol reveals the tumour as a high-density area. Uptake within the liver is not specific for HCC, since all hypervascular liver tumours, including focal nodular hyperplasia, adenoma, angioma and metastases, will retain Lipiodol. False-negative results may be observed with avascular, necrotic or fibrotic HCC.

Positron emission tomography

The contribution of FDG-positron emission tomography (PET) in the diagnosis of HCC remains limited because of low sensitivity (60%). FDG-PET can detect poorly differentiated but not well-differentiated HCC due to similarities between the metabolism of FDG in normal hepatocytes and hepatocellular cells. Recently, 18F-fluorocholine (FCH), a PET tracer of lipid metabolism, has been shown to be significantly more sensitive than 18F-FDG at detecting HCC, particularly in well-differentiated tumours.[29] Interestingly, in metastatic HCC, FDG-PET has a high sensitivity and is more suitable for the detection of bone metastases than CT or bone scintigraphy.[30]

Accuracy of imaging techniques

CT and MRI with contrast enhancement have the highest diagnostic accuracy (>80%) and the techniques can be combined. Nodules <1 cm need only a short-interval surveillance period, such as every 3 months for at least 2 years. Nodules >1 cm are suspicious. If CT and MRI show typical features of HCC, no further investigations are required. If the features are not typical, a percutaneous fine-needle biopsy should be performed.[31]

Requirement for and reliability of histological study

Pathological confirmation of HCC can be obtained by cytology, histology or a combination of these. The accuracy of pathological assessment is increased if a sample of non-tumourous tissue is available for comparison. Liver biopsy is limited by the potential for haemorrhage and pain, and may occasionally be responsible for neoplastic seeding and vascular spread. The reported incidence of needle tract seeding is 1–5%. Tumour involvement is generally limited to subcutaneous tissues, has a slow progression and it is possible to perform local excision without apparent impact on survival. Even if the false-positive rate is low, the risk of needle tract seeding is balanced by the risk of pursuing an aggressive treatment such as resection or transplantation in a patient without malignancy. Every attempt should be made not to puncture the nodule directly but to access the nodule through a thick area of normal liver. As described below, several studies have shown that expert pathological diagnosis of HCC can be reinforced by staining for GPC3, HSP70 and GS, particularly in biopsies of small lesions that are not clearly HCC.

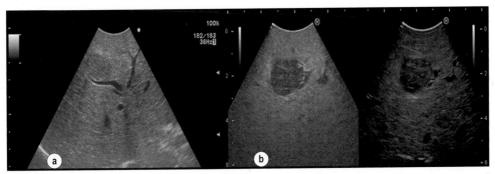

Figure 5.4 • Sonazoid CEUS of a patient with HCC located in segment 8. Image of the lesion in fundamental mode **(a)**. Kupffer image of the lesion **(b)**.

> ✅ There is a significant false-negative rate for fine-needle biopsy especially in small lesions, lesions that are difficult to access or those developing in a multinodular parenchyma. A negative result should therefore never rule out malignancy.

Diagnosis of HCC

The standard for the diagnosis of HCC is histology. This is particularly true for tumours <3 cm or when active treatment is required. Non-invasive diagnosis (using radiological imaging alone) requires rigorous technique and interpretation.

The first attempt to standardise the diagnostic criteria was considered in 2000 by the European Association for the Study of the Liver (EASL). Several studies reported that AFP determination lacked adequate sensitivity and specificity for effective surveillance and diagnosis.[27] The strategy advocated in the updated version of the diagnostic criteria in 2011[32] was based on imaging techniques and/or biopsy as follows.

- For nodules <1 cm found on US, it was considered that other imaging techniques would be unlikely to reliably confirm the diagnosis. Since the accuracy of liver biopsy for such small lesions and the likelihood of HCC is low, it was felt reasonable to repeat an US at 3–6 monthly intervals until the lesion disappeared, enlarged, or displayed characteristics of HCC. However, early HCC may take more than a year to reach this size. If there has been no growth over a period of up to 2 years, routine surveillance can be resumed.
- For nodules >1 cm found on US screening of a cirrhotic liver, diagnosis of HCC can be established by one contrast-enhanced imaging technique (multidetector CT or dynamic contrast-enhanced MRI). The specific imaging pattern of HCC is defined by intense contrast uptake during the arterial phase followed by contrast washout during the venous or delayed phases. The value of these non-invasive criteria for HCC in cirrhosis has been confirmed prospectively.[33-35] These typical imaging features have specificities and predictive positive values of approximately 100% and sensitivity of 71%.
- If the findings are not characteristic or the vascular features are not typical, and in other clinical settings (e.g. absence of cirrhosis), a diagnostic biopsy was recommended, although it was acknowledged that a negative biopsy did not exclude the diagnosis.

Subsequent to these recommendations, several studies reported that contrast-enhanced US may provide a false-positive HCC diagnosis and cannot selectively differentiate intrahepatic cholangiocarcinoma from HCC. This technique has therefore been withdrawn from the diagnostic algorithm initially proposed by the American Association for the Study of Liver Diseases (AASLD).

> ✅ Current guidelines for the positive diagnosis of HCC are:
> - For nodules >1 cm with cirrhosis, early uptake and delayed washout on a single dynamic imaging study (triphasic CT or MRI with gadolinium) is considered characteristic of HCC.
> - For nodules >1 cm without cirrhosis or if the vascular feature is not typical, a diagnostic biopsy should be recommended.
> - Biopsy of small lesions should be evaluated by expert pathologists. Tissue that is not clearly HCC should be stained with CD34, CK7, GPC3, HSP-70 and GS to improve diagnostic accuracy.
> - If the biopsy is negative for HCC, the lesion should be followed by imaging at 3–6-monthly intervals, for any interval change. If the lesion enlarges but remains atypical for HCC, a repeat biopsy is recommended.

Natural history of HCC and staging systems

Traditionally, the natural history of HCC is considered to be particularly grim, with a median survival of 6 months in symptomatic patients. However, the 3-year survival of asymptomatic untreated patients who are not end-stage at the time of presentation may be as high as 50%. These observations have important implications for HCC diagnosed at an early stage, particularly in patients with preserved liver function.

The aim of staging systems is to predict outcome. This can either be used to anticipate prognosis or, more recently, for selection of treatment. Survival of patients with HCC is mainly influenced by the morphological spread of tumour, the presence and severity of cancer-related symptoms, and the severity and evolution of the underlying cirrhosis. The most recent systems attempt to integrate all three groups of parameters.

- Although staging was determined initially by the TNM classification, the pathological staging of HCC has evolved in Eastern (Liver Cancer Study Group of Japan) and Western (American Joint Committee on Cancer, International Union Against Cancer) countries. These take into account the

Table 5.2 • Comparison of the tumour (T) staging in the Liver Cancer Study Group of Japan (LCSGJ) and American Joint Committee on Cancer (AJCC) staging systems

LCSGJ	
T1	Tumour <2 cm, unique *and* without vascular invasion
T2	Tumour <2 cm, multiple *or* with vascular invasion
	Tumour >2 cm single *and* without vascular invasion
T3	Tumour <2 cm, multiple *and* with vascular invasion
	Tumour >2 cm, multiple *or* with vascular invasion
T4	Tumour >2 cm, multiple *and* with vascular invasion
AJCC	
T1	Single tumour without vascular invasion
T2	Single tumour with vascular invasion or multiple tumours, none >5 cm
T3A	Multiple tumours, any >5 cm
T3B	Single tumour or multiple tumours of any size involving a major branch of the portal or hepatic vein
T4	Tumour(s) with direct invasion of adjacent organs other than gallbladder or with visceral peritoneum

AJCC/UICC and LCSGJ TNM classification of HCC.

number of tumours, vascular invasion and tumour size (Table 5.2). A limitation is that they are based on pathological findings and can only be applied accurately (retrospectively) in operated patients.

- Cancer-related symptoms have a detrimental impact on outcome that is assessed by the WHO performance status or the Karnofsky index. The presence of pain is a poor indicator of outcome.

- Liver damage induced by underlying liver disease has traditionally been assessed by the Child–Pugh score. This was, however, designed to assess the functional reserve of cirrhotic patients undergoing portocaval shunt surgery and is not entirely appropriate for HCC patients in whom therapeutic options may include liver transplantation and liver resection.

Several groups have attempted to combine these features within integrated staging systems. There are currently six such systems, designated as the CLIP (from Italy), GRETCH (from France), BCLC (from Spain), CUPI (from China), JSS and JIS (from Japan) scores. It is beyond the scope of this chapter to detail all of them (Table 5.3). It should be appreciated that these scores have been computed retrospectively by multivariate analysis of a specific patient population and not all have been externally validated.

Currently, the BCLC system is widely accepted, as it includes variables linked to tumour stage and function, physical status and cancer-related symptoms, and it combines each stage (very early stage: 0; early stage: A; intermediate stage: B; advanced stage: C; and end-stage: D) with a treatment algorithm. It has been externally validated and has been recently supported by both AASLD and EASL. However, validation in Eastern countries has not been achieved to date. One area of concern is regarding the definition of intermediate and advanced HCC; most Asian experts agree that early stage means that HCC can be controlled by curative treatment, but advanced stage (which includes portal vein invasion and distant metastasis) is hard to define in the BCLC system as it can be divided into two other

Table 5.3 • Main variables retained in prognostic models

	GRETCH		CLIP		CUPI	
Tumour morphology			Multinodular extension <50%	1	TNM I and II	−3
			Multinodular extension >50%	2	TNM III	−1
					TNM IV	0
Tumour biology	Portal thrombosis	1	Portal thrombosis	1		
	AFP >35 ng/mL	2	AFP >400 ng/mL	1	AFP >500 ng/mL	3
Liver function	Bilirubin >50 μmol/L	3	Child–Pugh A	0	Bilirubin <34 μmol/mL	0
	ALP >2N*	2	Child–Pugh B	1	Bilirubin 34–51 μmol/mL	3
			Child–Pugh C	2	Bilirubin >51 μmol/mL	4
					ALP >200 IU/L	3
General status	Karnofsky index <80	3			Asymptomatic	−4
Score range		0–11		0–6		−7 to 12

The numbers refer to the score given to each variable. A total score is obtained by adding each individual score. In the CLIP score, the median survivals according to the score in the initial[30] and prospective validations[32] were: score 0: 36–42 months; score 1: 22–32 months; score 2: 8–16 months; score 3: 4–7 months; score 4 or above: 1–3 months.
*2N = twice normal. AFP, α-fetoprotein; ALP, alkaline phosphatase.

different groups: locally advanced with portal vein invasion and advanced with extrahepatic metastasis. At present, most Asian countries have their own HCC staging system with different constituent variables.

> ✓ The BCLC system currently endorsed by the US and European clinical practice remains largely applied worldwide.

Screening for HCC

Screening is used routinely in countries where effective therapeutic interventions are available. HCC fulfils most of the criteria required for a surveillance or screening programme to be justified. HCC is common in highly endemic areas (and its incidence is growing in others) and it is associated with a high mortality. Furthermore, the survival is extremely poor by the time patients present with symptoms related to the tumour, and the population at risk is clearly defined (in particular – but not exclusively – patients with HCV- and HBV-related cirrhosis, especially when they are male and over 60 years of age). Acceptable screening tests with low morbidity and high efficacy exist that allow the tumour to be recognised in the latent/early stage. Finally, effective treatments exist in selected patients.

The two most common tests used for screening of HCC are US and serum AFP measurements, although many clinicians consider the latter investigation to be of little value for screening. However, an increase of AFP in patients who have a normal AFP at baseline should prompt a CT or MRI if US is negative. It should be underlined that US is difficult in obese patients with fatty liver disease and cirrhosis, but no alternative strategy for surveillance has been adequately tested.

No clear evidence is available to determine the optimal interval for periodic screening. Tumour doubling times vary widely with an average of 200 days. It has been estimated that the time taken for an undetectable lesion to grow to 2 cm is about 4–12 months, and that it takes 5 months for the most rapidly growing HCC to reach 3 cm. Because treatments are most effective for tumours <3 cm, screening programmes are usually performed at 6-monthly intervals. The efficacy of screening to improve the prognosis of HCC has mainly been demonstrated in China on HBV carriers.[36] These results require to be validated in other geographical areas. Until then, most rely on a 6-month interval (3–4 months in Japan) in high-risk patients. It has been reported that surveillance is cost-effective if the expected HCC risk exceeds 1.5% per year in patients with HCV and 0.2% per year in patients with HBV.[37]

There are limitations to screening programmes. Of patients presenting with HCC, 20–50% have previously undiagnosed cirrhosis and therefore escape surveillance. Access to medical care and compliance is a limitation in highly endemic areas, with 50% of patients with alcoholic cirrhosis defaulting from surveillance over 5 years. US is highly operator-dependent, and the cost and invasiveness of CT and MRI make them unsuitable for screening. However, these latter modalities are particularly suited in patients with irregular background liver parenchyma or obesity. Physicians should also take into account the presence of comorbid disease, severity of liver disease and available treatment options when deciding whether or not to screen a cirrhotic patient. Screening of Child–Pugh C patients in particular is inappropriate if they are not potential liver transplant candidates.

> ✓ Surveillance of at-risk patients is being used increasingly at 6-monthly intervals with US to detect HCC at an early stage.

> ✓ High-risk groups consist of those with established cirrhosis due to HBV, HCV and haemochromatosis. Male patients with alcohol-related cirrhosis abstaining from alcohol or likely to comply with treatment and those with chronic liver disease due to NASH should also be considered. Ultrasound is recommended as a screening tool whereas CT and MRI are most useful in confirming the diagnosis.

Treatment options

There is a wide range of treatment options for HCC (liver transplantation, liver resection, ablation, chemoembolisation, systemic treatments) and the decision should therefore be taken in a multidisciplinary team meeting involving a liver surgeon, interventional radiologist, oncologist and hepatologist, using predefined guidelines.

Liver transplantation, liver resection and ablation are traditionally defined as curative treatments. However, when underlying liver disease is present (typically cirrhosis), only transplantation is curative by simultaneously treating the aetiology of HCC. Recurrence is virtually constant with all other treatments.

In patients without cirrhosis, liver resection is the ideal treatment but this group accounts for only a small proportion of patients with HCC. In cirrhotic patients, management is more challenging and should take into account tumour extension, status of the non-tumoural liver and general condition of the patient.

Patients with HCC identified by surveillance usually present with smaller tumours and are more likely to benefit from a curative treatment. A recent population-based study raised a concern about the access to curative treatment in real-life practice. Despite full insurance coverage for all populations and standardised recommendations for HCC surveillance and management, only 22.8% of patients had curative treatment. Moreover, there were marked variations between areas in access to curative treatment.[38]

HCC in normal liver

The treatment of choice in patients with no or minimal coexisting fibrosis is partial liver resection. The non-tumourous liver has a high regenerating capacity allowing even major hepatectomies to be performed. Perioperative mortality and morbidity rates are less than 1% and 15%, respectively. Five-year survival is greater than 50%.[39] These results may, however, vary according to the population studied. Patients with a metabolic syndrome in particular, in whom most HCC are not associated with cirrhosis, are at increased risk of postoperative mortality. Lymphadenectomy is recommended as the prevalence of lymph node metastases is approximately 15%, compared to less than 5% in cirrhotic patients. Adjuvant chemotherapy is not recommended. Regular follow-up with throracoabdominal CT at 6-monthly intervals is recommended as early detection and treatment of recurrence may improve survival.

There is very little place for other invasive treatments. Percutaneous ablation, as a rule, has no role due to the usually large tumour size at diagnosis. Liver transplantation is associated with a perioperative mortality of 10%, a need for long-term immunosuppression, and long-term results are not significantly different from those of resection. In a recent multicentre study based on a collaboration of 38 European transplant centres, only 105 patients transplanted for an HCC occurring in a normal liver were identified.[40] Transplantation had been performed as the primary treatment because partial liver resection was precluded by anatomical factors or the need to preserve a sufficient volume of liver remnant, or as rescue treatment for intrahepatic tumour recurrence not amenable to repeat resection. The 5-year survival rate was 59% in patients without macrovascular or lymph node invasion, irrespective of tumour size and differentiation.

Liver resection of HCC in cirrhotic patients

Liver resection

Main limitations

Resection of HCC has four limitations in cirrhotic patients: (i) the tumour is multifocal in 20–60% of patients at the time of diagnosis and liver resection can normally only be considered in patients with unifocal tumours; (ii) cirrhosis is an important risk factor for the development of postoperative complications; (iii) oncological resections dictate wide margins whereas the diseased underlying liver usually requires parenchymal sparing; (iv) risk of recurrence is high because cirrhosis persists.

Risk of surgery and patient selection

The risk of hepatectomy is increased in cirrhotic patients due to coagulation defects, portal hypertension, liver failure and impaired regeneration. In-hospital death was 10% of patients in the 1990s (even higher in some subgroups) but has decreased since then as a result of improved patient selection, operative technique and perioperative management. Although some very large series report no mortality, the average mortality rates in national surveys or registries are 4–6% and are therefore higher than in non-cirrhotic patients or after resection of other malignancies.

Hepatectomy, as a rule, should only be performed in Child–Pugh A cirrhotic patients without clinically significant portal hypertension (defined by hepatic venous pressure gradient >10 mmHg or the presence of oesophageal varices or splenomegaly (>12 cm) and thrombocytopenia <100 000/mm^3). Child–Pugh B or C patients are at a prohibitive risk of early liver failure even after a minor hepatectomy or mere laparotomy. Child–Pugh A patients may, however, still be at increased risk of postoperative liver failure, in particular after major resections, due to impaired ability to regenerate. This correlates with the fibrosis grade, although it is only in patients with extensive fibrosis or cirrhosis that this impairment has clinical impact. Typically, following a major liver resection, there is an increase in prothrombin time (peak on postoperative day 1) and an increase in serum bilirubin (peak on postoperative day 3–5) that tend to normalise within 5–7 days. Recovery of both tests is in contrast delayed or absent in cirrhotic patients. When the prothrombin time is less than 50% of normal and serum bilirubin >50 μmol/L on postoperative day 5, the risk of postoperative mortality is close to 50%.

Additional selection criteria have therefore been proposed to select, among Child–Pugh A patients, those in whom surgery could be considered. In Japan, the indocyanine green (ICG) test is usually used. After injection of 0.5 mg ICG/kg bodyweight, retention of ICG is measured in peripheral blood, in particular 15 min after the injection (ICG-R15). Normal values of ICG-R15 are 10%. In cirrhotic patients, minor resections can be performed when it is 22% or less, but major resections only if it is less than 14–17%. In contrast, in Europe and the USA selection mainly relies on the absence of significant portal hypertension or cytolysis. This requires that patients have no evidence of oesophageal varices, splenomegaly, portosystemic shunts (including a patent umbilical vein) or ascites (even on imaging studies), and that they have a platelet count greater than 100×10^9/L. The BCLC group advocates that invasive measurement of the hepatic vein–portal vein pressure gradient should be <10 mmHg. Several studies have shown that a normal serum bilirubin and the absence of clinically significant portal hypertension are the best predictors of good outcomes after resection.[41,42] The MELD score and thrombocytopenia, irrespective of Child–Pugh grade and tumour features, have been shown to be associated not only with postoperative mortality and morbidity, but also with long-term survival.[43,44]

✔ In cirrhotic patients who have a single resectable lesion, hepatectomy should only be performed if they have well-preserved liver function, with a normal bilirubin and hepatic venous pressure gradient <10 mmHg (the so-called BCLC stage A).

There has been considerable interest in recent years in the optimal management of the remnant liver. This includes: (i) more selective use of inflow occlusion; (ii) avoiding excessive mobilisation of the liver; and (iii) measuring the future remnant liver volume (RLV) using CT reconstruction. In patients with chronic liver disease, a remnant liver volume of approximately 40% of the total liver volume is required before a major hepatectomy is performed. When this is not the case, preoperative portal vein embolisation (PVE) is indicated as a means of increasing the remnant liver volume and perhaps more importantly, preoperatively testing the ability of the liver to regenerate. When right hepatectomy is contemplated (the most frequent circumstance when there is a risk of small RLV), the right portal vein is percutaneously injected, under ultrasonographic guidance, with glue or ethanol. This should induce atrophy of the right liver within 2–6 weeks and compensatory hypertrophy of the left RLV. Due to its efficacy, PVE (alone or in association with TACE) has become almost routine before a right hepatectomy in cirrhotic patients.[45] The absence of hypertrophy of the left liver following a successful right PVE means that the liver is unable to regenerate and that hepatectomy is contraindicated. There is also increasing evidence that parenchymal size alone does not necessarily reflect function and there is therefore interest in the functional evaluation of the remnant liver volume.

✔ When major hepatectomy is contemplated, preoperative portal vein embolisation (PVE) of the lobe to be resected should be undertaken to test the ability of the future liver remnant to regenerate.

Technique

There is increasing evidence that both anatomical resections (as opposed to tumourectomies) and wide (as opposed to limited) margins may improve long-term survival without increasing the perioperative risk. The rationale is tumour spread through microvascular invasion, the incidence and extent of which is related to tumour diameter and poor differentiation. Several retrospective studies have reported an approximately 20% improvement in overall and disease-free survival following anatomical compared to limited resections.[46] The impact of the margin width has been evaluated in a prospective controlled trial.[47] A 2-cm margin was associated with a 75% 5-year survival as compared to 49% for 1-cm margins. Both concepts are not exclusive and should be taken into account, especially in tumours with a diameter between 2 and 5 cm.

✔ The concept of anatomical resections is to remove both the tumour and the adjacent segments that have the same portal tributaries. The aim should be to obtain margins >1–2 cm to ensure potential satellite nodules are also resected.

There is increasing interest in laparoscopic resection for HCC.[48] Although not formally proven yet, it may have the advantage of less intraoperative bleeding, fewer postoperative complications, reduced postoperative analgesic requirement and a shorter hospitalisation time. More specifically in the context of cirrhotic patients, it may also reduce the risk of postoperative ascites and its consequences as well as facilitate subsequent liver transplantation if required, because of fewer adhesions.[49]

Outcome after resection

The recent largest series using a US National Cancer Database has reported 5- and 10-year survival rates of 43.9% and 28.7% in 12 757 patients treated by resection between 1998 and 2011.[50] Independent predictors of survival were age, degree of liver damage, AFP level, tumour diameter, number of nodules, vascular invasion and surgical margins. Survival rates as high as 68% at 5 years have been reported in Child-Pugh A patients with well-encapsulated tumours of 2 cm diameter or less. These figures continue to improve, even when patients with larger tumours are included. Active treatment of recurrences has been a major reason for this improvement.

Treatment of recurrence

Tumour recurrence is the major cause of death following resection of HCC in the cirrhotic patient. Its incidence is 40% within the first year, 60% at 3 years and approximately 80% at 5 years. However, this is not unexpected as the precursor condition (cirrhosis) persists after surgery. It is frequently difficult to differentiate true recurrence from de novo tumours. The former tend to occur within the first 2 years and their main risk factors are vascular invasion, poor histological differentiation, presence of satellites and number of nodules. De novo recurrent tumours occur later and the main risk factors are the same as those of a primary HCC. Molecular analysis suggests that their respective proportions are 60–70% and 30–40%. Recurrence within the liver is multifocal in 50% of patients and is associated with distant metastasis in 15%, especially in the lungs, adrenal gland or bones. Extrahepatic recurrence without simultaneous intrahepatic recurrence is infrequent in patients with cirrhotic livers.

Evidence that neoadjuvant or adjuvant treatments reduce the risk of recurrence is currently lacking and these treatments are therefore not recommended. This applies to preoperative chemoembolisation, neoadjuvant or adjuvant chemotherapy, internal radiation with ^{131}I-labelled Lipiodol, adoptive immunotherapy, retinoic acid or interferon, although some of these strategies initially showed promising results. An update follow-up of the only randomised trial of adjuvant ^{131}I-labelled Lipiodol has shown that the improved overall and disease-free survivals in the treatment group persisted until the seventh postoperative year.[51] This study was characterised by a very high proportion of HBV-related HCC (88%). Three recent meta-analyses of published studies[52–54] favour the use of interferon to reduce the risk of HCC recurrence; however, the quality of the studies was low due to heterogeneity of the patient populations, interferon used, duration of the treatment regimen, and whether results were independent of the effect of viral suppression. No study has confirmed the potential efficacy of retinoic acid. Anti-angiogenic treatments are currently being evaluated.

The most effective strategy to prevent HCC recurrence is liver transplantation in selected patients (see below). However, there are two other important strategies. The first is management of the underlying chronic liver disease as this improves prognosis and it is possible that it also reduces tumour recurrence. The second is to actively screen operated patients and actively treat recurrences if they are confined to the liver, by repeat surgery or liver transplantation. There continues to be debate about whether repeat hepatectomy or secondary transplantation in patients with recurrent HCC is associated with a survival benefit.

✔ At present, the best way to improve survival is to monitor resected patients regularly as some may benefit from curative treatment of the recurrence if it is confined to the liver.

Liver transplantation (LT)

Rationale

HCC is the only tumour for which transplantation plays a significant role, and this is the most attractive therapeutic option because it removes both detectable and undetectable tumour nodules together with all the preneoplastic lesions that are present in the cirrhotic liver. In addition, it simultaneously treats the underlying cirrhosis and prevents the development of postoperative or distant complications associated with portal hypertension and liver failure.

Patient selection

LT is not readily available in most high endemic areas of HCC. Even when transplantation is available, there is a donor shortage; LT can therefore only be performed in a fraction (less than 5% in most Western countries) of HCC patients. HCC patients are considered potential candidates for LT if their anticipated survival is approximately the same as those patients transplanted for other indications. This may be achieved if strict selection criteria are applied; otherwise, HCC patients are at high risk of death from tumour recurrence. These include an HCC: (i) confined to the liver (i.e. no extrahepatic disease, including lymph nodes), (ii) without vascular extension and (iii) limited tumour burden.

Tumour burden was initially defined as a single tumour <5 cm or the presence of two or three tumours <3 cm (the so-called Milan criteria).[55] With the adoption of these criteria, the 5-year survival after LT ranges between 60% and 75%. There have subsequently been concerns that these criteria were too restrictive, which led to the proposal of expanded criteria. The most well-known and validated of these are the UCSF criteria – a single tumour <6.5 cm in diameter, or three or fewer tumours, the largest of which is <4.5 cm with the sum of the tumour diameters being <8 cm.[56] Others take into account poor tumour differentiation, or a high (or rapidly increasing) AFP serum concentration. An international consensus conference held in 2012 recommended a limited expansion of the listing criteria beyond the standard Milan criteria.[57] Predicting tumour biology through molecular profiling rather than tumour morphology is the aim of current research in this field.

Treatment on the waiting list

The average time from listing to transplantation in Europe and the USA is usually greater than 12 months. Up to 25% of patients may be excluded from the waiting list due to disease progression. Three approaches have been developed to avoid these drop-outs:

- Living-donor liver transplantation (LDLT) is an alternative source of grafts but has its own drawbacks, including the inherent risk for the donor, the risk of small-for-size grafts and the fact that only 25–30% of transplant candidates have a potential donor. It has the advantage of being performed rapidly, so avoiding drop-out on the waiting lists. The number of LDLT in Western countries has however decreased recently and the trend is to favour cadaveric transplantation through changes in allocation policies.

- New rules of graft allocation have been implemented, initially in the USA and subsequently in Europe. In the USA, the Model of End-stage Liver Disease (MELD) organ allocation policy implemented in 2002 has given priority to candidates with HCC within the Milan criteria. Waiting times have shortened, obviating the need for LDLT. Similar policies have been applied in other countries, such as France and the UK.

- Treatment of the tumour by resection, ablation or chemoembolisation is widely used while the patient is on the waiting list to avoid tumour progression beyond the oncological criteria. There is some evidence that these treatments may reduce drop-out rates on the waiting lists, but it is not clear if the outcome is the same for patients within or beyond the Milan criteria. The impact of these treatments on downstaging and post-transplantation survival is similarly uncertain. A specific advantage of resection over ablation or chemoembolisation is that it provides pathological details of the tumours. However, it is still unclear if the presence of poor prognostic factors should encourage or discourage transplantation.

✔ Liver transplantation is the key treatment option for patients with HCC who fulfil the Milan criteria.
- Reducing drop-out rates on the waiting list is dependent on changes in graft allocation policies and on treatment of the HCC while the patient is on the waiting list.
- Living donor liver transplantation can be proposed for HCC if the waiting list is expected to be so long that there is a high risk of drop-out because of tumour progression.

Transarterial chemoembolisation (TACE)
Technique
HCC, in contrast to the liver parenchyma, receives almost 100% of its blood supply from the artery. When the feeding artery is obstructed, the tumour experiences an ischaemic insult that results in extensive necrosis. With the development of more supraselective embolisation, greater attention is paid to accessory arteries that may contribute to tumour vascularity, such as the diaphragmatic or mammary arteries, that should also be embolised to achieve adequate control. Injection of iodised oil has been combined to improve the efficacy of embolisation. Iodised oil (Lipiodol), which is hyperdense on CT, is cleared from the normal hepatic parenchyma but retained in malignant tumours for periods ranging from several weeks to over a year. This accumulation, which is not associated with significant adverse effects, may be used for targeting cytotoxic drugs and increasing their concentration in the tumour cells. Recently, drug-eluting beads (DC-Beads) loaded with doxorubicin have been developed. This technique is much more expensive than conventional TACE but preliminary results show superior treatment response and delayed tumour progression.[58] Combination of TACE and anti-angiogenic treatments is under evaluation.[59]

Contraindications
TACE should not be performed in patients with liver decompensation, biliary obstruction, bilioenteric anastomosis and impaired kidney function. Portal vein thrombosis is also a contraindication unless it is limited to a section of the liver only and TACE can be performed in a highly selective manner on a limited tumour volume.

Morbidity and mortality
Mortality is less than 1% if these contraindications are applied. Overall, more than 75% of patients develop a post-embolisation syndrome characterised by fever, abdominal pain, nausea and raised serum transaminase levels. These symptoms, which are not prevented by antibiotics or anti-inflammatory drugs, are self-limiting and last for less than 1 week. More severe complications occur in less than 5% of patients and include, in decreasing order of frequency: cholecystitis or gallbladder infarction, gastric or duodenal wall necrosis, and acute pancreatitis. These, along with the post-embolisation syndrome, have become less frequent with the use of supraselective embolisation. Hepatic abscess formation is rare, occurring in 0.3%, but is associated with high mortality. The main risk factors are a previous history of bilioenteric anastomosis, large tumours and portal thrombosis.

Monitoring
The efficacy of TACE is assessed by CT (usually at 1 month) as the disappearance of the arterial vascular supply to the tumour and a decrease in its diameter. These features do not necessarily evolve in parallel. A decrease in tumour size may, for example, be associated with persistent vascularisation (i.e. residual tumour), whereas compact Lipiodol uptake without residual vascularisation may indicate complete tumour necrosis despite no significant decrease in size (**Fig. 5.5**).

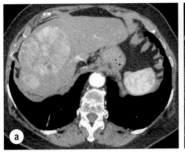
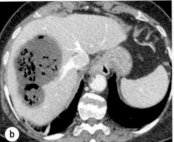
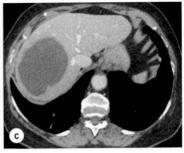

Figure 5.5 • HCC treated with microbeads chemoembolisation. **(a)** Pre-treatment; **(b)** 2 weeks after chemoembolisation: note the presence of necrosis. **(c)** 2 years after chemoembolisation: the image of the tumour remains, but it is avascular, indicating complete local control.

Efficacy

There is grade A evidence that TACE improves survival.[60] One of the largest studies is a prospective Japanese nationwide survey reporting median and 1-, 3-, 5- and 7-year survivals of 34 months, 82%, 47%, 26% and 16%, respectively, with a TACE-related mortality of 0.5%. Independent predictors of survival were, by decreasing order of influence: the degree of liver damage, portal vein invasion, maximum tumour size and number of lesions, and AFP levels. Two recent randomised controlled studies from Asia have reported data that are strongly supportive of surgical resection over TACE[61] or sequential TACE and radiofrequency ablation[62] in patients with multiple tumours.

> ✔✔ • TACE is one of the two non-curative treatment options (with sorafenib [Nexavar®]) that can improve survival.
> • TACE should be recommended as first-line palliative treatment for non-surgical patients with compensated Child–Pugh A and with large or multifocal HCC, without portal vein thrombosis or extrahepatic metastasis (so-called BCLC stage B).

Percutaneous local ablative therapy

Technique

Locoregional therapies are percutaneous treatment modalities that allow the injection of a damaging agent or the application of an energy source directly into the tumour. Damaging agents include chemicals such as ethanol or acetic acid. Energy sources either aim at increasing temperature by radiofrequency, microwave or interstitial laser photocoagulation or, alternatively, at decreasing temperature (cryoablation). Irreversible electroporation is a new non-thermal ablation therapy that uses a high-voltage direct electrical current to create nanopores in the cellular membrane that results in cell death via apoptosis. Radiofrequency ablation (RFA) has emerged as the most effective of these techniques. It exploits the conversion of electromagnetic

energy into heat via a needle electrode (15–18G), positioned in the tumour while the patient is made into an electric circuit by grounding pads applied to their thighs. The radiofrequency emitted from the tip causes ionic agitation and frictional heat, which leads to cell death from coagulation necrosis. The objective is to maintain a temperature of 55–100°C throughout the entire target volume for a sufficient period of time. Monitoring the impedance is important because excessive heating results in tissue charring, increased tissue impedance and decreased energy absorption.

> ✔✔ RFA is the first-line ablation technique. All randomised controlled trials comparing percutaneous ethanol injection (PEI) and RFA have suggested that the actuarial probability of local recurrence was significantly lower with RFA compared to PEI, and that RFA required fewer treatment sessions to achieve comparable anti-tumoural effects.[63,64]

Advantages and drawbacks

These ablative methods are minimally invasive, preserve the uninvolved liver parenchyma, have no systemic side-effects, and avoid the mortality and morbidity of major hepatic surgery. On the other hand, only tumours <5 cm are likely to be treated successfully and the smaller the diameter, the greater the probability of complete local control. The presence of multiple tumours (more than three) is also a limitation because of the need for repeated punctures. In addition, multiple tumours are either the result of multifocal carcinogenesis or vascular extension, and therefore a focal treatment is unlikely to be very effective. A key requirement is also the need to clearly visualise the tumour by US and access it safely. Hence, isoechoic HCC or tumours located in the upper part of segments 4, 7 and 8 or at the edge of the left lateral section if it extends behind the spleen may occasionally be unsuitable for treatment. Finally, whichever technique is used, the needle should not enter the tumour directly but pass through the hepatic parenchyma so as to prevent intraperitoneal bleeding or seeding of tumour cells. This may prove impossible for some superficial or protruding tumours. An experienced group reported that up to one-third of patients who were theoretically good candidates for ablation could not be treated due to non-visibility of the HCC on US, risk of thermal injury or absence of a safe path.[65]

Contraindications and limitations

Contraindications to ablation procedures include gross ascites, which favours intraperitoneal bleeding, coagulopathy that cannot be corrected, previous history of bilioenteric anastomosis or endoscopic sphincterotomy associated with bile bacterial contamination and therefore a risk of abscess formation. Additional contraindications (more specific to ablative techniques than ethanol injection) are the proximity of the tumour to the colon, duodenum, stomach or biliary confluence which may be injured or perforated by the heating process. RFA, unlike microwave ablation (MWA), is as a rule contraindicated in patients with a pacemaker. The efficacy of RFA also seems to be more impacted by the proximity of a vascular pedicle (the so-called cooling effect) than MWA. Whereas PEI is a short and very cheap procedure performed under light sedation, RFA is more costly, prolonged (20–90 minutes) and painful, and therefore generally performed under general anaesthesia. MWA is also performed under general anaesthesia but the procedure is quicker.

Mortality following ablation is less than 1% and morbidity less than 10% The most frequent complications are pleural effusion and segmental intrahepatic dilatation, which have no or limited impact. Severe complications include abscess formation, perforation of adjacent organs and intraperitoneal bleeding. Tumour seeding occurs in less than 5% of patients. Risk factors include subcapsular location and poor histological differentiation of the tumour. Coagulating the needle tract while removing the needle may reduce this risk.

Methods and margins

Ablation should not only target the tumour but also aim to achieve a safety margin so as to control satellite nodules. The incidence of these satellite nodules, as well as their distance from the main tumour increases as the main tumour enlarges and with poorly differentiated tumours. This safety margin should be 5 mm at least; hence, for an HCC measuring 3 cm in diameter, the diameter of the ablation should be 4 cm. This is best achieved with thermal rather than chemical ablation.

Methods to further improve tumour and margin control include multipolar ablation (several probes are placed around the tumour) and combining ablation with TACE.[66] Treatment response is assessed by CT or MRI at least 1 month after the procedure. RFA may result in a rim of fibrotic tissue (hypervascular on late phase MRI or CT) at the periphery of the tumour and should not be mistaken for residual tumour tissue. Follow-up thereafter relies on imaging studies at 3-monthly intervals to ensure that there is no recurrence of contrast enhancement.

Indication

Percutaneous ablative therapies have initially been performed in patients who were unsuitable for resectional surgery as recommended by EASL and AASLD. It has thereafter been used as neoadjuvant treatment in liver transplant candidates and for treatment of recurrence after liver resection.

As the results of ablation improve, due to improved technology and patient selection, it may also be considered as an alternative to surgery or even as a first-line treatment in selected situations. A large multicentre phase II trial reported a 97% sustained complete response rate and 68% actuarial 5-year survival following ablation in patients with HCC <2 cm.[67] The results of two RCTs comparing ablation and resection in patients with early HCC demonstrated no difference.[68,69]

> ✅ RFA is now considered by some centres as the first-line treatment for single nodules <2 cm in diameter.

However, meta-analyses still favour surgery compared to ablation in terms of 3-year survival and local control.[70,71] One additional concern is that both in the USA[72] and in Italy[73] there has been a recent temporal trend of increased use of ablation as a treatment for HCC with a simultaneous decrease in survival following this treatment, unlike what has been observed for other treatments. These observations suggest that the extension of indications for ablation should be strictly evaluated.

Other palliative treatments

Conventional systemic chemotherapy

Systemic chemotherapy has had very limited value in the past as only a very small number of patients obtained partial response or meaningful palliation using conventional drugs. Therefore, there is no rationale for using chemotherapy in patients with unresectable HCC outside of clinical trials.

Anti-angiogenic targeted therapies

✓✓ • One trial using molecularly targeted agents has, for the first time, demonstrated an improved overall survival in this disease and set a new standard as a first-line treatment of advanced HCC. These new agents target angiogenesis and epidermal growth factor (EGF) receptor pathways.
• Sorafenib (Nexavar®) is therefore recommended as first-line palliative option in patients not eligible for resection, liver transplantation, percutaneous ablation or TACE, if they still have preserved liver function.

Sorafenib exerts an anti-angiogenic effect by targeting the tyrosine kinases vascular endothelial growth factor (VEGF) receptors 2 and 3, and the platelet-derived growth factor receptor β. In an initial phase III trial, the median overall survival of Child–Pugh A cirrhotic patients with histologically proven and advanced HCC was 10.7 months in the treated group versus 7.9 months in the placebo double-blinded controlled arm of the study ($P = 0.00058$) and the median times to tumour progression were 24 weeks and 12 weeks, respectively ($P = 0.000007$).[74] This efficacy in advanced HCC (unresectable or metastatic) has been confirmed in an Asian randomised placebo-controlled trial that included mostly patients with HBV-related HCC[75] and in a large phase IV study with more than 3000 patients.[76] Side-effects included diarrhoea (39%), hand–foot syndrome (21%), anorexia (14%) and alopecia (14%). The anti-tumour effect, the pharmacokinetic profile and safety profile were similar in Child–Pugh A and B. These results have established sorafenib as the standard of treatment for advanced HCC in patients with Child–Pugh A (or B). Several trials assessing strategies including combination or sequential treatments are underway.

Other agents with comparable action pathways have been evaluated in phase II trials and include bevacizumab and sunitinib. Anti-EGF receptor agents, such as elotinib (Tarceva®) and cetuximab, also show promising results. Contraindications to these treatments include coronary artery disease, cardiac failure, systemic hypertension and Child B or C cirrhosis.

Radioembolisation

External beam radiation therapy has been of limited value in treating HCC because the normal liver parenchyma is very radiosensitive. Greater interest has therefore been placed on injecting radioisotopes such as ^{131}iodine-iodised oil or ^{90}Yttrium (^{90}Y)-labelled microspheres directly into the hepatic artery (radioembolisation), which offers the advantage of increased delivery within the tumour and decreased toxicity. The former agent has an efficacy comparable to that of chemoembolisation in patients with HCC

not complicated by portal thrombosis but is superior in patients with tumour portal extension. The use of ^{90}Y microspheres is recent and has been shown in a phase II trial to be safe and effective, in particular in patients with portal vein thrombosis.[77] One advantage of ^{90}Y-radioembolisation over TACE is that it may be indicated in patients with portal vein thrombosis, while TACE has been usually considered as a contraindication. These results have been reproduced in several studies, but without randomised controlled trials comparing ^{90}Y-labelled microspheres, TACE or other established treatments. To date, none of the retrospective studies have demonstrated an impact of radioembolisation on survival.[78]

Other treatments

Antiandrogenic, antioestrogenic and somatostatin analogues, once proposed, are currently considered ineffective.[25]

✓ New treatments such as radioembolisation and anti-angiogenics are promising, particularly in patients with vascular tumour invasion. The additional efficacy of radioembolisation over TACE, or of anti-angiogenics over no-treatment, requires strict assessment in the context of limited financial resources.

Defining a treatment strategy

Uncomplicated HCC associated with chronic liver disease

Treatment algorithms need to take account of availability of treatments.

• Liver transplantation, when available, is considered first and attention is therefore paid to the extent of liver disease, patient age and presence or absence of associated conditions. If a long waiting time (>6 months) is expected, resection, ablation or TACE are considered prior to liver transplantation.
• If transplantation is not available or not indicated, resection should be considered. Limiting factors are the number of nodules (ideally there should be only one) and the severity of underlying liver disease (patients should be Child–Pugh A and have neither cytolysis, portal hypertension nor impaired ICG tests). If a right hepatectomy is considered it should be preceded by PVE (with or without TACE).
• If resection is not considered due to the severity of the underlying liver disease and the nodule is single (or if there are fewer than three nodules),

ablation is the treatment of choice provided the tumour is <5 cm. For single tumours <2 cm, RFA is becoming a first-line treatment, as an alternative to resection.

- If neither resection nor RFA is considered, TACE is performed provided there is no ascites or liver failure (and in particular that serum bilirubin is <50 μmol/L) and that the tumour burden is not too extensive (no vascular invasion or extrahepatic metastases).
- Remaining patients are currently considered for anti-angiogenic treatments provided there is neither liver failure nor vascular disease.

According to this algorithm, it may be considered that the proportion of HCC patients who are candidates for transplantation is less than 5%, for resection 10–15%, for ablation 15–20% and for TACE 30–40%.

Treatment of complicated HCC

- *HCC with macroscopic portal vein invasion* is a contraindication for liver transplantation and ablative treatments. Traditionally TACE was also contraindicated (because of the risk of liver necrosis); it is today occasionally performed provided the thrombus is limited to a section of the liver and that embolisation is highly selective, with reduced doses and partial (rather than total) arterial occlusion as the endpoint. If thrombus does not extend into the main portal vein, surgical resection can be considered. Radioembolisation and anti-angiogenic therapy is otherwise indicated.
- *HCC with macroscopic invasion of hepatic veins* seems to carry an even worse prognosis as the tumour thrombus will extend into the inferior vena cava. When the thrombus is confined to the hepatic vein, resection if possible can be proposed. There is, however, a very high risk of pulmonary metastases developing within 6–12 months of surgery. Extension into the inferior vena cava or the right atrium is usually beyond any treatment.
- *Ruptured HCC* should be actively treated unless it occurs as a terminal presentation in patients with multiple tumours, portal thrombosis and end-stage liver failure. The primary aim of treatment is to stop bleeding, ideally by arterial embolisation. Subsequent hepatectomy can be associated with long-term survival. Indeed, (i) bleeding is not necessarily due to tumour

rupture, but occasionally due to rupture of an artery at the junction of the tumour and the adjacent parenchyma and (ii) even if the tumour has ruptured, this is not always associated with peritoneal seeding of tumour cells.

Fibrolamellar carcinoma (FLC)

FLC is a rare variant of HCC, defined as well-differentiated polygonal hepatic tumour cells with an eosinophilic granular cytoplasm surrounded by a fibrous lamellar stroma. It is most frequently observed in the Western hemisphere, where it accounts for approximately 1% of all HCCs. These tumours occur at a younger age than HCC (20–35 years), preferentially in women, and classically do not arise on a background of chronic liver disease.

- FLC are usually large at the time of diagnosis (8–10 cm), and the common revealing symptoms are a palpable mass, abdominal pain, weight loss, malaise and anorexia.
- Prognosis is better than that of HCC overall. Five-year survival following resection is 50–75%.[79]
- Resection is preferred to transplantation as the latter has very little or no place.

On imaging, FLC presents as a large solitary hypervascular heterogeneous liver mass with a central hypodense region due to central necrosis or fibrosis. On MRI, the central scar has low attenuation on T2 images, whereas the central scar of focal nodular hyperplasia has high attenuation. They have well-defined margins and calcification is present in 68%. Histology demonstrates deeply eosinophilic, polygonal neoplastic cells surrounded by a dense, layered fibrous stroma.

AFP levels are raised in less than 10% of patients.[79] Lymph node invasion within the hepatic pedicle is frequent (60%) and if resection is considered, simultaneous lymphadenectomy is recommended. There is a significant risk of recurrence, not only within the liver but also as lymph node or distant metastases. Close long-term follow-up is mandatory since recurrence and death beyond 5 years are common. Repeat surgery is a reasonable option in this younger patient population due to the relatively indolent course of the disease and the relative inefficacy of non-surgical treatments.

True FLC should be differentiated from mixed FLC–HCC, defined as conventional HCC displaying some distinct area with FLC features.[80] LT may be an alternative option in selected cases and survival rates of 48% can be obtained in patients transplanted for FLC–HCC.[81]

Intrahepatic cholangiocarcinoma (ICCA)

ICCA, also known as peripheral cholangiocarcinoma, is the second most frequent primary tumour of the liver after HCC. It arises from the peripheral intrahepatic biliary radicles, which differentiates them from hilar (Klatskin) tumours and common bile duct cholangiocarcinoma.

Until the very end of the 1980s there lacked immunohistological markers that could pinpoint the biliary origin of adenocarcinoma and ICCA were therefore probably frequently considered as being the liver metastasis of an adenocarcinoma of unknown origin. The diagnosis is currently ascertained through immunostaining.

This tumour has a poor prognosis overall and resection, sometimes at any cost, was the only therapeutic option. However, the recent implementation of a specific staging system and evidence that chemotherapy is effective pave the way for improved management.

Incidence

In the Western world, the incidence of ICCA is 0.3–3 per 100 000 per million, 10 times less than HCC. Recent reports suggest the incidence is increasing, particularly in the USA, UK, France, Italy, Japan and Australia. Although this increase may be real, it is probably mainly explained by improved identification of this tumour and changing rules on how they should be coded according to the International Classification of Diseases for Oncology (ICD).[82]

Risk factors

The traditional risk factors for cholangiocarcinoma include chronic biliary inflammation such as primary sclerosing cholangitis, chronic choledocholithiasis, hepatolithiasis, parasitic biliary infestation, Caroli's disease and choledochal cyst. However, in most patients with ICCA (more than 95%) none of these risk factors can be identified. The exception occurs in some areas of Asia and in particular north-eastern Thailand where the parasite *Opisthorcis viverrini* is particularly prevalent.

New risk factors are emerging, including chronic non-alcoholic liver disease, HBV infection, HCV infection, diabetes and the metabolic syndrome.[83] However, in contrast to HCC, most ICCAs develop without a background of liver disease. In surgical series, 75% of patients have normal livers, 16% have chronic hepatitis/liver fibrosis and 9% have cirrhosis.

Classification and staging

The Liver Cancer Study Group of Japan proposed a gross classification of ICCA into three types on macroscopic finding: mass-forming, which is by far the commonest type (75% in Asian series and probably more in the West); periductal-infiltrating, which spreads along the bile ducts; and intraductal-growth type with intraluminal spread. However, tumours may have mixed components, in particular a combination of mass-forming and periductal-infiltrating.

Whereas previously ICCA were staged using a similar system as HCC, the AJCC implemented a specific classification for ICCA in 2010.[84] The T staging takes into account the number of tumours and vascular invasion (the presence of either defines T2), rather than tumour size. The reason for this is that it is very unusual to diagnose ICCA early and size does not independently impact survival in published surgical series. T3 tumours are those perforating the visceral peritoneum or involving local extrahepatic structures by direct invasion, although this is fairly rare. The T staging also aims to take into account the periductal-infiltrating pattern of ICCA and, when present, defines T4. However, this infiltrating pattern may be difficult to identify on imaging studies or even on pathological specimens and there is no standardised definition yet. Lymph node involvement has a major impact on survival and when present, defines TNM stage III. Prevalence of lymph node extension is high and therefore lymphadenectomy should be routinely performed to achieve accurate staging. Median survival of patients with stage I is greater than 5 years (but these patients are very rare), whereas that of patients with stage II is 53 months and that of patients with stage III is 16 months.[85]

Pathology and progression analysis

Two distinct conditions that precede invasive cholangiocarcinoma have been identified. The first is a flat or micropapillary growth of atypical biliary epithelium, which has been called biliary dysplasia or biliary intraepithelial neoplasia. The second is an intraductal papillary neoplasm of the bile duct characterised by the prominent papillary growth of atypical biliary epithelium with distinct fibrovascular cores and frequent mucin overproduction. These preneoplastic conditions have mainly been analysed in hepatolithiasis and are observed more frequently in large bile ducts as hilar tumours than in small septal–interlobular bile ducts such as with ICCA. The dysplasia–carcinoma sequence therefore appears more obvious for hilar lesions than peripheral lesions. This suggests that an alternative source of ICCA could be the canals of Hering or hepatic progenitor cells, which are a target cell population for carcinogenesis in chronic liver disease.

Clinical presentation and laboratory tests

As a rule, ICCA tend to be diagnosed at an advanced stage because the tumour remains clinically silent for a long time. Symptoms, when present, include abdominal pain, malaise, night sweats, asthenia, nausea and weight loss. When they appear, the tumour is frequently unresectable.

ICCA typically occur with equal frequency in men or women between the age of 55 and 75 years. Liver function tests are non-specific even though an increase in liver enzymes (in particular GGT) may be the only initial finding in some patients. Although ICCA by definition excludes tumours arising from the biliary confluence or first-order branches, jaundice may be present if the tumour compresses or invades the biliary confluence.

Serum markers lack sensitivity and specificity. Carcinoembryonic antigen (CEA) exceeds 20 ng/mL in 15% and carbohydrate antigen (CA) 19–9 is >300 U/mL in 40% of cases. AFP exceeds 200 ng/mL in only 6% of patients.

Imaging studies

The main characteristic of mass-forming ICCA is that it is a fibrous tumour and therefore displays no enhancement on the arterial phase and delayed enhancement during the late phase. This may be seen both on CT and MRI. On MRI, lesions are hypointense on T1-weighted images and moderately to markedly hyperintense on T2-weighted images (**Fig. 5.6**). They are typically large, non-encapsulated, heterogeneous, associated with narrowing of adjacent portal veins and retraction of the liver capsule. As the tumour grows, satellite nodules frequently develop in the vicinity of the tumour, and subsequently in the contralateral lobe (**Fig. 5.7**). When superficial, these satellite nodules may not be visible on imaging. There

is a high propensity for lymph node invasion (present in 40% of resected patients if lymphadenectomy is performed routinely), but imaging studies have a sensitivity of only 50% and a specificity of 75% to predict this.

Diagnosis

The main differential diagnoses of ICCA are other fibrous tumours and in particular metastases from colorectal cancer. Both tumours may easily be confused on imaging studies. The diagnosis relies on a biopsy that shows an adenocarcinoma of biliary phenotype (CK7+ CK20–). Colorectal metastases are in contrast CK7–CK20+.

Treatment

Surgical resection is the only curative treatment. Unlike HCC, there is currently no place for liver transplantation.

As the tumour is usually diagnosed at an advanced stage, has ill-defined borders and occasionally extends to major portal branches or hepatic veins, surgery is frequently extensive. A major hepatectomy is required in 75–80%, with extension to segment 1 in 30% of cases and including the common bile duct in 20% of cases to achieve a complete resection. This surgery is therefore associated with significant postoperative mortality. This is estimated to be 6%, higher than following surgery for colorectal metastases and almost comparable to that of surgery for HCC despite the usual absence of chronic liver disease.

There is a significant risk (20–30%) that, despite adequate preoperative imaging, contraindications to a curative resection are identified at laparotomy. Staging laparoscopy has been advocated, but is also associated with high false-negative rates and, as a consequence, patients should be warned

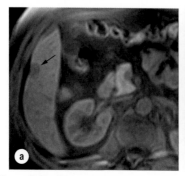 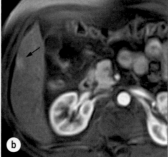 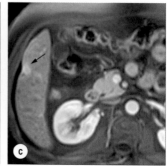

Figure 5.6 • Vascular kinetics of a small cholangiocarcinoma on MRI (*arrowed*). Note that the lesion is spontaneously hypointense **(a)**, that the uptake of vascular contrast is more pronounced in the late phase **(c)** than in the arterial phase **(b)** and that there is a retraction of the capsule.

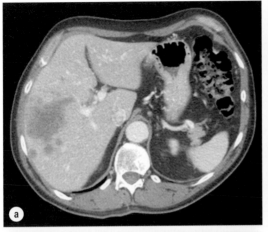

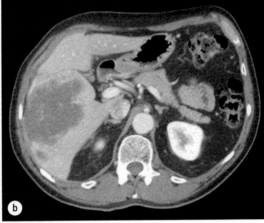

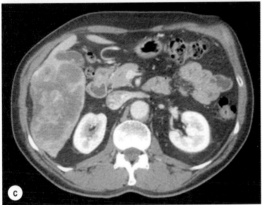

Figure 5.7 • CT of a patient with an intrahepatic/peripheral cholangiocarcinoma. Note the presence of typical satellite nodules at the periphery of the tumour **(a)**, the absence of vascular uptake **(b)** and the retraction of the capsule **(c)**.

preoperatively about this possibility. Furthermore, approximately 25% of resected patients will have an R1 or R2 resection. Survival following an R2 resection is usually comparable to, and occasionally worse than that of non-resected patients. Median survival following an R1 resection is typically 12 months and 3-year survival is nil.

According to the series published over the past decade, the 1-, 3- and 5-year survival rates following resection of ICCA are 67%, 38% and 27%, respectively. There are few data on survival beyond 5 years. Variables that influence postoperative survival most are the presence of lymph node invasion and an R1 resection.[86] Intraductal-growth-type ICCAs are rare but have a better long-term prognosis. Infiltrating-type ICCAs have a worse prognosis than the mass-forming type due to spread along Glisson's capsule and high incidence of lymph node involvement.

There is little evidence that these figures have improved over the past 10 years. However, recent studies have suggested that systemic chemotherapy may be effective in unresectable patients, which opens the possibility of combining surgery with either adjuvant and/or neoadjuvant chemotherapy.[87] One recent multicentre study reported that well-selected cirrhotic patients with

'very early ICCAs' (single tumours ≤20 mm) may become good candidates for liver transplantation with acceptable survival outcomes.[88]

> ✓ Surgical resection remains the only curative treatment for ICCA.
> Improvement in outcome will be dependent on multimodal treatment, including surgery and chemotherapy.

Epithelioid haemangioendothelioma (EHE)

EHEs are neoplasms of vascular origin that arise predominantly from soft tissues, bones and visceral organs, in particular the lung and the liver. Hepatic EHE develops from the endothelial cells lining the sinusoids and progresses along the sinusoids and vascular pedicles. It is extremely rare (no more than 200 cases have been reported) with an incidence of less than 1 per million population. It does not arise on a background of liver disease and there is no identified causative factor. Mean age at presentation is 42 years with a female to male ratio of 3:2.[89] Half present with right upper quadrant pain, a quarter incidentally and the remainder with severe symptoms such as ascites, jaundice, weakness and weight loss. Liver failure as a result of massive infiltration has been described.

These tumours are usually discovered at an advanced stage; almost 90% are multifocal and then usually involve both lobes. Approximately one-third of patients have extrahepatic spread to regional lymph nodes, peritoneum, lung and spleen.

Although the diagnosis is obvious when appropriate immunohistochemical staining is performed on tumour samples, it is frequently misdiagnosed on other investigations. Laboratory parameters are non-specific and tumour markers are normal. On imaging studies, the lesions are frequently confused with cholangiocarcinoma, metastatic carcinoma, sclerosing angioma or inflammatory pseudotumours. They are usually hypoechoic or heterogeneous on US, hypodense on CT with peripheral and/or central marginal enhancement on the arterial phase becoming isodense during the later phase and may display a halo or target pattern of enhancement. On MRI, they are hypointense on T1-weighted images, and heterogeneously hyperintense on T2-weighted images with similar contrast enhancement as that seen on CT. Multiplicity of lesions (especially if coalescent), their subcapsular location with liver capsule retraction and the presence of calcification (10–30%) or central necrotic and haemorrhagic areas should raise the suspicion of the diagnosis, especially in young patients. Histology shows a tumour composed of epithelioid and dendritic cells in variable proportions with a propensity for invasion of hepatic and portal veins, an overall ill-defined growth pattern and infiltrative margins. These features are difficult to identify or differentiate from other tumours on a percutaneous biopsy sample but immunostaining for factor VIII-related antigens is highly specific, demonstrating endothelial differentiation. Most tumours also stain positive for CD34 and CD31 endothelial markers. Epithelial markers including cytokeratins are negative.

The natural history of this tumour is highly variable. Although exceptional, prolonged survival of more than 10 years has been reported without treatment, and both partial and complete spontaneous tumour regression has even been described. On the other hand, some patients die within 2 weeks of diagnosis and 20% are dead within 1 year. Overall, only 20–40% survive more than 5 years. Because of the rarity of this tumour and its highly variable course, there is no widely accepted therapeutic strategy.

Partial hepatectomy is rarely feasible due to the invariable multifocal involvement of the liver. Palliative resection is not advocated as some have raised concerns that liver regeneration could promote a flare-up of residual tumours. Reports of favourable outcome with an estimated 5-year survival of 75% probably represent a highly selected subgroup.

The place of liver transplantation has recently been clarified by a multi-institutional analysis.[90] In 59 patients reported to the European Liver Transplant Registry, impressive 5- and 10-year survival rates of 83% and 74%, respectively, were reported. Invasion of lymph nodes and presence of restricted extrahepatic involvement had limited impact on survival and should therefore not be considered as contraindications to transplantation.[91] The current shortage of liver grafts and the prolonged waiting time may dictate that liver transplantation is indicated only in highly selected patients. Experience with locoregional or systemic chemotherapy is small and of limited value, especially as first-line therapy. Neoadjuvant combination therapies using anti-VEGF antibodies, however, deserve investigation.

Angiosarcoma

Angiosarcomas of the liver are rare tumours with a dismal prognosis. A recent European survey estimated its incidence as being 0.1 per million/year, being less than 1% of primary liver tumours. The 1-, 3- and 5-year survival rates were 20%, 8% and 5%, respectively. Despite its rarity, it has received attention because of its frequent association with environmental carcinogens. There is clear association with prior exposure to thorium dioxide (Thorotrast), arsenicals and vinyl chloride. Association with androgenic anabolic steroids, oestrogens, oral contraceptives, phenelzine and cupric acid has also been reported. Overall, up to 50% of angiosarcomas are associated with previous exposure to a chemical carcinogenic agent.

These environmental risk factors may account for the male predominance (gender ratio of 3:1) and age at the time of diagnosis (50–70 years). Patients usually experience non-specific symptoms such as abdominal pain, weakness, fatigue, anorexia and weight loss, but an acute abdomen related to tumour rupture is a classical presentation. Biological abnormalities may include haemolytic anaemia and thrombocytopenia, which are related to microangiopathic haemolysis and intravascular coagulation respectively.

Morphologically, angiosarcoma may present as a large solitary mass or as multinodular lesions. On CT, they are usually hypodense and remain so after contrast injection except for occasional focal areas of central or peripheral ring-shaped enhancement (**Fig. 5.8**). On delayed imaging, the lesion continues to enhance compared with that of the early-phase images. On MRI, the lesions tend to be hyperintense on T2-weighted images and heterogeneous on T1-weighted images, with focal hyperintensity on a background of hypointensity. Enhancement on the arterial and portal phases is heterogeneous.

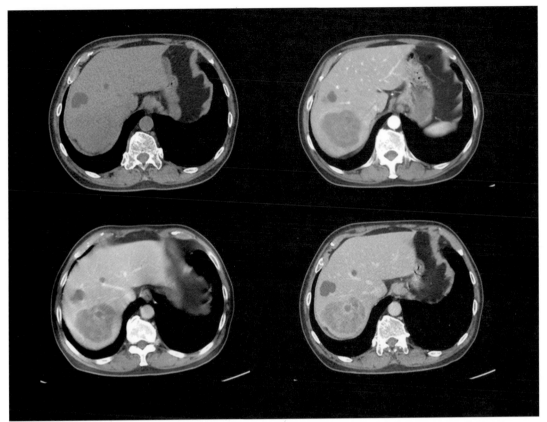

Figure 5.8 • CT of a patient with an angiosarcoma located in the right liver. Note that the lesion is spontaneously hypodense and remains so after contrast injection except for occasional focal areas of central or peripheral ring-shaped enhancement.

Although the progressive enhancement could mimic that of angioma, angiosarcomas clearly differ in that they are usually multiple and more heterogeneous, and enhancement is of lower intensity compared to the aorta, whereas it is the same for angioma.

The tumour develops from endothelial cells lining the hepatic sinusoids, and grows along these and the blood vessels. Disruption of hepatic plates may result in the development of cavities filled with tumour debris or haematoma, which favours the invasion of hepatic and portal veins. These tumours have ill-defined borders and typically involve the entire liver.

Angiosarcomas are rapidly growing and median survival is 6 months. Most patients have metastases at presentation, most notably in the lung and spleen. The latter may be involved in up to half of patients. Death may also result from liver failure or intraperitoneal bleeding due to tumour rupture.

It is considered reasonable to attempt resection when possible and to administer chemotherapy, although it is still poorly effective. Radiation therapy may have some value in this particular tumour. Transplantation has not been associated with survival beyond 3 years due to tumour recurrence, and is therefore not indicated.

Other sarcomas, including leiomyosarcoma, tend to have a better prognosis and should be resected if feasible.[92]

Primary hepatic lymphoma

Although malignant lymphoma frequently involves the liver, primary hepatic lymphomas are rare. Gross examination reveals a single large tumour mass, multiple masses or diffuse infiltration in approximately a third of cases each. Most primary hepatic lymphomas are classified as diffuse large-cell lymphomas of B-cell lineage. Some cases of primary hepatic lymphomas have been reported in association with AIDS or with chronic liver disease. On imaging, they appear as hypodense lesions (**Fig. 5.9**), not always homogeneous. Rim enhancement and calcifications may be present. They are hypointense on T1-MRI and slightly enhanced on T2 sequences. The primary treatment is chemotherapy. However, some solitary lesions are resected without a preoperative diagnosis and chemotherapy is then administered postoperatively.

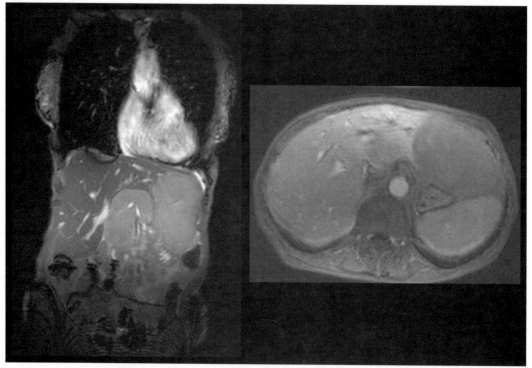

Figure 5.9 • CT of patient with a primary hepatic lymphoma of the left liver. Note that the lesion appears as hypodense lesion.

Key points

- Epidemiological studies indicate that both incidence and mortality of HCC are increasing worldwide, but have stabilised in some Western countries.
- Development of HCC is linked to the presence of an underlying liver disease. Major risk factors for HCC include viral infection, alcohol ingestion and metabolic syndrome.
- Surveillance of cirrhotic patients and at-risk populations is recommended to detect HCC at an early stage provided treatment is feasible.
- US is recommended as a screening tool, while CT and MRI are useful to confirm the diagnosis. Liver biopsy is recommended in selected cases.
- Patients with HCC should be managed in multidisciplinary settings including hepatologists, liver surgeons, liver transplant teams, oncologists, pathologists and interventional radiologists.
- The level of evidence for most treatment options for HCC is limited to cohort investigations with few randomised controlled trials, most of which deal with treatment of advanced disease.
- Five treatments are available on the basis of evidence-based data: transplantation, resection, radiofrequency ablation, chemoembolisation and sorafenib.
- Liver transplantation is the treatment of choice in cirrhotic patients with limited tumour involvement, as it removes both tumour and the preneoplastic liver.
- Liver resection is the treatment of choice in patients with normal liver parenchyma and is indicated in cirrhotic patients with preserved liver function and no clinically significant portal hypertension.
- Percutaneous treatments are effective in patients with small tumours.
- Transarterial chemoembolisation and radioembolisation are effective in selected non-surgical patients with preserved liver function.
- Sorafenib is effective in selected palliative patients who still have preserved liver function.

Key references

1. Ferlay J, Soerjomataram I, Dikshit R, et al. Cancer incidence and mortality worldwide: sources, methods and major patterns in GLOBOCAN 2012. Int J Cancer 2014;136(5):E359–86. PMID: 25220842.

3. Poordad F, Hezode C, Trinh R, et al. ABT-450/r-ombitasvir and dasabuvir with ribavirin for hepatitis C with cirrhosis. N Engl J Med 2014;370(21):1973–82. PMID: 24725237.

4. Belli LS, Berenguer M, Cortesi PA, et al. Delisting of liver transplant candidates with chronic hepatitis C after viral eradication: a European study. J Hepatol 2016;65(3):524–31. PMID: 27212241.

9. Rinella ME. Nonalcoholic fatty liver disease: a systematic review. JAMA 2015;313(22):2263–73. PMID: 26057287.

13. Siegel AB, Zhu AX. Metabolic syndrome and hepatocellular carcinoma: two growing epidemics with a potential link. Cancer 2009;115(24):5651–61. PMID: 19834957.

14. Cauchy F, Zalinski S, Dokmak S, et al. Surgical treatment of hepatocellular carcinoma associated with the metabolic syndrome. Br J Surg 2012;100(1):113–21. PMID: 23147992.

15. Vigano L, Conci S, Cescon M, et al. Liver resection for hepatocellular carcinoma in patients with metabolic syndrome: a multicenter matched analysis with HCV-related HCC. J Hepatol 2015;63(1):93–101. PMID: 25646890.

16. Wong RJ, Cheung R, Ahmed A. Nonalcoholic steatohepatitis is the most rapidly growing indication for liver transplantation in patients with hepatocellular carcinoma in the U.S. Hepatology 2014;59(6):2188–95. PMID: 24375711.

22. Laurent A, Dokmak S, Nault JC, et al. European experience of 573 liver resections for hepatocellular adenoma: a cross-sectional study by the AFC-HCA-2013 study group. HPB (Oxford) 2016;18(9):748–55. PMID: 27593592.

42. Berzigotti A, Reig M, Abraldes JG, et al. Portal hypertension and the outcome of surgery for hepatocellular carcinoma in compensated cirrhosis: a systematic review and meta-analysis. Hepatology 2014;61(2):526–36. PMID: 25212123.

60. Llovet JM, Bruix J. Systematic review of randomized trials for unresectable hepatocellular carcinoma: Chemoembolization improves survival. Hepatology 2003;37(2):429–42. PMID: 12540794.
This meta-analysis of randomised controlled trials (RCTs) demonstrates that TACE should be recommended as first-line non-curative option for intermediate HCC (as defined by the BCLC staging system) as it improved survival.

61. Yin L, Li H, Li AJ, et al. Partial hepatectomy vs. transcatheter arterial chemoembolization for resectable multiple hepatocellular carcinoma beyond Milan criteria: a RCT. J Hepatol 2014;61(1):82–8. PMID: 24650695.
This is the first RCT to demonstrate an improved survival benefit of resection in patients with multiple HCC.

62. Liu H, Wang ZG, Fu SY, et al. Randomized clinical trial of chemoembolization plus radiofrequency ablation versus partial hepatectomy for hepatocellular carcinoma within the Milan criteria. Br J Surg 2016;103(4):348–56. PMID: 26780107.
This RCT demonstrates an improved survival benefit of resection in patients with HCC within Milan criteria.

63. Lopez PM, Villanueva A, Llovet JM. Systematic review: evidence-based management of hepatocellular carcinoma –an updated analysis of randomized controlled trials. Aliment Pharmacol Ther 2006;23(11):1535–47. PMID: 16696801.
This meta-analysis of four RCTs shows the efficacy of radiofrequency ablation (RFA) in terms of better local control in patients with HCC >2cm, as compared to percutanenous ethanol injection (PEI).

64. Cho YK, Kim JK, Kim MY, et al. Systematic review of randomized trials for hepatocellular carcinoma treated with percutaneous ablation therapies. Hepatology 2009;49(2):453–9. PMID: 19065676.
This meta-analysis of four RCTs demonstrates that RFA significantly improves survival for patients with HCC, as compared to PEI.

74. Llovet JM, Ricci S, Mazzaferro V, et al. Sorafenib in advanced hepatocellular carcinoma. N Engl J Med 2008;359(4):378–90. PMID: 18650514.
This RCT demonstrates an improved survival benefit for sorafenib in patients with advanced HCC.

78. Vente MA, Wondergem M, van der Tweel I, et al. Yttrium-90 microsphere radioembolization for the treatment of liver malignancies: a structured meta-analysis. Eur Radiol 2009;19(4):951–9. PMID: 18989675.

88. Sapisochin G, Facciuto M, Rubbia-Brandt L, et al. Liver transplantation for 'very early' intrahepatic cholangiocarcinoma: international retrospective study supporting a prospective assessment. Hepatology 2016; 64(4):1178–88. PMID: 27481548.

91. Lai Q, Feys E, Karam V, et al. Hepatic epithelioid hemangio-endothelioma and adult liver transplantation: proposal for a prognostic score based on the analysis of the Eltr-Elita Registry. Transplantation 2017101:555–564. PMID: 27926594.

6

Colorectal liver metastases

Amir A. Rahnemai-Azar
Mary E. Dillhoff
Carl Schmidt
Timothy M. Pawlik

Introduction

Despite recent advances in screening, diagnosis and management, colorectal cancer (CRC) remains the second leading cause of cancer death in Western countries. In 2012, 1.4 million new CRC cases with close to 694 000 deaths were estimated to have occurred worldwide.[1] Almost two-thirds of patients with CRC develop distant metastases. The liver is the most frequent site of metastases, with liver disease being detected either at the time of CRC diagnosis (synchronous; 20–25%) or subsequently (metachronous; 40%). The extent of liver disease is a key determinant of survival in patients with isolated colorectal liver metastases (CRLM).[2]

✅✅ While the median survival of patients with advanced CRLM has improved over the last several decades with the introduction of more efficacious chemotherapy, surgical resection remains the cornerstone of potentially curative therapy.[2–4]

Diagnosis

The diagnosis of CRLM is usually based on imaging during evaluation of patients with CRC. Rarely, depending on clinical presentation, percutaneous fine-needle aspiration (FNA) biopsy may be used to confirm the diagnosis. While the risk of tract seeding following FNA biopsy for CRLM is low, typically there is no need for biopsy.[5–7] Most often

a thorough history and physical examination, as well as laboratory tests (e.g. CEA [carcinoembryonic antigen] level) and characteristic imaging of the lesion are adequate to substantiate a diagnosis of CRLM. Imaging is important to stage adequately the extent of disease, which in turn will help tailor subsequent therapy. Multiple different imaging modalities can be utilised to assess patients with CRLM (Table 6.1).

Transabdominal ultrasonography (US) is a relatively inexpensive test that can provide general information about the number, location and extent of liver metastases. The addition of duplex can increase US sensitivity to define the proximity of lesions to adjacent vital structures such as the portal vein and inferior vena cava.

✅✅ US is **not** a sensitive diagnostic test for CRLM and can fail to identify over 50% of metastatic lesions.[8,9]

One of the major limitations is reliance on the skill and knowledge of the operator. In addition, other factors such as the patient's body habitus, presence of steatosis and the inability to detect extrahepatic disease hampers the diagnostic yield and utility of US. In contrast to transabdominal US, intraoperative US (IOUS) has a much higher sensitivity to detect CRLM through high-resolution imaging of the liver.[8] However, with the increasing use of magnetic resonance imaging (MRI) and positron emission tomography–computed

Table 6.1 • Advantages and limitations of various imaging modalities in evaluating liver metastases

Modality	Advantages	Pitfalls

US	Low cost
	Availability
		High operator dependence
		Body habitus dependence
		Low sensitivity in
		  Liver steatosis
		  Small lesions
		  Extrahepatic spread

IOUS	Localisation of deep-seated lesion Mapping vasculature Real-time guidance for surgical plane Guiding RFA	Increases duration of surgery

CT	Availability
	Relatively low cost
	High sensitivity and specificity
	Extrahepatic spread evaluation
	Vascular mapping
	Liver volume estimation
	Planning targeted therapies
	Therapy monitoring
		Poor confidence in
		  Detecting < 1 cm lesions
		  Lesion detection in chemotherapy-induced liver steatosis
		  Distinction of malignant from benign
		Not suitable for
		  CM allergies
		  Compromised renal function

MRI	Increased sensitivity and specificity for
	  Detection of small lesions (<1 cm)
	  Detection of lesions after chemotherapy-induced fatty changes
	  Lesion characterisation
	Treatment planning
	Therapy response monitoring
		Not suitable for patients with
		  Claustrophobia
		  Implants (pacemaker, stents, etc.)
		  Impaired renal function (CE-MRI)
		  Non-compliance

PET	Accurate extrahepatic site detection Superior sensitivity and specificity when combined with CT/CE-CT Therapy response monitoring Detection of residual or recurrent disease	Limited accessibility High cost Poor detection of lesions < 1 cm After chemotherapy

Reproduced from Sahani DV, Bajwa MA, Andrabi Y, et al. Current status of imaging and emerging techniques to evaluate liver metastases from colorectal carcinoma. Ann Surg 2014;259(5):861–72.

tomography (PET-CT), detection of new unsuspected lesions by IOUS has decreased.[10,11] Nonetheless, IOUS does help identify new lesions in a subset of patients and also enables surgeons to perform hepatectomy more safely by providing real-time guidance of the resection plane. In a series of 60 patients with liver metastases, Leen et al. demonstrated that the addition of contrast improved diagnostic accuracy of IOUS up to 96%.[12] Other studies have noted that the diagnostic yield of contrast-enhanced US in the detection of liver metastases is comparable to contrasted-enhanced MRI.[13–15]

At most centres, triple-phase contrast multidetector computed tomography (MDCT) is the modality of choice for CRC staging and screening for liver metastases. CRLM typically appear as hypoattenuating lesions and are best identified in the portal venous phase of scanning (Fig. 6.1).[16] Arterial phase images are typically used to distinguish metastatic disease from benign vascular lesions and also to identify the liver vascular anatomy for pre-surgical planning or if placement of a hepatic arterial infusion pump is being considered (Fig. 6.2).[17] Additionally, extrahepatic metastases may be detected by obtaining chest, abdomen and pelvic images. The major disadvantage of CT is its lower sensitivity in recognising small liver lesions (<1 cm), especially in patients with background liver parenchymal disease, such as steatosis.[18,19]

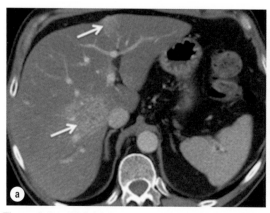
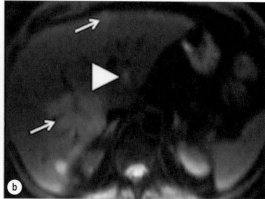

Figure 6.1 • **(a)** Axial contrast-enhanced portal phase CT of the liver shows the presence of two metastases (*thin arrows*); **(b)** diffusion MRI (b = 100 s/mm^2): discovery of an additional metastasis in segment 2 (*arrowhead*). Legou F. et al. Diagn Interv Imaging. 2014 May;95(5):505-12. Copyright © 2014 Elsevier Masson SAS. All rights reserved.

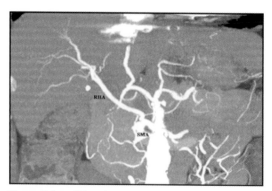

Figure 6.2 • CT angiogram. A maximum intensity projection rendered coronal 3-dimensional image demonstrating a replaced right hepatic artery from superior mesenteric artery in a patient scheduled for right lobe resection for liver metastases from CRC. Sahani DV. et al. Current status of imaging and emerging techniques to evaluate liver metastases from colorectal carcinoma. Ann Surg. 2014 May;259(5):861-72.

MRI provides high-resolution assessment of the liver and can be superior to CT in detecting and characterising indeterminate small lesions (Figs 6.1, **6.3**),[8] with sensitivity rates of 91–97%, compared to 71–73% for CT.[20,21] MRI is also more accurate in differentiating benign and malignant subcentimetre liver lesions, with a specificity of 97.5%, compared to 77.3% for MDCT.[22] More notably, MRI tends to be more accurate in detecting and characterising CRLM if there is underlying liver parenchymal disease.[8,23] Recent advances in MRI techniques, including the introduction of tissue-specific contrast agents such as gadobenate dimeglumine and gadoxetate (Gd-EOB-DTPA; Primovist in Europe and Eovist in the USA), as well as diffusion-weighted imaging (DWI), have further enhanced diagnostic yield of CRLM (**Figs 6.4, 6.5**).[24–26]

Positron emission tomography (PET) is another commonly used imaging modality. PET utilises an intravenously administered radioactive tracer, fluorodeoxyglucose (FDG), to identify metabolically active metastatic lesions. The use of PET can supplement CT. For example, Strasberg et al. showed that in 43 patients with CRLM, laparotomy was avoided in six patients based on FDG-PET findings that initially were not detected on CT.[27] Another randomised control study of 150 patients with CRLM noted that the number of futile laparotomies was reduced from 45% to 28% by the addition of preoperative FDG-PET.[28] In a meta-analysis, FDG-PET was reported to have superior results in preoperative staging of CRC compared with CT alone, especially for detecting extrahepatic disease (sensitivity and specificity of 91.5% and 95.4% versus 60.9% and 91.1%, respectively).[29] According to the National Comprehensive Cancer Network (NCCN) guidelines, FDG-PET should be considered in patients with CEA elevation and suspected disease recurrence. The use of PET in CRC staging is limited due to insufficient anatomic detail, poor sensitivity for lesions smaller than 1 cm, and false-positive results in the setting of inflammation (**Fig. 6.6**). However, integration of FDG-PET imaging and CT addresses some of these limitations, particularly with regard to anatomic detail and it is particularly useful in detecting extrahepatic disease (**Fig. 6.7**).[30]

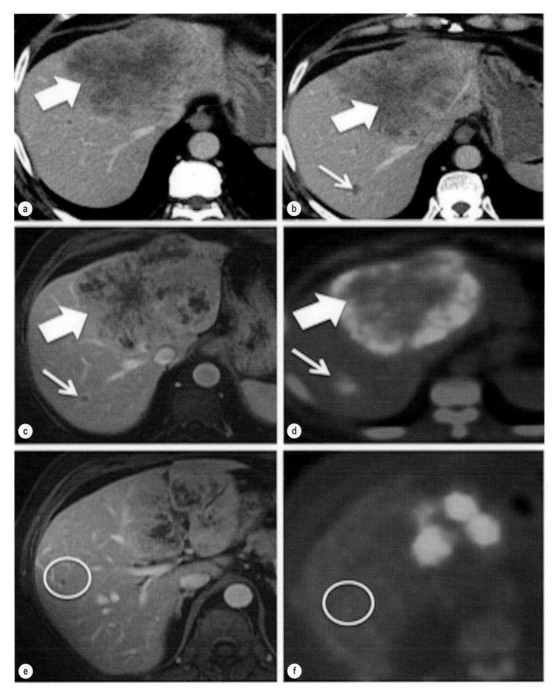

Figure 6.3 • **(a)** Portal venous phase contrast-enhanced liver CT: necrotic mass, with fibrous enhancement centred on segments 2–4 (*thick arrow*); **(b)** a second hypodense lesion on CT scan is visible in segment 7 (*thin arrow*); **(c)** MRI shows peripheral enhancement of both lesions (*arrows*); **(d)** both lesions are hypermetabolic on PET-CT (*arrows*); **(e)** discovery of an additional lesion on portal venous phase contrast enhanced MRI (*circle*); **(f)** this third lesion was not seen on CT or PET-CT (*circle*).

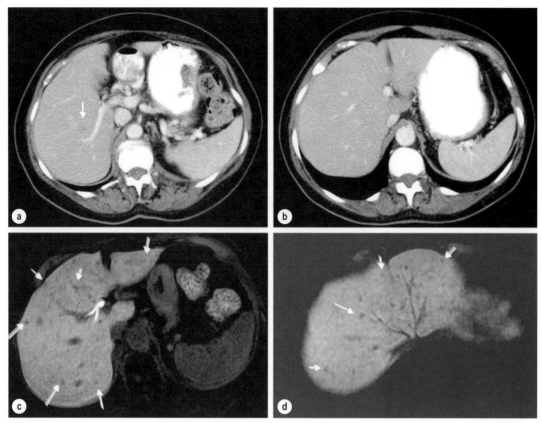

Figure 6.4 • A 44-year-old man, with stage III colon cancer resected 1 year previously and treated with chemotherapy. Follow-up restaging CE-CT examination **(a, b)** showed reduced liver attenuation in comparison to spleen due to steatosis and a possible lesion in the right lobe (*arrow*). Liver MRI was performed with hepatobiliary contrast agent Eovist to evaluate for surgical resection. Ten-minute delayed hepatobiliary phase, T1-weighted fat saturation MR images **(c, d)** demonstrate enhancing liver parenchyma and numerous non-enhancing, small metastases scattered within the right and left lobe of liver (*arrows*).
Sahani DV. et al. Current status of imaging and emerging techniques to evaluate liver metastases from colorectal carcinoma. Ann Surg. 2014 May;259(5):861-72.

Surgical resection

Patient selection

Surgical resection with negative microscopic margins (R0 resection) offers patients with CRLM the best chance for long-term survival. The optimal selection of patients for hepatic resection is evolving and in recent years the paradigm of surgical resectability has shifted from surgeon-based technical issues to a patient-disease-focused multidisciplinary approach.

In 1989, Steele et al. introduced several factors including the number of metastatic lesions (≤3), maximum lesion dimension (<5 cm), timing of metastases (metachronous), adequate free margin (>1 cm), and absence of extrahepatic metastases as determinants of the best outcome following surgical resection for CRLM.[31] However, with recent advances in multidisciplinary management of CRLM patients, the relevance of many of these factors has been challenged.[32–36]

> ✔✔ According to the Americas Hepato-Pancreato-Biliary Association (AHPBA) most recent expert consensus statement and also the NCCN guidelines, CRLM is considered resectable as long as the tumour can be removed completely (R0 resection), the predicted future liver remnant (FLR) function is adequate to prevent postoperative liver failure, extrahepatic sites of the disease are controllable, and the primary tumour can be resected for cure.[37,38]

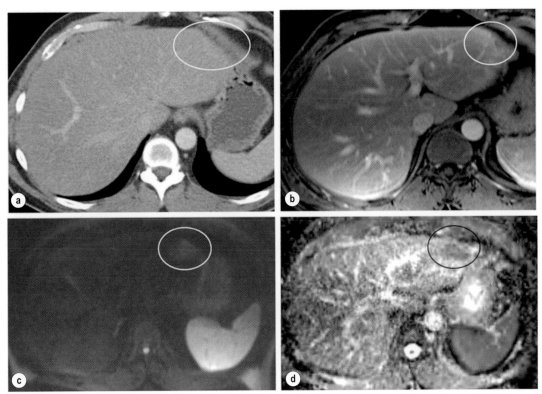

Figure 6.5 • A 51-year-old man with CRLM being treated with chemotherapy. Follow-up CE-CT **(a)** and CE-MRI **(b)** failed to demonstrate left lobe metastasis that is more obvious on DW-MRI **(c)** as a focal bright area in the left lobe (*arrow*) with associated restricted diffusion on apparent diffusion coefficient image **(d)** (*arrow*).
Sahani DV. et al. Current status of imaging and emerging techniques to evaluate liver metastases from colorectal carcinoma. Ann Surg. 2014 May;259(5):861-72.

Issues in management of CRLM

Current practice for margin status

Several studies have demonstrated that resection margin width is not a determinant of long-term survival.[39,40] Achieving R0 resection, regardless of its width, is enough to define the resectability of a metastatic tumour.

Role of the FLR in resection of CRLM

The focus of current liver surgery practice is on preserving adequate liver remnant function to prevent post-resection liver failure, rather than the volume of disease. Previously, the anticipated ability to preserve a minimum of two contiguous segments of hepatic parenchyma with adequate vascular inflow and outflow, and adequate biliary drainage was sufficient to consider a hepatic resection.[41] However, recent advances in accurate prediction of FLR volume and function have optimised the selection of patients with CRLM for surgery (**Fig. 6.8**).

A patient with a normal underlying liver requires at least a 20% FLR to prevent postoperative liver failure. The percentage increases to 30% for patients who have steatosis or steatohepatitis, often after receiving preoperative chemotherapy, and to 40% in patients with underlying cirrhosis.[42]

> ✓✓ Patients who do not meet FLR requirements may benefit from additional preoperative procedures to induce hypertrophy of the FLR, such as portal vein embolisation (PVE) or associating liver partition and portal vein ligation for staged hepatectomy (ALPPS).[43–46]

Extrahepatic metastatic disease and role of surgery

The lungs, intra-abdominal lymph nodes (LNs) and peritoneum are the most common sites of CRC metastases after the liver. The presence of extrahepatic metastases has been associated with

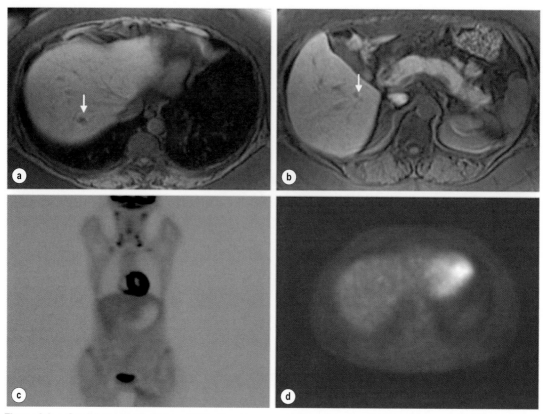

Figure 6.6 • Small liver metastasis from CRC without increased FDG uptake in a 47-year-old woman. CE-MRI of the liver shows two small metastatic deposits (*arrow*) in the right lobe **(a, b)**. Representative coronal and axial images from a whole-body FDG-PET examination **(c, d)** show no corresponding focal increased FDG uptake in the liver.
Sahani DV. et al. Current status of imaging and emerging techniques to evaluate liver metastases from colorectal carcinoma. Ann Surg. 2014 May;259(5):861-72.

poor outcomes and traditionally considered a contraindication for hepatic resection. However, with recent advances in surgical techniques and systemic medical treatment, hepatic resection can be considered in patients with extrahepatic disease amenable to surgical resection or long-term oncologic control with adjuvant chemotherapy. Patients with extrahepatic disease who are being considered for resection should be managed in a multidisciplinary setting and generally should be treated with preoperative therapy to help define the tumour biology.

Role of diagnostic laparoscopy before CRLM resection

Diagnostic laparoscopy may prevent unnecessary laparotomy in patients with occult intraperitoneal metastases. In general, considering that many patients will have undergone surgical exploration of the peritoneum at the time of primary tumour resection and because of the accuracy of current imaging modalities, diagnostic laparoscopy is typically reserved for only high-risk patients (i.e. very high CEA, indeterminate imaging for peritoneal disease, etc.).

Current surgical strategy in management of patients with bilateral CRLM

The choice of surgical strategy for patients with bilateral CRLM depends on the burden and location of the tumour. One-stage simultaneous multiple atypical hepatic resections, with preservation of adequate FLR, is a safe and effective technique in management of small and favourably positioned bilateral CRLM. For patients with extensive bilobar metastases, several strategies including parenchymal-sparing hepatectomy (PSH), combination of ablation with repeat PSH and two-stage hepatectomy, can be applied.

PSH has been shown to be safe and effective for the management of CRLM without compromising oncological outcomes. Furthermore, with

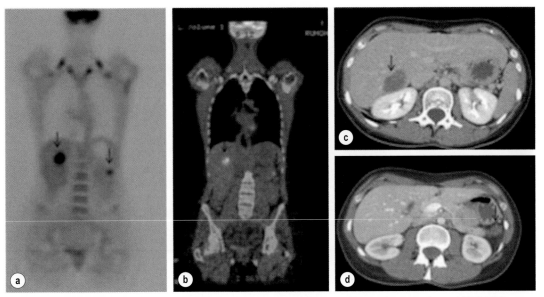

Figure 6.7 • Whole-body PET-CT was performed on a 49-year-old woman with rectal cancer. Coronal FDG-PET **(a)** and fused PET-CT **(b)** images from whole-body PET-CT show a focus of intense FDG uptake in the liver (*arrows*). Corresponding axial image **(c)** acquired during CT shows the metastatic deposit in the right lobe of liver (*arrow*). Another discrete extrahepatic peritoneal metastatic deposit is evident in the left side of upper abdomen on the FDG-PET and fused PET-CT image (*arrow*) that on corresponding axial CT image **(d)** is located adjacent to the tail of pancreas (*arrow*). (FDG indicates 18-fluoro-deoxyglucose.)
Sahani DV. et al. Current status of imaging and emerging techniques to evaluate liver metastases from colorectal carcinoma. Ann Surg. 2014 May;259(5):861-72.

preservation of liver parenchyma, PSH increases the potential of salvage repeat hepatectomy for patients with recurrent intrahepatic disease. The combination of multimodal therapies is another approach to treat patients with multiple lesions when complete resection of all metastases is not feasible. In this approach, hepatectomy addresses the main tumour mass while the residual tumour is extirpated with local tumour-ablative therapy. Combination resection-ablative therapy does not compromise disease-specific survival when compared with major resections and two-stage hepatectomies. In certain circumstances, combination resection-ablation can be associated with decreased blood loss, shorter hospital stay and less morbidity.

Patients with inadequate FLR may be considered for two-stage hepatectomy. In this approach, removal of a portion of metastatic disease is combined with occlusion of the contralateral portal vein, either by surgical ligation or subsequent percutaneous embolisation. A second curative-intent stage of the operation is performed after hypertrophy of the contralateral liver when there has been adequate increase of the FLR volume. Although the choice between minor or major liver resection at the first stage hepatectomy remains

debatable, most centres proceed with initial resection of tumours within the FLR contralateral to the planned PV occlusion, and then perform the subsequent ipsilateral second-stage resection. The long-term survival of patients who complete both stages is comparable to patients with more limited disease treated by a conventional single-stage strategy.

Preoperative chemotherapy

The role of preoperative chemotherapy in management of CRLM can be discussed in three categories of patients – those with resectable metachronous, unresectable and synchronous disease.

Resectable metachronous CRLM

Current data regarding neoadjuvant chemotherapy in patients with resectable metachronous CRLM are conflicting. The potential advantages of preoperative chemotherapy in this group are in facilitating resection of large tumours and assessment of tumour response to chemotherapy. In contrast, progression of disease and the possible increased risk of post-resection complications and liver insufficiency are considered potential

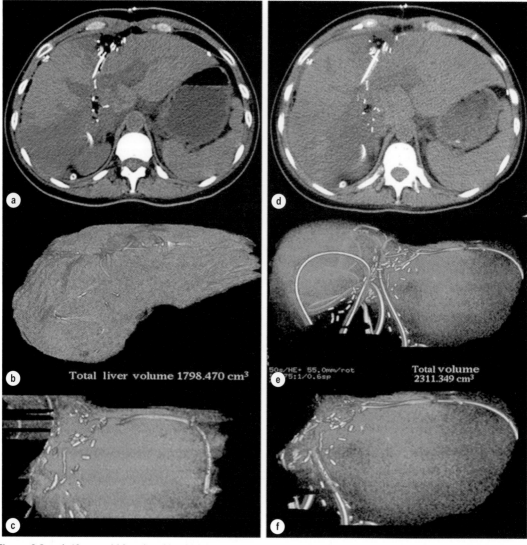

Figure 6.8 • A 48-year-old female, with a history of rectal cancer and liver metastases underwent right portal vein ligation and in situ liver-splitting surgery. The postoperative axial **(a)** and volumetric CT images of the liver (b, c) show TLV = 1798 cm^3 **(b)**, and left lobe volume **(c)** = 612 cm^3. Axial **(d)** and volumetric CT images obtained after 1 week **(e,f)** show an increase in TLV to 2311 cm^3 **(e)** and left lobe volume to 908 cm^3 **(f)**, corresponding to 35% increase in volume. (TLV indicates total liver volume.)
Sahani DV. et al. Current status of imaging and emerging techniques to evaluate liver metastases from colorectal carcinoma. Ann Surg. 2014 May;259(5):861-72.

drawbacks. The EORTC 40983 phase III trial investigated the efficacy of neoadjuvant chemotherapy.[47] In this study, 364 patients with up to four CRLM were randomly assigned to liver resection with or without perioperative FOLFOX4 chemotherapy. In the chemotherapy group, patients received a median of six cycles with an average delay of 16 weeks before surgical resection, with six cycles delivered in the postoperative setting. Disease progression was observed in 11 of the 182 patients assigned to chemotherapy, with the majority being new extrahepatic lesions. As it is likely that these new lesions would have occurred even after immediate resection, it is reasonable to consider that chemotherapy helped to avoid surgery in patients with aggressive tumour biology. While the number of patients who underwent liver resection was similar between the two groups, only eight patients (5%) in the chemotherapy group had a non-therapeutic laparotomy because of extensive disease compared with 18 patients (11%) in the surgery group.[47]

✔✔ These data strongly suggest that delaying surgery would not result in resectable liver metastases becoming unresectable. Of note, the rate of postoperative complications (25%) and liver insufficiency (8%) were higher among patients treated with perioperative chemotherapy compared with surgery alone (16% and 4%, respectively). Postoperative mortality was not significantly different between the two groups. After 3 years, the absolute increase in progression-free survival (PFS) with chemotherapy was 8.1% in eligible patients (from 28.1% in the surgery alone group to 36.2% in the chemotherapy group; HR 0.77; $P = 0.041$).[47] In the latest update of the trial, 5-year PFS still remained higher in eligible patients who received perioperative chemotherapy, while 5-year overall survival (OS) was not significantly different between the two groups.[48]

While more studies are required to investigate the role of preoperative chemotherapy in patients with resectable CRLM, selection of neoadjuvant therapy needs to be based on factors that include tumour biology, risk of underlying liver insufficiency and difficulty of the resection.

✔✔ The recommended duration of neoadjuvant therapy is typically 4–6 cycles and liver resection is typically delayed for at least 4 weeks after completion of chemotherapy. Although using FOLFOX, FOLFIRI, or XELOX chemotherapy regimens are all acceptable, the optimal regimen has not been established.[38,49]

✔✔ Current data from randomised trials evaluating the benefit of adding novel targeted therapies like cetuximab, panitumumab (both EGFR inhibitors) or bevacizumab (VEGFR inhibitor) to a front-line oxaliplatin-containing regimen are mixed and necessitate future investigation.[50–53]

Unresectable metachronous CRLM

Preoperative systemic chemotherapy has the potential to downsize unresectable CRLM and convert initially inoperable lesions to resectable tumours. Such conversion has been reported in 3–36% of patients with unresectable disease and may vary due in part due to the subjective definition of unresectability.[54–57] FOLFOX and FOLFIRI are two suggested regimens for induction therapy, with a high objective response rate.[38] Higher resectability rates have been reported for regimens that contain both oxaliplatin and irinotecan, such as FOLFOXIRI.[56,58]

✔ Despite conflicting data, the addition of biologic agents such as cetuximab, panitumumab, or bevacizumab to the induction chemotherapy regimens has been recommended in selected patients.[38,49]

When employing preoperative 'conversion' chemotherapy, liver resection should be performed when the metastases become clearly resectable, but typically delayed at least 4 weeks after completion of chemotherapy. According to NCCN guidelines, response to conversion therapy should be evaluated every 2 months.[38]

✔✔ Traditionally, the RECIST criteria are used to assess changes in tumour size.[59,60]

Although novel CT-based morphologic criteria and PET functional imaging have been proposed as indicators of a response for targeted therapies, their application as standard measures requires further validation and confirmation.[61–63] It is also important to note that complete radiological response is not always equivalent to complete pathological response. Benoist et al. showed that 83% of 66 CRLM that disappeared on CT after chemotherapy had viable tumour.[64] More recently, with more advanced chemotherapy, the incidence of viable tumour after a complete radiological response is probably lower, and in the range of 40–50%.

Synchronous CRLM

In patients with resectable synchronous CRLM, preoperative systemic chemotherapy has the potential to identify patients with aggressive tumour biology. The size of the majority of metastatic lesions and the primary tumour either decreases or remains stable with the administration of modern systemic chemotherapy.[47,65] Widespread tumour progression on chemotherapy may be a contraindication to subsequent liver resection, as such a procedure may provide no benefit.[34,66] In patients with unresectable synchronous CRLM, preoperative chemotherapy should be given in an attempt to convert the lesions to being resectable.

For patients with synchronous CRLM, the timing of hepatic resection is another controversial topic. Although there is no randomised cohort trial to compare staged and simultaneous approaches, simultaneous resection of the primary with the liver metastases tends to be associated with a shorter total length of hospital stay and less morbidity, but with comparable 5-year survival.[67,68]

✔✔ In a recent meta-analysis of 18 studies, Kelly et al. reported that there were no clear perioperative or survival advantages for any given surgical approach.[69]

Rather, colectomy may be safely combined with curative resection of CRLM for most patients, except perhaps those with multiple bilateral metastases, inadequate FLR, or when extensive operations are anticipated either for the primary or metastatic disease. For these patients, many can be treated with resection of the primary colorectal tumour together with the first part of a two-stage hepatectomy. At a subsequent date, a second hepatectomy is undertaken to extirpate the residual disease in the contralateral liver. For patients who are presenting with symptoms related to the primary tumour such as bleeding, obstruction, or perforation, colorectal-first staged hepatectomy is recommended.[68,70]

Adjuvant chemotherapy

The main goal of adjuvant chemotherapy is to reduce the disease recurrence that can occur in up to 60–70% of patients following resection of CRLM.

Systemic chemotherapy

Two phase III trials with similar design, FFCD and EORTC/NCIC, investigated the benefit of 5-fluorouracil (5FU)-based chemotherapy following resection of CRLM.[71,72] Although preliminary results demonstrated a trend toward better disease-free survival (DFS) and overall survival (OS) in the group of patients who received adjuvant chemotherapy, both trials were closed prematurely due to slow accrual. In a pooled analysis of both trials ($n = 278$), Mitry et al. showed that adjuvant chemotherapy was associated with better median progression-free survival (PFS) (27.9 months vs 18.8 months, $P = 0.058$) and OS (62 months vs 47 months, $P = 0.095$) compared with surgery alone.[73] In another randomised clinical trial of 180 patients who underwent curative CRLM resection, the 3-year DFS was improved with uracil-tegafur/leucovorin adjuvant therapy; however, OS remained the same.[74]

Several studies have explored the efficacy of modern chemotherapy regimens as adjuvant therapy after resection of liver metastases. Adding irinotecan to 5-fluorouracil-leucovorin (5FU-LV), FOLFIRI regimen, has not been associated with a significant improvement in DFS or OS compared with 5FU-LV alone.[75] Although there are no randomised studies comparing FOLFOX (oxaliplatin-5FU-LV) with 5FU-LV, perioperative FOLFOX4 chemotherapy was associated with a trend toward improved 3-year PFS relative to surgical resection alone.[47] However, 5-year OS was not significantly different between the two groups (51.2 months in FOLFOX4 perioperative chemotherapy group vs 47.8% in surgery alone).[48] The benefit of novel molecular-targeted therapies in management of CRLM also has been investigated. In the new EPOC trial, addition of cetuximab, an epidermal growth factor receptor (EGFR) inhibitor, to FOLFOX chemotherapy in patients with initially resectable CRLM resulted in improved PFS.[50]

Hepatic artery infusion (HAI) chemotherapy

The main rationale for HAI chemotherapy is that liver metastases derive their blood supply predominantly from the hepatic artery. A few small randomised trials have demonstrated a benefit with HAI chemotherapy alone in patients with CRLM in terms of OS and intrahepatic recurrence-free survival (RFS).[76,77] However, these findings have not been validated in larger studies.[78] In contrast, several studies have demonstrated the therapeutic advantage of adjuvant HAI combined with systemic chemotherapy.[79–81] Kemeny et al., in a randomised trial of 109 patients with potentially resectable CRLM reported that combined systemic and regional HAI therapy was associated with a better 4-year intrahepatic RFS (67%) and overall RFS (46%) compared with surgery alone (43% and 25%, respectively).[80] In another study, 2-year intrahepatic RFS and 2-year OS of patients treated with combined therapy after hepatic resection were superior to patients who received systemic therapy alone.[79] The benefit persisted long-term at 10-year follow-up.[81] Recent studies have also demonstrated the survival benefit of adjuvant HAI-floxuridine in addition to modern systemic chemotherapy using oxaliplatin or irinotecan.[82,83]

Because of lack of long-term OS benefit, potential hepatobiliary toxicity associated with HAI chemo-therapy, possible surgical complications of pump placement, and the improved effectiveness of modern systemic chemotherapy regimens, HAI has not gained universal acceptance. However, HAI chemotherapy with or without systemic FU-LV is a reasonable approach in the management of CRLM following liver resection at institutions with experience.

Portal vein infusion chemotherapy

Because of aforementioned risks of HAI, the efficacy of portal vein infusion as an alternative regional chemotherapy has been investigated.[84] Despite a lower incidence of hepatic toxicity, portal vein infusion chemotherapy was associated with lower OS and DFS compared with HAI and is not utilised in the treatment of CRLM.

Survival and prognosis

✅ Prior to availability of current chemotherapeutic agents, the 5-year OS of patients with CRLM ranged from 30% to 40%.[85]

However, with ongoing advancements in the multidisciplinary management of CRLM and the advent of new systemic chemotherapies, the 5-year OS of many patients with CRLM has now improved to 50–60%.

Several studies have identified perioperative clinicopathological factors including primary tumour stage, CEA level, number of CRLM, size of the largest lesion, presence of extrahepatic disease and margin status as predictors of postoperative prognosis.[85–88] However, other investigators have failed to validate the correlation of these factors with outcome.[89–91] Similarly, different scoring systems, which were developed by combining these factors, have been inconsistent in accurately predicting prognosis following surgical resection.[85,87] In one of the earliest efforts, Nordlinger et al. developed a scoring system composed of age, size of largest metastasis, CEA level, stage of the primary tumour, disease-free interval, number of liver nodules and resection margin status.[87] By giving one point to each of these factors, the authors classified patients into three risk groups with different 2-year survival. Subsequently, in analysis of 1001 patients with CRLM who underwent liver resection, Fong et al. identified seven criteria as independent predictors of poor outcome: positive margin ($P=0.004$), extrahepatic disease ($P=0.003$), node-positive primary ($P=0.02$), disease-free interval from primary to metastases <12 months ($P=0.03$), number of hepatic tumours >1 ($P=0.0004$), largest hepatic tumour >5 cm ($P=0.01$), and CEA >200 ng/ml ($P=0.01$).[85] The authors used the last five factors to create a clinical risk score that was predictive of outcome (Table 6.2). Although several other predictive systems have been developed, the clinical value of most scoring systems is undetermined. In a study by Nathan et al., only poor-to-moderate prognostic

discriminatory ability of the Fong, Nordlinger and MSKCC predictive scoring systems was reported with C-statistics of just 0.57, 0.56 and 0.57, respectively.[92]

✔✔ A study by Roberts et al. assessed the prognostic value of eight different scores and noted that only the Rees postoperative index was a significant predictor of DFS and disease-specific survival.[93]

Nodal status of the primary tumour, differentiation degree of the primary tumour, presence of extrahepatic disease, tumour diameter, CEA level, and resection margin status are the six main components of the Rees postoperative index.[86]

✔✔ Sasaki et al. recently introduced an externally validated 'Metro-ticket' tumour burden score model as an accurate tool to predict long-term survival of patients with CRLM undergoing resection with excellent prognostic discriminatory power.[94]

Scoring systems might provide useful clues toward disease prognosis and guide patient selection and surveillance, but should not be relied upon to exclude patients from being considered for curative-intent resection.

Tumour biology is one of the strongest predictors of prognosis in patients with CRLM.[95] With increasing use of preoperative chemotherapy, tumour response assessed by imaging modalities can be used as a marker of tumour biology. Several investigators have

Table 6.2 • Fong et al. prognostic clinical risk score

Cumulative score	1 yr	2 yr	3 yr	4 yr	5 yr
0	93	79	72	60	60
1	91	76	66	54	44
2	89	73	60	51	40
3	86	67	42	25	20
4	70	45	38	29	25
5	71	45	27	14	14
Prognostic factor	**Score 0**	**Score 0**	**Score 0**	**Score 1**	**Score 1**
Node-positive primary	Negative	Negative	Negative	Positive	Positive
Disease-free interval	≥12 mth	≥12 mth	≥12 mth	<12 mth	<12 mth
Number of liver metastases	1	1	1	>1	>1
Size of major liver metastases	≤5 cm	≤5 cm	≤5 cm	>5 cm	>5 cm
CEA (ng/mL)	<200 ng/mL	<200 ng/mL	<200 ng/mL	>200 ng/mL	>200 ng/mL

Reproduced from Spolverato G, Ejaz A, Azad N, et al. Surgery for colorectal liver metastases: the evolution of determining prognosis. World J Gastrointest Oncol 2013;5(12):207–21.

shown that tumour response was associated with RFS and OS.[66,96] However, with the advent of novel biologic therapies, better modalities than traditional CT images are required for this purpose.

✅✅ Recently, molecular biomarkers such as *KRAS* and *BRAF V600E* mutations have gained popularity not only as prognostic factors but also as a guide for personalising treatment in patients with CRLM. Some studies have demonstrated an independent association between *KRAS* mutation and worse OS and RFS.[97–99]

Furthermore, *KRAS* status might predict the pattern of recurrence and hence guide surveillance strategies.[100,101] *BRAF* mutations have been consistently reported to be associated with poor prognosis.[102,103]

Surveillance

Although surgery is the best option for cure in patients with CRLM, the majority of patients ultimately die from recurrent disease. The liver and lung are the most common sites of tumour recurrence, with the liver being the only site in 35–40% of cases.[104–106] Repeat resection can be considered in selected patients. The 5-year survival of patients who undergo repeat hepatic resection for recurrent liver metastases is reported to be 40–50% with acceptable perioperative morbidity and mortality.[107–109] The duration of relapse-free interval and the number of lesions are the main predictors of prognosis.[106,107]

✅ Post-hepatectomy monitoring is recommended to identify early and potentially resectable recurrences. There is no definitive consensus regarding the extent and frequency of follow-up after surgery for CRLM. However, repeat physical examination, serum CEA measurement and CT of chest, abdomen and pelvis every 3–6 months for the first 2 years, and then every 6 months for up to 5 years seems to be a reasonable approach.[38,106,110]

Management of unresectable CRLM

The management of unresectable CRLM has improved over time, with the median survival approaching 3 years in some of the current trials.

Chemotherapy

Systemic chemotherapy

Palliative chemotherapy in patients with unresectable CRLM can relieve symptoms, improve quality of life and prolong survival. Several combinations of available antitumour medications can be used in patients with inoperable CRLM. The advent of targeted molecular therapies has further improved the efficacy of current regimens (Table 6.3).

Either irinotecan- or oxaliplatin-based regimens (e.g. FOLFOX, FOLFIRI, or XELOX) can be administered as a first-line therapy with relatively similar efficacy.[38,49] Several studies have failed to show the superiority of FOLFOX over FOLFIRI, and selection is usually made based on the regimen toxicity profile as well as patient fitness.[111,112] However, if the patient has already received adjuvant oxaliplatin-containing therapy in the previous 12 months, FOLFIRI is the preferred treatment. The substitution of capecitabine for short-term FU plus leucovorin infusion, XELOX, increases convenience with comparable response rate (RR), PFS and OS.[113,114]

Triple-regimen therapy, FOFOXIRI, is recommended in young patients with severe symptoms, high tumour burden, or contraindications to biologic agents such as *RAS/BRAF* mutations.[38,49] In a phase III trial of 244 patients with unresectable CRLM, FOLFOXIRI was associated with improved RR, PFS and OS compared with FOLFIRI.[115] Similarly, Cremolini et al. demonstrated that median OS in patients treated with FOLFOXIRI plus bevacizumab was longer than FOLFIRI plus bevacizumab (29.8 months vs 25.8 months, respectively; HR 0.8; $P = 0.03$).[116]

The addition of molecular-targeted therapies to a first-line chemotherapy regimen can also be a reasonable approach. In a pooled analysis of seven randomised controlled trials, Hurwitz et al. demonstrated that the addition of bevacizumab to chemotherapy was associated with an increase in OS (HR, 0.80; 95% CI, 0.71–0.90) and PFS (HR, 0.57; 95% CI, 0.46–0.71).[117] In a phase III study of 1401 patients with metastatic colorectal cancer, Saltz et al. concluded that bevacizumab in combination with oxaliplatin-based chemotherapy improved PFS. There was no difference in RR and OS with combination therapy.[118] In contrast, other studies have challenged the therapeutic benefit of bevacizumab.[119] Furthermore, several trials have confirmed the efficacy of adding anti-EGFR medications like cetuximab or panitumumab to first-line chemotherapy regimens in the palliation of patients with inoperable wild-type *KRAS* metastatic colorectal cancer.[120,121]

The choice of bevacizumab or anti-EGFR agents depends upon several factors. In patients with *RAS/BRAF* mutated tumours or patients who have markers of anti-EGFR resistance, bevacizumab is the preferred medication. Likewise, patients with right-sided primary tumours are less likely to benefit from cetuximab. The administration of bevacizumab should be carefully considered in elderly patients with

Table 6.3 • Most commonly used chemotherapy regimens in patients with colorectal liver metastasis and their components

Regimen	Irinotecan	Oxaliplatin	Leucovorin	Fluorouracil/capecitabine
FOLFIRI	✓		✓	✓
FOLFOX		✓	✓	✓
XELOX		✓		✓
FOLFOXIRI	✓	✓	✓	✓

a history of intra-arterial thromboembolic events or patients with recent major surgical intervention.

HAI chemotherapy

The role of HAI chemotherapy in management of advanced inoperable CRLM is typically limited to patients with isolated liver lesions that are not amenable to surgical resection or ablation. The infusion catheter is usually inserted into the gastroduodenal artery; as such, hepatic artery thrombosis, biliary toxicity, incomplete perfusion of the liver, and misperfusion to the stomach or duodenum with ulcers are all possible complications.[122] Floxuridine is the most thoroughly studied agent used in HAI therapy, but recently some investigators demonstrated the safety of delivering modern chemotherapy agents such as oxaliplatin and irinotecan via this route.[123–126] Although several studies have demonstrated the superiority of HAI chemotherapy in improving RR over FU-based systemic therapies, its survival advantage has been inconsistent.[127,128] Considering that irinotecan- or oxaliplatin-based systemic therapy was not used in most of these trials, the actual value of HAI chemotherapy in the management of patients with unresectable CRLM remains uncertain.

Other hepatic-artery based therapeutic strategies, including Yttrium-90 transarterial radioembolisation (Y-90 TARE) and transarterial chemoembolisation (TACE), have shown promising early results in palliation of patients (**Fig. 6.9**). However, establishing their role as standard therapy requires larger randomised trials, which are ongoing.

Ablation therapy

Tumour ablation is an alternative to systemic chemotherapy in patients with unresectable isolated liver metastasis. Radiofrequency ablation (RFA) is the most common method of local ablation therapy and can be performed by open, laparoscopic, or percutaneous approaches. Despite the lack of

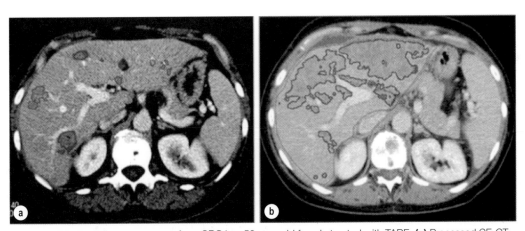

Figure 6.9 • Multifocal liver metastases from CRC in a 50-year-old female treated with TARE. **(a)** Processed CE-CT image before TARE shows segmentation of metastatic lesion and liver for estimation of tumour burden and liver volume, respectively. **(b)** Processed CE-CT image from the same patient approximately 2 months after TARE shows substantial interval increase in tumour.
Sahani DV. et al. Current status of imaging and emerging techniques to evaluate liver metastases from colorectal carcinoma. Ann Surg. 2014 May;259(5):861-72.

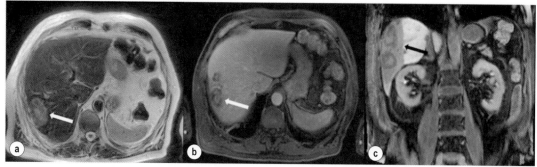

Figure 6.10 • A 56-year-old man with liver metastases from CRC **(a)** (*white arrow*) who underwent proton therapy. Images from follow-up MRI **(b, c)** show reduced enhancement on the dynamic contrast-enhanced images indicating response to therapy on 10-minute delayed hepatobiliary phase (*white arrow*). A sharp demarcation between treated liver from uninvolved left lobe (*black arrow*) is evident (c).
Sahani DV. et al. Current status of imaging and emerging techniques to evaluate liver metastases from colorectal carcinoma. Ann Surg. 2014 May;259(5):861-72.

randomised trials, multiple retrospective studies have demonstrated the superiority of surgical resection over RFA in patients with potentially resectable CRLM, with lower local recurrence rates and longer PFS and OS.[129–131] In a systematic review of the literature, Wong et al. concluded that there was not sufficient evidence to recommend RFA in patients with potentially resectable CRLM.[132]

Considering its limitations in treatment of tumours located in proximity to major blood vessels and other vital structures, as well as the decreased efficacy at tumour size >3 cm, RFA is not recommended as a first-line therapy in management of patients with unresectable CRLM, especially in the presence of extrahepatic disease. More recently, microwave ablation (MWA) has become more popular and is utilised in many centres. MWA still has the same limitations of RFA in treating patients with inoperable disease.

Radiation therapy

The effective antitumour dosage of traditional external beam radiation therapy (EBRT) is very toxic to the normal liver parenchyma. Development of radiation techniques utilising

targeted radiation such as stereotactic body radiotherapy (SBRT) has provided a new opportunity for local control of CRLM (**Fig. 6.10**). In a phase II trial of 42 patients with inoperable CRLM, SBRT was associated with a promising median OS of 29.2 ± 3.7 months.[133] Van der Pool et al. have also advocated SBRT as a treatment option for lesions not amenable for resection or RFA.[134] However, future randomised trials are required to confirm these findings.

Conclusion

The treatment of CRLM has evolved over the last several decades. The cornerstone of potentially curative therapy remains surgical resection. Multidisciplinary care that involves thoughtful utilisation of perioperative chemotherapy is also critical to optimise the chance of long-term survival. Options for patients with advanced unresectable disease have expanded and now include more effective combined systemic chemotherapy with possible targeted biologic therapy, as well as locoregional liver-directed catheter-based therapy.

Key points

- The liver is the most frequent site of metastases in patients with colorectal cancer and the extent of liver disease is a key determinant of patient survival.
- The diagnosis of CRLM is usually based on imaging findings; however, rarely percutaneous fine-needle aspiration biopsy may be used to confirm the diagnosis.
- Surgical resection with negative microscopic margins (R0 resection) offers patients with CRLM the best chance for long-term survival. With recent advancements in multidisciplinary management of patients,

CRLM may be considered resectable as long as the tumour can be removed completely (R0 resection), the predicted future liver remnant (FLR) function is adequate to prevent postoperative liver failure, extrahepatic sites of the disease are controllable, and the primary tumour has been resected for cure.

- The advent of portal vein embolisation (PVE), staged hepatectomy with portal vein ligation, parenchymal-sparing hepatectomy with serial liver resections, and combining surgery with ablation has increased the number of patients with CRLM who might benefit from surgical resection.
- The selection of neoadjuvant therapy in management of patients with resectable CRLM needs to be considered individually, based on tumour biology, risk of liver insufficiency, and difficulty of any potential resection.
- In patients with unresectable CRLM, preoperative systemic chemotherapy has the potential to downsize lesions and convert initially unresectable disease to resectable disease.
- The main goal of adjuvant chemotherapy is to reduce the risk of disease recurrence that can occur in up to 60–70% of patients following resection of CRLM.
- Either irinotecan- or oxaliplatin-based regimens (e.g. FOLFOX, FOLFIRI, or XELOX) can be administered as a first-line systemic chemotherapy in patients with unresectable CRLM with relatively similar efficacy. The benefit of additional molecular-targeted therapies to first-line chemotherapy regimens requires further investigation.
- A multidisciplinary approach involving a medical oncologist, surgeon, radiologist and pathologist is the key in management of CRLM.

▶ Toronto HPB video atlas – http://pie.med.utoronto.ca/TVASurg/all-cases/

🌐 Full references available at **http://expertconsult.inkling.com**

Key references

3. Stangl R, Altendorf-Hofmann A, Charnley RM, et al. Factors influencing the natural history of colorectal liver metastases. Lancet 1994;343(8910):1405–10. PMID: 7515134.
   Provided natural outcome of patients with CRLM who did not receive any treatment and introduced six factors (percentage liver volume replaced by tumour [LVRT], grade of malignancy of the primary tumour, presence of extrahepatic disease, mesenteric lymph-node involvement, serum carcinoembryonic antigen [CEA], and age) as independent determinants of survival.

8. Sahani DV, Bajwa MA, Andrabi Y, et al. Current status of imaging and emerging techniques to evaluate liver metastases from colorectal carcinoma. Ann Surg 2014;259(5):861–72. PMID: 24509207.
   A review of the role of current imaging modalities in diagnosis and management of CRLM.

37. Adams RB, Aloia TA, Loyer E, et al. Selection for hepatic resection of colorectal liver metastases: expert consensus statement. HPB (Oxford) 2013; 15(2):91–103. PMID: 23297719.
   Expert consensus about the criteria of resectability and selection of patients with CRLM for hepatic resection.

43. Abdalla EK. Portal vein embolization (prior to major hepatectomy) effects on regeneration, resectability, and outcome. J Surg Oncol 2010;102(8):960–7. PMID: 21165999.
   Described the role of PVE in liver regeneration and prevention of hepatic insufficiency after hepatectomy.

45. de Santibanes E, Clavien PA. Playing Play-Doh to prevent postoperative liver failure: the 'ALPPS' approach. Ann Surg 2012;255(3):415–7. PMID: 22330039.
   The ALPPS procedure and its role in prevention of post-hepatectomy liver failure.

47. Nordlinger B, Sorbye H, Glimelius B, et al. Perioperative chemotherapy with FOLFOX4 and surgery versus surgery alone for resectable liver metastases from colorectal cancer (EORTC Intergroup trial 40983): a randomised controlled trial. Lancet 2008;371(9617):1007–16. PMID: 18358928.
   The randomised trial demonstrated the role of perioperative chemotherapy in management of patients with CRLM who underwent liver resection.

48. Nordlinger B, Sorbye H, Glimelius B, et al. Perioperative FOLFOX4 chemotherapy and surgery versus surgery alone for resectable liver metastases from colorectal cancer (EORTC 40983): long-term results of a randomised, controlled, phase 3 trial. Lancet Oncol 2013;14(12):1208–15. PMID: 24120480.
   Long-term follow-up results of previous study.

49. Van Cutsem E, Cervantes A, Adam R, et al. ESMO consensus guidelines for the management of patients with metastatic colorectal cancer. Ann Oncol 2016;27(8):1386–422. PMID: 27380959.

Guidelines of European society for medical oncology in comprehensive management of patients with metastatic colorectal cancer.

50. Primrose J, Falk S, Finch-Jones M, et al. Systemic chemotherapy with or without cetuximab in patients with resectable colorectal liver metastasis: the New EPOC randomised controlled trial. Lancet Oncol 2014;15(6):601–11. PMID: 24717919.
Addition of cetuximab to chemotherapy and surgery for resectable CRLM in *KRAS* exon 2 wild-type patients results in shorter progression-free survival.

59. Eisenhauer EA, Therasse P, Bogaerts J, et al. New response evaluation criteria in solid tumours: revised RECIST guideline (version 1.1). Eur J Cancer 2009; 45(2):228–47. PMID: 19097774.
Provided guidelines for assessment of treatment response.

69. Kelly ME, Spolverato G, Le GN, et al. Synchronous colorectal liver metastasis: a network meta-analysis review comparing classical, combined, and liver-first surgical strategies. J Surg Oncol 2015;111(3):341–51. PMID: 25363294.
This meta-analysis demonstrated that there is no clear statistical surgical outcome or survival advantage towards any of three available approaches in management of patients with synchronous CRLM.

85. Fong Y, Fortner J, Sun RL, et al. Clinical score for predicting recurrence after hepatic resection for metastatic colorectal cancer: analysis of 1001 consecutive cases. Ann Surg 1999;230(3):309–18; discussion 18–21. PMID: 10493478.
Provided a clinical score to predict outcome of patients with CRLM following surgical resection.

93. Roberts KJ, White A, Cockbain A, et al. Performance of prognostic scores in predicting long-term outcome following resection of colorectal liver metastases. Br J Surg 2014;101(7):856–66. PMID: 24817653.
Compared the value of different prognostic scores in predicting long-term outcome of patients with CRLM following hepatic resection.

94. Sasaki K, Morioka D, Conci S, et al. The tumor burden score: a new 'Metro-ticket' prognostic tool for colorectal liver metastases based on tumor size and number of tumors. Ann Surg 2016; Oct 19. [Epub ahead of print]. PMID: 27763897.
Introduced a prognostic tool based on maximum tumour size and number of lesions for patients undergoing hepatic resection of CRLM.

99. Andreatos N, Ronnekleiv-Kelly S, Margonis GA, et al. From bench to bedside: clinical implications of KRAS status in patients with colorectal liver metastasis. Surg Oncol 2016;25(3):332–8. PMID: 27566041.
This systematic review showed that mut-*KRAS* status predisposed to worse RFS and OS in patients with CRLM.

110. Meyerhardt JA, Mangu PB, Flynn PJ, et al. Follow-up care, surveillance protocol, and secondary prevention measures for survivors of colorectal cancer: American Society of Clinical Oncology clinical practice guideline endorsement. J Clin Oncol 2013;31(35):4465–70. PMID: 24220554.
Practice guideline about follow-up care of patients with CRLM.

7

Non-colorectal hepatic metastases

Nathan Zilbert
Carol-anne Moulton
Steven Gallinger

Introduction

Colorectal cancer (CRC) is the most common source of secondary hepatic tumours, although almost any solid malignancy can metastasise to the liver. Tumour cells from gastrointestinal tract malignancies may reach the liver directly via the portal circulation and liver metastases may occur in apparent isolation, as is sometimes seen with CRC. In contrast, metastases from non-gastrointestinal tumours may seed the liver via the systemic circulation and are generally indicative of disseminated disease.

The development of liver metastases was historically considered a preterminal event with treatment limited to palliation; however, the success of hepatectomy in improving outcomes in metastatic CRC has generated renewed enthusiasm in considering resection of liver metastases for non-colorectal primary cancers. Liver resection has become the standard of care for colorectal liver metastases (CRLM) and many centres have adopted an increasingly aggressive approach, with reported 5-year survival rates exceeding 50% in selected cases.[1,2] The complementary use of portal vein embolisation (PVE), radiofrequency ablation (RFA) and staged resection strategies has increased the proportion of patients eligible for resection. At the same time, advances in surgical technique and knowledge of liver anatomy have significantly reduced the morbidity and mortality associated with liver resection to less than 20% and 5%, respectively.[2,3]

Liver metastases of non-colorectal origin constitute a diverse group of tumours, most commonly arising from gastrointestinal sites. These tumours can be broadly divided into neuroendocrine and non-neuroendocrine malignancies, encompassing unique and markedly varied natural histories. Neuroendocrine tumours (NETs) have historically been described as indolent malignancies with hepatectomy for NET liver metastases associated with 5- and 10-year survival rates of 77.4% and 50.4%, respectively.[4] While hepatectomy is an accepted management strategy for NETs, it is performed less frequently for non-neuroendocrine tumours.

Evidence regarding hepatectomy for non-colorectal metastases originates largely from retrospective reviews spanning several decades of experience.[5–8] Many studies fail to distinguish between NET and non-NET metastases, and when that distinction is made, the non-NET metastases are usually considered a single entity despite comprising a heterogeneous set of pathologies. Reports focusing on a single tumour type are usually based on small case series. With advances in surgical techniques, and promising results observed for CRC and NET hepatic metastases, the role of surgical treatment for non-NET liver tumours has once again become an area of active interest.

✅ Due to the paucity of prospective, controlled data, the appropriate indications for hepatectomy for non-CRC metastases are unclear. Factors routinely associated with improved long-term outcomes include a long disease-free interval between treatment of the primary tumour and development of liver metastases, little or no extrahepatic disease, the projected future liver remnant and well- to moderately-differentiated cancer.[9] Unfortunately, no single measure of tumour biology yet exists though intensive research on molecular classification will lead to improved selection over the next decade.[10–12]

Pathophysiology and molecular basis of liver metastases

Achieving cancer cure requires the complete eradication of all tumour cells. Thus, for most solid tumours, complete surgical excision is the cornerstone of treatment, often with adjuvant systemic treatment to treat microscopic disease. In the presence of metastases there is an apparent contradiction in using a local therapy – surgery – to treat what is considered disseminated disease.

The rationale behind a surgical approach to metastatic disease is based on the concept of site-specific metastases. First proposed by Paget in 1889, this 'seed and soil' hypothesis argues that solid tumours have a distinct pattern of distant organ involvement created by the target organ microenvironment. Ewing proposed a 'mechanical' theory in which the metastatic pattern is determined by the venous drainage of the primary tumour.[13] Neither theory takes into account the complexity of the metastatic process, which requires that a cancer cell gains specific invasion and metastatic potential before it can disseminate. The clonal selection model of the metastatic process suggests that heterogeneity develops within a population of cancer cells through mutational events, allowing a subpopulation to randomly acquire the necessary traits to disseminate successfully.[14] Alternatively, it has been argued that within cancers of the same pathological type, i.e. breast cancer, some tumours are a priori more likely to develop metastases than others. This is supported by gene expression data where specific molecular signatures have been found to accurately predict prognosis in breast cancer,[15] ovarian cancer[16] and melanoma.[17] Similarly, in CRC the genotype of microsatellite instability correlates with a decreased likelihood of metastatic spread.[18]

A recent refinement to Paget's hypothesis, based on molecular genetic research, suggests that the primary tumour is itself capable of preparing the 'soil' by creating a 'premetastatic niche'.[19] Every cancer has a type-specific pattern of cytokine expression that appears to direct both malignant and non-malignant cells to specific distant organs. The influx and clustering of bone-marrow-derived haematopoietic cells is one of the earliest events in the development of a metastatic deposit. This is closely followed by local inflammation and the release of matrix metalloproteinases. These local events appear to mediate remodelling of the extracellular matrix, creating a more permissive microenvironment for the eventual deposition and growth of malignant cells.[20] Thus, the primary tumour both chooses and alters the sites to which it metastasises. For reasons not yet understood, many solid tumours preferentially metastasise to the liver.

If the site-specific hypothesis of metastatic spread is correct, complete surgical excision of liver metastases can remove the only site of disease and offer a chance for cure. Nonetheless, residual micrometastatic disease may exist within the liver, and hepatic recurrences are a common cause of treatment failure following hepatectomy. Even in the presence of micrometastases, the removal of all macroscopic disease may have immunological benefits. The immune-suppressing effects of cancers are well accepted: malignant cells can induce both adaptive and innate immune suppression, facilitating tumour growth.[21] The degree of immune suppression correlates with the tumour burden[22] and if all gross metastatic disease can be removed, host defences may attack micrometastatic deposits more effectively. The use of neoadjuvant or adjuvant chemotherapy may improve cure rates by controlling micrometastases.[23,24]

The advent of next generation sequencing technologies and high-density oligonucleotide arrays has further deepened our understanding of the metastatic process. Whereas the ability of a cancerous cell to metastasise was once believed to occur following the accumulation of multiple somatic mutations in many cancer-causing genes, new findings, specifically in pancreatic cancer, have challenged this belief. Studies by Yachida et al.[25] and Campbell et al.[26] describe the existence of multiple subclones within a primary pancreas cancer tumour, each containing a unique genetic signature corresponding to an eventual site of metastatic spread. These subclones are present many years before an eventual metastasis is clinically detected, when disease is at an early stage. Furthermore, metastases seen in different organs share many common genetic mutations as well as site-specific changes that confer a selective growth advantage in the respective tissue. Alternatively, Notta et al. have recently challenged the timing of tumour evolution of pancreas cancer whereby a 'single cataclysmic' event, such as chromothripsis, spawns a highly metastatic clone capable of seeding multiple organs very rapidly.[27]

Studies investigating single nucleotide polymorphisms in genes associated with tumour dormancy and immune response checkpoints have associated certain mutations with survival outcomes in patients undergoing resection of CRLM.[28,29] These findings could assist oncology teams in better risk-stratifying patients for surgical resection and theoretically similar studies could be performed on patients with non-CRLM, though at present there are few validated data available. Future studies on the biology of metastases are likely to improve our understanding of this complex process, translating into more effective therapy.

Clinical approach to non-colorectal liver metastases

Routine clinical, radiological and serological assessments for liver metastases should be guided by the propensity for liver metastases of each specific tumour type and the ability of potential treatments to alter the outcome of the metastatic disease. In imaging the liver, the choice of transabdominal ultrasound (US), contrast-enhanced ultrasound (CEUS), contrast-enhanced triphasic computed tomography (CT), magnetic resonance imaging (MRI) and positron emission tomography (PET) will be dictated by tumour type as well as local availability and expertise.

Some patients can be assessed for recurrence using more targeted techniques and biochemical markers (e.g. CA-125 for epithelial ovarian cancer, chromogranin A for NETs). Nuclear imaging (octreotide scans) can detect NETs expressing somatostatin receptors with 80–90% sensitivity. Whole-body PET using a new somatostatin analogue, [^{68}Ga]DOTA-TOC, has been found to be accurate for the detection of new metastases in NETs following radionuclide therapy.[30] Occasionally, the original presentation of a NET will be a liver metastasis from an unidentified primary, and the investigative focus is aimed at localisation of the primary tumour. Novel biomarkers, such as circulating tumour cells and cell-free DNA will soon be used to guide decision-making.[31,32]

✅ When a patient is considered for hepatic metastasectomy, the most critical component of the clinical assessment is an accurate determination of the extent of metastatic spread, including a thorough assessment for extrahepatic disease. The anatomical areas targeted for investigation (brain, lung, bone) will be determined by the known metastatic pattern of the primary tumour. Multidisciplinary input from specialists with expertise in hepatic surgery and management of the primary cancer is essential.

Certain tumours, such as gastric, breast and ovarian cancer, have a predilection for intraperitoneal spread. Although CT is the preferred modality for diagnosing peritoneal carcinomatosis, its accuracy is still limited by histological type, the anatomical site of spread and the size of tumour deposits.[33] For many of these equivocal cases, diagnostic laparoscopy has been recommended. Routine laparoscopy with laparoscopic ultrasound for patients with potentially resectable non-CRLM has been found to result in a change in management in 20% of cases and may be used selectively in preoperative staging.[34]

While the discussion that follows will review management and outcomes of liver resection for hepatic metastases based on primary tumour type, general considerations as proposed by Adam et al. in 2006 remain relevant.[5] In their review of 1452 patients from 41 centres undergoing liver resection for non-colorectal and non-neuroendocrine primary tumours, age >60 years, presence of extrahepatic disease, R2 resection and major hepatectomy were associated with decreased overall survival. These factors should be considered when contemplating liver resection for these patients.

Treatment strategies

Several treatment modalities exist for metastatic disease, and the therapeutic approach must be tailored to the tumour type, the performance status of the patient and the extent of disease. Treatment decisions in this context can only be determined properly by a multidisciplinary oncology team. Non-surgical ablative strategies and systemic or locally delivered chemotherapy can be used as adjuncts to resection.

Radiofrequency ablation (RFA) has been reported to be safe and successful at achieving local control in patients with liver metastases from breast cancer,[35] ovarian cancer[36] and NETs.[37] The major limitation of RFA is the difficulty in achieving complete necrosis for tumours >3 cm, as well as limited utility when tumours are close to major vascular or biliary structures. Novel techniques such as microwave ablation (MWA), stereotactic radiotherapy and irreversible electroporation (IRE), need to be assessed in prospective randomised trials as they may supplant surgical resection in some cases.[38–40]

Transarterial embolisation (TAE) takes advantage of the differential blood supply of liver metastases, which depends mainly on the hepatic arteries, and the normal parenchyma, which relies more heavily on the portal vein. Transarterial chemoembolisation (TACE) involves the local delivery of a drug prior to occluding the artery and allows prolonged exposure of the tumour to the agent without increasing systemic toxicity. Both TAE and TACE have been well described for the treatment of unresectable hepatocellular carcinoma[41] and the symptomatic relief of NETs.[42]

Finally, it behooves the surgical oncologist to keep abreast of the explosion of recent advances in systemic therapy, such as immunotherapy, to ensure proper selection of patients who will benefit from resection.[43]

Management of liver metastases by primary tumour

Neuroendocrine tumours

NETs represent a diverse group of tumours originating throughout the gastrointestinal tract. They are classified by site of origin and include gastrointestinal and pancreatic histological subtypes.[44] Neuroendocrine tumours arise most commonly in the midgut and may secrete serotonin and other bioactive amines. Pancreatic NETs (PNETs) can be non-functional or hormonally active (e.g. insulinoma, glucagonoma, gastrinoma, VIPoma), manifesting varied clinical syndromes.

NETs are graded based on mitotic rate and Ki67 proliferative index on a scale from 1 to 3.[44] Grade 1 and 2 tumours are considered to have indolent growth patterns. Despite this benign description, 46–93% of patients with NETs will have liver involvement at the time of diagnosis, with 5-year untreated survival of 0–20%.[45] Systemic chemotherapy with platinum-based regimens has shown a response rate of up to 67% in grade 3 NETs. Nevertheless, the survival benefit of chemotherapy is limited and associated with significant toxicity.[46]

Somatostatin analogues such as octreotide and lanreotide can achieve symptomatic relief in 70–80% of patients with functional tumours.[47–49] Both have also been shown to confer improvement in progression-free survival compared to placebo.[47,49] There is emerging evidence that pasireotide, a somastatin analogue that binds more somatostatin receptors than octreotide or lantreotide, may have an even greater antiproliferative effect.[50] Furthermore, agents such as the receptor tyrosine kinase inhibitor sunitinib, the mammmalian target of rapamycin (mTOR) inhibitor everolimus, and the antivascular endothelial growth factor (anti-VEGF) bevacizumab have shown promise in metastatic NETs.[46,51]

NETs metastasise preferentially to the liver, and in many patients the liver remains the only site of metastatic disease for a prolonged period of time. The majority of patients have multifocal, bilobar disease, of which less than 20% are candidates for surgery[45] (**Fig. 7.1a,b**). Liver resection may be

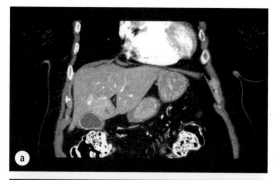

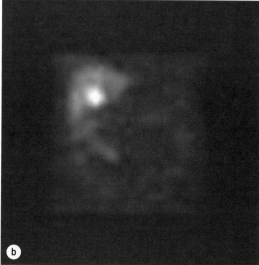

Figure 7.1 • **(a)** A 67-year-old female with a node-positive distal jejunal carcinoid tumour and synchronous solitary liver metastasis in segment 4B. **(b)** Octreotide scan of the same patient. Transaxial single-photon emission computed tomography (SPECT) demonstrates abnormal activity in segment 4B corresponding to known metastasis on CT.

performed with curative intent, symptom control or prolongation of survival in the palliative setting.

The choice of treatment for NET hepatic metastases is largely dependent on underlying tumour biology and pattern of metastatic spread.[52] The metastatic pattern of spread in the liver for NETs also has prognostic implications and is categorised into three morphological subtypes:[52,53] (I) 'restricted metastases' involving one lobe or two adjacent segments; (II) 'dominant lesion with bilobar metastases' whereby a single major focus is accompanied by multiple contralateral satellite lesions; (III) diffuse, multifocal liver metastases affecting multiple segments within and between lobes. Patients with type I or II disease (25% and 15% of cases, respectively), in the absence of extrahepatic metastases, can be considered for curative surgical resection.[52,53] The aim of liver resection with curative intent in NETs is to leave no residual disease (R0 resection) in both primary and secondary sites, and this may be associated with 5-year survival rates of up to 85%.[42,45]

✅ Hepatic resection for metastatic NETs results in improved overall survival compared to those receiving supportive care. Furthermore, R1 and R2 resections result in 5-year survival rates of 70% and 60%, respectively, challenging the dogma that surgery should be reserved only for patients most likely to have an R0 resection. Cytoreduction aims to reduce tumour volume by at least 90% in situations where R0 resection is not feasible. Although there are no data from randomised trials, large series using historical controls or contemporary cases matched for stage have demonstrated that liver resection with optimal cytoreduction results in improved survival.[54–56] Cytoreduction can also offer effective and durable palliation from symptoms for patients with functional tumour syndromes.[55–57] As a result, surgical debulking has been advocated for both functional and non-functional tumours.[58] An aggressive approach, sometimes combining liver resection with other ablative strategies, is warranted (**Fig. 7.2a,b**). Liver transplantation is an emerging option for NET liver metastases that are otherwise unresectable but is controversial.

Despite resection, hepatic recurrence occurs in up to 84% of patients at 5 years post-surgery.[56] Recurrence is suspected by the elevation of tumour markers such as 5-hydroxyindoleacetic acid (5-HIAA) and chromogranin A. Chromogranin A is more sensitive than 5-HIAA in identifying disease progression and high levels have been shown to predict poorer outcomes. A reduction in chromogranin A levels of >80% predicts a good outcome following cytoreductive hepatectomy, even when complete resection has not been achieved.[59]

Non-surgical treatment modalities used for NET metastases include RFA, TAE and TACE. RFA in isolation can achieve symptomatic relief and local control of variable duration in up to 80% of NET patients with hepatic metastases. Although studies comparing RFA to other modalities are limited, RFA has been advocated in patients with bilobar disease with up to 14 hepatic lesions of <7 cm in diameter, involving up to 20% of liver volume.[46,56] TAE and TACE appear to deliver comparable results and thus one modality is not favoured over the other. Embolisation is usually indicated for more extensive hepatic disease or for tumours in close proximity to biliary structures precluding RFA.[56] Duration of response is routinely short as the tumour rapidly develops collaterals and thus repeat treatments are often required.[58] Embolisation is contraindicated in patients with 50–75% liver involvement due to the risk of precipitating acute hepatic failure. In general, aggressive multimodal therapy with embolic, ablative and systemic strategies is recommended to debulk or downstage metastatic NETs.[58] Symptom control with non-surgical approaches, recognising that repeat treatments may be required, can limit the need for cytoreductive surgery in many patients.

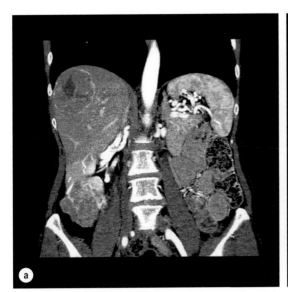
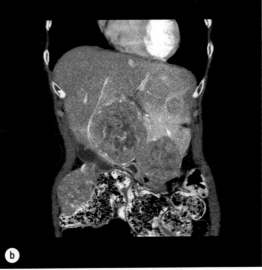

Figure 7.2 • **(a)** A 59-year-old female with an incidental finding of multiple NET metastases. There was no evidence of primary tumour on octreotide scan and endoscopy. Note multiple hypervascular, large metastases with central necrosis. **(b)** Same patient as in **(a)**. A debulking operation to remove 90% of tumour burden would be possible by performing an extended right hepatectomy with wedge resections from segment 2.

Liver transplantation has been advocated for patients with extensive, unresectable liver metastases with no extrahepatic disease. A retrospective study of 150 patients who underwent transplantation for metastatic NET reported 5-year survival comparable to patients with hepatocellular carcinoma.[60] Of those transplanted, patients under the age of 55 without the need for concurrent major resection of the primary tumour had the best overall survival.[9] Concerns remain regarding tumour recurrence in the context of immunosuppression, so while liver transplantation does appear to confer long-term survival in carefully selected patients, optimal patient selection criteria remain in evolution.[61,62].

Gastrointestinal stromal tumours

Gastrointestinal stromal tumours (GIST) are the most common gastrointestinal mesenchymal malignancies and originate from the interstitial cells of Cajal.[63] Approximately 70–80% of GISTs harbour a mutated c-Kit proto-oncogene, which results in the constitutive activation of this receptor tyrosine kinase leading to unregulated cell growth. Two-thirds of c-Kit mutations are located on exon 11.[64] C-Kit exon 9 and PDGFRA mutations, encompassing a wild-type kinase domain that modulates receptor inhibitor sensitivity, account for another 5–10% of GISTs.[65]

Primary GISTs represent 1% of all gastrointestinal malignancies, and arise in the stomach (55–60%), small intestine (30–35%), colon/rectum (5–10%) and oesophagus (5%).[66,67] The primary tumour can be classified into four prognostic categories ranging from very low risk to high risk, according to site of the primary lesion, size of the primary lesion, and the number of mitotic figures identified on histology.[68] Resection remains the standard treatment of primary GIST.

Imatinib mesylate is a selective tyrosine kinase inhibitor that has revolutionised the treatment of GIST.[68] Despite complete surgical resection with microscopic negative margins, recurrence (local or distant) occurs in 50% of patients.[68] The use of imatinib in the adjuvant setting was investigated in the phase III ACOSOG placebo-controlled trial (Z9001) for patients with resected GIST >3 cm in size. A statistically significant 1-year recurrence-free survival (RFS) of 98% in the treatment group versus 83% in the placebo group was observed, prompting the inclusion of imatinib as an adjuvant treatment modality in patients with moderate to high-risk primary tumours.[68] Response to imatinib is greatest in tumours that harbour the c-Kit exon 11 mutation, with resistance rates higher in patients harbouring exon 9 or platelet-derived growth factor receptor α mutations.[68]

The treatment of metastatic and recurrent GIST has similarly been transformed by imatinib. Recurrence of GIST most commonly occurs with one of two metastatic patterns: local recurrence with peritoneal disease or liver metastases.[69] Most patients with recurrent or metastatic GIST will receive imatinib as first-line treatment, with a clinical response demonstrated in 80%. This response is durable with a median survival of 48 months.[70] However, many patients develop imatinib resistance and disease progression caused by the development of secondary mutations.[71] Second- (e.g. sunitinib) and third-line agents (e.g. nilotinib and masitinib) have shown promise in patients resistant to imatinib.[72]

The efficacy and low side-effect profile of imatinib prompted initial enthusiasm for the combined use of surgery and imatinib in the management of metastatic GIST. Although evidence guiding surgical management in metastatic GIST is limited, a study combining neoadjuvant imitanib with surgery and adjuvant imitanib in patients with previous R0 resection of the primary tumour has shown a favourable 3-year survival.[73] A recent Dutch study evaluated 48 patients who underwent liver resection for GIST metastases, 36 of whom received TKI therapy either pre- or postoperatively. Median survival was 7.5 years and 5-year overall survival was 76%. Multivariate analysis demonstrated that R0 resection of the liver metastasis was the only significant predictor of survival.[74] A multicenter European study retrospectively evaluated 239 patients undergoing hepatic metastectomy, all of whom received adjuvant imatinib. R0/R1 resection was found to be a significant predictor of survival and median survival in this group was 8.7 years. Other significant predictors of survival were female gender and metastases confined to the liver (compared to liver plus peritoneum).[75]

> ✓ GIST liver metastases are usually unresectable and therefore imatinib is generally accepted as first-line treatment for metastatic disease. The efficacy and low side-effect profile of imatinib has promoted enthusiasm for the combined use of surgery and imatinib in the management of metastatic GIST. High-quality evidence is lacking but retrospective series studying the combination of surgery with imatinib in patients with resectable metastases demonstrate good results with 5-year survival rates of over 70%.

Disease progression is managed by imatinib dose escalation followed by second- and third-line agents. In the event of tumour rupture or haemorrhage, surgery or hepatic artery embolisation may be performed in an emergency setting. Six to twelve months of imatinib therapy is recommended for patients with unresectable hepatic metastases and if the tumour responds, resection can be considered if an R0 resection can be anticipated.[67]

Breast cancer

The liver is the third most common site of breast cancer metastases after bone and the lungs.[76] The widely held concept that liver metastases in breast cancer reflects diffuse systemic disease has led to a nihilistic view of the role of liver resection in this setting. However, an aggressive surgical approach has been proposed for patients presenting with the liver as the sole site of involvement. The data are mostly retrospective and are based on heterogeneous indications, making it difficult to provide strong evidence-based guidelines.

Although metastatic breast cancer is common, isolated liver lesions in metastatic breast cancer are seen in less than 10% of patients.[77,78] In a Japanese series of 11 000 breast cancer patients treated over an 18-year period only 34 patients had resectable liver metastases.[79] Selection criteria for such metastases are inconsistent in surgical series, with some centres considering resection only for disease confined to the liver while others advocate a more liberal approach. In short, there are no clear selection criteria for resection. Oestrogen receptor-positive primary tumours and a prolonged disease-free interval of >48 months before development of metastases have been associated with improved survival.[76] Response to chemotherapy also appears to be an important predictor of survival. In one study, patients who progressed during prehepatectomy chemotherapy had a 5-year survival rate of 0% compared to 11% in responders.[80] Therefore, surgery should only be considered in patients who have responded to preoperative chemotherapy or hormonal therapy, or both.

> ✅ Isolated liver metastases from breast cancer are rare. Previous response systemic therapy appears to be an important predictor of survival following liver resection for metastatic breast cancer.

A meta-analysis of 36 studies including 1025 patients undergoing liver resection for breast cancer metastases showed a median overall survival of 41 months (data from 25 studies) after curative intent surgery with a median time to recurrence of 11.5 months (from 6 studies).[76,81] Five-year overall survival rates range from 25-60%.[76,79,82–84] Five-year disease-free survival rates are lower than overall survival rates, suggesting that liver resection may function as a cytoreductive rather than curative procedure in these highly selected patients.[76,81]

Most of these data come from retrospective surgical case series. A recent study of patients with isolated hepatic metastases from the Memorial Sloan Kettering Cancer Center compared the outcomes of 69 patients treated with resection or ablation with 98 patients treated with systemic therapy. In this series the median overall survival of the surgical cohort was 50 months, which was similar to the 45 months for the chemotherapy cohort. This finding persisted after propensity score matching of 49 patients in each group. However, 10 (15%) of the surgically treated patients had a disease-free survival of >5 years, indicating there are selected patients who benefit from an aggressive surgical approach.[78] This is reinforced by a French report of 19 patients who underwent repeat hepatectomy for breast cancer metastases with 5-year overall survival (following the second liver resection) of 46% and median survival of 41 months.[85]

Ovarian cancer

Epithelial ovarian cancer represents the most common malignancy of the ovary and cytoreductive surgery and platinum-based chemotherapy are the mainstays of treatment. Unfortunately, most patients develop chemoresistance after 24–36 months and the median survival for advanced disease is 3.5 years.[86–88] Aggressive surgical debulking is advocated in advanced cases, with optimal cytoreduction targeted at <1 cm of residual disease.[89] Intraperitoneal chemotherapy has been demonstrated to further improve survival compared to intravenous therapy and requires optimal debulking in order to be effective.[90] Successful cytoreduction is thus a crucial step in the management of advanced ovarian cancer.

Although the liver is rarely the only site of metastatic disease in ovarian cancer, hepatectomy can be an important component of a primary cytoreduction strategy. Ovarian cancer can involve the liver through the development of peritoneal lesions on the surface of the liver (stage III – **Fig. 7.3**) or intraparenchymal metastases (stage IV – **Fig. 7.4**). Survival is improved for patients with stage IV disease who have undergone adequate debulking surgery including hepatectomy.[91,92] Peritoneal metastases that invade the liver parenchyma may be difficult to distinguish from parenchymal metastases that spread haematogenously and can reflect different disease biology and response to therapy, including liver resection.[87,88] If this distinction can be made preoperatively those with haematogenous liver metastases can be considered to have advanced disease (similar to those with pulmonary metastases) and are treated with palliative systemic therapy rather than surgery.[87,88]

Survival following primary surgical debulking is inversely correlated with volume of residual disease, disease stage and tumour differentiation. Similarly, survival following hepatectomy for recurrent disease is dependent on optimal cytoreduction, negative margin status, greater pelvic than abdominal disease and a longer recurrence-free interval.[93] It has been demonstrated that when complete cytoreduction of

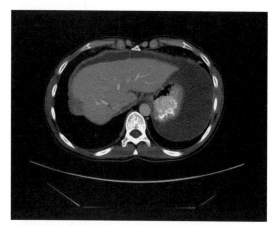

Figure 7.3 • Stage III ovarian cancer with hepatic involvement. Note direct invasion of liver capsule by peritoneal tumour plaque.

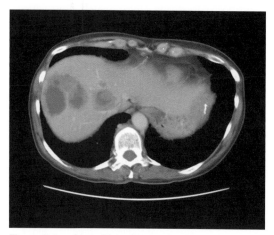

Figure 7.4 • Stage IV ovarian cancer with intraparenchymal liver metastases.

recurrent disease is possible hepatic resection should be considered as the median survival is improved.[87] TACE and RFA offer potential alternative therapeutic options in achieving local control in patients with contraindications to resection or as adjuncts to systemic therapy.[87,94]

Renal cell carcinoma

Approximately 20–30% of patients with renal cell carcinoma (RCC) present with synchronous metastatic disease and another 20–40% of patients with previous nephrectomy will develop metastatic disease.[95,96] Fewer than 5% of patients have metastases restricted to the liver and liver metastases portend a poor prognosis of 7–12 months.[97,98] Systemic therapy options for RCC are limited. Interleukin-2 and interferon-α were previously used as first-line therapy for metastatic

RCC and were not found to be active against liver metastases.[98,99] Current regimens employ tyrosine kinase inhibitors like sunitinib, which is associated with an improved progression-free survival in phase III trials, and emerging data suggest that immune checkpoint inhibitors are effective in metastatic RCC.[99,100]

The available data on hepatic resection for RCC metastases are limited to retrospective reports. A study from the Netherlands examined 33 patients who underwent resection or ablative therapy for RCC hepatic metastases. The study documented no operative mortality, with 5-year disease-free and overall survival of 11% and 43%, respectively. The median overall survival was 33 months.[95] A second retrospective study compared 68 patients who underwent surgery to a cohort of 20 patients who were eligible but refused an operation. Disease in these patients was mostly confined to the liver. Overall 5-year survival in the treatment arm was 62% in comparison to 29% in the control group.[101] A review of six studies including 140 patients who underwent liver resections reported 5-year overall survival rates ranging between 34% and 43% and a median survival of 16–48 months.[96] Factors associated with better survival included metachronous metastases, R0 metastectomy and non-sarcomatoid histology.[95,96,98,101]

More contemporary series have examined liver resection for RCC metastases in the context of TKI use. In one series of 39 patients undergoing liver resection (37 patients) or ablation (2 patients) the overall median survival was 42 months. During a median follow-up period of 2.2 years, 74% of patients who received no targeted therapy recurred, compared to 40% of patients, maintained on postoperative treatment. Multivariate analysis identified postoperative TKI therapy as a predictor of survival.[102] Preoperative TKI therapy has also been shown to downsize unresectable RCC liver metastases in order to facilitate safe liver resection.[103]

Melanoma

The prognosis for patients with metastatic melanoma is poor and the median survival for patients with stage IV disease has historically been 6–9 months.[104] Gastrointestinal and liver metastases occur in 2–4% of individuals with stage IV disease,[105] and palliative radiotherapy and systemic chemotherapy have largely been ineffective in conferring a survival advantage. Biological agents such as interferon-α and interleukin-2 have yielded modest response rates that are rarely durable and are associated with significant toxicity.[104] Favourable results in patients undergoing metastasectomy in the lung, soft tissues or abdomen have provided some enthusiasm for surgery in a selected patient population.

The available evidence for hepatectomy for metastatic melanoma is limited and consists largely of subset analyses from larger series of patients with non-CRLM. One retrospective study evaluated all patients who presented with metastatic melanoma over the last decade at a single Australian institution. In this series, 13 patients underwent resection for liver metastases. Median disease-free interval from resection of the primary was 49 months, median disease-free survival was 14 months and median overall survival was 21 months.[105] An American series of 24 patients undergoing liver resection had similar results with a reported median disease-free survival of 12 months and median overall survival of 28 months.[106]

The biological behaviour of metastatic melanoma depends in part on the site of origin of the primary tumour.[107] Cutaneous melanoma is more common than ocular melanoma.[108] While both metastasise to the liver, they appear to do so with distinct patterns and natural history. Ocular melanoma metastasises to the liver more frequently, and is more likely to be associated with isolated liver metastases than cutaneous melanoma.[107,108] Survival following hepatectomy appears to be more favourable in this highly selected but rare group of patients with melanoma of ocular origin. Pawlik et al. reported a 5-year survival rate of 21% for liver resection for ocular melanoma, with a 0% 5-year survival rate for cutaneous melanoma. However, 75% of resected patients in this study developed recurrent disease, and the rate of recurrence was similar between the ocular and cutaneous groups.[108]

Liver resection with postoperative tumour infiltrating lymphocyte (TIL) therapy has been explored. TIL involves resection of metastatic lesions followed by extraction and culture of infiltrating lymphocytes ex vivo with interleukin-2. A direct comparison was performed between patients with complete surgical resection versus those with residual hepatic disease receiving postoperative TIL. The observed 3-year overall survival was 53% in the TIL cohort, with prognosis largely favoured by lack of extrahepatic disease and a single hepatic metastasis.[109]

New molecular therapies have become standard of care in treatment of metastatic melanoma. BRAF and MEK inhibitors (e.g. vemurafenib and trametinib, respectively) are used for patients with tumour mutations in the *BRAF* gene. Imatinib has been used in patients with tumours harbouring mutations in the *KIT* gene. Immunomodulators targeting CTLA-4 (e.g. ipilimumab) and PD-1 (e.g. nivolumab) are used increasingly in all patients with advanced melanoma. These agents collectively have improved overall survival for patients with advanced melanoma compared to interleukin-2 and conventional cytotoxic chemotherapy.[110] The widespread use of these agents may lead to an increased number of patients referred for consideration for resection of isolated hepatic metastases. It is difficult to estimate the impact that liver resection will have on these patients, but it seems reasonable to adopt a resectional approach in highly selected patients, i.e. those with a long disease-free interval from treatment of the primary tumour to development of metastases, and patients who can be rendered disease-free following surgery.

Non-colorectal gastrointestinal adenocarcinoma

Liver metastases from non-colorectal gastrointestinal (GI) adenocarcinomas can arise from the oesophagus, stomach, pancreas, gallbladder, ampulla of Vater, small bowel and bile duct. Hepatic resection has generally been considered to be contraindicated in these cases.

Oesophagus

Metastatic oesophageal cancer is usually widely disseminated and is associated with a 5-year survival of 3–5% when multiple sites of disease are present and 7–8% when disease is limited to the liver.[111] Two case reports in the English-language literature describe hepatectomy for isolated, synchronous liver metastases.[112,113] In both cases hepatectomy was performed simultaneously with oesophagectomy and was followed by hepatic arterial chemotherapy. Both patients developed multiple liver metastases at 6 and 7 months postoperatively. These recurrences responded partially to systemic chemotherapy, and the patients were alive with disease at 14 and 18 months following hepatectomy. A report of four cases of liver resection for metachronous oesophageal cancer metastases has also been published. All patients received chemotherapy before liver resection. Two patients died at 10 and 21 months following liver resection, one was alive at 22 months, and one patient had prolonged survival of 92 months after chemotherapy and liver resection.[114] Thus, although rarely feasible, hepatectomy may provide a limited survival benefit in chemosensitive oesophageal cancer with isolated liver metastases. Given the small number of cases in the literature, liver resection in this context should be offered rarely and only in highly selected patients.

Stomach

Gastric adenocarcinoma is the second most common cause of cancer-related death worldwide, and the liver is a major site of spread in 9–40%, though in most cases the metastatic pattern is diffuse involving the peritoneum and distant lymph nodes.[115-118] Overall 5-year survival in patients with liver metastases ranges from 0 to 10% and surgery has historically been contraindicated. There is some emerging literature that liver resection or ablation may provide a therapeutic benefit in the rare situation when hepatic metastases are isolated. A meta-analysis of 23 retrospective studies including 802 patients reported a 5-year overall survival of 23.8% and a median survival of 22 months.[117] Size and number of hepatic metastases correlated with overall survival. A subsequent meta-analysis of 39 studies (many the same as in the previous study) including 909 patients had similar findings: 27.8% overall 5-year survival and median overall survival of 29 months with better outcomes seen in Asian studies compared to Western series.[119]

A Japanese group reported on their experience using an aggressive approach to gastric cancer liver metastasis, adopting the same patient selection criteria as for CRLM. Median recurrence-free survival was similar between both groups (15.2 months for CRLM versus 16.4 months for gastric cancer metastases), while the 5-year overall survival in patients with CRC (193 patients) was 55% compared to 14% in patients with gastric cancer (26 patients). Metachronous metastases, solitary metastasis and moderate or well-differentiated tumours were associated with longer survival in the gastric cancer group.[118] A second Japanese group restricted liver resection to those patients with three or fewer metastases. In their series of 28 patients, overall 5-year survival was 32% and median survival was 49 months.[120] A contemporary series of 94 patients from 28 Japanese hospitals used a mix of resection and ablation for liver-only gastric metastases. They reported a 5-year overall survival rate of 42.3% with no differences between resection, ablation, or combined approaches for the liver metastases. Patients with solitary liver metastases and <3 positive lymph nodes had an improved survival.[121]

The Italian Research Group for Gastric Cancer has recently advocated resection of synchronous hepatic metastases if an R0 resection can be performed of both the primary and the metastases.[116,122] A cohort of 53 patients who underwent curative intent synchronous R0 resection had a median survival of 13 months and a 5-year overall survival rate of 9.3%. This was significantly improved compared to a median survival of 6.6 months in 98 contemporary patients undergoing palliative gastrectomy and a 3-month median survival for 44 patients who underwent surgical bypass.

These results suggest that a highly selected subset of patients with gastric cancer liver metastases can achieve long-term survival with an aggressive surgical approach. Whether Asian results can be extrapolated to Western populations remains unclear.

Small bowel

Primary small-bowel malignancies represent an exceedingly rare but histologically diverse subgroup accounting for 2% of all GI malignancies.[123] Small-bowel adenocarcinoma (SBA) represents the majority of these tumours and is seen in up to 5% of patients with familial adenomatous polyposis (FAP). By virtue of its non-specific clinical presentation and the limitations of radiological and endoscopic diagnostic modalities to examine the small bowel, approximately 80% of patients present with advanced disease. In addition, the low prevalence of SBA limits our understanding of the natural history of tumour spread, restricting the development of clear treatment guidelines. A multicentre retrospective French study examining the efficacy of chemotherapy in 93 patients with advanced SBA, compared various chemotherapeutic regimens for progression-free survival (PFS) and overall survival (OS). Median PFS and OS were 6.6 and 15.1 months, respectively, with best outcomes seen with FOLFOX.[85] Negative prognostic factors include a poor baseline WHO performance status, elevated carbohydrate antigen (CA) 19-9/carcinoembryonic antigen (CEA) levels and the presence of a duodenal primary. The ability of surgery to prolong PFS in hepatic SBA metastases has only been described in a single case report of an FAP patient with a PFS of 3 years following neoadjuvant chemotherapy and surgery.[123] Future studies examining liver resections in metastatic SBA will provide further guidance as to its role in this disease. At present metastectomy should be considered contraindicated.

Pancreas

Pancreatic ductal adenocarcinoma (PDAC) accounts for 90% of all histological subtypes of pancreatic cancer and confers a poor overall prognosis.[124] Over the last 50 years, PDAC has continued to rank as the tenth most common cancer in the Western world and the fourth leading cause of cancer death. PDAC presents in a non-specific manner, often when disease is already at an advanced stage. Improvements in chemotherapy, surgical technique and knowledge of tumour biology have translated into marginal improvements in survival. Currently, only 15–20% of patients present with disease amenable to curative resection, of whom 20% are alive at 5 years.[124] The overall average 5-year survival for unresectable PDAC is 5%, with a median survival of 8–11 months for patients with metastatic disease receiving chemotherapy.[124–126] Due to the dismal prognosis in patients with localised resectable disease, surgery for metastatic PDAC has been contraindicated. Yamada et al. examined the role of hepatectomy in non-neuroendocrine pancreatic cancer, including five patients with PDAC, one with adenosquamous carcinoma and one with cystadenocarcinoma.[127] Patients were chosen for surgery if complete excision of hepatic disease was deemed feasible, reliable control of the primary disease was possible and the liver was the only site of spread. Overall 5-year survival in this cohort was 16.7%; however, five patients developed recurrence and subsequently died of their disease within 4–52 months. Prognostic factors appear to correlate with disease-free interval from primary to metastases and the presence of negative surgical margins at metastasectomy.[127] A study of 69 patients from six European centres evaluated synchronous pancreas and liver resections for patients with PDAC and isolated hepatic metastases. Outcomes were compared with 69 matched patients who did not undergo resection and median survival was greater in the resection group (14.5 months vs 7.5 months). Four patients were alive longer than 5 years in the resection group compared to none in the non-resection group.[128] Although these authors highlight the potential role of liver resection in metastatic PDAC there is need for future studies to clarify the true benefit of this approach and identification of factors that can assist clinicians in selecting patients appropriately. Molecular stratification biomarkers may prove useful in this rare setting.[10,129]

The available evidence for hepatectomy in the management of metastases from non-colorectal, non-neuroendocrine GI primaries is limited, and few meaningful statements can be made as to the utility of this treatment strategy. Gastric cancer specifically may be the exception to this with some encouraging reports from Asia of acceptable survival after liver resection from multiple centres. With improvements in safety of liver resection coupled with encouraging results from other malignancies metastasising to the liver, future prospective studies will shed light on the role of hepatic resection for non-colorectal, non-neuroendocrine GI cancers.

> ✅ The available evidence for hepatectomy in the management of metastases from non-colorectal, non-neuroendocrine GI primaries is limited, and few meaningful statements can be made as to the utility of this treatment strategy. There is emerging evidence from both Asia and Europe that acceptable results can be achieved for highly selected patients undergoing liver resection for gastric cancer metastases.

Testicular cancer

Metastasectomy is well established in the management of disseminated non-seminomatous germ cell testicular carcinoma that does not completely respond to chemotherapy, though isolated liver metastases are rare.[130] One series of 15 patients reported an overall 10-year survival of 62% after resection of hepatic metastases.[131]

A single institution experience of 57 liver resections performed over the last two decades demonstrated that surgery for hepatic metastases is safe and efficacious. Based on the presence and histological type of tumour in the liver, 40–70% of patients remain disease-free at 20 months.[132] Negative prognostic indicators included viable tumour in the resected specimen, metastases >3 cm in diameter and pure embryonal carcinoma in the primary lesion.

Urothelial cancer

Data for metastasectomy in the management of disseminated urothelial cancer are sparse, and no studies specifically address the role of hepatectomy. Of those patients treated for primary urothelial cancer, 30% will recur, of which 75% will have distant spread. Five-year survival of 28% has been reported following resection of lung, brain, adrenal, small-bowel or lymph node metastases with variation in the use of adjuvant chemotherapy.[133] Metastasectomy has also been employed for palliation.

Lung cancer

The management of metastatic lung cancer is largely restricted to radiation and chemotherapy. Although the surgical management of hepatic metastases remains controversial, most cases have been reviewed within the broader context of non-colorectal, non-neuroendocrine GI tumours. Hepatic metastases appear most commonly in right-sided non-small-cell lung tumours with concomitant bone metastases. A small case series of highly selected patients with one or two liver lesions has shown that surgery may confer a marginal survival benefit.[134] Nevertheless, the role of surgery as well as other treatment modalities (RFA, TAE/TACE) cannot be definitively made with current evidence. Recent advances in targeted therapy and immunotherapy may guide decision-making in the future in this context.[135]

Adrenocortical tumours

Adrenocortical tumours with liver metastases are rare, and literature on the management of this disease scenario is mostly anecdotal. Case reports have provided no clear guidance regarding the role of surgical or ablative strategies but disease control after resection of hepatic metastases has been reported.[136] Metachronous liver metastases with a disease-free interval >1 year from primary to metastasis may derive benefit from metastectomy.[137]

Endometrial cancer

Metastatic endometrial cancer is usually multifocal and rarely managed operatively. A single-centre report described the results of five patients who developed metastatic disease to the liver ranging from 11 months to 10 years after primary resection. All patients underwent hepatic surgery, with disease-free survival of 8–66 months. Based on these results, the authors advocate referral to a hepatobiliary specialist with the intent of pursuing surgery.[138] Other isolated reports of long-term survivors exist within the context of larger studies focused on NCRNNET hepatic metastases.

Conclusion

The success of an aggressive surgical approach in the management of CRLM has, in part, provided the impetus for liver resection for non-CRLM. As experience with liver resection has increased, with an improved safety profile, enthusiasm for performing metastectomy for non-colorectal primaries has also increased. Extrapolating surgical strategies from one malignancy to another is reasonable in some cases; however, fundamental biological differences between various neoplasms require thoughtful consideration of differences in the natural history and non-surgical treatment modalities that are available for each tumour site. Unfortunately, strong evidence-based data are lacking and it is therefore necessary for the treating surgeon to have a good working knowledge of the biology and management of various malignancies. In most cases, this is augmented by the multidisciplinary tumour board and a critical mass of subspecialists to assist in decision-making. Multidisciplinary review with experts in both hepatectomy and management of the primary tumour type should therefore be considered mandatory before performing liver resection for non-CRLM.

It is worth emphasising that, in most cases, liver metastasectomy should be performed with curative intent. The case for resection of breast cancer metastases is evolving, with some liver surgeons advocating resection in a selected patient population responsive to preoperative chemotherapy. There is no strong evidence that non-curative intent surgery is helpful for patients with liver metastases from gastrointestinal tract primaries, with the possible exception of gastric cancer as discussed above.

The presence of extrahepatic disease is almost always a contraindication to liver resection, except within the context of a prospective trial or for specific malignancies such as ovarian cancer and neuroendocrine tumours. The critical variables that usually predict cure after liver resection of secondary cancer of almost all types include prolonged disease-free interval from resection of the primary tumour, negative resection margins, additional complementary systemic treatment options and performance status.

Future efforts should be directed toward the conduct of randomised trials designed to test the role of liver surgery for the common non-colorectal malignancies, and the discovery of genetic signatures and other biomarkers.

Key points

- The majority of patients with non-CRLM have disseminated disease and are not candidates for hepatectomy.
- Treatment decisions must take into account clinical surrogates of tumour biology. Patients with synchronous liver metastases, a short disease-free interval and extrahepatic disease are believed to have more aggressive tumours and are less likely to gain significant survival benefit from liver resection.
- With few exceptions, liver resection for metastatic disease should be performed with curative intent. The ability to achieve negative resection margins is a significant prognostic factor.
- Debulking surgery including liver resection has been shown to significantly improve survival in metastatic NETs. Aggressive cytoreduction, often using a multimodality approach, is indicated in most cases of metastatic NETs.
- Cytoreduction including hepatectomy, followed by intraperitoneal chemotherapy, appears to improve survival in stage III/IV ovarian adenocarcinoma.
- Patients with breast cancer liver metastases that respond to preoperative chemotherapy appear to gain a survival benefit from hepatectomy.
- Level I and II evidence regarding hepatectomy for the treatment of non-CRLM is lacking, and the indications for surgery are evolving.
- It behooves the surgical oncologist to keep abreast of the explosion of recent advances in systemic and biologic therapies, such as immunotherapy, to ensure proper selection of patients who will benefit from liver resection for non-traditional indications.

References available at **http://expertconsult. inkling.com**

8

Portal hypertension and liver transplantation

Stephen O'Neill
Gabriel C. Oniscu

Introduction

In recent years the surgical management of portal hypertension and its complications has largely been replaced by less invasive endoscopic and radiological treatments. Surgery, however, still has a role for patients with extrahepatic portal hypertension and those who are suitable candidates for liver transplantation (which can cure the underlying liver disease).

Acute variceal bleeding can also present to surgical teams either directly as an undifferentiated gastrointestinal haemorrhage or following referral from gastrointestinal bleeding services. It is therefore crucial that all surgeons have an understanding of portal hypertension pathophysiology and the management options for various presentations and complications.

Pharmacotherapy, endoscopic band ligation (EBL) and radiological treatment with transjugular intrahepatic portosystemic shunt (TIPSS) are the most common treatment modalities for variceal bleeding. However, where adequate surgical expertise exists, portosystemic shunts can still be considered an option for refractory bleeding in patients without significant liver failure, particularly when less invasive modalities are unavailable or contraindicated. Liver transplantation is the definitive treatment for portal hypertension but is restricted to patients with chronic liver disease who fulfil listing criteria and reflects the severity of underlying liver pathology rather than the extent of portal hypertension and the impact of previous therapy options.

This chapter will discuss the aetiology, pathophysiology, presentation, evaluation and management of portal hypertension as well as its complications. There will be a specific focus on treating varices and the surgical options for portal hypertension (including shunts and liver transplantation). Evidence-based guidance will be provided for key clinical scenarios as well as less common presentations such as portal hypertensive gastropathy, segmental portal hypertension, Budd–Chiari syndrome and portal vein thrombosis.

Aetiology

Portal hypertension is initiated by an increased vascular resistance to the blood flow within the portal system that leads to an increase in portal blood pressure (normal pressure range 5–10 mmHg). Depending on the anatomical location within the portal system where the resistance to portal flow occurs, the aetiology of portal hypertension is traditionally subdivided into prehepatic (at the level of the splenic, mesenteric or prehepatic portal vein), intrahepatic (within the liver) or posthepatic (at the level of the hepatic venous outflow). Sinusoids are low-pressure channels within the liver that receive blood flow from portal venous and hepatic artery tributaries. Intrahepatic conditions that lead to portal hypertension can be further subdivided into presinusoidal, sinusoidal and postsinusoidal causes (**Fig. 8.1**). However, this division is an oversimplification as many liver conditions are associated with high portal pressure at more than one level. Notable exceptions are schistosomiasis, sarcoidosis and congenital hepatic fibrosis that affect the presinusoidal sector and have preserved

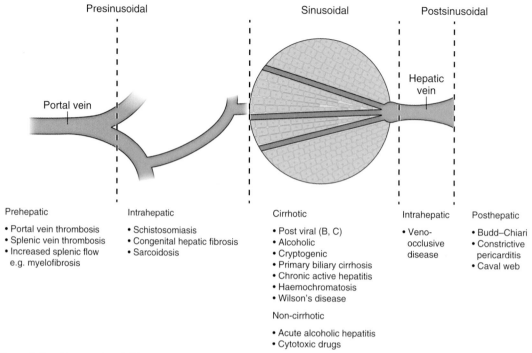

Figure 8.1 • Causes of portal hypertension.

hepatocellular architecture and therefore normal liver function.

The prehepatic causes of portal hypertension include thrombosis of the portal, mesenteric and splenic veins or extrinsic compression of the portal vein itself (e.g. by tumour or lymph nodes). Posthepatic causes of portal hypertension are rare and include thrombosis of the hepatic veins (Budd–Chiari syndrome) or inferior vena cava, as well as cardiac causes such as right heart failure and constrictive pericarditis.[1] Intrahepatic causes of portal hypertension are by far the most common. In the Western world, liver cirrhosis resulting in sinusoidal obstruction and increased vascular resistance is responsible for portal hypertension in 90% of cases. Viral hepatitis and alcoholic liver disease are the principal causes of liver cirrhosis, but other common causes include haemochromatosis, primary biliary cirrhosis and primary sclerosing cholangitis. The main cause of postsinusoidal portal hypertension is veno-occlusive disease, which can occur following treatment with oxaliplatin-based chemotherapy agents (e.g. for colorectal liver metastases) or following cytoreductive therapy for haematopoietic stem cell transplantation.

Definition of portal hypertension

The pressure gradient between the hepatic and portal vein is known as the hepatic venous pressure gradient (HVPG) (normal range 3–5 mmHg).[1] Measurement of the HVPG is an indirect measure of portal pressure but presently is the best available technique to assess the presence of portal hypertension and its severity.[2] The HPVG is not routinely measured in clinical practice because it is an invasive interventional radiological procedure that requires both resources and experienced staff to perform hepatic vein catheterisation.[3] However, a HPVG of >5 mmHg defines the presence of portal hypertension.[1] Complications of portal hypertension start to occur once the HPVG is >10 mmHg.[2]

✅ An HVPG >12 mmHg is the threshold for variceal bleeding and ascites.[4] Studies demonstrate that when treatment reduces HVPG to <12 mmHg, variceal bleeding is prevented and varices may decrease in size or disappear altogether.[5] When this target is not reached, a substantial reduction in HPVG by more than 20% still offers protection against variceal bleeding.[6]

Therefore, these two parameters are regarded as the endpoints of therapeutic strategies to lower portal pressure. Patients meeting these parameters are said to be 'HVPG responders'. Current evidence suggests that these therapeutic endpoints may also minimise the risk of other complications of portal hypertension, including ascites, spontaneous bacterial peritonitis and hepatorenal syndrome.[7,8]

Pathophysiology

Portal hypertension arises from (a) an increase in resistance to portal blood flow and (b) an increase in the inflow of portal blood.[9] Distortion of liver architecture by cirrhosis primarily causes a passive increase in the resistance to portal blood flow. Secondly, there is an associated rise in hepatic vascular tone that dynamically increases hepatic vascular resistance to portal blood flow.[10] Increased intrahepatic tone is believed to be a result of imbalances between elevated endogenous vasoconstrictors and a relative decrease in the endogenous vasodilator nitric oxide.[11] An increase in the inflow of portal blood is caused by progressive splanchnic vasodilatation, which is also associated with hyperdynamic systemic circulation. Pharmacological therapy for portal hypertension, such as terlipressin and non-selective beta-blockers, is aimed at reducing the increased splanchnic blood flow.[12]

Decompression of the increased pressure in the portal vein results in shunting of up to 90% of portal blood flow back to the heart through portosystemic collaterals.[13] Potentially troublesome collaterals develop at various watershed areas between the portal venous and systemic venous circulation.[1] These areas include the cardia (between intrinsic and extrinsic gastro-oesophageal veins); the stomach (from enlargement of peripheral venous tributaries of the left gastric, short gastric and gastroepiploic veins); the falciform ligament (through paraumbilical veins, which are recanalised remnants of the umbilical circulation of the fetus); the retroperitoneal tissues (through mesenteric or peritoneal venous tributaries communicating with retroperitoneal veins, e.g. gonadal, lumbar, or paraduodenal veins); and the anal canal (where the superior haemorrhoidal vein belonging to the portal system anastomoses with the middle and inferior haemorrhoidal veins which belong to the caval system).[1,14]

Of relevance to the surgeon, oesophageal and gastric varices can rupture leading to acute gastrointestinal bleeding. Periumbilical collaterals of enlarged veins in the falciform ligament ('caput medusae') may bleed during abdominal surgery. Stomal and parastomal varices can develop secondary to venous communications between the surgically relocated mesenteric veins of the bowel and the cutaneous veins that drain into the inferior epigastric veins.[1] Finally, anorectal varices can be identified during the course of lower gastrointestinal investigations and although they rarely cause bleeding, can be life-threatening in severe cases.[15]

Natural history

Gastro-oesophageal varices are present in approximately half of cirrhotic patients.[9,16] In patients with portal hypertension, gastric varices are less prevalent (5–33% of patients).[17] After the initial diagnosis of cirrhosis, varices occur with an incidence of 5% per year[18] and the incidence is higher in decompensated (60%) versus compensated liver disease (40%).[19]

In unselected patients, the incidence of variceal bleeding is roughly 20–30% after 2 years of follow-up.[20] The risk of bleeding from oesophageal varices is higher if the HVPG is >12 mmHg and in larger varices (defined by a diameter of >5 mm on endoscopic assessment).[4,21,22] The rate of progression from small to large varices is approximately 10–15% per year.[18]

Initial mortality from uncontrolled bleeding is 6–8% but in the 6 weeks following the primary bleed the mortality rate increases to 25–30%.[20] Mortality from variceal bleeding is associated with liver function; patients with a more advanced liver failure having a mortality risk of 30–50% at 6 weeks.[23]

After an initial variceal bleed when no treatment has been instigated, the risk of re-bleeding is 60% and mortality risk is 40–50% after 1–2 years.[20] Therefore, surveillance and treatment to prevent re-bleeding are mandatory and supported by current guidance.[14] Re-bleeding risk reduces substantially in 'HVPG responders'. These patients also have a lower risk of spontaneous bacterial peritonitis, ascites and reduced mortality.[24]

Severity of liver disease

The incidence of varices, the risk of bleeding and mortality risk following a variceal bleed are associated with the severity of liver disease.[19,23,25] Liver dysfunction has traditionally been classified using the Child–Pugh score, which along with bilirubin, albumin and prothrombin includes subjective interpretation of the grading of ascites and encephalopathy (both of which can be altered by therapy)[26] (Table 8.1).

The Model for End-stage Liver Disease (MELD) includes only objective measures of total serum bilirubin, serum creatinine and prothrombin time and may be a superior prognostic indicator[27] (Box 8.1). Initially developed as a predictor of short-term post-TIPSS survival in patients with variceal bleeding, MELD scoring is now widely used to list and rank patients for liver transplantation.[28] In the UK, the UKELD score (which includes sodium in addition to the MELD variables) is used for similar purposes and is more discriminative with regards

Table 8.1 • Child–Pugh classification

Measure	Points		
	1	**2**	**3**
Bilirubin (mmol/L)*	<34	34-50	>50
Albumin (g/L)	>35	28-35	<28
Prothrombin time (s prolonged)	<4	4-6	>6
Encephalopathy	None	Mild	Marked
Ascites	None	Mild	Marked

Grade A 5–6 points; Grade B 7–9 points; Grade C 10–15 points.
*In primary biliary cirrhosis, the point scoring for bilirubin level is adjusted as follows: 1 = <68, 2 = 68–170, 3 = >170.

to mortality 1-year post-liver transplant. Therefore, candidates for transplantation must have an expected mortality without transplantation >9%, which corresponds to a UKELD score >49 in order to be waitlisted.[29] Liver transplantation is discussed further at the end of the chapter.

Presentation

Portal hypertension can present with acute and life-threatening variceal bleeding. Varices are usually diagnosed at endoscopy. A classification of the grading of gastro-oesophageal and gastric varices is detailed in Table 8.2. Non-emergency presentation of patients with portal hypertension is variable and ranges from non-specific malaise, anorexia and weight loss associated with chronic liver disease to advanced encephalopthy with decompensation. Dysarthria, characterised by imprecise articulation and confusion or aggression, may point to encephalopathy and is secondary to an increased level of toxins such as ammonia in the systemic circulation. Predisposing or exacerbating factors for encephalopathy include portosystemic shunts (spontaneous and surgically or radiologically created), constipation and gastrointestinal haemorrhage (with resultant increases in the absorption of nitrogenous products).

On clinical examination, signs of advanced liver disease may include jaundice, spider naevi, palmar

Box 8.1 • Model for End-stage Liver Disease (MELD)

MELD is calculated for patients over the age of 12 based on the following variables:
- Serum creatinine (mg/dL)
- Total bilirubin (mg/dL)
- INR (international normalised ratio)

The formula incorporates these variables as:

$$MELD = 3.78 \left[Ln \, serum \, bilirubin \, (mg/dL) \right] + 11.2 \left[Ln \, INR \right] + 9.57 \left[Ln \, serum \, creatinine \, (mg/dL) \right] + 6.43$$

The following rules must be observed when using this formula:

1. 1 is the minimum acceptable value for any of the three variables.
2. The maximum acceptable value for serum creatinine is 4.
3. The maximum value for the MELD score is 40. All values higher than 40 are given a score of 40.
4. If the patient has been dialysed twice within the last 7 days, then the value for serum creatinine used should be 4.0.

In being considered for liver transplantation, patients with a diagnosis of liver cancer are assigned a MELD score based on how advanced the cancer is, using the TNM staging system.

Table 8.2 • Classification of oesophageal and gastric varices

Oesophageal varices	Grade 0 (absent)	
	Grade 1 (small)	Varices that collapse on insufflation of oesophagus with air
	Grade 2 (medium)	Varices that do not collapse on air insufflation
	Grade 3 (large)	Varices that are large enough to occlude the lumen
Gastric varices	GOV1	Gastro-oesophageal varices extending <5 cm from the oesophagus across gastro-oesophageal junction
	GOV2	Gastro-oesophageal varices extending into the fundus across gastro-oesophageal junction
	IGV1	Isolated gastric varices in the fundus
	IGV2	Isolated non-fundic varices

erythema and ascites. Ascites is due to increased formation of hepatic and splanchnic lymph, hypoalbuminaemia, as well as retention of salt and water due to increased aldosterone and antidiuretic hormone levels. Some patients may have dilated umbilical vein collaterals ('caput medusae'). Splenomegaly can also occur as a result of vascular engorgement. An important but rare form, segmental (also known as left upper quadrant or' 'sinistral') portal hypertension, occurs in patients with splenic vein thrombosis. This should be suspected in patients with bleeding varices but normal liver function, particularly if there is a history of either acute or chronic pancreatitis. On initial blood investigations, serum bilirubin may be elevated and serum albumin decreased. Haematological consequences of hypersplenism include anaemia, thrombocytopenia and leucopenia.

Evaluation

The American Association for the Study of Liver Diseases (AASLD) and British Society of Gastroenterology (BSG) recommend screening endoscopy as the gold standard investigation for varices once diagnosis of cirrhosis is established.[9,14] Doppler ultrasonography is a useful initial imaging modality, which can determine spleen size as well as liver structure together with portal vein patency, hepatic vein patency and flow velocity. Transient elastography (FibroScan, Echosens, Paris, France) is a non-invasive technique that uses the principles of ultrasound to derive tissue stiffness in the liver by measuring the speed of propagation of a low-frequency wave, which then correlates with liver fibrosis. A low liver stiffness on transient elastography combined with a platelet count >120000/μL is reported as having a negative predictive value for oesophageal varices approaching 100%.[30,31] However, there is a lack of consistent results with this technique and recent guidelines suggest that transient elastography may be more useful for predicting decompensation in patients with cirrhosis.[14] Capsule endoscopy is not considered an alternative to standard endoscopy but it could have a role in patients who cannot tolerate endoscopy.[14] Invasive angiography is no longer required to delineate vascular anatomy as sufficient clarity can be provided non-invasively by computed tomography (CT) and magnetic resonance imaging (MRI) angiography.

Management

The management of portal hypertension and gastro-oesophageal varices includes first-line (pharmacotherapy and endoscopy) and second-line (TIPSS and surgical shunts) options. The following section will discuss the role of these options (with supporting evidence) in the context of three key clinical scenarios:

1. the prevention of bleeding in patients with varices who have never bled;
2. the emergency management of an acute variceal bleeding episode;
3. prophylaxis against further bleeding episodes in those with a history of bleeding.

It should be noted that while the emergency management of many patients could initially begin in a district general hospital setting, patients may require referral to specialist centres with expertise in liver diseases and access to interventional radiology.

First line therapy options

Pharmacotherapy

Pharmacological treatment can be used for primary prophylaxis of bleeding or to treat active haemorrhage.

> ✅✅ A meta-analysis has indicated that ongoing treatment with non-cardioselective beta-blockers (propanolol or nadolol) significantly reduces the bleeding risk from 25% to 15% over a median follow-up period of 24 months but with no significant reduction in mortality.[18] The benefit of therapy was only proven in patients with grade II (or larger) varices and there was no evidence to support the use of primary prophylactic therapy in patients with grade I varices.

In the primary prophylaxis of variceal bleeding, currently propranolol is the favoured option followed by carvedilol or nadolol as alternatives.[14] A single-centre randomised controlled trial (RCT) of carvedilol versus EBL for primary prophylaxis reported significantly reduced bleeding with carvedilol (10% vs 23%, $P = 0.04$), with no effect on survival; however, a second multicentre RCT did not show any differences in bleeding or mortality.[32,33] Further studies comparing the efficacy of carvedilol and propranolol have been suggested.[14] Assessment of the success of primary prophylactic therapy is ideally undertaken by measurement of the HVPG before and after initiating prophylaxis, the aim being to induce a 'HVPG response' (HVPG <12 mmHg or reduction by >20%).[5] In practice, however, measurement of HVPG is invasive, requires specific training and is probably not cost-effective for assessing primary prophylactic treatment. Therefore the dose of beta-blocker is titrated to the maximum tolerated or a heart rate of 50–55 beats per minute. Nitrates are not recommended for prophylaxis either alone or in combination with beta-blockers.[14]

In terms of acute bleeding, a number of RCTs have demonstrated that early administration of vasoactive drugs facilitates endoscopy, improves control of bleeding and reduces the 5-day re-bleeding rate.[34,35] Therefore, all patients with acute variceal bleeding should receive splanchnic vasoconstrictors (terlipressin or somatostatin) as soon as variceal bleeding is suspected and this should be continued until haemostasis is achieved or for up to 5 days following the index bleed.[14]

> ✔✔ Antibiotics providing Gram-negative cover are recommended for all patients with suspected or confirmed variceal bleeding as a Cochrane meta-analysis of 12 placebo-controlled trials found improved survival (relative risk=0.79, 95% CI 0.63–0.98), reduced bacterial infections (relative risk=0.43, 95% CI 0.19–0.97) and decreased early re-bleeding (relative risk=0.53, 95% CI 0.38–0.74).[36]

The selection of antibiotics should be guided by local protocols but evidence from a RCT indicated that intravenous ceftriaxone was more effective than oral norfloxacin in the prophylaxis of proven infections (26% vs 11%, $P=0.03$), spontaneous bacteraemia or spontaneous bacterial peritonitis (12% vs 2%, $P=0.03$) in patients with advanced cirrhosis and haemorrhage.[37] Proton pump inhibitors are not indicated unless there is associated peptic ulcer disease.[14]

Endoscopy

As an alternative to pharmacotherapy, EBL repeated every couple of weeks until obliteration of varices can be used for the primary prophylaxis of bleeding.[14] It is the preferred option when there are contraindications to the use of non-cardioselective beta-blockers.EBL is also the procedure of choice for initial assessment and primary control of variceal haemorrhage.[9,14]

> ✔✔ In oesophageal varices EBL is the standard of care over endoscopic sclerotherapy, as a result of a meta-analysis of seven RCTs comparing the two techniques. EBL and endoscopic sclerotherapy have almost equal rates of immediate haemostasis (89% vs 88 %, respectively) but sclerotherapy is associated with higher rates of re-bleeding (31% vs 47%), mortality (24% vs 3 %) and stricture formation (0% vs 11%).[38,39]

In contrast to oesophageal varices, tissue adhesives (e.g. N-butyl-cyanoacrylate, isobutyl-2-cyanoacylate, or thrombin) are more effective at achieving haemostasis and preventing re-bleeding in patients with GOV2, IGV1 and IGV2 gastric varices.[39,40]

> ✔ Evidence from a RCT confirmed that endoscopic sclerotherapy with cyanoacrylate was more effective and also safer than EBL in the management of bleeding gastric varices.[40]

The use of cyanoacrylate is therefore recommended in GOV2 and IGV for both the treatment of acute bleeding and endoscopic surveillance treatment.[14]

Second-line therapy options

Second-line therapies for varices can be considered in two scenarios. The first is to control ongoing active haemorrhage following unsuccessful attempts with first-line therapy or to address re-bleeding, and the second is to provide more conclusive prevention of re-bleeding. Balloon tamponade is considered under second-line therapy but must be viewed as a temporising measure to offer time until definitive second-line therapy can be arranged. Liver transplantation is the definitive treatment option for portal hypertension (as it addresses underlying disease) and is discussed at the end of this chapter.

Balloon tamponade

Balloon tamponade is a temporary measure of achieving haemostasis by direct compression of bleeding varices and should be considered only as a bridge to more definitive treatment (either TIPSS or surgery). A recent series reported effective haemostasis with oral-gastric tube placement in 79% of patients.[41]

The Sengstaken–Blakemore tube (3 lumen tube) and Minnesota tube (4 lumen tube) are the two types of oral-gastric tubes most often encountered in clinical practice. The Linton–Nachlas tube (2 lumen tube) has just a gastric balloon and has a more limited use. Intubation and airway protection should be considered early in the management of any massive gastrointestinal haemorrhage but it is mandatory prior to oral-gastric tube insertion. Placement of the tube endoscopically or over a guide wire may also reduce the risk of complications, particularly oesophageal rupture.[14] Alternatively, a laryngoscope can be used to aid insertion.

The oral-gastric tube may have some utility for controlling bleeding from junctional gastric (GOV1 or GOV2) varices but has little effect on controlling bleeding gastric varices in the fundus or further down the stomach. Inflation of the oesophageal balloon is delayed and should be undertaken only if the gastric balloon alone does not achieve haemostasis, as there is an increased risk of necrosis at the gastro-oesophageal junction. The oesophageal balloon must be deflated every 12 hours to prevent necrosis and for similar reasons the gastric balloon should not be inflated for more than 48 hours. Upon deflation of the balloons re-bleeding occurs in 50% of patients with oesophagogastric varices.[42] Re-bleeding is the rule for gastric varices unless more definitive control of bleeding is established.[14]

Oral-gastric tube insertion is associated with a complication rate of 20–30% which includes aspiration pneumonia, oesophageal rupture, asphyxia from balloon migration, oesophageal ulcers, pressure necrosis (tongue or lips), arrhythmia and chest pain.[43,44] Currently, balloon tamponade is only accepted as a bridge treatment for bleeding varices to definitive rescue therapy.[45] However, recently a dedicated self-expandable covered oesophageal metal stent has been introduced as an alternative to oesophageal balloon tamponade. In a recent small RCT comparing oesophageal stenting to balloon tamponade in 28 patients, improved results were seen with oesophageal stenting in terms of adverse-event-free survival with haemostasis (66% vs 20%, $P=0.025$), control of bleeding (85% vs 47%, $P=0.037$), transfusional requirements (2 vs 6 units, $P=0.08$) and adverse events (15% vs 47%, $P=0.077$).[43]

TIPSS (Transjugular intrahepatic portosystemic shunt)

TIPSS is an interventional minimally invasive radiological procedure that has largely replaced surgical portocaval shunts.[46] The procedure is performed by image-guided needle puncture from a hepatic vein to an intrahepatic branch of the portal vein. The track is maintained by a stent so blood flow to the liver is preserved and decompression of the hypertensive portal system is achieved.

> ✅ TIPSS was previously performed with open bare metal expandable stents but polytetrafluoroethylene (PTFE) covered stents are now recommended as they have less need for revision due to increased patency rates at 2 years (76% vs. 36%) with no associated increase in post-procedural encephalopathy.[14,47,48]

TIPSS can be used for various complications of portal hypertension including refractory ascites, hepatic hydrothorax, portal hypertensive gastropathy and hepatorenal syndrome. However, TIPSS (with or without embolisation of varices) is principally used as a rescue therapy for treating active variceal bleeding not controlled by first-line therapies. It is successful in 95% of cases with a re-bleeding rate of 18%.[49] TIPSS is also more effective at preventing recurrent variceal bleeding than endoscopic therapy but this comes at the expense of worsening encephalopathy and procedure-related complications such as perforation of the liver capsule, inadvertent biliary puncture, hepatic artery

injury, intraperitoneal bleeding, hepatic infarction, fistulisation, haemobilia and haemolysis.[50,51]

The early post-procedural complications of TIPSS are secondary to the direct shunting of portal flow into the venous system, which reduces the clearance of toxins and can worsen encephalopathy. After TIPSS, the reported incidence of new onset or worsening hepatic encephalopathy ranges from 13% to 35%.[52] Post-TIPSS encephalopathy appears more frequently in cirrhotic patients with refractory ascites.[53] Other risk factors for developing encephalopathy include age >65 years, Child–Pugh score >12, prior encephalopathy, placement of a large-diameter stent (>10 mm), and low post-TIPSS portosystemic pressure gradient (<5 mm Hg).[54] An increased venous return with subsequent heart failure or liver failure secondary to ischaemic injury from reduced portal perfusion have also been reported.

In the longer term, stent infection, stent thrombosis or stenosis, and stent migration may occur.[51] As such, patients require regular follow-up by Doppler ultrasound with further intervention needed to address stent-related complications before re-bleeding occurs.

Absolute contraindications to TIPSS include primary prevention of variceal bleeding, severe heart failure, tricuspid regurgitation, multiple hepatic cysts, uncontrolled sepsis, unrelieved biliary obstruction and severe pulmonary hypertension. Relative contra-indications include centrally placed hepatomas, obstruction of all hepatic veins, significant portal vein thrombosis, severe un-correctable coagulopathy (INR >5), thrombocytopenia (platelet count <20 000/cm^3) and moderate pulmonary hypertension.[53]

> ✅ In previous studies the MELD score has been shown to be better than the Child–Pugh score at predicting post-TIPSS mortality.[55] In a further study, the technical success rate of elective TIPSS was 100% with a 30-day mortality rate of 11%, but in a sub-analysis, patients with a MELD score of >24 demonstrated the highest risk of 30-day mortality.[56]

Surgical shunts (**Fig. 8.2**)

There are numerous surgical options for the treatment of portal hypertension and its complications. These include the direct portocaval shunt, selective distal splenorenal shunt and interposition 'C' or 'H' graft portocaval shunts. There remain indications for these procedures in select candidates but the caveat is that few surgeons have retained the expertise to perform the techniques.[46]

The direct portocaval shunt is a technique that completely redirects portal blood flow from the portal vein to the vena cava thus bypassing the liver. It is still utilised by the University of California group with excellent results (control of bleeding

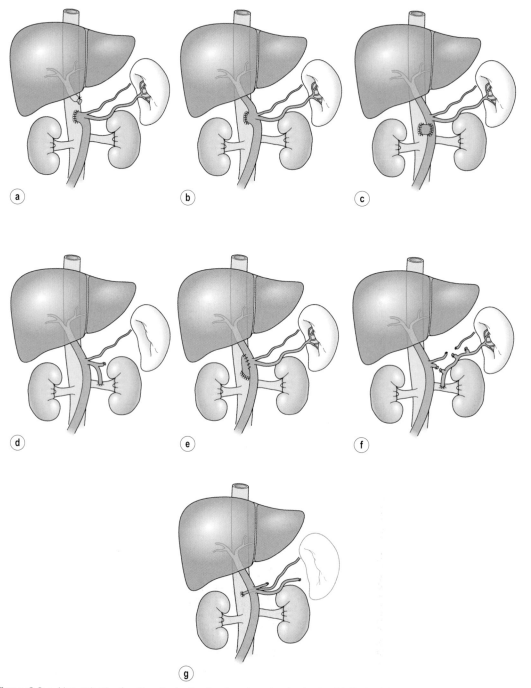

Figure 8.2 • Non-selective **(a–d)** and selective **(e–g)** portosystemic shunts. **(a)** End-to-side portocaval. **(b)** Side-to-side portocaval. **(c)** Mesocaval (jugular vein graft or prosthesis). **(d)** Proximal splenorenal. **(e)** Small-diameter PTFE H-graft portocaval. **(f)** Distal splenorenal (Warren). **(g)** Left gastric-to-IVC (Inokuchi). (IVC, inferior vena cava.)

in 99–100%), reflecting their extensive experience with the procedure and excellent organisation.[57–59] However, the results have never been replicated (or refuted) in other centres and direct primary portocaval anastomosis, while producing the most effective reduction in portal pressure, carries the highest encephalopathy rates for surgical shunt procedures.[46]

The selective distal splenorenal shunt selectively decompresses the oesophagogastric and splenic area while allowing mesenteric portal blood flow to the liver. However, the main disadvantage of this technique is loss of selectivity and late function as a total shunt.[46]

☑ A multicentre RCT involving 140 patients with Child–Pugh A or B cirrhosis with refractory variceal bleeding showed no significant difference with selective distal splenorenal shunting compared to TIPSS with regards to the re-bleeding rate (5.5% vs 10.5%) or survival at 2 years (81% vs 88%) and 5 years (62% vs 61%). In both groups half of the patients developed hepatic encephalopathy. However, the combined rate of thrombosis, stenosis and need for re-intervention was much lower for the distal splenorenal shunt compared with TIPSS (11% vs 82%).[60]

Interposition 'C' or 'H' graft portocaval shunts are small-diameter portocaval shunts that act as partial portosystemic shunts, thus reducing portal pressure while preserving blood flow to the liver with the intention of minimising the risk of encephalopathy and liver failure. In one study of non-transplantation candidates with Child–Pugh A and B disease and refractory variceal bleeding there was good long-term survival with the use of the small-diameter portocaval H-graft but results were poor in a small number of Child–Pugh C class patients (1-year survival in Child–Pugh A 83%, Child–Pugh B 90% and Child–Pugh C 0%).[61] In a previous study of a single surgeon's 18-year experience with operations for variceal haemorrhage using various types of shunt surgery, the operative mortality rate progressively worsened with increasing Child–Pugh score (Child–Pugh A 3%, Child–Pugh B 8% and Child–Pugh C 26%).[62]

☑☑ A Cochrane review in 2006 assessed 22 trials with 1409 patients to compare total surgical shunt, selective distal splenorenal shunt and TIPSS with endoscopic therapy (sclerotherapy and/or banding). Shunts reduced re-bleeding but had a higher incidence of acute and chronic encephalopathy with no differences in short-term mortality or long-term survival. The shunt occlusion rate was 3% overall, 8% for distal splenorenal shunt and 59% for TIPSS.[63]

Overall, when assessing these data, Child–Pugh C patients carry a high perioperative risk and have a poor 1-year survival following surgical shunting.[53,61,62] However, because fewer postoperative interventions are required to ensure patency of a surgical shunt than with TIPSS, surgery may be preferred in some patients with Child–Pugh A and B disease.[53] This is particularly the case in areas where TIPSS and transplantation are not as readily available. Depending on local expertise, surgical shunting

can also be considered if TIPSS is not possible (e.g. centrally placed tumour).[14] Indeed, a recently published retrospective study suggested better results with surgical shunting compared to TIPSS in patients with a MELD of 14 or less, including favourable survival at 5 years (100% vs 40%, P <0.001).[64] There are other specific situations when surgery may be preferred including in those with 'normal' livers (e.g. patients with schistosomiasis).[46]

In terms of choice of operation, if portal vein thrombosis is present, a selective distal splenorenal shunt is advocated and allows for splenic conservation. For patients without cirrhosis and with a patent portal vein, options include a direct portocaval and selective distal splenorenal shunt, depending on local expertise. Shunts should be avoided in liver transplantation candidates as the presence of a portocaval shunt significantly increases the risk of transplantation in terms of higher transfusion requirements, longer intensive care unit and hospital stay and greater short- and long-term mortality. TIPSS rather than shunt surgery is the preferred option prior to considering liver transplantation if an intervention is required (e.g. unsuccessful attempts at endoscopic treatment of variceal bleeding). If TIPSS is not possible in transplantation candidates, surgery at a site distant from the liver hilum should be considered, either as a selective distal splenorenal or interposition mesocaval shunt.[65]

Clinical scenarios

Prevention of variceal bleeding

All patients should be screened for varices at the time of diagnosis of cirrhosis.[9,14,16] If no varices are seen on initial endoscopy then plans should be made to repeat the endoscopy in 2–3 years.[14] If grade I varices are seen, then annual endoscopy is recommended unless decompensation occurs and in this case endoscopy should be repeated immediately.[14]

First-line therapy for primary prophylaxis of bleeding in oesophageal varices comprises non-selective beta-blockers or EBL.[9] A meta-analysis comparing beta-blockers to EBL for primary prophylaxis reported that EBL was associated with a small reduction in the incidence of first variceal bleed but no difference in overall mortality.[66,67] Though EBL was associated with lower incidence of adverse events, these events included bleeding from ligation ulcers and were considered more severe since the adverse events requiring withdrawal of beta-blocker resolved after discontinuing therapy.[66,67]

Recent guidance from the BSG suggests that for primary prophylaxis of bleeding in grade II oesophageal varices and grade I oesophageal varices with 'red signs' on endoscopy, the use of non-selective beta-blockers or EBL is appropriate irrespective of the severity of liver disease. Pharmacological treatment with propranolol is first-line option in these guidelines, with EBL utilised in those with a contraindication or intolerance to beta-blockers, taking into account the preferences of the patient. If a beta-blocker is started there is no indication to repeat endoscopy.[14] Due to cost and risk of sedation, the AASLD offers pragmatic advice that endoscopy can be avoided in patients who are already taking non-selective beta-blockers for other reasons at the time of their diagnosis of cirrhosis.[9]

Once prophylactic therapy is commenced it should be continued indefinitely, although it is suggested that beta-blockers are discontinued at the time of spontaneous bacterial peritonitis, renal impairment and hypotension.[14,68]

✅ On cessation of treatment, the patient assumes the same bleeding risk as untreated patients (25%), and there may also be an associated increased risk of mortality over untreated patients in those who withdraw from treatment.[69]

It has been suggested that EBL may be preferred for large varices, with high-risk stigmata (e.g. red wale marks), and Child–Pugh B and C cirrhosis.[16] If EBL is selected, it should be repeated every couple of weeks until obliteration of varices is confirmed with follow-up endoscopy repeated for assessment of recurrent disease.[9,70] Nitrates, TIPSS and sclerotherapy are not recommended treatments for primary prophylaxis of variceal bleeding.[9,14,16] An algorithm for the primary prevention of variceal bleeding is provided in **Fig. 8.3**.

Treatment for bleeding varices

As is the case with all major upper gastrointestinal bleeds, the initial concern in the management of acute variceal bleeding should be airway protection, with a low threshold for endotracheal intubation if required. Resuscitation should be undertaken in a high-dependency or intensive care unit with appropriate blood products according to local protocols, correction of coagulopathy, prophylactic antibiotics and vasoactive agents (terlipressin or somatostatin).[14] Endoscopic therapy has been considered first-line treatment for the management of acute variceal haemorrhage since guidelines were released in 1995 and should be offered to unstable patients immediately after resuscitation and within 24 hours in all other stable patients.[14,45,71] First-line therapy is successful in 80–85% of patients.[72]

In the event of failure of first-line endoscopic therapy or if a second re-bleeding event occurs, a further endoscopy can be considered but guidelines from the AASLD suggest that an alternative treatment modality should be attempted next.[9,45] If bleeding is difficult to control, an oral-gastric tube should be inserted until further endoscopic treatment, TIPSS or (less frequently) surgery can be undertaken depending on local resources and expertise.[14] Specialist input should be sought at this time and transfer to a specialist centre that provides a 24-hour emergency TIPSS service should be urgently considered.[14]

The delay between the initial bleed and TIPSS placement, the number of endoscopic attempts and need for balloon tamponade correlate with increased mortality when using TIPSS as a rescue therapy.[44] The strongest predictor of negative outcome is a HVPG >20 mmHg. Although HVPG measurement

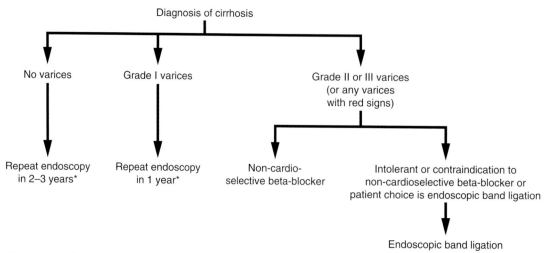

Figure 8.3 • Algorithm for the primary prevention of variceal bleeding. *If there is clear evidence of disease progression this interval can be adjusted by the treating clinician. Endoscopy should also be offered at time of decompensation.

is not routinely undertaken in clinical practice, risk factors suggestive of a HVPG >20 mmHg include Child–Pugh C cirrhosis, non-alcohol-related cause of cirrhosis, systolic blood pressure at the time of bleeding <100 mmHg or active bleeding at the time of endoscopy.[73,74]

Initial reports on the use of TIPSS for the management of recurrent variceal bleeding were favourable with a 92% haemostatic success rate, and an overall 1-year survival rate of 75–100%, 68–86% and 49–73% for Child–Pugh A, B and C, respectively.[75,76]

✔✔ Two subsequent RCTs have shown that early TIPSS (within 24–72 hours of admission) compared with continued medical management including endoscopic therapy (sclerotherapy or band ligation) is associated with significant improvement in survival among high-risk patients (Child–Pugh B patients, Child–Pugh C patients with a score <14, and those with HVPG >20 mmHg).[41,77]

After satisfactory haemostasis with first-line therapy, and depending on local resources, early TIPSS (<72 hours after index variceal bleed) can therefore be considered in selected patients with Child–Pugh B cirrhosis and active bleeding or Child–Pugh C cirrhosis with a score <14.[14]

Despite the results of these RCTs and subsequent recommendations, TIPSS is still not considered a first-line therapy since there is better access to endoscopy, which is also needed to prove variceal haemorrhage as the source of gastrointestinal bleeding. If TIPSS is unavailable or not feasible due to contraindications, and local expertise permits, surgical shunting can be considered in Child–Pugh A patients with minimal comorbidity.[14]

Gastric varices

Gastric varices are categorised based on their relationship with oesophageal varices as well as their site in the stomach[17] (see Table 8.2). GOV1 are considered extensions of oesophageal varices and should be managed in a similar fashion.[14] The presence of IGV1 should prompt investigation for the presence of splenic vein thrombosis,[9] and if present splenectomy is curative.[78] The management of gastric varices is challenging and the threshold to place a TIPSS for bleeding gastric varices is much lower compared with oesophageal varices. The AASLD practice guidelines recommend TIPSS when cyanoacrylate injection or thrombin are unavailable, when there is operator unfamiliarity with these adhesives or in cases of failure of single endoscopic treatment.[9] Balloon tamponade is suggested as a temporising treatment for GOV and IGV1 but is unlikely to be effective for varices more distal in the stomach.[14]

Another viable radiological alternative for non-TIPSS candidates is balloon-occluded retrograde transvenous obliteration. This procedure involves insertion of a balloon catheter via the femoral or internal jugular vein into the spontaneous gastro-renal outflow shunt followed by embolisation of the veins draining the gastric varices. By blocking the decompressive gastrorenal shunt the procedure could aggravate portal hypertension but it may preserve hepatic function better than TIPSS.[79]

It is recommended that patients with GOV1 are entered into an endoscopic surveillance programme. Endoscopic surveillance with cyanoacrylate injection as needed is recommended for GOV2 and IGV.[14] An algorithm for the management of acute variceal bleeding is illustrated in **Fig. 8.4**.

Portal hypertensive gastropathy

Portal hypertensive gastropathy is an abnormality of the gastric mucosa characterised endoscopically by a mosaic-like pattern resembling 'snake-skin', with or without red spots.[80] The overall prevalence of portal hypertensive gastropathy in cirrhosis is roughly 80% and it is strongly correlated with the severity of cirrhosis.[81] Currently, definitive recommendations for treatment of asymptomatic portal hypertensive gastropathy are lacking.[82] During an 18-month follow-up period, the incidence of acute bleeding was 3%, the bleeding-related mortality rate was 13% and the incidence of chronic bleeding was 11%.[81] Octreotide and terlipressin are advocated for the treatment of acute bleeding from portal hypertensive gastropathy based on their ability to decrease portal blood flow. Non-selective beta-blockers are the foundation of treatment for chronic bleeding.[82] In a previous RCT, propanolol reduced recurrent bleeding from portal hypertensive gastropathy.[83] Although endoscopy is key in establishing the diagnosis, the role of endoscopic therapy for portal hypertensive gastropathy is contentious and its utility is felt to be minimal due to the diffuse nature of the bleeding.[80,82,84] When medical management is unsuccessful, rescue therapy with TIPSS or surgical shunting may be required. Liver transplantation is a last resort in cases of refractory bleeding.[82]

Segmental portal hypertension

Segmental portal hypertension resulting from splenic vein thrombosis should always be considered as the potential cause of bleeding gastric varices in patients with pancreatic pathology. Those with advanced malignancy of the pancreas can usually be controlled with medical management or endoscopic treatment. Patients with chronic pancreatitis who develop variceal bleeding as a result of thrombosis of the splenic vein should be considered for splenectomy, which is often curative. An alternative option to splenectomy is splenic artery embolisation.[14]

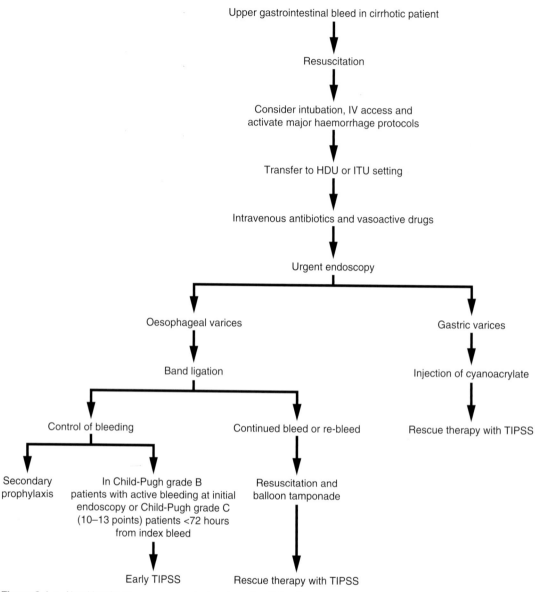

Upper gastrointestinal bleed in cirrhotic patient

Resuscitation

Consider intubation, IV access and activate major haemorrhage protocols

Transfer to HDU or ITU setting

Intravenous antibiotics and vasoactive drugs

Urgent endoscopy

Oesophageal varices

Gastric varices

Band ligation

Injection of cyanoacrylate

Control of bleeding

Continued bleed or re-bleed

Rescue therapy with TIPSS

Secondary prophylaxis

In Child-Pugh grade B patients with active bleeding at initial endoscopy or Child-Pugh grade C (10–13 points) patients <72 hours from index bleed

Resuscitation and balloon tamponade

Early TIPSS

Rescue therapy with TIPSS

Figure 8.4 • Algorithm for the management of acute variceal bleeding.

Budd–Chiari syndrome

Budd–Chiari syndrome is an uncommon condition with an estimated incidence of 0.8 per million per year.[85] It results from obstruction of venous outflow from the liver, usually as a result of thrombotic occlusion of the hepatic veins. Presentation can be fulminant, acute, subacute or chronic. The classic presentation of Budd–Chiari syndrome is a triad of abdominal pain, ascites and hepatomegaly,[86] although it can be asymptomatic in up to 20% of patients, usually in the presence of large collaterals from the hepatic veins.[87] Hypercoagulable states and an underlying myeloproliferative neoplasm are present in approximately 50% of cases.[87] It is therefore worth considering the diagnosis in all patients with liver dysfunction and a background history of either a prothrombotic tendency or myeloproliferative disorder.[86] Ultrasonography will demonstrate absent or reduced hepatic venous outflow, with CT demonstrating abnormal liver perfusion.

Referral to an expert centre with hepatology specialists, radiology expertise and surgical skills is advised. An experienced haematologist should also be involved in the care of the patient. Initial management (successful in two-thirds) focuses on anticoagulation, initially with low-molecular-weight heparin.[87] Life-long anticoagulation is supported by guidelines from the British Committee for Standards in Haematology.[88]

Endovascular therapy in the form of angioplasty with stenting may be required if anticoagulation is unsuccessful.[89] TIPSS is now considered standard of care for Budd–Chiari syndrome if initial anticoagulation and angioplasty are unsuccessful and although there are no randomised data, the results from published case series are beneficial.[86]

✅ A multicentre retrospective study of 124 patients that underwent TIPSS for Budd–Chiari syndrome reported 12- and 60-month liver transplant-free survival of 88% and 78%, respectively.[90] In a further multicentre study of 62 patients the 12- and 60-month liver transplant-free survival following TIPSS was 88% and 72%, respectively.[91] Recent data from a large single-centre study of 67 patients reported survival rates of 92%, 80% and 72% at 12, 60 and 120 months, respectively.[86]

Interestingly, hepatic encephalopathy is less of a concern with TIPSS for Budd–Chiari syndrome as the reduction in hepatic congestion generally improves liver function.[86] An alternative to TIPSS is surgical shunting, but the decision to proceed to a surgical shunt should be made at a specialist liver transplant centre, generally when TIPSS has failed and in patients who have no liver dysfunction and are not candidates for liver transplantation.[87] In a small subgroup of patients, TIPSS is unsuccessful and liver transplantation needs to be considered, particularly if there is evidence of hepatic decompensation and jaundice. The relationship between hepatocellular carcinoma and Budd–Chiari syndrome is uncertain but in one study that included 97 patients with Budd–Chiari syndrome, hepatocellular carcinoma occurred in 4% of patients after 5 years of follow-up.[92] The AASLD practice guidelines suggest 6-monthly hepatocellular carcinoma surveillance in chronic Budd–Chiari syndrome.[93] Overall, however, prognosis is good, with 5-year survival approaching 90%.[94]

Portal vein thrombosis

Portal vein thrombosis is a rare condition that is associated with a range of precipitating factors, including cirrhosis, cancer, surgery, intra-abdominal infection, hypercoagulable states, myeloproliferative conditions and extrinsic compression of the vein. Often it is a combination of these factors that leads to portal vein thrombosis.[95] The incidence of portal vein thrombosis is estimated to be 0.7 per 100 000 per year and in the absence of underlying malignancy and cirrhosis, survival at 1 year and 5 years is 92% and 76%, respectively.[96] Portal vein thrombosis can present acutely or chronically, with the latter more likely to result in variceal bleeding due to portal hypertension.[1]

Treatment of portal vein thrombosis depends on the overall clinical picture of the patient and takes into consideration the presence of symptoms, the degree of reversibility of the precipitating causes, malignancy and cirrhosis. Medical management may involve observation with no active therapy (particularly if the patient is asymptomatic and has an obvious reversible precipitating cause, e.g. abdominal infection or pancreatitis) or anticoagulation (with a low threshold in malignancy and thrombosis extending into mesenteric veins or progressing on imaging without treatment). Conventional anticoagulant drugs such as low-molecular-weight heparin and warfarin may be used in cirrhotic patients with portal vein thrombosis, particularly in those eligible for liver transplantation as this may mitigate propagation of the clot, thus facilitating or even permitting transplantation.[97] The presence of portal vein thrombosis is not a contraindication to liver transplantation, but the procedure may not be feasible if the thrombus extends into the entire portomesenteric system.[98] Thrombectomy or thrombolysis may be considered if there is progressive abdominal pain suggestive of an emergency presentation with mesenteric ischaemia.[99]

Endovascular options in the setting of acute portal vein thrombosis include mechanical recanalisation, local targeted thrombolysis, or a combination of these treatments.[1] Radiological interventions have extended into the portal venous system by percutaneous transhepatic, transjugular and even the transplenic routes in selected cases.[100] Acute portal vein thrombus can also be treated by TIPSS combined with a combination of techniques for thrombolysis (e.g. clot disruption by balloon, suction embolectomy, basket extraction of clot and mechanical thrombectomy) but these carry the risk of vascular trauma.[95]

Prevention of re-bleeds

In the context of variceal haemorrhage, re-bleeding is defined as any bleed that arises >48 hours after the initial admission (as long as the patient has been free of bleeding for at least 24 hours). 'Early' re-bleeding is defined as re-bleeding within 6 weeks of the initial bleed, while 'late' re-bleeding is defined as re-bleeding after 6 weeks.[45] When haemostasis is initially achieved with endoscopic therapy, re-bleeding occurs in up to 30% of patients.[101] Recurrent variceal haemorrhage requiring salvage TIPSS is associated with a high mortality.[41]

Bleeding gastric varices, active bleeding at the time of endoscopy, low serum albumin, renal failure and a HVPG >20 mmHg have been described as predictive factors for early re-bleeding.[102–104] Risk factors associated with late re-bleeding include liver decompensation, presence of ascites, underlying hepatocellular carcinoma, active alcohol use and high-risk stigmata on endoscopy (e.g. red wale sign).[105]

✔✔ Meta-analyses of studies using beta-blocker therapy to prevent re-bleeding have demonstrated both a significant reduction in mortality (27% vs 20%) and a decreased incidence of re-bleeding (63% vs 42%).[18]

Beta-blockers and EBL combination therapy are recommended as the optimal secondary prophylaxis strategy against re-bleeding.[14] It is suggested that varices are banded at 2–4-weekly intervals until eradication. After successful eradication of varices, patients should be followed up by repeat endoscopy at 3 months, then 6-monthly intervals thereafter, with any recurrent varices being treated with further EBL.[14]

In the early TIPSS trial, patients randomised to receive early TIPSS (<72 hours after index variceal bleed) had a 1-year probability of remaining free of re-bleeding that was significantly lower compared with those randomised to medical therapy with EBL (50% vs 97 %, $P < 0.001$).[41]

✔✔ In a meta-analysis published before this early trial, a decreased incidence of recurrent variceal bleeding and decreased mortality due to re-bleeding were also reported with TIPSS, but at the expense of an increased rate of encephalopathy and no overall reduction in mortality.[50]

TIPSS is therefore reserved for those who re-bleed despite combined beta-blocker and EBL therapy.[14] Shunt surgery can also be recommended where local expertise and resources are available in Child–Pugh A and B patients when TIPSS is not feasible.[14]

Liver transplantation

The gold standard treatment for end-stage liver disease is liver transplantation. In 2013, across seven transplant units in the UK (three of which perform paediatric liver transplantation), 871 liver transplants were performed. In April 2014, there were 512 patients registered on the liver transplant waiting list. Current waiting time on the adult liver transplant list is 142 days while paediatric patients wait on average 78 days.[98]

Living donor liver transplantation is technically challenging and has a 38% risk of morbidity to the donor with an estimated donor mortality rate of 0.18%.[106] Therefore, the vast majority of liver transplants performed (particularly in the Western world) are from whole livers obtained from deceased donors. An important variation is split liver transplantation. Most commonly the graft is split between an adult and a child and the liver is divided into an extended right lobe graft (segments IV–

VIII) (for the adult recipient) and a partial left graft that includes segments II and III (for the paediatric recipient). Both in situ and ex situ liver splitting has been described. Split liver for two adults has also been described, although results are less good.

With a greater demand for transplantation, extended criteria liver grafts are increasingly utilised. However, these grafts are much more vulnerable to ischaemic injury due to pre-existing pathology.[107,108] There is no uniform classification of an extended criteria liver graft, but risk factors such as increased donor age, high serum sodium, low blood pressure, liver steatosis and prolonged cold ischaemic times are recognised as being harmful to graft function.[109]

✔ An objective donor liver index including duration of cold ischaemia, cause of donor death, donor race and height and type of donor correlates with outcome following transplantation.[110] Recently, a UK donor liver index has been described that takes into account donor age, sex, type of donor, height, bilirubin, smoking history and whether the liver was split.[111]

Donation after circulatory death (DCD) represents nearly 50% of the donor population in the UK but only 36% of the livers are utilised. Compared to liver grafts from donation after brainstem death (DBD) donors, DCD grafts suffer prolonged warm ischaemic times and this contributes to an increased incidence of biliary complications, ischaemic cholangiopathy, graft loss and mortality following transplantation.[112]

Indication

Patients should be considered for liver transplantation if they have a projected life expectancy (without transplantation) of <1 year or an unacceptable quality of life (e.g. secondary to persistent intractable pruritis or chronic encephalopathy) and providing that they have a 50% predicted 5-year post-transplant survival. The major indications for liver transplantation are acute liver failure, end-stage liver disease in patients in whom transplantation would extend life expectancy and hepatocellular carcinoma (usually on a background of liver dysfunction that precludes liver resection). In practical terms, patients should be referred for transplant assessment when major complications of cirrhosis develop, such as variceal haemorrhage, ascites, hepatorenal syndrome and encephalopathy. Other 'variant' syndromes that fulfil criteria for elective listing include diuretic resistant ascites, hepatopulmonary syndrome, familial amyloidosis, primary hyperlipidaemias and polycystic liver disease.[98]

The Milan criteria outline when liver transplantation should be considered for hepatocellular carcinoma (HCC) and include solitary HCC with a diameter <5 cm, or up to three nodules with a diameter <3 cm and no evidence of extrahepatic spread or vascular invasion.[113] Recently. extension of the Milan criteria was adopted by NHS Blood and Transplant in the UK with up to five lesions <3 cm permitted, or a solitary 5–7 cm lesion downstaged with local therapy and chemotherapy, provided there is <20% growth and no new nodules appearing over a 6-month period. An alpha-fetoprotein (AFP) level >10 000 ng/mL was previously considered a contraindication as it correlates with vascular invasion and loss of tumour differentiation. However, more recent evidence from Duvoux and colleagues suggests that an AFP level >1000 ng/mL may correlate with recurrence of HCC.[114] This work led to the adoption of the Duvoux criteria when considering downstaged HCC (Table 8.3). This combines AFP level with tumour size and number of nodules. A score of ≤2 points following downstaging treatment is now used to determine eligibility for liver transplantation in the UK. Other criteria for transplanting HCC are considered elsewhere and include the San Francisco criteria (single lesion ≤6.5 cm, or 2–3 lesions of ≤4.5 cm with a total tumour diameter ≤8 cm).[115]

Donor hepatectomy

The liver is assessed at the time of retrieval for consistency, colour and sharpness of the edges, which can all give an indication regarding quality of the graft and whether there is steatosis. It is important to accurately estimate the size of the liver and relay this to the implanting surgeon as the weight of the liver graft may influence recipient selection. The graft-to-recipient weight ratio should be at least 0.8% and more formal weighing of the graft can be performed following completion of the donor hepatectomy.[98]

After donor checks are performed and relevant paperwork is reviewed, a midline laparotomy is performed in the donor. The round ligament and the falciform ligament are divided. The chest is opened, adhesions to the liver taken down and the left triangular ligament is divided. The hepatogastric ligament is inspected for the presence of an aberrant left hepatic artery. The presence of an aberrant right hepatic artery is initially assessed by palpation for an arterial pulsation lateral and posterior to the portal vein.

The common bile duct is divided above the duodenum, ligating the distal end. To minimise biliary injury due to stagnant bile, the gallbladder is incised and irrigated until clear fluid drains from the cut end of the bile duct. The amount of dissection in the liver hilum depends on the surgeon's experience, but in general identification and control of the gastroduodenal artery and splenic artery are sufficient in the warm phase. Intravenous heparin is administered, the distal aorta is ligated and then the infra-renal aorta is cannulated in preparation for cold perfusion. Dual liver perfusion via the portal vein is useful particularly in DCD.

The supracoeliac aorta is clamped, the venous drainage is achieved by venting the suprahepatic inferior vena cava and cold perfusion is commenced. The entire abdominal cavity is packed with slush ice to allow rapid in situ cooling of the liver, including above the diaphragm in the costodiaphragmatic angles. In the DCD setting after treatment withdrawal, asystolic arrest and verification of death, the donor is transferred to the operating theatre and a rapid laparotomy is carried out, followed by immediate perfusion with cold preservation fluid.[116]

During the cold phase of the operation, the infrahepatic inferior vena cava (IVC) is divided above the renal veins. The cold dissection commences in the hilum by dividing the previously identified gastroduodenal artery. The portal vein is divided approximately 1 cm above the duodenum. The common hepatic artery is followed towards the coeliac axis. The origin of the splenic artery is then divided leaving a 5-mm stump to allow for arterial reconstruction if required. The coeliac trunk is then taken with a patch of aorta. The diaphragm is divided around the suprahepatic cava, starting on the left side of the inferior vena cava, continuing posteriorly and completing the division by taking a patch of the right hemidiaphragm around the right lobe of the liver. The right lobe is separated from the right adrenal gland and the right kidney, and the retroperitoneal tissue at the back of the inferior vena cava. The aorta is fully divided, and the liver is removed.

Table 8.3 • Duvoux criteria scoring system

Variable	Points
Largest diameter tumour (cm)	
≤3	0
3–6	1
>6	4
Number of nodules	
1–3	0
≥4	2
Alpha-fetoprotein level (ng/mL)	
≤100	0
100–1000	2
>1000	3

Once removed, the liver is placed on ice before being perfused on the back table at the donor centre. The liver should be kept at 4°C throughout the bench procedure by submerging it in slushy iced water. The liver is checked for injuries, size and degree of steatosis. The vena cava is dissected and the phrenic and adrenal veins stumps are ligated to avoid bleeding on reperfusion. The portal vein is dissected for an adequate length. The hepatic artery is then dissected and check made for aberrant or missed arteries. The right hepatic artery is reconstructed if required and all the vessels are flushed to assess for integrity and leaks.

Recipient hepatectomy

The recipient hepatectomy aims to safely remove the diseased liver with preservation of the venous outflow into the IVC, portal venous inflow and hepatic artery inflow. The bile duct is preserved to enable a duct–duct anastomosis. A portal–caval anastomosis is not mandatory during the recipient hepatectomy, but when performed it preserves mesenteric outflow and can minimise bowel oedema and bleeding.

Implant

Three major techniques for liver implantation have been described, which differ according to the type of venous outflow of the graft. If the recipient IVC has been excised with the cirrhotic liver, implantation involves an end-to-end anastomosis between the supra- and infrahepatic donor cava and the respective ends of the recipient IVC (**Fig. 8.5**).

If the recipient vena cava has been preserved and the hepatic veins (either middle and left or all three) have been preserved, the liver can be implanted using a 'piggy-back' technique whereby the suprahepatic IVC is anastomosed to the middle

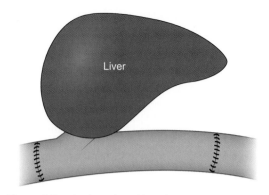

Figure 8.5 • Implantation with end-to-end anastomosis between the supra- and infrahepatic donor cava and the respective ends of the recipient IVC.

and left of all three recipient hepatic veins (**Fig. 8.6**). A third option is a 'modified piggy-back technique', which involves preservation of the native inferior vena cava and a side-to-side anastomosis with the donor's inferior vena cava (**Fig. 8.7**).

The advantage of the 'piggy-back' technique is the preservation of the systemic venous return from the lower body and mesenteric venous return (if a portocaval shunt has been created). The caval anastomosis is followed by reconstruction of the portal vein in an end-to-end manner (after which the liver is reperfused) and then reconstruction of the hepatic artery. Biliary drainage is usually fashioned with an end-to-end anastomosis between the donor and recipient common bile duct. Alternatively, a biliary reconstruction with Roux-en-Y hepatico-jejunostomy can be performed.

Complications

The risk of graft primary non-function is approximately 1% for DBD liver transplants and 2% for DCD liver transplants. There is a relatively low incidence of

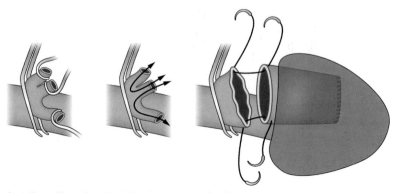

Figure 8.6 • Implantation with a 'piggy-back' technique whereby the suprahepatic inferior vena cava is anastomosed to the middle and left or all three recipient hepatic veins.

biliary infection and anastomotic strictures requiring intervention or surgery.[117] A previous meta-analysis included 25 studies with 62 184 liver transplant recipients (DCD = 2478 and DBD = 59 706) and reported that in comparison to DBD, there was a significant increase in biliary complications [OR = 2.4 (1.9, 3.1); P <0.00001] and ischaemic cholangiopathy [OR = 10.5 (5.7, 19.5); P <0.00001] following DCD liver transplantation. The overall incidence of biliary complications was 26% following DCD liver transplantation compared to 16% following DBD liver transplantation. The overall incidence of ischaemic cholangiopathy was 16% following DCD liver transplantation compared to 3% following DBD liver transplantation.[112] Acute rejection can occur in as many as 40% of the patients during the first 3 months post-transplantation. Liver biopsy may be required to distinguish between rejection and viral infection. Pulse steroids, antithymocyte globulin, or other adaptions of the immunosuppressive regimen usually manage rejection episodes. Re-transplantation is the last option when therapy fails and the patient re-develops hepatic failure.

Immunosuppression

Triple immunosuppression therapy with tacrolimus in combination with either azathioprine or mycophenolate mofetil and a short period of steroids (usually 3 months) is the backbone of immunosuppression regimens after liver transplantation. Side-effects of long-term immunosuppression include raised blood pressure, renal dysfunction, diabetes and an increased risk of malignancy, such as skin cancer and lymphoproliferative disorders.

Results

According to the European Liver Transplant Registry, since 2000, survival at 1-, 3- and 6-months post-liver transplantation is 94%, 91% and 88%, respectively. When considering only patients who survive beyond 6 months, patient survival rates are excellent (96% at 1 year, 83% at 5 years, 71% at 10 years, 61% at 15 years and 52% at 20 years).[106]

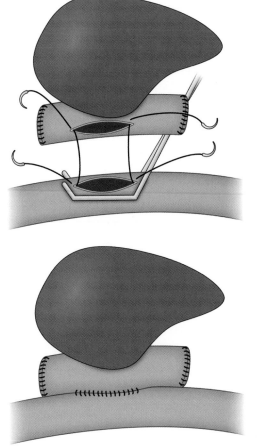

Figure 8.7 • 'Modified piggy-back' technique, with preservation of the native inferior vena cava and a side-to-side anastomosis with the donor's inferior vena cava.

hepatic artery thrombosis (1–7%, depending on the graft type) but this leads to a roughly 50% chance of graft loss and if it occurs within 21 days it is considered an indication for super-urgent re-transplantation.[98] Outflow obstruction caused by stenosis at the caval anastomosis is a rare but serious complication, with a reported incidence of 1–6%. Portal vein thrombosis occurs with an incidence of 2–26%.[98] Biliary complications include ischaemic cholangiopathy, as well as bile leak, bile duct necrosis, biliary casts,

---

Key points

- Patients with grade II varices or worse who have not bled should be treated with beta-blockers unless there are medical contraindications.
- Endoscopic band ligation (EBL) is the initial treatment of choice for acute variceal bleeding.
- After bleeding, patients should enter a programme of variceal ligation or beta-blockade to prevent recurrent bleeding.

- Transjugular intrahepatic portosystemic systemic shunt (TIPSS) should be considered in patients in whom endoscopic therapy is unsuccessful.
- After satisfactory haemostasis with first-line therapy, and depending on local resources, early TIPSS (<72 hours after index variceal bleed) can also be considered in selected patients with Child–Pugh B cirrhosis and active bleeding at initial endoscopy, or Child–Pugh C cirrhosis with Child–Pugh score <14.
- Liver transplantation should be considered in appropriate cases once variceal bleeding is problematic.
- Shunt surgery should be considered for non-cirrhotic patients with recurrent variceal bleeding and for Child–Pugh A and B patients who do not have access to TIPSS or transplantation.
- Liver transplantation offers the definitive treatment for portal hypertension secondary to cirrhosis.
- Due to the scarcity of organs the trend to use DCD donors as a source of livers continues to increase but these livers have a higher incidence of biliary complications.

🌐 Full references available at **http://expertconsult. inkling.com**

Key references

18. D'Amico G, Pagliaro L, Bosch J. Pharmacological treatment of portal hypertension: an evidence-based approach. Semin Liver Dis 1999;19(4):475–505. PMID: 10643630.

Meta-analysis demonstrating decreased bleeding risk with beta-blockers and grade II varices.

36. Chavez-Tapia NC, Barrientos-Gutierrez T, Tellez-Avila FI, et al. Antibiotic prophylaxis for cirrhotic patients with upper gastrointestinal bleeding. Cochrane Database Syst Rev 2010;(9):CD002907. PMID: 20824832.

Cochrane meta-analysis showing reduced mortality, infections and decreased re-bleeding with antibiotics in patients with variceal bleeding.

38. Laine L, Cook D. Endoscopic ligation compared with sclerotherapy for treatment of esophageal variceal bleeding: a meta-analysis. Ann Intern Med 1995;123(4):280–7. PMID: 7611595.

Meta-analysis reporting lower rates of re-bleeding, mortality and stricture formation with band ligation versus sclerotherapy in patients with variceal bleeding.

41. Garcia-Pagan JC, Caca K, Bureau C, et al. Early use of TIPS in patients with cirrhosis and variceal bleeding. N Engl J Med 2010;362(25):2370–9. PMID: 20573925.

RCT demonstrating better survival in early TIPSS in Child–Pugh B patients and Child–Pugh C patients with a score <14.

50. Zheng M, Chen Y, Bai J, et al. Transjugular intrahepatic portosystemic shunt versus endoscopic therapy in the secondary prophylaxis of variceal rebleeding in cirrhotic patients: meta-analysis update. J Clin Gastroenterol 2008;42(5):507–16. PMID: 18344888.

Meta-analysis reporting decreased incidence of recurrent variceal bleeding and decreased deaths due to re-bleeding with TIPSS compared to medical therapy with band ligation but increased rates of encephalopathy and no survival benefit.

63. Khan S, Tudur Smith C, Williamson P, et al. Portosystemic shunts versus endoscopic therapy for variceal rebleeding in patients with cirrhosis. Cochrane Database Syst Rev 2006;(4):CD000553. PMID: 17054131.

Cochrane review comparing surgical shunts with TIPS with endoscopy for variceal bleeding reported a lower risk of re-bleeding and occlusion with surgery but a higher incidence of encephalopathy and no mortality benefit.

77. Monescillo A, Martinez-Lagares F, Ruiz-del-Arbol L, et al. Influence of portal hypertension and its early decompression by TIPS placement on the outcome of variceal bleeding. Hepatology 2004;40(4):793–801. PMID: 15382120.

RCT demonstrating better survival in early TIPSS in patients with HVPG >20 mmHg.

9

Pancreas and islet transplantation

Andrew Sutherland
John Casey

Introduction

The discovery of insulin by Banting and Best in the early part of the 20th century saw type I diabetes become a treatable chronic illness rather than a rapidly fatal diagnosis. Since then, patients with diabetes have been able to lead relatively normal lives thanks to ongoing refinements in insulin therapy. Despite this, many patients will suffer from the secondary complications of diabetes, including retinopathy, neuropathy, nephropathy and premature cardiovascular disease. The prognosis for a patient who has diabetic nephropathy is poor and the 10-year survival for a 45-year-old on dialysis is <10%.[1] These patients can benefit from simultaneous pancreas and kidney transplantation (SPK). This not only removes the need for dialysis, but also results in normoglycaemia without the need for insulin in >85% of patients.[2] Pancreas transplant alone (PTA) is reserved for patients in the absence of renal disease with life-threatening complications of diabetes, principally intractable impaired awareness of hypoglycaemia (IAH). For this set of patients, the risk of the surgery and life-long immunosuppression outweighs the risk associated with IAH and coma.

Unfortunately the morbidity and mortality associated with pancreas transplantation means that only a limited number of patients are deemed fit enough for surgery. An alternative treatment for these patients is islet transplantation. Many of the complications of whole pancreas transplantation are associated with the exocrine portion of the pancreas (pancreatitis, pancreatic fistula). The islets of Langerhans account for only 1% of pancreatic mass but contain the beta and alpha cells responsible for insulin and glucagon production necessary for glycaemic control. Islet cell isolation and transplantation has emerged over the last decade as an excellent treatment option for intractable hypoglycaemic awareness and offers a much lower risk alternative to PTA. Together pancreas transplant and islet transplant come under the banner of 'beta-cell replacement therapy'.

Pancreas transplantation

History of pancreas transplantation

The first pancreas transplant was performed over 50 years ago in the University of Minnesota in 1966.[3] Early experience with pancreatic transplantation was disappointing and remained so for many years. Difficulties were related to the management of the exocrine secretions and septic complications, a high incidence of thrombosis, acute rejection and pancreatitis. For the first half of its 50-year history, less than 1200 pancreas transplants were performed worldwide. Even after the introduction of ciclosporin in 1983, 1-year patient and graft survival rates were only 75% and 37%, respectively. Understandably, in the 1970s and 1980s enthusiasm for pancreas transplantation was scarce; the predominant sentiment was scepticism. Throughout the 1990s significant changes occurred. These came about as a consequence of improvements in organ retrieval and preservation methods, refinements in surgical techniques, advances in immunosuppression, progress in the prophylaxis and treatment of infection, and the experience gained in donor and recipient selection. Success rates following pancreas transplantation are now comparable with other forms of organ transplantation. There have now been over 42 000 pancreas transplants performed worldwide.[4]

Interestingly, pancreas transplantation has never been compared with insulin therapy in a prospective controlled trial and it is very unlikely that such a trial will ever be performed. However, considerable experience and a substantial body of evidence has accumulated, which now favours the viewpoint of the enthusiasts rather than the sceptics.

Indications for pancreas transplantation

Pancreas transplantation aims to replace beta cell function, reduce short- and long-term complications of diabetes and increase long-term survival. There are two main scenarios when transplantation is considered in diabetic patients:

1. *Diabetic patients with renal failure:* Simultaneous pancreas and kidney transplant (SPK) is the treatment of choice in patients with type I diabetes and an estimated glomerular filtration rate of <20 mL/min/1.73 m^2. Transplantation can also be considered in type II diabetics with renal failure who have a BMI of <27. In patients who have already received a living or deceased kidney transplant, pancreas after kidney transplant (PAK) can be considered. In those patients that are deemed not fit enough for an SPK, simultaneous islet kidney transplant (SIK) can be considered.

2. *Diabetic patients in the absence of renal failure:* Patients with diabetes complicated by frequent, severe metabolic complications despite optimum insulin therapy may be suitable for PTA. These patients are often at risk of IAH and coma, or severe hyperglycaemia that requires hospital admission. For patients with severe IAH, an alternative and lower risk option to PTA is islet transplantation. The risks and benefits of simultaneous kidney pancreas transplant and contraindication and risks for transplant are summarised in Boxes 9.1 and 9.2. A treatment algorithm for beta-cell replacement is given in **Fig. 9.1**.

Box 9.1 • Potential risks and benefits of simultaneous pancreas–kidney (SPK) transplantation

Risks
- Perioperative morbidity and mortality
- Potential for pancreas transplant to adversely affect kidney transplant outcome
- Consequences of higher immunosuppression

Benefits
- Improved quality of life, insulin independence
- Potential benefits on diabetic complications
- Improved life expectancy

Box 9.2 • Contraindications and risk factors for pancreas transplantation

- Inability to give informed consent
- Active drug abuse
- Major psychiatric illness or non-compliant behaviour
- Recent history of malignancy
- Active infection
- Recent myocardial infarction
- Evidence of significant uncorrectable ischaemic heart disease
- Insufficient cardiac reserve with poor ejection fraction
- Any other illness that significantly restricts life expectancy
- Age > 60 years
- Significant obesity (BMI > 30)
- Severe aortoiliac atherosclerosis

Pancreas retrieval operation

The pancreas is a close neighbour of the liver and shares important vascular structures. During multiorgan retrieval procedures, priority needs to be given to the liver. Specific arterial anomalies of the blood supply to the liver that preclude successful liver or pancreas transplantation are very rare. Although a detailed description of the surgical procedure for pancreas retrieval is not given, several pertinent points are highlighted below.

University of Wisconsin (UW) solution was first developed as a pancreatic preservation solution[5] and remains the benchmark for pancreas preservation. The cold ischaemia tolerance of the pancreas is somewhere between that of the liver and the kidney. In pancreas allografts perfused with UW solution, 20 hours was thought to be the limit for successful preservation, beyond which a time-dependent deterioration in outcome occurred.[6] Although earlier data failed to demonstrate a clear benefit from a preservation time of <20 hours, most surgeons intuitively aimed for shorter preservation times. More recent data now suggest that ischaemia time is of greater importance in recipients of suboptimal

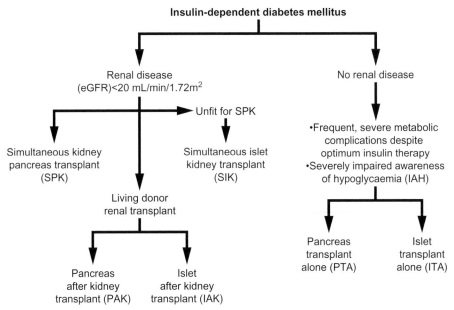

Insulin-dependent diabetes mellitus

Renal disease
(eGFR)<20 mL/min/1.72m²

Unfit for SPK

Simultaneous kidney
pancreas transplant
(SPK)

Simultaneous islet
kidney transplant
(SIK)

Living donor
renal transplant

Pancreas
after kidney
transplant (PAK)

Islet
after kidney
transplant (IAK)

No renal disease

•Frequent, severe metabolic
complications despite
optimum insulin therapy
•Severely impaired awareness
of hypoglycaemia (IAH)

Pancreas
transplant
alone (PTA)

Islet
transplant
alone (ITA)

Figure 9.1 • Beta cell replacement treatment algorithm.

grafts. In such cases ischaemia times >12 hours are likely to be associated with poorer outcomes, and in the USA median cold ischaemia time for all pancreas transplants has been <12 hours since 2006.[7,8]

The pressure gradient between mean arterial pressure and portal venous pressure that maintains blood flow through the pancreas can be significantly diminished during the perfusion of the abdominal organs in retrieval operations. Particular attention is required to maintain an adequate gradient if a cannula for perfusion is placed in the portal venous system as well as the aorta. Many transplant units perfuse abdominal organs with an aortic cannula only, and there is some evidence that supports the view that additional portal perfusion is unnecessary.[9] For the interests of the pancreatic allograft, aortic perfusion alone is the most 'physiological' state that allows satisfactory perfusion and adequate drainage of the effluent.

It is common practice to flush the donor duodenum using a nasogastric tube with an antiseptic or antibiotic solution during the retrieval operation. No evidence exists to demonstrate the superiority of any solution used for duodenal decontamination, and povidone–iodine during cold storage may be toxic to duodenal mucosa.[10] Donor duodenal contents should be submitted for bacterial and fungal culture. The results may be important in guiding the management of infection in pancreas transplant recipients.[11]

Careful and minimal handling of the pancreas during retrieval is important. Removal of the spleen and the pancreatico-duodenal graft en bloc with the liver is the quickest and safest method for both

organs. The organs are then easily and quickly separated on the back table at the retrieval centre.

Further back-table preparation of the pancreas, which takes place in the recipient centre, is a crucial part of the procedure and takes a minimum of 2 hours. The short stumps of the gastroduodenal artery (GDA) and the splenic artery should be marked with fine polypropylene sutures at the time of retrieval. Demonstration of good collateral circulation within the pancreatico-duodenal arcade (between the superior mesenteric artery [SMA] and the GDA) by flushing the arteries individually at the back table is reassuring. An iliac artery 'Y' graft of donor origin anastomosed to the SMA and the splenic artery is the most common method of reconstruction for the graft arterial inflow (**Fig. 9.2**). Meticulous dissection and ligation of the lymphatic tissue and small vessels around the pancreas is important to prevent haemorrhage upon reperfusion of the graft in the recipient. Particular attention should be paid to secure the duodenal segment staple lines by inversion with further sutures.

The pancreas transplant operation

General considerations

In SPK transplantation, pancreatic implantation is usually performed first because of the lower ischaemia tolerance of the pancreas. It is easier to implant the pancreatic graft on the right side. The renal allograft can also be placed intra-abdominally with anastomoses to the left iliac vessels. Alternatively, an extraperitoneal renal

Pancreatico-duodenal graft excised with an aortic patch

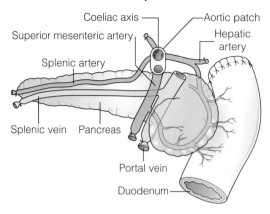

Reconstruction of arterial vessels

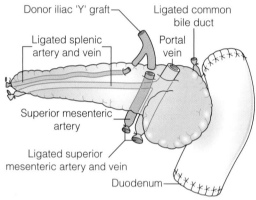

Figure 9.2 • In the absence of an aortic patch containing hepatic artery and the gastroduodenal artery, the pancreatic graft reconstruction requires a donor iliac 'Y' graft.

transplant on the left side can be performed using the same incision or through a separate left iliac fossa incision. A further alternative is to implant the renal graft ipsilaterally, using more caudal segments of the recipient right iliac vessels.

Severely atherosclerotic and calcified vessels in some diabetic recipients can be a challenge during pancreatic implantation. Iliac 'Y' grafts used for reconstruction offer greater flexibility in choosing a suitable arterial anastomotic site in the recipient vessels. The most common technique used for pancreas transplantation has been intra-abdominal implantation of the whole pancreas together with a donor duodenal segment. Currently the choices available to the surgeon are related to the management of the exocrine secretions and venous drainage, as discussed below.

Management of exocrine secretions

Drainage of the exocrine secretions of pancreatic grafts into the recipient's bladder was the most common technique, accounting for 90% of US pancreas transplants during the 1980s and early 1990s. The popularity of this technique was due to its perceived safety, primarily less serious consequences of anastomotic leak (compared with enteric drainage) in the days of higher doses of corticosteroids and unrefined immunosuppression. The ability to monitor amylase levels in the urine has been considered an additional advantage of bladder drainage. However, the unphysiological diversion of pancreatic exocrine secretions into the urinary bladder causes frequent complications, often leading to chronic and disabling symptoms. As a consequence, conversion of the urinary diversion to enteric drainage is required in many patients. It is for this reason that enteric drainage has largely replaced bladder drainage as the method of choice for the management of exocrine secretions in the USA and in most European centres.

Any part of the recipient's small bowel can be used for anastomosis with the allograft duodenum. No data exist to demonstrate the superiority of one particular site over another. Roux-en-Y loops, which were commonly used, are becoming rare and a simple side-to-side entero-enterostomy is preferred.[12]

Delayed endocrine function from the transplanted graft is uncommon and insulin infusion should be discontinued at the time of reperfusion. Recipients achieving insulin independence for the first time in many years is a gratifying consequence for the surgeon; however, patients can become hypoglycaemic at this stage. Blood sugar levels should be checked frequently and a low rate of dextrose infusion is often required.

Management of the venous drainage

Drainage of the venous outflow from pancreas grafts into the portal circulation was first described by Calne in 1984.[13] This complex surgical technique using a segmental graft and gastric exocrine diversion in a paratopic position has never gained popularity. Drainage of the venous outflow into the systemic circulation at the level of the lower inferior vena cava has now become the norm in pancreatic transplantation. However, some units still use portal venous (PV) drainage via the superior mesenteric vein (SMV).[14] Several studies, including prospective randomised comparisons, have shown that this offers at least equivalent outcome to that of systemic venous (SV) drainage, with no compromise in safety.[15–17] The impetus for PV drainage was to achieve a more physiological delivery of insulin. A theoretical benefit was considered to be avoidance of hyperinsulinaemia, which has been linked with atherogenesis.[18] However, none of the studies of metabolic function after PV drainage have shown a clear benefit in terms of glucose metabolism, lipid profiles or atherogenesis, but some studies have observed a reduction in acute rejection rates.[15–17]

Immunosuppression in pancreas transplantation

Historically, there is ample evidence that the incidence of acute rejection is higher after pancreas transplantation compared with kidney transplantation.[6,19] The reasons for this difference are not clear. Nevertheless, there has been general acknowledgement of the higher immunological risk of pancreas transplantation. This has resulted in the evolution of strategies that use more intense immunosuppressive protocols for pancreas transplantation compared to kidney transplantation.

In Europe, immunosuppressive protocols in solid-organ transplantation in general have been less aggressive compared to US protocols. In the evolution of immunosuppression for pancreas transplantation, tacrolimus has largely replaced ciclosporin and mycophenolate mofetil (MMF) has replaced azathioprine based on sound evidence from prospective randomised trials showing improved outcomes.[20–24]

Steroid withdrawal or avoidance has been a focus of study in the last decade. As yet there is no evidence demonstrating a significant benefit from steroid avoidance or withdrawal, but experience reveals that it is feasible without adversely affecting outcome in pancreas transplant patients.[25,26]

Induction therapy with biological agents is part of the immunosuppressive protocol in nearly all pancreas transplants.[27] This is based on prospective multicentre trials that demonstrated a reduced incidence and severity of rejection episodes with biological induction therapy.[28–30] A comparison of different induction therapies (OKT3, ATG, basiliximab or daclizumab) compared to no induction showed a reduction in acute rejection with induction therapy, but no consistent pattern has emerged to demonstrate the superiority of any one specific biological agent when used in conjunction with tacrolimus-based immunosuppression.[31] More recent evidence from a single-centre randomised comparison suggests that alemtuzumab induction is associated with similar graft and patient survival rates compared to ATG induction, but results in a lower incidence of acute rejection and better safety profile, with a significantly lower incidence of CMV infection.[32]

Diagnosis and management of acute rejection following pancreas transplantation

One of the notable features about pancreas transplantation over the last 15 years has been the considerable reduction in the incidence of acute rejection. In 1992, 74% of SPK transplant recipients and 50% of solitary pancreas transplant recipients (this probably underestimates the true incidence) were reported to have received anti-rejection therapy.[6,19] This had reduced to 19% and 17%, respectively, by 2000.[12]

An important feature of pancreatic graft rejection, for the purposes of patient management, is the lack of a reliable early marker. In SPK transplants, diagnosis of acute rejection almost completely relies on monitoring of renal allograft function by measuring serum creatinine levels and undertaking renal biopsy when indicated. Discordant rejection of allografts only occurs rarely following SPK transplantation, with isolated pancreas rejection in 5–10% of acute rejection episodes.[19] Monitoring for acute rejection and patient management in the early postoperative period is a particular challenge in patients following solitary pancreas transplantation.

Acute rejection of the pancreas affects the exocrine pancreas first. The inflammation may cause pain and a low-grade fever associated with a rise in serum amylase. These symptoms and signs are non-specific, can be subtle and do not distinguish between acute rejection and other causes of graft inflammation (such as ischaemia–reperfusion injury or allograft pancreatitis). Islets of Langerhans are scattered sparsely throughout the exocrine pancreas and beta cells have considerable functional reserve. Therefore, dysfunction of the majority of islets resulting in hyperglycaemia as a consequence of rejection occurs only very late in the course of pancreatic rejection. Imaging modalities such as computed tomography (CT) or magnetic resonance imaging (MRI) visualise the pancreas and are helpful to exclude other pathology (such as lack of perfusion which may be segmental, or intra-abdominal collections). There are no specific radiological signs of acute rejection. Detection of urinary amylase in bladder-drained grafts is a sensitive indicator of exocrine function. However, detection of hypoamylasuria lacks specificity. A >25% reduction in urinary amylase correlates with acute rejection in no more than half of the cases when assessed by biopsy.[33] A stable urinary amylase may therefore be helpful in excluding acute rejection, but detection of hypoamylasuria is non-specific and unhelpful.

Pancreas allograft biopsy has recently become established as a reliable and safe technique, and is the gold standard in the diagnosis of acute rejection in solitary pancreas transplants. Percutaneous biopsy under ultrasound or CT guidance is the most common method. Histological criteria for the diagnosis and grading of rejection have been standardised.[34]

Histological examination of pancreas graft biopsies correlates with clinical and serological findings and has revealed two distinct pathways of rejection (similar to the more widely recognised pattern in kidney transplantation): T-cell-mediated rejection and antibody-mediated rejection.

✅ A recent article by Papadimitriou and Drachenberg[35] provides an authoritative and up-to-date review of the histological criteria for these two subtypes of acute pancreas allograft rejection, as well as mechanisms leading to graft injury and differential diagnosis.

The recognition of antibody-mediated rejection as a distinct entity in pancreas transplantation explains conflicting results in published data from earlier years, as some cases of treatment-resistant acute pancreas allograft rejection were thought to be cell-mediated rejection. It also partially explains the improved success rates in solitary pancreas transplantation as a consequence of liberal surveillance biopsies.[32] Finally, the increasing utilisation of pancreas allograft biopsies has cast doubt on the validity of the assumption that isolated rejection of the kidney or the pancreas graft in SPK recipients is uncommon. Monitoring of donor-specific antibodies has become routine. In a multivariate analysis of 433 pancreas transplants at the Oxford Transplant Centre, development of de novo donor-specific antibodies (DSA) emerged as a strong independent predictor of pancreas graft failure (hazard ratio 4.66, $P < 0.001$).[36]

Early or mild cell-mediated acute rejection of the pancreas allograft concurrent with kidney rejection can be succesfully treated with high-dose corticosteroids. Recurrent acute rejection or moderate to severe rejection episodes require treatment with anti-T-cell agents. International Pancreas Transplant Registry (IPTR) data show that steroids were used in 85% of SPK and 80% of solitary pancreas transplant recipients diagnosed with acute rejection.[12] However, 48% of SPK recipients and 80% of solitary pancreas recipients with acute rejection were also given anti-T-cell agents, suggesting that many patients were treated with both. There are not enough data to make evidence-based recommendations on the optimum treatment for acute antibody-mediated rejection. Experience with the management of antibody-mediated rejection in kidney transplantation would suggest a potential role for plasma exchange with or without intravenous immunoglobulin and/or rituximab.

Acute rejection in pancreas allografts is not life-threatening and caution is advised against overimmunosuppression. If diagnosed before the onset of hyperglycaemia, most rejection episodes are reversible. The UNOS data for 4251 patients who received SPK transplants between 1988 and 1997 were analysed by Reddy et al. in order to determine the influence of acute rejection on long-term outcome.[37] Acute rejection of either graft increased the relative risk of pancreas and kidney graft failure at 5 years. The relative risks, adjusted for other risk factors, were 1.32 and 1.53 for pancreas and kidney, respectively, if acute rejection occurred. The worst outcome was in patients who had both kidney and pancreas rejection.

Complications of pancreas transplantation

Pancreas transplantation is associated with a higher incidence and a greater range of complications than kidney transplantation. Furthermore, postoperative patient management constitutes a greater challenge (Box 9.3). Between a quarter and a third of patients require re-laparotomy following pancreas transplantation to deal with complications. Part of the reason for the increased incidence of complications is the higher level of immunosuppression in a high-risk diabetic population who already exhibit impaired infection resistance, poor healing and a high prevalence of comorbidity. Other factors relate to the allograft, which unlike kidney or liver

---

Box 9.3 • Complications of pancreas transplantation

Vascular complications
- Thrombosis: allograft venous or arterial thrombosis
- Haemorrhage: early haemorrhage from allograft vessels and late haemorrhage (rupture of pseudoaneurysms)

Infective complications
- Systemic infection: opportunistic infections associated with immunosuppression
- Local infections: peritonitis, localised collections, enteric or pancreatic fistulas

Allograft pancreatitis
- Ischaemia–reperfusion injury or reflux pancreatitis (especially after bladder drainage)

Complications specific to bladder drainage
- Chronic dehydration, acidosis, recurrent urinary tract infections, haematuria, chemical cystitis, urethral strictures or urethral disruption

allografts is not sterile and uniquely possesses rich proteolytic enzymes, making it susceptible to specific complications such as secondary haemorrhage, pancreatitis, leaks and fistula formation. The blood flow to the pancreas is much lower than that to the kidney and this is a further risk factor, specifically for thrombotic complications. Finally, bladder drainage of the exocrine secretions is associated with a high incidence of complications unique to this unphysiological diversion. Increasing donor age, prolonged preservation time, recipient obesity and donor obesity are risk factors for complications and early graft loss.

Vascular complications

Thrombosis

Allograft venous or arterial thrombosis occurs more commonly following pancreatic transplantation compared to kidney transplantation. Venous thrombosis is more common than arterial thrombosis by a factor of 2:1.[38] Graft thrombosis is by far the most common cause of early graft loss following pancreas transplantation. An analysis of US pancreas transplants performed until the end of 2008 revealed that 5% of SPK transplants and 7% of solitary pancreas transplants failed as a result of thrombosis[37] (Table 9.1). Among the recognised risk factors for thrombosis, donor-related factors have the greatest impact. These include donor age, donor BMI, cardiovascular and cerebrovascular cause of donor death, prolonged preservation time, excessive flush volumes and pressure, and the type of preservation solution. A technical factor predisposing to thrombosis could be the use of venous extension grafts for the portal vein anastomosis, which should be only very rarely required. Concern about a potentially higher incidence of thrombosis following portal venous drainage has not been borne out by clinical experience.

Graft thrombosis, once diagnosed, requires prompt laparotomy and graft pancreatectomy. There are reports of surgical, radiological and pharmacological interventions in small numbers of cases.[39–41] Virtually all of these refer to highly selected cases of segmental, incomplete thrombosis.

Routine use of heparin for prophylaxis against allograft vascular thrombosis is used by some but is not standard practice in many units and is associated with increased risk of haemorrhage.

Table 9.1 illustrates the relative prevalence of early complications of pancreas transplantation leading to graft loss from the IPTR database.

Haemorrhage

Release of the vascular clamps and reperfusion of the pancreatic allograft during the recipient operation can be tricky, with potential for bleeding from multiple points on the allograft. The key to avoiding this is meticulous preparation of the allograft on the back table prior to implantation.

Haemorrhage in the early postoperative hours is often a result of the proteolytic and fibrinolytic activity of the pancreatic exocrine secretions leaking from the surface of the pancreas and coming into contact with thrombus-sealed small vessels or vascular anastomoses. Early postoperative bleeding is the most common indication for re-laparotomy after pancreas transplantation. Unlike graft thrombosis however, bleeding has little impact on ultimate outcome and <1% of pancreas grafts are lost to bleeding[42] (Table 9.1).

Late haemorrhage following pancreas transplantation is an uncommon but catastrophic complication, often due to the rupture of a pseudoaneurysm or direct erosion of one of the anastomoses secondary to a leak. Any unexplained fever, tachycardia, leucocytosis or abdominal pain in recipients of pancreas transplants should lead to investigation for a leak or intra-abdominal collection.

Infective complications

Pancreas transplantation, in common with all transplant procedures that require immunosuppression, is associated with an increased risk of mostly opportunistic infections. CMV disease is more common after pancreas transplantation compared with kidney or liver transplantation. Antiviral prophylaxis in CMV-mismatched donor/recipient pairs is mandatory. Unique to pancreatic transplantation are intra-abdominal septic complications, which occur as a consequence of bacteria or fungi transmitted from the donor via the allograft, or as a consequence of an anastomotic leak. Patients on peritoneal dialysis at the time of transplantation have a higher rate of intra-abdominal infection compared with those on haemodialysis.[6]

Table 9.1 • Causes of early graft loss after pancreas transplantation in USA primary deceased donor pancreas transplants (January 2004 to January 2009)

Causes of early graft loss	SPK	PAK	PTA
	n = 4320	n = 1148	n = 494
Thrombosis	5.1%	7.4%	6.6%
Infection	0.6%	0.8%	0.4%
Pancreatitis	0.6%	0.4%	0.4%
Anastomotic leak	0.4%	0.2%	0.3%
Bleeding	0.2%	0.3%	0.3%
Total graft loss	6.9%	9.1%	7.9%

SPK, simultaneous pancreas–kidney transplants; PAK, pancreas after kidney transplants; PTA, pancreas transplantation alone.

Allograft pancreatitis

Cold storage and ischaemia–reperfusion injury inevitably result in a degree of oedema of the pancreatic allograft. This is a commonly encountered finding if a re-laparotomy becomes necessary in the first few postoperative days, and it is not always associated with an elevation in serum amylase. There is no universally agreed definition of allograft pancreatitis. Bladder drainage (especially in the presence of autonomic neuropathy affecting bladder function and causing high intravesical pressures) can be associated with recurrent episodes of allograft pancreatitis due to reflux. Catheter drainage of the bladder for at least 7–10 days is usually adequate for the management of the acute episode but ultimately enteric conversion may be required.

During the pancreas transplant operation, allograft exocrine function starts very promptly upon revascularisation and the duodenal segment quickly fills with pancreatic juice. Excessive distension of the stapled duodenal segment and consequent reflux may cause postoperative pancreatitis. Donor age, donor obesity and prolonged preservation times are other factors associated with allograft pancreatitis. The distinction between allograft pancreatitis and acute rejection in the presence of an oedematous pancreas, abdominal pain and a slightly raised serum amylase is a difficult clinical diagnosis.

Complications specific to bladder drainage

The most common consequence of the diversion of the exocrine pancreatic secretions into the bladder is a chemical cystitis, which predisposes patients to infection, persistent haematuria and troublesome dysuria. Dysuria is more troublesome in men, with urethritis that can progress to urethral disruption. Failure of reabsorption of the exocrine secretions results in chronic dehydration and acidosis. Urinary tract infections are much more common compared to intestinal drainage. Persistent haematuria may necessitate repeated blood transfusions. As mentioned above, reflux allograft pancreatitis is another potential complication. As a consequence of one or more of these complications, enteric conversion of the exocrine drainage may become necessary. The enteric conversion rate in bladder-drained pancreas transplants increases with increasing follow-up and can be as high as 40% at 5 years.[19]

Outcome following pancreas transplantation

Patient and graft survival rates following pancreas transplantation continue to improve. The most recent analysis of IPTR data reveals excellent short- and medium-term results, with 1-year and 3-year patient survival rates of 95% and 92%, respectively, in all three pancreas transplant categories.[43]

Factors influencing pancreas transplantation outcome

Recipient age

Increasing recipient age is a small but significant risk factor in the outcome of pancreas transplantation. Historically, patient and graft survival rates have been higher in younger recipients. However, in recent years more careful patient selection has resulted in improved outcome in older recipients, to the extent that the short-term outcome following pancreas transplantation is no different for patients older than 45 years at the time of transplantation compared to younger patients.[44] Five-year patient survival after SPK transplantation is 86% for recipients aged 35–49 years at the time of transplantation compared with 81.7% for those aged 50–64 years.[44]

Re-transplantation

Re-transplantation appears as a consistent and significant risk factor for graft survival in all categories. One-year pancreas graft survival after re-transplantation in the SPK category is 70.8% (±9.3%) compared to 85.4% (±0.9%) in primary SPK transplants.[44]

HLA matching

Analyses of US registry data have inconsistently shown limited evidence for the influence of HLA matching on pancreas transplant outcome.[45] The effect of HLA matching, when present, has been small and seemed to affect different categories during different eras or was confined to different classes of HLA mismatches. The likely explanation is that HLA matching has negligible or no influence on the outcome of pancreas transplantation, as is suggested by the most recent analysis of the IPTR database.[43]

Management of exocrine secretions and management of venous drainage

The surgical technique employed for exocrine diversion has no influence on outcome in pancreas transplantation. Pancreas graft survival rates at 1 year following SPK transplantation for the 2000–2004 cohort in the US were 87% and 85% for bladder-drained and enteric-drained grafts, respectively. More recent analyses confirm that the method of exocrine diversion has no influence on patient or graft survival rates.[27] Similarly, outcomes are similar comparing systemic and portal venous drainage.[44]

Immunosuppression

Immunosuppressive therapy has a major influence on the outcome following pancreas transplantation. In the last decade, tacrolimus and MMF have been the basis of maintenance immunosuppression in the large majority of patients. Multivariate analyses reveal that the tacrolimus/MMF combination is associated with significant reductions in pancreas graft loss (relative risk (RR) = 0.74, P = 0.08 for SPK; RR = 0.51, P = 0.001 for PAK; and RR = 0.46, P = 0.014 for PTA). In a cohort of transplants undertaken between 2006 and 2010, antibody induction was associated with lower risk of pancreas graft failure following SPK, but not PAK or PTA, and only when depleting antibodies were used.[27]

Donor factors

Donor age, donor obesity and donor cause of death have been linked with the outcome of pancreas transplantation. Whilst all of these variables may be independently associated with outcome, they are likely to be inter-related; for instance, younger donors are more likely to have died of trauma, whilst older and obese donors are more likely to have died of a cerebrovascular cause.

An analysis of all SPK transplants performed in the USA during a 12-year period between 1994 and 2005 (n = 8850) has conclusively shown increasing donor age to be a risk factor in pancreas transplantation.[46] Pancreas and kidney graft survival and patient survival at 1 year were significantly inferior in the old donor group (>45 years) compared to the young donor group <45 years (77% vs 85%, 89% vs 92% and 95% vs 93%, respectively). Five-year pancreas graft survival was 72% versus 60% for young versus old donor transplants, respectively.

Humar et al.[47] reported the outcome of 711 deceased donor pancreas transplants performed between 1994 and 2001. The outcomes were analysed for three groups based on donor BMI. Patients who received grafts from obese donors (BMI >30) had a higher incidence of complications and inferior graft survival. The incidence of technical failure was 9.7% in the BMI <25 group, 16.3% in the BMI 25–30 group and 21% in the BMI >30 group (P = 0.04). More recently, the same group of authors published an analysis in a slightly larger cohort of pancreas transplant patients in order to determine risk factors for technical failure following pancreas transplantation.[48] Technical failure, defined as thrombosis, bleeding, leaks, infections or pancreatitis, was responsible for the loss of 13.1% of transplants (131 of 973). On multivariate analysis the following were significant risk factors: recipient BMI >30 (RR = 2.42, P = 0.0003), preservation time >24 hours (RR = 1.87, P = 0.04) and cause of donor death other than trauma (RR = 1.58, P = 0.04). Donor obesity had borderline significance.

Pancreas grafts from paediatric donors (aged >4 years) can be used with excellent results.[25] Organs from DCD (donation after circulatory/cardiac death) donors constitute an increasing proportion of the deceased donor pool. University of Wisconsin experience and the pooled US data suggest that the outcome of pancreas transplantation using DCD grafts is equivalent to that achieved with DBD (donation after brain death) donor organs.[49,50] More recent data from Oxford, one of the world's largest pancreas transplant programmes, reveal a higher risk of pancreas graft failure with DCD grafts. The poorer outcome was confined to solitary pancreas transplant recipients with prolonged preservation times.[7,8]

It is evident that donor selection has a major influence on the outcome of pancreas transplantation. Therefore, other risk factors such as preservation time, recipient BMI and comorbidity need to be considered when using suboptimal grafts for pancreas transplantation.

Long-term outlook following pancreas transplantation

Pancreas transplantation and life expectancy

Clearly, one of the most important issues for patients considering pancreas transplantation is whether their life expectancy will be influenced by the transplant. Numerous studies and analyses of databases have consistently shown that successful pancreas transplantation is associated with improved survival prospects in diabetic patients. No prospective controlled study has ever been carried out that compares pancreas transplantation with insulin therapy and hence all available evidence is subject to selection bias.

Several studies have addressed the question of the impact of pancreas transplantation on long-term mortality in a number of different ways. The University of Wisconsin experience in 500 SPK transplant recipients published in 1998[51] simply quotes a 10-year patient survival rate of 70%. This is matched in their experience only by recipients of living-donor kidney transplants. Unsurpassed as they are, these results were obtained in a highly selective group of young patients with a relatively short duration of diabetes and kidney failure and strict eligibility criteria excluding those with ischaemic heart disease.

A large US registry analysis published in 2001 looked at the outcome in 13 467 adults with type I diabetes registered on kidney and SPK transplant waiting lists between 1988 and 1997.[52] Adjusted 10-year patient survival was 67% for SPK transplant recipients, 65% for living-donor kidney (LKD) transplant recipients and 46% for cadaveric kidney (CAD) transplant recipients. Taking the mortality of patients who remained on dialysis as a reference, the adjusted relative risk of 5-year mortality was 0.40, 0.45 and 0.74 for SPK, LKD and CAD recipients, respectively. Another large review of the UNOS database published in 2003 analysed long-term survival in 18 549 type I diabetic patients transplanted between 1987 and 1996.[53] There was a long-term survival advantage in favour of pancreas transplant recipients (8-year crude survival rates: 72% for SPK, 72% for LKD and 55% for CAD). This diminished but persisted after adjusting for donor and recipient variables and kidney graft function.

Influence of pancreas transplantation on diabetic complications

Nephropathy

There is convincing evidence that successful pancreas transplantation can stop the progression of diabetic nephropathy and reverse associated histological changes. This evidence largely comes from studies that have assessed the course of diabetic nephropathy in kidney allografts in SPK or PAK transplant recipients.[54,55] Fioretto et al. have shown that established lesions of diabetic nephropathy in native kidneys can be reversed with successful pancreas transplantation (PTA).[56] In the setting of clinical transplantation the beneficial effect of the pancreas graft is counterbalanced by the nephrotoxicity of the immunosuppressive drugs.

Retinopathy

✔✔ Patients with type I diabetes often quote preservation of eyesight as one of the main reasons for considering pancreas transplantation. There is good evidence that better blood glucose control reduces the risk of progression of retinopathy.[57] However, in practice the large majority of patients undergoing pancreas transplantation will have advanced proliferative retinopathy. Hence prevention of retinopathy is seldom a major factor in the consideration of the risks and benefits of pancreas transplantation.[58]

Retinopathy needs to be treated prior to transplantation with laser photocoagulation, which is an effective treatment. For the minority of patients who present with non-proliferative retinopathy or those who have recently undergone treatment for proliferative retinopathy, there is a risk of rapid progression of the retinopathy following transplantation. Such patients require close ophthalmic follow-up within the first 3 years of transplantation. Stabilisation of retinopathy after pancreas transplantation takes 3 years.[58–60] During this time, any patient who has an indication or develops an indication for laser treatment should undergo treatment.

Patients often report improved vision soon after pancreas transplantation. Improvement in macular oedema is demonstrable soon after transplantation and can result in early improvement of vision. It is unclear whether this is a consequence of euglycaemia or a consequence of the kidney transplant improving fluid balance. It is probable that euglycaemia offered

by pancreas transplantation, over and above the benefits of the non-uraemic environment, results in better elimination of osmotic swelling of the lens, hence improving fluctuations in vision that diabetic patients experience.[58]

Neuropathy

Patients with end-stage renal failure and type I diabetes almost universally exhibit an autonomic and peripheral (somatic) diabetic polyneuropathy as well as uraemic neuropathy. Improvement in neuropathy following SPK transplantation using objective measures of nerve function has been demonstrated by several transplant centres.[61,62] For individuals with intractable and distressing symptoms of neuropathy the clinical benefit may be considerable. Reversal of neuropathic symptoms takes many months and a clinically relevant benefit may not be evident for 6–12 months after transplantation. Obesity, smoking, the presence of advanced neuropathy and poor renal allograft function are predictors of poor recovery in nerve function after SPK transplantation.[63]

Cardiovascular disease

Pancreas transplantation has demonstrable benefits on microangiopathy in diabetics.[64] Some of its effects on retinopathy, nephropathy and neuropathy may be mediated through this mechanism. It has been more difficult to demonstrate any improvement in macroangiopathy. The enhanced survival prospects after pancreas transplantation ought to be, at least in part, due to improvement in the cardiovascular risk profile. Evidence to support this is accumulating. Fiorina et al. demonstrated favourable influences of pancreas[65] and islet[66] transplantation on atherosclerotic risk factors, including plasma lipid profile, blood pressure, left ventricular function and endothelial function. This translates into reduced cardiovascular death rate.[67,68] Similar improvements occur in early non-uraemic diabetics after PTA.[69]

Islet transplantation

The concept of extracting and transplanting islets is not new and was initially attempted in 1893 in Bristol when a fragmented sheep's pancreas was transplanted subcutaneously into a 15-year-old boy dying of ketoacidosis.[70] This early xenograft was, not surprisingly, unsuccessful but predated the discovery of insulin by nearly 30 years. The era of experimental islet research began in 1911, when Bensley stained islets within the guinea-pig pancreas using a number of dyes, and was able to pick free the occasional islet for morphological study.[71] Mass isolation of large numbers of viable islets from the human pancreas has proven to be a challenge ever since. The average adult human pancreas weighs 70 g, contains an average of 1–2 million islets of average diameter 157 μm, constituting between 0.8 and 3.8% of the total mass of the gland.[72] It was almost 100 years after the work of Bensley that Scharp et al. reported insulin independence after islet transplantation; however, even this was short-lived and difficult to reproduce.[73]

✅✅ In 2000, the Edmonton group reported a series of seven consecutive patients in whom insulin independence was achieved after islet transplantation.[74]

The remarkable outcome in the Edmonton patients was achieved by transplanting at least two islet preparations from different donors and using a novel steroid-free immunosuppression regimen of tacrolimus, sirolimus and induction with daclizumab. This regimen has been termed 'the Edmonton protocol' and many units worldwide have attempted to replicate these outcomes, with variable success.[75,76] In the aftermath of the Edmonton protocol, islet transplantation is considered in many countries as 'standard of care' for a select group of patients with type I diabetes and is funded through the healthcare system in Canada and the NHS in the UK. The results of combined islet and kidney transplantation now match those of islet transplantation alone,[77,78] and recent data suggest that islets transplanted with a kidney may prolong the patient and kidney graft survival and protect against diabetic vascular complications.[79,80]

Patient selection and assessment

There are two principal indications for islet transplantation:

1. *Severely impaired awareness of hypoglycaemia (IAH) despite optimum insulin therapy.* IAH occurs in 20–25% of patients with type I diabetes and is potentially life threatening. These patients have a defective counter-regulatory hormonal response to hypoglycaemia, are unable to identify low blood sugars and therefore institute corrective measures.[81] Defective recognition of hypoglycaemia increases the risk of severe hypoglycaemic episodes that can result in coma and death. The impact on quality of life for these patients is substantial, and social activities and employment can be severely restricted; indeed, in the UK, patients with IAH cannot hold a UK driving licence.

2. *Patients with type I diabetes and a functioning kidney allograft who are unable to maintain their HbA1c below 7%.* In this patient group it is not necessary to demonstrate IAH as they are already taking immunosuppression and it has been shown that the improved glycaemic control after islet transplantation in this setting is associated with a reduction in long-term diabetic complications.

Impaired awareness of hypoglycaemia can be assessed by patient history and by asking the patient to keep a diary of insulin usage, dietary intake and hypoglycaemic events, in particular those events requiring assistance from relatives or those requiring hospitalisation. The use of a continuous glucose monitoring sensor (CGMS) can be very useful in assessing daily glucose profiles pre- and post-islet transplantation (**Fig. 9.3**).[82] Scoring systems such as the Gold or Clark scores allow numerical documentation of the degree of IAH. The Gold score asks the question 'do you know when your hypos are commencing?' and the patient completes

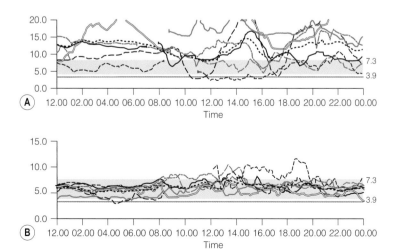

Figure 9.3 • CGMS profiles before **(a)** and after **(b)** islet transplantation.

a linear scale from 1 to 7 (always aware to never aware). A score of 4 or above suggests IAH. The Clark method asks eight questions to document the patient's exposure and responses to moderate and severe hypoglycaemia, and again a score of 4 or more suggests IAH.[81] Ryan et al. have described a composite HYPO score based on 4 weeks of glucose values.[83] They suggest that this provides a more objective assessment of the metabolic instability of an individual patient and allows pre- and post-transplant comparison. Patients should be assessed by a multidisciplinary team consisting of a diabetologist, transplant surgeon, dietician and a diabetes nurse specialist. This will ensure an optimum insulin regimen and dietary compliance and that the patient is fully informed about the likely outcome of islet transplantation and the risks involved, principally post-transplant immunosuppression.

Islet isolation

Donor factors contributing to successful islet isolation have been documented by Lakey et al. (Table 9.2).[84] This paper suggests that pancreases from older donors with a higher body mass index (BMI) should result in a significantly higher islet yield. O'Gorman et al. have suggested a scoring system from 1 to 100 to give a numerical assessment of the likelihood of successful isolation from a specific donor pancreas.[85] These studies, however, only predict successful isolation and do not take into consideration data that suggest that islets isolated from younger donors are functionally better.[86] In the UK, a sharing scheme was introduced in December 2010 where patients for SPK transplantation and islet transplantation are placed on a common waiting list and pancreases offered on a named patient basis. Multiple donor and recipient factors are taken into consideration, allowing islet and whole pancreas recipients equal access to suitable organs.

Most of the outcome data on islet transplantation are based on organs from brain-dead donors (DBD); however, there is growing evidence that pancreases from donation after circulatory death (DCD) can produce transplantable preparations and good outcomes. Most of the data on DCD islet transplantation are from the Kyoto group and although long-term graft survival is obtained, insulin independence is less common.[87-91]

It is critical that the pancreas for islet isolation is retrieved with the same care as that for whole pancreas transplantation and that cold ischaemia time is minimised, ideally to under 8 hours.[92] Pancreases should be transported rapidly and the staff in the isolation laboratory should be ready to begin the isolation immediately. It has been demonstrated that suspending the explanted pancreas in a bilayer of oxygenated perfluorocarbon (PFC) and University of Wisconsin (UW) solution during or after transport allows satisfactory islet preparations to be obtained from suboptimal pancreases and may even increase yields from pancreases with long ischaemia times.[93,94] PFC-based preservation may also help expand the donor pool by improving islet isolation from DCD pancreases and older donors.[95]

The semi-automated process for islet isolation that is used in most laboratories was described by Ricordi et al. in 1989.[96] This involves digestion of the pancreas using a combination of collagenase enzyme and mechanical dissociation of the pancreas in the Ricordi chamber (**Fig. 9.4**). A number of new enzyme blends have been developed for human isolation, including collagenase NB1 (Serva), Liberase MTF (Roche) and C1 collagenase HA (Vitacyte). Each of these differs slightly in the enzyme blend and manufacturing process but promises to deliver more consistent, better-quality islet yields. The preparation is then

Table 9.2 • Donor-related variables predicting isolation success

Variable	P value	R value	Odds ratio
Donor age (yr)	<0.05	0.18	1.10
Body mass index	<0.01	0.19	1.30
Local vs distant procurement team	<0.01	0.21	7.04
Min. blood glucose	<0.01	−0.24	0.68
Duration of cardiac arrest	<0.01	−0.17	0.81
Duration of cold storage	<0.05	−0.13	0.86

Reproduced from Lakey JR, Warnock GL, Rajotte RV, et al. Variables in organ donors that affect the recovery of human islets of Langerhans. Transplantation 1996;61(7):1047–53. With permission from Lippincott, Williams & Wilkins.

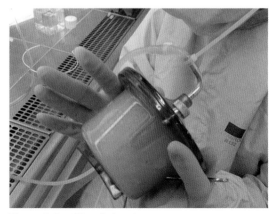

Figure 9.4 • Ricordi chamber.

purified on a continuous density gradient using a COBE 2991 cell separator, resulting in a packed cell volume of only 1–2 mL (**Fig. 9.5**).[97] Although unpurified preparations can be used (particularly in autotransplants), the risk of portal vein thrombosis, portal hypertension and disseminated intravascular coagulation (DIC) is increased.[98–101]

After isolation and purification, it is now standard practice to place the islet preparation in culture for 12–48 hours. There are compelling data that this does not adversely affect islet graft function and does in fact increase purity of the preparation.[102] Extended culture up to 48 hours can also be used to assess the viability of an islet graft, particularly after DCD isolation.

The number of islets in the preparation is documented in terms of islet equivalents (IEQ). This counting method adjusts for the fact that islets vary greatly in size, and cell viability stains such as fluorescenediacetate/propidium iodide and SytoGreen/ethidium bromide are used to determine the viable beta-cell mass.[103]

The minimum release criteria in the UK for an islet preparation are:

- >200 000 islet equivalents
- >70% viability
- >30% purity
- Gram-stain negative
- Endotoxin-negative

It is accepted that these criteria are subjective and open to observer variation and error. Some assessment of the 'quality' of the preparation should also be made. Experienced islet laboratory staff can comment on the morphology of the cells, the integrity of the islets and whether or not there is evidence of central necrosis within the islets. Islet oxygen consumption rate and beta-cell ATP content show good correlation between product testing and in vivo islet function in animal studies, and may be useful in the future, but are time-consuming and expensive. The Minnesota group has demonstrated good correlation between marginal mass islet transplants in diabetic nude mice and outcome of human islet transplants from the same donor.[104]

Modern islet isolation facilities must comply with current good manufacturing practice (cGMP). The facility must be purpose-built to comply with regulatory authorities, which in the UK comprise the Human Tissue Authority (HTA) and the Medicines and Healthcare products Regulatory Authority (MHRA). These regulations are designed to ensure that each laboratory produces a safe, consistent and traceable product, by influencing the structural design of the laboratory, the documentation of standard operating procedures and of individual isolations, and training of members of the isolation team. Modern islet isolation is therefore expensive and requires a large number of staff to cover a 24/7 on-call rota. In the UK, a hub-and-spoke model exists, whereby three isolation facilities provide islets for transplantation in seven centres.

The islet transplant

In the original Edmonton protocol, >11 000 IEQ/kg were required to achieve insulin independence and therefore at least two islet infusions are normally required.[74] Islet preparations are blood group matched with the potential recipient, but the need for close tissue matching is not clear. There is no evidence that closely matched preparations have a better outcome; however, it is likely to be beneficial to avoid repeated common mismatches as recipients may, in the event of graft rejection, become sensitised to multiple common alloantigens.

The islets are normally infused into the portal vein of the recipient under local anaesthetic and sedation in the radiology suite.[105] A 4-Fr cannula is introduced under ultrasound and videofluoroscopy

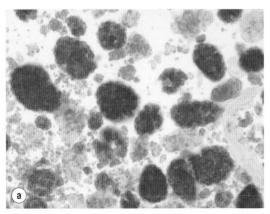
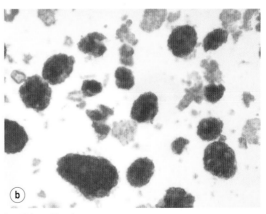

Figure 9.5 • Islets stained red with dithizone before **(a)** and after **(b)** purification.

into the main portal vein and the islet preparation infused under gravity feed over a period of 15–20 minutes (**Fig. 9.6**). Portal venous pressures are measured during the infusion process and if there is a significant rise, the infusion should be stopped until the portal pressure falls. The islet preparation is heparinised (35 U/kg patient body weight) to reduce the risk of portal vein thrombosis. This should ideally be done by experienced interventional radiologists and the track of the cannula occluded on withdrawal to reduce the risk of bleeding. The infusion into the portal vein can also be carried out by surgical cannulation of an omental vessel or the umbilical vein. The intraportal site for islet embolisation was recognised to be the most efficient location for islet implantation in the rodent, with the benefit of high vascularity, proximity to islet-specific nutrient factors and physiological first-pass insulin delivery to the liver.[106] While many different sites have been tried for islet implantation, the optimal site appears to be through portal venous embolisation. Attempts to embolise the spleen have led to significant life-threatening complications of splenic infarction, rupture and even gastric perforation.[107,108] More recently, reports of experimental implantation of islets into the gastric submucosa have shown improved vascularisation of the graft.[109] Recent developments in encapsulation technology have stimulated interest in using alternative sites. Encapsulation devices protect the islets from immunological attack while allowing insulin to be secreted.[110] Such devices have been implanted subcutaneously, intramuscularly and into the omentum, but with limited clinical application to date.

After infusion into the liver, the islets undergo a process of angiogenesis, which takes 14–21 days. Interestingly, this is often reflected in the reduced need for insulin in islet graft recipients around 3–4 weeks post-transplant.

Immunosuppression and outcomes

All seven patients in the original Edmonton experience were insulin-independent at 1 year post-transplant; however, follow-up of this cohort revealed that only 10% remained free of insulin at 5 years.[111] Alternative immunosuppression strategies have been reported in an attempt to improve these long-term outcomes. T-cell-depleting agents such as antithymocyte globulin (ATG), anti-CD3 and alemtuzumab (campath/anti-CD52) have been used as alternative induction therapy and combined with agents such as etanercept/tumour necrosis factor (TNF)-α or mycophenolate mofetil/tacrolimus as maintenance therapy.[112] Barton et al. have published data from the Collaborative Islet Transplant Registry on 677 patients receiving 1375 islet infusions between 1999 and 2010.[113] These data demonstrated a significant improvement in long-term insulin independence in the 2007–2010 era compared to earlier years (**Fig. 9.7**), with 3-year insulin independence approaching 50%. This report also documented that patients who received T-cell-depleting agents combined with TNF-α inhibition had better 3- to 5-year insulin independence rates (62% vs 43%). More recently, data from the UK and the US clearly demonstrate that islet transplantation provides protection from severe hypoglycaemic episodes, restores awareness of hypoglycaemia and improves glycaemic control.[114–116]

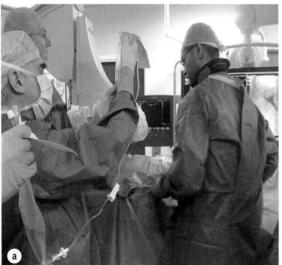
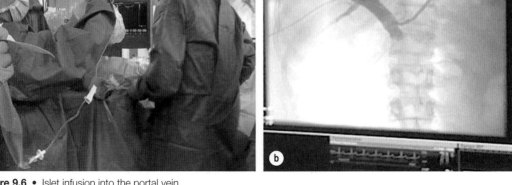

Figure 9.6 • Islet infusion into the portal vein.

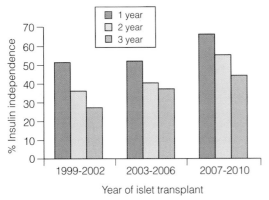

Figure 9.7 • Improvement in long-term insulin independence after islet transplantation from 1999 to 2010.[113]

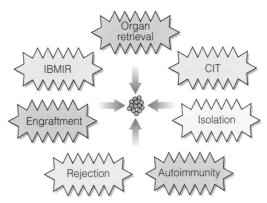

Figure 9.8 • Barriers to long-term islet graft function.

Serious adverse events after islet transplantation are either related to the infusion procedure or the immunosuppression. The more serious procedure-related complications of segmental portal vein thrombosis and bleeding have been reported in 4% and 10%, respectively.[117,118] The risk of portal vein thrombosis can be minimised by heparinisation of the recipient and by using only low-volume, high-purity preparations. Bleeding from the liver puncture can be avoided by using a fine-bore cannula and by ablating the track in the liver using coils, thrombostatic agents or a coagulative laser.[105] Leucopenia, neutropenia and sepsis have all been described after islet transplantation.[119] A reduction in estimated glomerular filtration rate has been described in islet transplant recipients in the long term post-transplantation, but reports of clinically significant renal impairment are rare.[113]

One of the biggest challenges in islet transplantation is monitoring the graft. No reliable investigations exist to monitor graft function or detect acute rejection. Experimental studies in rats suggest that islets labelled with superparamagnetic iron oxide (SPIO) nanoparticles can be monitored using magnetic resonance imaging (MRI) scanning and that loss of the islet-related MRI spots correlates with rejection.[120] Metabolic studies such as the C-peptide response to a glucose challenge may give an indirect indication of ongoing graft mass but as yet cannot aid in predicting acute rejection.[121]

Barriers to long-term function

Figure 9.8 illustrates the multiple factors that contribute to islet death and subsequent graft failure. The organ retrieval process and subsequent cold ischaemia time (CIT) have a significant negative impact on the outcome of islet isolation. The increasing use of pancreases from DCD donors where there have not been the physiological changes associated with brain death may be beneficial for islet isolation, and techniques such as using extracorporeal membrane oxygenation (ECMO) circuits in the donor may result in islets that are protected from ischaemic change. There is no doubt that minimising the time between cross-clamp in the donor and beginning the isolation process in the laboratory improves the islet yield and long-term graft function, requiring that pancreases must be transported rapidly to the laboratory and the isolation process started immediately. Improvements in isolation techniques have seen an increase in the average number of islets that can be produced per isolation with resultant improvements in graft survival.

There is an immediate blood-mediated inflammatory reaction (IBMIR) to the islet graft as soon as the islets are infused into the portal vein. Platelets bind to the surface of the islets and leucocytes infiltrate the graft. This contributes largely to the early loss of islets post-transplantation, which can be as high as 60% of the graft.[122] Strategies such as heparinisation of the recipient and ongoing insulin therapy may help to abrogate this process.[123] Little is known about the engraftment process of human islets within the liver. Transient elevation of liver enzymes is very common post-islet transplantation and it is interesting that the use of anti-inflammatory agents such as TNF-α blockers appears to improve graft survival.

Islets as a cell therapy

The shortage of organ donors coupled with the increased demand for islets has led to much research into alternative sources of insulin-producing cells that would be renewable and not depend solely on the availability of human cadaveric donors. The use of fetal or adult porcine islets for human xenotransplants has been explored; however, the high levels of immunosuppression required and the risk of transmission of porcine endogenous infections means that xenotransplantation is still some way in the future.

Stem cells are capable of both self-renewal and multilineage differentiation. They have the potential to proliferate and differentiate into any type of cell and to be genetically modified in vitro, thus providing a renewable source of cells for transplantation. Several potential strategies exist for developing a replenishable supply of beta cells. One of these is through directed differentiation of human embryonic stem cells (hESCs).[124] Functioning beta cells have been produced using this technology but concerns have been raised around the reproducibility of these processes and the potential for these cells to develop into teratomas. In 2006, Takahashi and Yamanaka described a technique whereby adult somatic cells could be de-differentiated and then induced to develop into different cell types.[125]

They used a cocktail of four transcription factors to produce these induced pluripotent stem cells (iPS cells), and many groups have now reproduced this work and developed cells of multiple lineages using this technology. The Melton group from Cambridge demonstrated that, in vivo, three transcription factors are required for beta-cell development, namely Ngn3, Pdx1 and MafA.[126] These are encouraging steps forward in the development of stem-cell-derived islets but there are still issues around upscaling of cell numbers and the potential for residual de-differentiated cells to produce tumours in the recipient. Recent developments in large-scale beta cell production in vivo are grounds for optimism and an exciting prospect is the potential existence of stem cells within the pancreas that could develop into new beta cells or with the potential to transdifferentiate non-endocrine tissue into functioning islets.[127–129]

Key points

- As of the end of 2010, over 35 000 pancreas transplants have been performed worldwide. In the USA alone there are more than 100 000 patients with functioning transplants; around 10 000 of these are pancreas allografts.
- The outcome following pancreas transplantation has improved considerably in the last 10–15 years. It is now comparable to the outcome for other solid-organ transplants.
- The number of pancreas transplants reached a peak in 2004. Activity has been declining in the USA since then in all three categories. An overall decrease of 20% was observed in 2010, compared with 2004. The largest decrease was observed in the PAK category (55%), followed by PTA (30%) and SPK (8%).
- Pancreas transplantation activity in the UK has followed a different pattern, with a much sharper increase in activity between 2000 and 2007, followed by a more modest decline since then.
- Despite the reduction in activity, pancreas transplant outcomes have remained at least as good in the last decade.
- Induction immunosuppression with biological agents is used in pancreas transplantation more often than any other solid-organ transplant. Tacrolimus/MMF combination is the basis of the most commonly used maintenance immunosuppression protocols. Steroid minimisation or avoidance is gaining momentum.
- Over the last 15 years, enteric drainage has gradually replaced bladder drainage as the preferred technique for the management of exocrine secretions in pancreas transplantation.
- Portal venous drainage, introduced in the mid-1990s, has not gained increasing popularity. It is used in just under a fifth of SPK and PAK transplants, and in 10% of PTA transplants.
- Evidence regarding the influence of pancreas transplantation on diabetic complications and life expectancy is not available from prospective controlled trials. Nevertheless, accumulating evidence from many studies strongly suggests that successful pancreas transplantation has a favourable influence on diabetic complications and survival prospects for patients.
- Islet transplantation is now considered as 'standard of care' for patients with type I diabetes and severely impaired awareness of hypoglycaemia.
- The long-term outcomes of islet transplantation have improved significantly over the last 10 years, with insulin independence at 3 years approaching that of whole pancreas transplantation.
- Immunosuppression with T-cell-depleting agents appears to give the best long-term graft survival.

Recommended video:
- Pancreas and islet cell transplant – https://youtu.be/z_mb9_FHdgI

🌐 Full references available at http://expertconsult.inkling.com

Key references

35. Papadimitriou JC, Drachenberg CB. Distinctive morphological features of antibody mediated and T-cell mediated acute rejection in pancreas allograft biopsies. Curr Opin Organ Transplant 2012;17:93–9. PMID: 22227719.

This publication provides an authorative review of the histological criteria for acute pancreas allograft rejection and the mechanisms leading to graft injury.

36. Mittal S, Page SL, Friend PJ, et al. De novo donor-specific HLA antibodies: biomarkers of pancreas transplant failure. Am J Transplant 2014;14(7):1664–71. PMID: 24866735.

In a multivariate analysis of 433 pancreas transplants at the Oxford Transplant Centre, development of de novo donor specific antibodies (DSA) emerged as a strong independent predictor of pancreas graft failure (hazard ratio 4.66, P < 0.001).

57. The Diabetes Control and Complications Trial Research Group. The effect of intensive treatment of diabetes on the development and progression of long-term complications in insulin dependent diabetes mellitus. N Engl J Med 1993;329:977–86. PMID: 8366922.

This paper provides good evidence that better blood glucose control reduces the risk of progression of retinopathy.

74. Shapiro AM, Lakey JR, Ryan EA, et al. Islet transplantation in seven patients with type 1 diabetes mellitus using a glucocorticoid-free immunosuppressive regimen. N Engl J Med 2000;343(4):230–8. PMID: 10911004.

This publication from the Edmonton group demonstrated that long-term insulin independence can be achieved with islet transplantation and paved the way for the modern era of islet transplantation.

96. Ricordi C, Lacy PE, Scharp DW. Automated islet isolation from human pancreas. Diabetes 1989;38(Suppl. 1):140–2. PMID: 2642838.

This paper was the first to describe the semi-automated technique of human islet isolation – a technique that is still used by islet laboratories worldwide.

113. Barton FB, Rickels MR, Alejandro R, et al. Improvement in outcomes of clinical islet transplantation: 1999–2010. Diabetes Care 2012;35(7):1436–45. PMID: 22723582.

Data from the CITR is presented in this paper that demonstrates improved outcomes after islet transplantation over three eras, with a 3-year insulin independence rate after islet transplantation of >40% in the current era.

The spleen and adrenal glands

Brendan Visser
Geoffrey W. Krampitz

Introduction

The spleen is a wedge-shaped secondary lymphoid organ present in all vertebrates. The word spleen originated from the Greek language, which was then translated into Latin and Middle English and then into its current English form. The Roman anatomist Galen identified the spleen as the source of black bile, one of the major humors of the body, and a major subsidiary organ of the liver. In antiquity, the spleen was thought to be the seat of spirit and courage or such emotions as melancholy and anger. The immunological and haematopoietic functions of the spleen have only recently been appreciated. Given the immunological consequences of asplenism, the indications for complete surgical resection have evolved and given rise to spleen-preserving and spleen-conserving approaches.

Anatomy and embryology

The spleen is the largest reticuloendothelial organ, being approximately the size of a clenched fist and normally weighting 150–250 grams.[1] The spleen is shaped like a cupped hand situated in the left hypochondrium. It has two surfaces, the diaphragmatic surface that is smooth and convex and is in contact with the diaphragm, and visceral surface that is irregular and concave and has impressions contacting the fundus of the stomach, left kidney, splenic flexure of the colon and tail of the pancreas. The spleen is an intraperitoneal organ that is suspended by multiple ligamentous folds of peritoneum, namely, the gastrosplenic connecting the hilum of the spleen with the greater curvature of the stomach, the splenorenal connecting the hilum of the spleen to the left kidney and containing the splenic vessels and tail of the pancreas, and the phrenicocolic connecting the left colic flexure and diaphragm to the diaphragmatic surface of the spleen.[2] The spleen forms from the cephalic aspect of the lateral plate mesoderm during the fifth week of gestation. Multiple aggregations of mesodermal cells condense to form a single organ. In up to 11% of individuals, one or more of these aggregates of splenic tissue fails to condense, and instead forms an accessory spleen, or splenule.[3] The haemopoietic function of the spleen results from infiltration of cells from the yolk sac wall and near dorsal aorta that continues to produce red blood cells into the second trimester. Although the haematopoietic function of the spleen normally ceases in the fifth month of gestation, lymphocyte and monocyte generation persists throughout life.

The spleen derives its major blood supply from the splenic artery, which emanates from the abdominal aorta as a branch of the coeliac trunk, traverses a tortuous course along the superior border of the pancreas, giving rise to the left gastroepiploic artery and short gastric arteries before dividing into multiple branches that enter the hilum of spleen (**Fig. 10.1**). The arteries ramify throughout the organ radially into splenic arterioles that branch into penicillar arterioles that ultimately terminate in splenic cords (**Fig. 10.1**). Here, the reticuloendothelial cells and splenic macrophages come in intimate contact with blood and its contents as it percolates through the splenic cords and across walls of the splenic sinuses. Owing to the large amount of infiltrating blood, the red pulp is a principal site of blood filtration, where

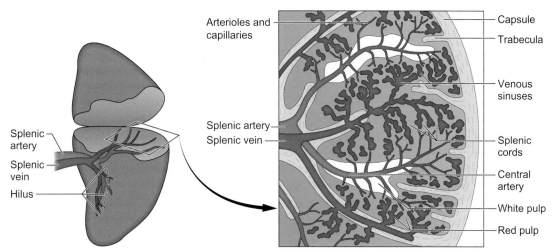

Figure 10.1 • Gross anatomical features of the spleen. The spleen is a cupped hand-shaped retroperitoneal organ with diaphragmatic and visceral surfaces. The spleen derives its major blood supply from the splenic artery, which divides before entering the hilum of spleen into multiple branches that ramify throughout the organ radially into splenic arterioles that branch further into penicillar arterioles that ultimately terminate in splenic cords. The major vascular outflow from the spleen occurs via coalescence of the open sinuses via reticular trabeculae into the splenic vein, which exits via the hilum of the spleen.
Modified from © 2006 Pearson Education, Inc., publishing as Benjamin Cummings, In: Elaine N. Marieb, Katja Hoehn, Human Anatomy & Physiology, 7th edition. Fig. 20.6a,b.

ageing blood cells are destroyed via programmed cell removal.[4] Scattered throughout the red pulp are local expansions of lymphocytes that appear as white pulp (**Fig. 10.2**). White pulp is closely associated with central arterioles that are surrounded by periarterial lymphatic sheaths containing T lymphocytes. Surrounding the T lymphocytes are follicles that contain B lymphocytes. In response to antigen presentation, these B lymphocytes become activated and produce antibodies that play a significant role

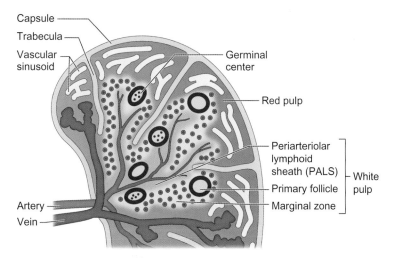

Figure 10.2 • Microscopic anatomical features of the spleen. The red pulp of the spleen is the principal site of blood filtration where reticuloendothelial cells and splenic macrophages come into intimate contact with the blood and its contents as it percolates through the splenic cords and across walls of the splenic sinuses. The white pulp of the spleen is local expansions of lymphocytes scattered throughout the red pulp. White pulp is closely associated with central arterioles and their surrounding periarterial lymphatic sheaths that contain T lymphocytes, which are surrounded by clusters of B lymphocytes. Between the red and white pulps is a marginal zone that contains antigen-presenting cells crucial for initiating lymphocyte activation.

in opsonisation of extracellular organisms including encapsulated bacteria. Between the red and white pulps is a marginal zone that contains antigen-presenting cells crucial for initiating lymphocyte activation. The association of lymphoid and myeloid cells in the red and white pulp makes the spleen a principal site of intersection between the innate and adaptive immune systems.[1] The major vascular outflow from the spleen occurs via coalescence of the open sinuses via reticular trabeculae into the splenic vein, which exits via the hilum of the spleen and courses medially to converge with the superior and inferior mesenteric veins to form the portal vein.

The spleen is invested by two fibrous capsules, the outer tunica serosa that is derived contiguous with the peritoneum and invests the organ except at the hilum, where the peritoneum reflects into the phrenicocolic and gastrosplenic ligaments, and the tunica albuginea that invests the entire organ and at the hilum is reflected inward along the vessels to form sheaths from which the trabecular framework of the spleen emanates.

Indications for splenectomy

Trauma

The spleen's juxtaposition in the left upper abdomen to the 9th, 10th and 11th ribs renders it extremely vulnerable to injury during blunt or penetrating trauma. Haemodynamically unstable patients should undergo emergency laparotomy and splenectomy without delay. Patients who are haemodynamically stable should undergo abdominal computed tomography (CT) with intravenous contrast to evaluate the extent of splenic injury, which will guide further management. The grading criteria for splenic injuries is shown in Table 10.1.[5,6] Non-operative management, including bedrest, telemetry

monitoring, haemoglobin/haematocrit laboratory monitoring every 6 hours, and documented hourly serial abdominal examination for 24 hours following injury, has become the standard of care for haemodynamically stable patients with low to moderate grade injuries (grade I–III) in the absence of evidence of active extravasation on initial contrast-enhanced CT.[7] Failure of non-operative management, defined as hypotension or evidence of ongoing haemorrhage requiring operative intervention, is associated with hypotension on presentation, grade III injury with contrast blush, or grade IV/V injuries.[8] Ninety-five per cent of non-operative management failures occur within 72 hours of injury.[9] Increasingly, spleen-preserving selective angioembolisation is used following failure of non-operative management.[10] All patients undergoing splenectomy or at high risk for splenectomy should receive vaccinations for encapsulated bacteria prior to discharge from hospital.

Haematological

The most common indication for splenectomy is for patients with immune thrombocytopenic purpura (ITP). ITP is an autoimmune disorder characterised by antibody-induced platelet destruction by splenic macrophages.[11,12] ITP is initially treated with glucocorticoids or intravenous immunoglobulin and platelet transfusions. More recently, rituximab and thrombopoietin-receptor agonists have been introduced into the traditional armamentarium.[13,14] Splenectomy is indicated for medically refractory ITP.[15] Thrombotic thrombocytopenic purpura (TTP) is an autoimmune disorder caused by antibodies to ADAMTS13 that results in altered von Willebrand factor homeostasis leading to thrombotic microangiopathy.[16] TTP classically has been defined as the pentad of fever, thrombocytopenia,

Table 10.1 • Spleen injury scale (1994 revision)

Grade	Injury type	Description of injury
I	Haematoma	Subcapsular, <10% surface area
	Laceration	Capsular tear, <1 cm parenchymal depth
II	Haematoma	Subcapsular, 10–50% surface area; intraparenchymal, <5 cm in diameter
	Laceration	Capsular tear, 1–3 cm parenchymal depth that does not involve a trabecular vessel
III	Haematoma	Subcapsular, >50% surface area or expanding; ruptured subcapsular or parenchymal haematoma; intraparenchymal haematoma ≥5 cm or expanding
	Laceration	>3 cm parenchymal depth or involving trabecular vessels
IV	Laceration	Laceration involving segmental or hilar vessels producing major devascularisation (>25% of spleen)
V	Laceration	Completely shattered spleen
	Vascular	Hilar vascular injury with devascularised spleen

Advance one grade for multiple injuries up to grade III.

microangiopathic haemolytic anaemia, renal dysfunction and neurologic symptoms, although presentation of these symptoms is highly variable. Acutely, TTP is treated with plasmapharesis, which results in remission in more than 80% of cases. Patients who are refractory to plasmapharesis or who develop recurrence of disease require splenectomy.[17]

Hereditary spherocytosis (HS) is an autosomal dominant or recessive abnormality of erythrocytes caused by mutations in membrane structural proteins. These mutations lead to cytoskeletal instability that results in altering the normal biconcave erythrocytes into pathognomonic spherocytes that are osmotically fragile and prone to rupture. Cells with these dysfunctional proteins are degraded in the spleen leading to anaemia, jaundice, and splenomegaly.[16] A common complication of HS is cholelithiasis from pigmented stones. Splenectomy is curative, and concurrent cholecystectomy should be performed if indicated.

Other disorders of erythrocyte structure include sickle cell anaemia and thalassaemia. Sickle cell anaemia (SCA) is an autosomal recessive disease caused by mutations in haemoglobin subunit beta-globin, which leads to reductions of the elasticity of the protein under conditions of low oxygen tension that result in deforming of the erythrocyte into a sickle shape. A major feature of SCA is painful episodes of sickle cell crisis complicated by vaso-occlusive phenomena, aplastic or haemolytic anaemia, as well as splenic sequestration. Splenic sequestration can lead to hypersplenism and ultimately splenic infarction. Treatments include blood transfusion and hydoxycarbamide with splenectomy for refractory cases.[18] Thalassaemias are a group of genetic disorders that lead to abnormal ratios or absence of haemoglobin subunits. Beta-thalassaemia results in an excess of alpha-globin that forms insoluble tetramers that precipitate within the erythrocyte interfering with erythropoiesis, cell maturation and function, leading to anaemia. Alpha-thalassaemia results in an excess of beta-globin that also forms tetramers, which, under conditions of stress, precipitate leading to anaemia. Treatment of thalassaemia includes blood transfusion and iron chelation therapy.[19] Splenectomy is indicated in high transfusion-dependent patients with hypersplenism.

Autoimmune haemolytic anaemia (AIHA) is a disorder caused by antibodies directed against erythrocytes leading to Fc or complement-mediated haemolysis in the spleen. AIHA can be primary, idiopathic or secondary to another underlying illness (lymphoproliferative disorders and other autoimmune disorders) or drug reactions. Treatment includes immunosuppressive therapies (corticosteroids, rituximab, azathioprine) and splenectomy in refractory cases.

Felty syndrome comprises a triad of rheumatoid arthritis, splenomegaly and neutropenia. Approximately 1–3% of all patients with rheumatoid arthritis are affected by Felty syndrome. Increased mortality is associated with recurrent infections due to neutropenia secondary to decreased granulogenesis and increased peripheral destruction of granulocytes. Although the exact cause of Felty syndrome is unknown, it is thought to be an autoimmune disorder associated with HLA-DR4, rheumatoid factor and antinuclear antibody. Neutropenia can be effectively treated with disease-modifying anti-rheumatic drugs. Splenectomy results in immediate improvement of neutropenia in 80% of patients.[20]

Neoplastic

A number of neoplasms may require splenectomy. Traditionally, Hodgkin's lymphoma was staged by laparotomy and splenectomy, although this is no longer routine. Haematological malignancies such as non-Hodgkin's lymphoma, hairy cell, chronic myelogenous leukaemia and chronic lymphocytic leukaemia may present with symptomatic splenomegaly and pancytopenia that may require splenectomy in selected patients. Primary splenic angiosarcoma is a rare and aggressive malignant neoplasm arising from splenic vascular endothelium. It is associated with a very poor prognosis, and splenectomy is the only chance of cure.[21] The most common primary sources of splenic metastasis are breast, lung, colorectal, ovarian and melanoma. Splenectomy may be indicated in the event of oligometastatic disease. Although metastases to the spleen are usually asymptomatic, they may occasionally lead to splenomegaly or spontaneous rupture.

Infectious

Infectious diseases involving the spleen may require splenectomy. Hydatid disease caused by *Ecchinococcus granulosus* in the spleen has been reported. Hydatidosis is treated with albendazole and en bloc resection of the parasitic cysts. Splenectomy must be performed without rupturing the cyst to avoid disseminated disease and potential anaphylactic reaction. Albendazole is an effective adjuvant therapy in the treatment of hydatid cyst.[22] Bacterial splenic abscesses that are multiloculated, not amenable to percutaneous drainage, or that have failed to resolve with percutaneous drainage and antibiotics may require splenectomy.

Splenectomy

Open

Open splenectomy can be performed with the patient in the supine position with arms extended and using a midline or left subcostal incision depending on the indication. Packs are placed behind the spleen to elevate and bring it towards the midline. The colon is retracted inferiorly and the stomach is retracted superiorly to expose the gastrocolic ligament. The gastrocolic ligament is divided in the avascular plane to open the lesser sac and expose the splenic artery coursing along the superior border of the pancreas. In patients with splenomegaly, early isolation and ligation of the splenic artery and vein are recommended at this point. The gastrosplenic ligament containing the short gastric arteries and the phrenicocolic ligament are divided to mobilise the spleen medially and allow elevation to expose the splenorenal ligament. If the spleen is normal in size, ligation and division of the splenic artery and vein using clamps and ties or a vascular linear stapling device is performed at this point. Once the specimen is removed, the abdomen is inspected for accessory spleens, which are removed if found.

Laparoscopic

Since the first report of the procedure in 1991 by Delaitre and Maignein,[23] laparoscopic splenectomy has become the standard approach for removal of the spleen for most indications. The patient is positioned in the right lateral decubitus position flexed at the hip, which allows for maximum exposure of the left hypochondrium and gravity, to reveal the ligamentous attachments. The right arm is extended and the left arm suspended. The surgeon and assistant face the patient. Video monitors are positioned at the head of the bed. Four trocars are generally placed along a linear curve situated below the left costal margin once pneumoperitoneum is achieved using a Hassan technique. The optical trocar is usually inserted in the anterior axillary line below the left costal margin. Lateral working ports at the mid-axillary line and posterior-axillary line, as well as a medial working port at the mid-clavicular line below the left costal margin are placed under direct vision. The next step involves freeing the splenic flexure and mobilising the colon inferiorly and medially. This facilitates the division of the gastrosplenic ligament and short gastric vessels, which mobilises the stomach medially to reveal the hilum of the spleen and splenorenal ligament containing the splenic artery and vein. The spleen is rotated medially and the lateral peritoneal attachments are divided. The posterior peritoneum is opened to reveal the vessels, which are then divided using a vascular endoscopic stapling device while protecting the pancreas. The freed specimen is placed in a bag, morcellated and removed. Once the specimen is removed, the abdomen is inspected for accessory spleens, which are removed if found.

Partial splenectomy

A major long-term risk of total splenectomy is overwhelming infection, particularly in children younger than 5 years. Consequently, partial splenectomy has gained popularity, initially in the paediatric population, but increasingly in adult patients. Partial splenectomy may be done open or laparoscopically, although a minimally invasive technique is usually the preferred method. The indications for partial splenectomy include benign tumours (hamartoma, epidermoidal cyst, or localised lymphangioma or haemangioma) and haematologic conditions leading to hypersplenism. Partial splenectomy may not be performed for tumours that are centrally located due to the terminal blood supply of the spleen. The operating room set-up, patient positioning, trocar placements and initial dissection are the same as for laparoscopy. However, careful control of the individual vessels that supply the different pedicles of the spleen is the most critical difference. The hilar vessels, leading to an anterior artery and posterior vein, terminating in the splenic parenchyma, are meticulously dissected. Depending on the location of the tumour, the vessels terminating in the pole or region containing the abnormality are isolated. Placing a temporary clamp will create an area of demarcation to confirm the appropriate selection. The artery and vein are then divided in sequence (if the upper pole is selected, the short gastrics will be divided as well). The line of demarcation is then used to guide the transection along the surface of the parenchyma. The parenchyma is then cauterised and divided. The omentum can be placed in contact with the cut section of the spleen. The remainder of the procedure is similar to the laparoscopic approach.

Splenectomy vaccinations

Because the spleen is particularly important in the immune response to encapsulated bacteria, vaccinations against *Haemophilus influenza* B, *Streptococcus pneumoniae* and *Neisseria meningitidis* should be administered perioperatively. For all elective cases, vaccinations should be administered at least 2 weeks preoperatively. For emergency cases, vaccinations should be administered 2–4 weeks postoperatively, although for trauma patients, just prior to discharge is acceptable due to a high incidence of loss to follow-up. The purpose of perioperative vaccination is to avert overwhelming postsplenectomy infection (OPSI). OPSI is the development of a fulminant, rapidly fatal bacterial infection following splenectomy. OPSI is the most feared complication after removal of the spleen, and the incidence in the first 2 years postsplenectomy is estimated at 0.9% for adults and 5% for children.[24]

Adrenal

Introduction

The adrenal glands are bilateral neuroendocrine organs that are situated superiorly in relation to the kidneys. The word adrenal originated from the Latin *ad renalis*, meaning 'of the kidneys'. The Roman anatomist Galen is believed to be the first to describe 'loose flesh' in relation to what is now known as the left adrenal vein. The 16th century anatomist Bartolomeus Eustachius gave a more definitive description and illustration of the adrenal glands in his work *Opuscula Anatomica*.[25] Knowsley-Thornton performed the first successful adrenalectomy in 1889 on a 36-year-old woman with a 20-pound adrenal tumour.[26] Since that time, there have been significant advances in understanding the function of the adrenal glands and improvements in assessing the indications and techniques for performing adrenalectomy.

Anatomy and embryology

The adrenal glands are retroperitoneal endocrine organs situated above and slightly medial to the kidneys within the renal fascia on both sides of the abdomen (**Fig. 10.3**). The right adrenal gland has a pyramidal shape while the left adrenal gland is semilunar. The left adrenal gland is bounded anteriorly by the peritoneum, tail of the pancreas and splenic artery, posteriorly by the left crus of the diaphragm and kidney, and medially by the left inferior phrenic artery and left gastric arteries. The right adrenal gland is bounded anteriorly by the inferomedial angle of the bare area of the liver, posteriorly by the diaphragm and superior pole of the right kidney, and medially by the inferior phrenic artery and vena cava. The adrenal glands are composed of two heterogenous types of tissue that are arranged into distinct components. The cortex is the outermost component of the adrenal gland and is derived from intermediate mesoderm. The cortex is subdivided into different layers, namely the zona glomerulosa, zona fasciculata and zona reticularis (**Fig. 10.4**). The medulla is the innermost component of the adrenal gland and is derived from neural crest cells (**Fig. 10.4**). The adrenal glands are highly vascular organs that receive their blood supply from the superior adrenal artery (a branch of the inferior phrenic artery), the middle adrenal artery (a direct branch from the aorta), and inferior adrenal artery (a branch of the ipsilateral renal artery) (**Fig. 10.3**). Venous drainage is different for the right and left adrenal glands. The right adrenal drains via a shorter right adrenal vein directly into the inferior vena cava, while the left adrenal gland drains via a longer left adrenal vein that is often joined by the left inferior phrenic vein before emptying into the

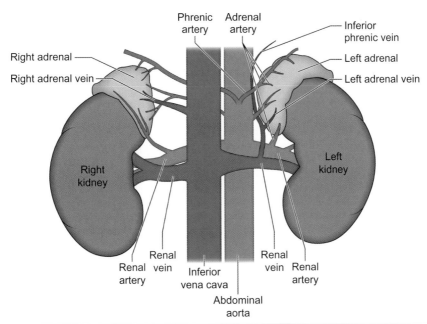

Figure 10.3 • Gross anatomical features of the adrenals. The adrenal glands are retroperitoneal endocrine organs situated above and slightly medial to the kidneys, which receive their blood supply from the superior, middle, and inferior adrenal arteries. The right adrenal drains via a shorter right adrenal vein directly into the inferior vena cava, while the left adrenal gland drains via a longer left adrenal vein that is often joined by the left inferior phrenic vein before emptying into the left renal vein.

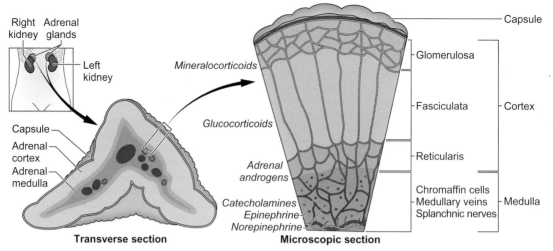

Figure 10.4 • Microscopic anatomical features of the adrenals. The adrenal glands are composed of an inner medulla and outer cortex. The adrenal medulla produces catecholamines. The adrenal cortex is divided into the zona glomerulosa, where mineralcorticoids are produced, zona fasciculata, where glucocorticoids are produced, and the zona retularis, where androgens are produced.

left renal vein. Lymphatic drainage from the adrenal glands flows directly into adjacent periaortic and paracaval nodes.

Physiology

Two separate endocrine organs, namely the cortex and medulla, comprise the adrenal gland. The adrenal cortex metabolises cholesterol to produce different steroid hormones in each zone (**Fig. 10.4**). In all three zones, the rate-limiting step is the conversion of cholesterol to pregnenolone by cholesterol desmolase, which is directly regulated by adrenocorticotropic hormone (ACTH) from the pituitary, which in turn is regulated by corticotropin-releasing (CRH) hormone from the hypothalamus. The zona glomerulosa is the main site for the production of mineralocorticoids that regulate salt balance and blood volume. In this zone, 3-beta-hydroxysteroid dehydrogenase, 21-alpha-hydroxylase, 11-beta-hydroxylase, and aldosterone synthase to convert pregnenolone to aldosterone. Aldosterone is the principal mineralocorticoid that acts by binding nuclear receptors in cells of the distal convoluted tubules and collecting duct of the kidneys and drives transcription of genes that activate basolateral Na/K pumps to increase reabsorption of sodium and excretion of potassium and acid. The Na/K pumps create a concentration gradient that results in water reabsorption into the blood, thereby expanding intravascular volume and increasing blood pressure. The zona fasciculata is the main site for production of glucocorticoids that have many effects on metabolism. Pregnenolone and

progesterone are modified by 17-alpha-hydroxylase, which can be further modified by 21-hydroxylase and 11-beta-hydroxylase to produce cortisol, the major glucocorticoid in humans. Cortisol is secreted directly into the circulation immediately upon its synthesis and circulates in both bound and free unbound state. The free form passes into target cells by diffusion and binds to cytosolic receptors found in virtually all cells in the body. Once bound to its receptor, cortisol not only has glucose-regulating properties but also exerts a myriad of effects on gluconeogenesis, glycogenesis, protein synthesis, lipolysis, mineral homeostasis, vascular tone, immunosuppression and wound healing. In addition, cortisol acts on cells of the hypothalamus and anterior pituitary to negatively regulate production of CRH and ACTH. The zona reticularis is the principal site for androgen production. A series of hydroxylase and dehydrogenase enzymes convert pregnenolone to androstenedione and testosterone. These androgens can be modified by aromatases resulting in oestrone and oestradiol, and by 5-alpha-reductase to produce dihydrotestosterone, resulting in male and female steroid effects during development.

There are a number of enzyme defects that can lead to adrenal dysfunction and congenital adrenal hyperplasia. The most common form of congenital adrenal hyperplasia is caused by a 21-hydroxylase deficiency that leads to excess androgen and mineralocorticoid, and deficient glucocorticoid resulting in salt-wasting dehydration and ambiguous genitalia or virilisation. Dysfunctional 11-beta-hydroxylase leads to excess mineralocorticoid and androgen production, which leads to virilisation and hypertension. Defects in the enzyme 17-alpha-hydroxylase cause a rare form of congenital adrenal hyperplasia characterised by glucocorticoid and androgen deficiency and mineralocorticoid excess. This condition may lead to ambiguous genitalia at birth or delayed puberty, as well as hypokalaemic hypertension.

Like the peripheral sympathetic ganglia, the adrenal medulla is embryologically derived from neural crest cells. The medullary chromaffin cells have rudimentary nerve fibres and the ability to synthesise, store, and secrete catecholamines, primarily epinephrine.[27] The rate-limiting step is the formation of dopa from tyrosine via the enzyme tyrosine hydroxylase, which is principally regulated by ACTH. Although peripheral nerve terminals and the adrenal medulla both have the ability to produce norepinephrine, only the adrenal medulla contains the enzyme phenylethanolamine-N-methyltransferase (PNMT) that converts norepinephrine to epinephrine, which constitutes 80–85% of the adrenal medulla secretion. Catecholamines released by the adrenal medulla bind a large family of transmembrane-signalling adrenoreceptors to exert a variety of effects associated with acute stress responses, including tachycardia, hypertension, increased peripheral vascular resistance, gastrointestinal inactivation, bronchodilatation, and increased metabolism.[28]

Indications for adrenalectomy

Adrenal masses may be benign or malignant and functional or non-functional. The systematic work-up of any suspected adrenal pathology should begin with a thorough history and physical examination investigating the possibility of functional symptoms and assessment for the rare possibility of a genetic syndrome. The history should query for poorly controlled hypertension, diabetes, oedema, palpitations, diaphoresis, headaches, flushing or ecchymosis. The physical examination should inspect for central obesity, peripheral wasting, oedema, weakness, dorsocervical lipodystrophy, striae, atrophic skin and facial plethora. Initial laboratory studies should include biochemical evaluation of plasma sodium, potassium, bicarbonate and glucose levels.

Aldosteronoma (primary hyperaldosteronism)

Primary aldosteronism was first described as a clinical syndrome by Conn in 1955.[29] The signs and symptoms of primary hyperaldosteronism are non-specific and include resistant hypertension and hypokalaemia, although patients may also complain of polydipsia, polyuria, muscle weakness and cramping. Hyperaldosteronism may occur more commonly than originally thought, with increasing prevalence in patients with more severe forms of essential hypertension.[30] In addition, hyperaldosteronism may occur in the absence of hypokalaemia, as electrolyte abnormalities may be a late manifestation of the disease.[31,32] The most common causes of primary aldosteronism are a solitary aldosterone-producing adenoma (APA) and idiopathic hyperaldosteronism (IHA). Other less common forms include primary adrenal hyperplasia, familial hyperaldosteronism and aldosterone-producing adrenocortical carcinoma. Mutations of the potassium channel gene *KCNJ5* have been identified as the cause in APA.[33–35] Other less common somatic mutations in *ATP1A1*, *ATP2B3*, *CACNA1D* and *CTNNB1* have also been identified in aldosterone-producing lesions. Biochemical studies that can aid diagnosis are plasma aldosterone to renin ratio, as a means to increase the diagnostic accuracy of either laboratory value alone. In addition, demonstrating that endogenous aldosterone secretion is not inhibited by exogenous saline infusion has been used to confirm the diagnosis. CT can then be used for localisation.

Cushing syndrome

In 1932, Harvey Cushing attributed the syndrome of truncal obesity, facial plethora, hypertension, polyphagia and polydipsia to pituitary adenomas discovered upon autopsy of patients with these physical findings. The most common cause of this syndrome is iatrogenic administration of exogenous glucocorticoids. Thus, thorough medical and pharmacological histories are crucial. The most common non-iatrogenic cause of this syndrome is Cushing's disease, adrenal glucocorticoid excess caused by ACTH-producing pituitary adenoma. Although the pituitary adenomas of Cushing's disease secrete excessive amounts of ACTH, they generally retain some negative feedback responsiveness to high doses of glucocorticoids. In contrast, ectopic ACTH-producing tumours can also cause the syndrome but are insensitive to negative feedback by high doses of glucocorticoids. The major cause of ACTH-independent Cushing's syndrome is a glucocorticoid-producing adrenal adenoma. Because these tumours secrete excessive cortisol, production of ACTH is suppressed in an otherwise normal hypothalamus–pituitary–adrenal axis. The initial step in the diagnosis of Cushing's syndrome is to confirm the presence of elevated cortisol levels by measuring night-time serum or salivary cortisol, 24-hour urinary cortisol and/or undertaking an overnight low-dose dexamethasone suppression test. The next step is to determine whether the cause of hypercortisolaemia is an ACTH-dependent or independent process. If serum

ACTH levels are suppressed, an ACTH-independent process originating from the adrenal glands is the likely cause of the syndrome. If serum ACTH levels are elevated, a high-dose dexamethasone suppression test is required. If ACTH levels are suppressed with high-dose dexamethasone, the likely aetiology is a pituitary tumour. However, if ACTH levels are unaffected by high-dose dexamethasone, an ectopic source of ACTH is the likely cause. If an adrenal cause is suspected, an abdominal CT should be performed to localise the tumour. Cortisol-secreting adrenal tumours, particularly those with overt Cushing's syndrome and high cortisol levels, have been associated with somatic activating mutations in protein kinase A (PKA) catalytic subunit (*PRKACA*) and the Gs alpha subunit (*GNAS*).[36,37]

Pheochromocytoma

Pheochromocytoma is a catecholamine-secreting tumour that arises from the neuroectodermally derived chromaffin cells of the adrenal medulla. Paragangliomas are related tumours that arise from similar cells of the sympathetic ganglia. These tumours are rare, occurring in <0.2% of patients with hypertension.[38] The majority of pheochromocytomas are benign, solitary and unilateral, and occur in adults. Pheochromocytomas are usually sporadic, although they can accompany genetic syndromes including multiple endocrine neoplasia (MEN) 2a and 2b caused by a number of somatic mutations in the gene *RET* that encodes a transmembrane receptor tyrosine kinase involved in a number of signalling pathways,[39] von Recklinghausen's syndrome caused by mutations in the *NF1* gene that encodes neurofibrin 1, a negative regulator of the ras signal transduction pathway, and von Hippel–Lindau syndrome caused by a mutation in the tumour suppressor *VHL* gene. Patients typically present with refractory hypertension, palpitations, headaches and diaphoresis. Symptoms are usually episodic with variable frequency and duration. The diagnosis of pheochromocytoma is dependent on demonstrating elevated catecholamines in the plasma or urine. Initially, plasma metanephrine and normetanephrine levels should be obtained. In addition, 24-hour urine vanillylmandelic acid, metanephrines, and fractionated catecholamines may be obtained. Once a biochemical diagnosis has been made, the tumour can be localised by CT, magnetic resonance imaging (MRI) or ^{123}I meta-iodobenzylguanidine (MIBG) scan.

Patients with pheochromocytoma have chronic hypersecretion of catecholamines that causes volume-contraction as well as haemodynamic and glycaemic instability. Thus, they must be pre-medicated with a selective alpha-adrenergic receptor-blocker (phenoxybenzamine) for several weeks before proceeding to adrenalectomy.

Postoperatively, patients are susceptible to vasoplegia and hypoglycaemia, and should be monitored closely.

Primary adrenocortical carcinoma

Adrenocortical carcinomas are rare tumours that can be functional and cause hyperaldosteronism, hypercortisolism, and/or virilisation, or non-functional and present as an abdominal mass or incidental finding. Most adrenocortical carcinomas are sporadic, but some occur as part of several hereditary cancer syndromes, including Li–Fraumeni syndrome caused by inactivating mutations of the *TP53* tumour suppressor gene,[40] Beckwith–Wiedemann syndrome caused by a mutation in the insulin-like growth factor 2 (*IGF2*) gene,[41,42] and MEN1 caused by inactivating mutations of the *MEN1* tumour suppressor gene.[43] The majority of patients with adrenocortical carcinomas present with tumours >4 cm that produce a clinical syndrome of hormone excess. A significant number have distant metastases at presentation, usually to liver, lungs, lymph nodes and bone.[44] Initially, a biochemical work-up similar to those described above must be pursued. Imaging characteristics on CT can distinguish adenomas from carcinoma and MRI can accurately evaluate the extent of vascular or adjacent organ involvement. Positron emission tomography (PET)/CT is also useful for determining distant sites of disease. Adrenocortical carcinoma is staged using the TNM staging criteria. T1 tumours are <5 cm with no local invasion, while T2 tumours are >5 cm with no local invasion. T3 tumours are of any size with invasion into the surrounding fat, while T4 tumours are any size with invasion into adjacent organs. N0 indicates no positive lymph nodes, while N1 designates lymph node involvement with tumour. M0 indicates the absence of distant metastases, while M1 specifies that the cancer has spread to distant sites. The 5-year survival disease-specific survival rate for American Joint Commission on Cancer (AJCC) stage I tumours (T1N0M0) is 82%, stage II tumours (T2N0M0) is 58%, stage III tumours (T1/2N1M0 or T3N0M0) is 55% and stage IV tumours (T3N1M0 or T4N0M0 or TxNxM1) is 18%. The 5-year disease-specific survival for the European Network for the Study of Adrenal Tumours stage I tumours (T1N0M0) is 82%, stage II tumours (T2N0M0) is 61%, stage III tumours (T3/4N0M0 or TxN1M0) is 50% and stage IV tumours (TxNxM1) is 13%.[45] Complete surgical resection is the only potentially curative treatment for adrenocortical carcinoma, although mitotane, an adrenocorticolytic drug, has been used in the adjuvant setting or for unresectable or recurrent disease.[46]

Incidentaloma

Adrenal incidentalomas are tumours that are incidentally discovered on imaging performed during the work-up of unrelated conditions. Autopsy studies suggest a prevalence of clinically unapparent adrenal masses of 1–9%, which increases with age. Moreover, with the widespread use of cross-sectional imaging in clinical practice, adrenal masses are serendipitously discovered in 4–10% of patients.[47,48] The work-up of adrenal incidentalomas must address functionality and malignant potential of the mass that will guide treatment or observational approaches. A thorough history and physical examination must be performed to evaluate for potential subtle clues about functionality or malignancy that may have been overlooked during prior assessments. Biochemical evaluations as described above should be performed to rule out aldosterone, cortisol or catecholamine-producing adrenal masses. Although most adrenal incidentalomas are non-functional, approximately 10–15% secrete excess adrenal hormones.[49,50] Malignancy is a rare cause of adrenal incidentalomas. Fewer than 5% of adrenal incidentalomas are primary adrenocortical carcinoma or non-adrenal metastases. The size and imaging characteristics are useful in determining whether an adrenal mass is benign or malignant. Non-contrast CT, contrast-enhanced CT with delay and MRI are useful in evaluating incidentalomas. PET/CT can also be used in cases where imaging is equivocal and tissue diagnosis by fine-needle aspiration (FNA) should only be pursued in selected cases and only after pheochromocytoma has been ruled out.[51] Adrenalectomy is recommended for functional lesions, masses >4cm, or tumours with imaging characteristics concerning for malignancy. For masses with benign appearances (<10 HU, washout >50%), small (<4cm), and completely non-functional, imaging and biochemical surveillance between 3 and 12 months is reasonable.[48–50]

Secondary adrenal metastases

Metastases should be suspected in patients with adrenal masses and a history of extra-adrenal malignancy. Renal cell carcinoma, melanoma, non-small-cell lung cancer, breast cancer, colorectal cancer and lymphoma have a predilection for spread to the adrenal glands. Most adrenal metastases are asymptomatic, and are discovered on surveillance imaging for cancer. They are usually unilateral, although a significant percentage may be bilateral.[52] Although chemotherapy is usually the treatment for disseminated cancer, open or laparoscopic adrenalectomy may be performed in patients with otherwise well-controlled disease with either synchronous or metachronous oligometastases to the adrenal gland.[53–57]

Adrenalectomy

Open

Left

The patient is placed in a slight right lateral decubitus position. The abdomen is accessed via an extended subcostal incision. The splenic flexure of the colon is mobilised and the omental attachments along the transverse colon are divided allowing access to the lesser sac. The splenorenal, splenophrenic and retroperitoneal attachments of the spleen are divided and the tail of the pancreas is rotated medially, exposing the adrenal gland in the retroperitoneum. Gerota's fascia and the upper border of the left kidney are identified and divided. The left renal hilum is dissected to reveal the left renal vein and its confluence with the left adrenal vein, which is ligated and divided just cephalad to its confluence with the inferior phrenic vein. The retroperitoneal fat and suprarenal tissue are elevated and dissected off the superior pole of the left kidney, lateral abdominal wall and left quadratus lumborum muscle. The three main arterial branches from the left renal artery, aorta and left phrenic artery are ligated during the dissection. The medial dissection is carried as far as necessary to obtain a negative margin. For oncologic adrenalectomy, para-aortic lymph nodes are dissected and removed en bloc with the specimen. The pitfalls of left adrenalectomy are injury to the spleen, pancreas or diaphragm, rupture of the capsule of the gland and misidentification of the vascular anatomy.

Right

The patient is placed in a slight left lateral decubitus position. The abdomen is accessed via an extended subcostal incision. The liver is mobilised medially by dividing the triangular ligament to allow exposure of the inferior vena cava and the right adrenal gland. The right border of the vena cava is dissected caudally to the diaphragm to allow the right adrenal vein to be identified, ligated and divided. The right border of the vena cava is dissected rostrally to reveal the right renal hilum. Gerota's fascia and the upper border of the right kidney are identified and divided. The retroperitoneal fat and suprarenal tissue are elevated and dissected off the superior pole of the right kidney, lateral abdominal wall and right quadratus lumborum muscle. The three main arterial branches from the right renal artery, aorta and right phrenic artery are ligated during dissection of the right suprarenal tissues. If performed for oncological purposes, an en bloc dissection of the associated lymph nodes is also performed as part of the medial extent of the dissection of the suprarenal tissue. The major pitfalls of a right adrenalectomy are tumour rupture, injury to the vena cava and right diaphragmatic injury.

Laparoscopic

Gagner and his colleagues performed the first laparoscopic adrenalectomy in 1992.[58] Since then, minimally invasive approaches have become the gold standard for benign adrenal tumours. Minimally invasive approaches offer a magnified view of the operative field, improved control of the vascular pedicles and smaller incisions that result in reduced postoperative discomfort, hospital stay and wound morbidity compared to open approaches. Open approaches are still considered the standard surgical management in primary adrenal malignancy. Although laparoscopic approaches for clinically unsuspected adrenocortical carcinoma were initially associated with a high recurrence rate,[59] recent data suggest that laparoscopic approaches may be an option in carefully selected cases that minimise jeopardising oncological outcomes.[60]

Left

The patient is placed in a right lateral decubitus position flexed at the hip. The right arm is extended and the left arm suspended. The surgeon faces the patient and the assistant is behind the patient. Video monitors are positioned at the head of the bed. Four trocars are generally placed along a linear curve situated below the left costal margin once pneumoperitoneum is achieved using a Hassan technique. After exploration of the abdomen, the spleen is mobilised by dividing the splenorenal ligament starting at the inferior pole and extending up to the left crus of the diaphragm. The medial reflection of the spleen and pancreas is dissected along the splenic vein exposing the left renal and adrenal veins. The left adrenal vein is dissected cephalad to reveal its convergence with the inferior phrenic vein, where it is ligated and divided. Next, the inferior, middle and superior adrenal arteries are ligated and divided. The superior, posterior and lateral aspects of the gland are dissected free. Cephalad retraction allows dissection of the gland along its inferior adrenal pedicle, which frees it from the superior pole of the kidney. The gland is then placed in a plastic bag and removed.

Right

The patient is placed in a left lateral decubitus position flexed at the hip. The left arm is extended and the right arm suspended. The surgeon faces the patient and the assistant is behind the patient. Video monitors are positioned at the head of the bed. Four trocars are generally placed along a linear curve situated below the right costal margin once pneumoperitoneum is achieved using a Hassan technique. The right adrenal gland is situated behind the liver, necessitating its medial mobilisation by dividing the triangular ligament. An atraumatic liver retractor is introduced through the lateral port to hold the liver out of the way. Mobilisation of the liver allows for identification of the vena cava, which is the main anatomical landmark for identifying and dissecting the right adrenal gland. The right border of the vena cava is dissected caudally to expose the renal vein, which constitutes the inferior landmark of the operating field. The vena cava is then dissected cephalad to the diaphragm, to expose the main adrenal vein and, if present, the accessory adrenal vein. Both are ligated and divided. The arterial blood supply is then identified, ligated and divided. The gland is then freed from its fatty and inferior ligamentous attachments along the superior pole of the kidney. The gland is then placed in a plastic bag and removed.

Key points

- The spleen is a highly vascularised organ located in the upper left abdomen with important haematopoietic and immunological functions.
- A number of traumatic, haematologic or neoplastic causes, or infectious disease, require surgical intervention to remove all or part of the spleen.
- Splenectomy can be performed with open or laparoscopic approaches.
- The adrenal glands are bilateral retroperitoneal neuroendocrine organs situated above the kidneys.
- The adrenal glands are the site for steroid hormone and catecholamine production that have a variety of tissue targets and physiological functions.
- A number of benign and malignant diseases require surgical intervention to remove one or both adrenal glands.
- Adrenalectomy can be performed with open or laparoscopic approaches.

🌐 Full references available at **http://expertconsult. inkling.com**

Key references

5. Moore EE, Shackford SR, Pachter HL, et al. Organ injury scaling: spleen, liver, and kidney. J Trauma 1989;29(12):1664–6. PMID: 2593197.

   The Organ Injury Scaling (OIS) committee was commissioned at the 1987 meeting of the American Association for the Surgery of Trauma to devise injury severity scores for individual organs to facilitate clinical research. The organ injury scaling has led to validated algorithms for operative management and clinical decision-making based on injury severity.

13. Kuter DJ, Rummel M, Boccia R, et al. Romiplostim or standard of care in patients with immune thrombocytopenia. N Engl J Med 2010;363(20): 1889–99. PMID: 21067381.

    An open-label, prospective, randomised, double-arm trial showing improved primary endpoints for patients who received romiplostim compared to standard of care for ITP.

14. Godeau B, Porcher R, Fain O, et al. Rituximab efficacy and safety in adult splenectomy candidates with chronic immune thrombocytopenic purpura: results of a prospective multicenter phase 2 study. Blood 2008;112(4):999–1004. PMID: 18463354.

    A multicentre, prospective, open-label, single-arm, phase II trial demonstrating rituximab as a safe and effective splenectomy-avoiding option in some adults with chronic ITP.

24. Mourtzoukou EG, Pappas G, Peppas G, et al. Vaccination of asplenic or hyposplenic adults. Br J Surg 2008;95(3):273–80. PMID: 18278784.

    Provides evidence-based guidelines for vaccination for prevention of overwhelming sepsis in asplenic patients.

35. Choi M, Scholl UI, Yue P, et al. K+ channel mutations in adrenal aldosterone-producing adenomas and hereditary hypertension. Science 2011;331(6018): 768–72. PMID: 21311022.

    Identified mutations in the adrenal potassium channel KCNJ5 that result in constitutive aldosterone production and cell proliferation leading to aldosterone producing tumours.

36. Goh G, Scholl UI, Healy JM, et al. Recurrent activating mutation in PRKACA in cortisol-producing adrenal tumors. Nat Genet 2014;46(6):613–7. PMID: 24747643

37. Sato Y, Maekawa S, Ishii R, et al. Recurrent somatic mutations underlie corticotropin-independent Cushing's syndrome. Science 2014;344(6186):917–20. PMID: 24855271.

    Identified genetic mutations resulting in cyclic adenosine monophosphate (cAMP)-independent protein kinase (PKA) activation that led to the development of cortisol-producing adrenal tumours.

11

Gallstones

Ian J. Beckingham

Introduction

The gallbladder serves as a reservoir to hold bile and release it in a bolus when fat is ingested (Fig. 11.1). Fat in the stomach results in the release of cholecystokinin (CCK) which causes contraction and emptying of the gallbladder as food enters the duodenum. Bile helps to emulsify fat within the small bowel and aid its absorption. Whilst in the gallbladder, bile is concentrated by the absorption of up to 70% of the water content.

Many animals do not have gallbladders – all members of the deer family (except the musk deer), all of the equine family, camels, giraffes, elephants, rhinoceroses, whales, some birds (such as doves, pigeons and parrots), rats and some fish, do not have gallbladders. It is thought that the presence of a gallbladder is related to the interval of food intake. Thus animals, like humans, cats and dogs, which take in food at intervals, require a larger amount of bile acids to aid digestion of fats arriving in a bolus, rather than in a more constant stream.

In some societies the gallbladder is attributed with more than just physical properties. In Korea, the flighty nature of deer is blamed on its lack of a gallbladder, and when a person acts eccentrically or irrationally Koreans say the person lacks a gallbladder. Conversely, when someone is brave, bold and daring, they say the person has a big gallbladder.[1] The Chinese proclaim the calming influence of bile and use powdered bovine gallstones in their traditional medicines as an antipyretic and to aid sleep and cure diseases of the liver and epilepsy. Ox gallstones are also used as an aphrodisiac and bovine gallstones can fetch up to $14000 a kilo on the commercial market.

Pathogenesis of gallstones

Bile is composed of a complex solution of bilirubin (the byproduct of effete red blood cells), cholesterol, fatty acids and various minerals. If one or more of the major components is present in excess, then the solution becomes supersaturated and cholesterol crystals form within the bile (Fig. 11.2). These eventually coalesce to form cholesterol or 'mixed' (cholesterol/bilirubin) gallstones. Cholesterol supersaturation can result from either excessive hepatic secretion of cholesterol, or decreased hepatic secretion of bile salts or phospholipids with relatively normal cholesterol secretion. In >90% of patients, supersaturation results from altered hepatic cholesterol metabolism.[2,3] For stones to form there is a need for a nidus, and mucin that is secreted by the gallbladder wall may serve as a nidus and act as a pro-nucleating (crystallisation-promoting) protein. Variations in mucin composition and decreased degradation of mucin by lysosomal enzymes are associated with a higher incidence of stone formation.[4]

Loss of gallbladder motility and excessive sphincteric contraction are also associated with gallstone formation (Fig. 11.3). Hypomotility leads to prolonged bile stasis (delayed gallbladder emptying) and decreased reservoir function. If the situation persists for long enough, crystals coalesce with formation of biliary sludge and subsequently stones.[5]

Patients with Crohn's disease, or who have undergone intestinal resection or total colectomy, are also more prone to develop cholesterol stones. This is due to impaired enterohepatic circulation leading to reduced hepatic secretion of bile salts in the bile (Fig. 11.4). This results in higher concentration

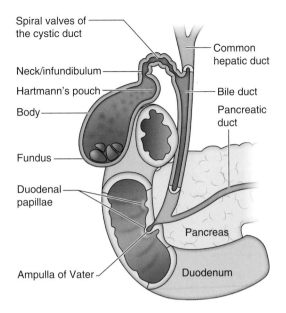

Spiral valves of the cystic duct

Neck/infundibulum

Hartmann's pouch

Body

Fundus

Duodenal papillae

Ampulla of Vater

Common hepatic duct

Bile duct

Pancreatic duct

Pancreas

Duodenum

Figure 11.1 • Anatomy of the gallbladder and bile ducts.

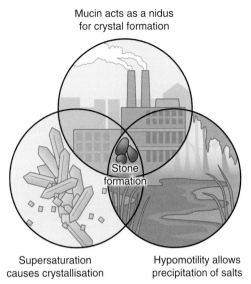

Mucin acts as a nidus for crystal formation

Stone formation

Supersaturation causes crystallisation

Hypomotility allows precipitation of salts

Figure 11.3 • Components required for gallstone formation.

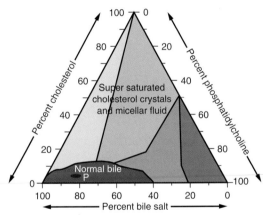

Figure 11.2 • Triangular coordinate equilibrium phase diagram of the cholesterol–phospholipid–bile salt system in the gallbladder. Bile composition at point P (normal, non-lithogenic bile); bile salts (80%); phospholipids acids (15%); cholesterol 5%.

and decreased solubilisation of cholesterol and its precipitation as crystals, with eventual stone formation.

Risk factors

As with most diseases, the development of gallstones is caused by a mixture of genetic and environmental factors. Patients with cholelithiasis often have a strong family history, with gallstones occurring three times more frequently in first-degree relatives than in spouses or unrelated controls.[6] It has been estimated that genetic factors account for

approximately 25% of gallstones.[7] Gallstones are most common in white European and American populations and least common in black Africans (Fig. 11.5). Intermediate rates are found in Asian populations. The highest prevalence is seen in native American populations with a prevalence of 60% in the Pima Indian population of Southern Arizona.

Female gender (10:1 female to male ratio), previous pregnancy and a family history of gallstone disease are highly correlated with cholelithiasis (Box 11.1).[8] Oestrogen increases cholesterol secretion and diminishes bile salt secretion, increasing the cholesterol saturation within bile. Diminished gallbladder motility is commonly seen during pregnancy, with a 10–15 times higher incidence of cholelithiasis seen in women who have had children.[8] Biliary sludge is found in 5–30% of pregnant women and definitive gallstones become established in 5%.[9]

A number of disease processes can result in the supersaturation of cholesterol in bile, including rapid weight loss in the morbidly obese patient (due to excess cholesterol within the bile), total parenteral nutrition (which induces gallbladder hypomotility in the presence of high lipid levels), and drugs that promote cholesterol secretion into the bile, e.g. fibrates.

Other risk factors include a high dietary intake of fats and carbohydrates, a sedentary lifestyle, type 2 diabetes mellitus and dyslipidaemia (increased triglycerides and low HDL). A diet high in fats and carbohydrates predisposes a patient to obesity, which increases cholesterol synthesis, biliary secretion of cholesterol, and cholesterol supersaturation. Patients with a BMI >45 have a 7-fold higher incidence of gallstones compared with non-obese women.[10]

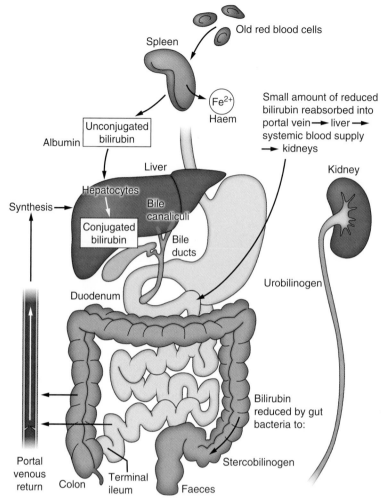

Figure 11.4 • Enterohepatic bile circulation.

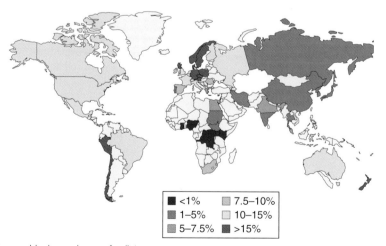

Figure 11.5 • Geographical prevalence of gallstones.
Adapted from Figge A, Matern S, Lammert F. Molecular genetics of cholesterol cholelithiasis: identification of human and murine gallstone genes. Z Gastroenterol 2002;40(6):425–32.

- Female
- Fair (Caucasian)
- Fat (high cholesterol excreters, rapid weight loss, obesity)
- Fertile (post pregnancy and gallbladder stasis)
- Forties (requires several years to develop from crystals to stones)

The old adage acts as a good mnemonic and still holds more than a modicum of truth.

However, a direct correlation between high dietary intake of fats and cholelithiasis risk has not been directly established.

Pigment stones

Black pigment stones account for approximately 10% of gallstones. They are formed when there is an excess of unconjugated bile as a result of increased enterohepatic circulation of bilirubin caused by excessive breakdown of red blood cells. The increased bilirubin concentration within the bile results in precipitation of calcium bilirubinate to form black pigmented stones. These stones are most frequently seen in patients with chronic haemolytic anaemias (e.g. hereditary spherocytosis, sickle cell disease, B thalassaemia), ineffective erythropoiesis (e.g. pernicious anaemia) and liver cirrhosis.

Patients with ileal disease (e.g. Crohn's disease), total colectomy or extended ileal resections have impairment of intestinal bile salt absorption and an increased incidence of gallstones. These may be cholesterol stones due to loss of specific bile salt transporters in the terminal ileum resulting in excessive bile salt excretion in faeces and a diminished bile salt pool. However, in some patients these changes may also lead to formation of pigment gallstones because increased bile salt delivery to the colon enhances solubilisation of unconjugated bilirubin, thereby increasing bilirubin concentrations in bile (Fig. 11.4). Patients with cystic fibrosis also have bile acid malabsorption and approximately 20–30% of patients will develop gallstones.

Brown pigment stones differ from other types of gallstone in that they predominate within the other areas of the biliary tract, particularly the intrahepatic ducts, as well as within the gallbladder. They are mostly seen in South-East Asia and are usually associated with parasite infestation and *Escherichia coli* infection (see later section – Intrahepatic stone disease).

Presentation

Gallstones are very common, with an incidence of 10–15% of the adult population.[11] The majority of people with gallstones are asymptomatic and therefore unaware of their presence. In post-mortem studies, approximately 90% of people with gallstones had no attributable symptoms during their lifetime.

Biliary pain

Gallstones cause symptoms when the cystic duct is occluded during the attempted expulsion of bile from the gallbladder. The resulting contraction of the gallbladder smooth muscle results in activation of visceral nerve fibres in the gallbladder wall and the sensation of referred pain in the associated dermatome (T9) in the epigastrium and radiation round or through to the back. Viscerally innervated pain is often poorly localised and may be accompanied by nausea or vomiting. Local cytokine release can cause irritation of the adjacent parietal peritoneum resulting in pain in the right upper quadrant. The pain lasts for a significant period of time (typically 30 minutes to several hours) and may be related in part to ischaemia within the gallbladder wall as a result of muscular occlusion of the gallbladder microcirculation. The severity of the pain is sufficient to interfere with performance of daily activities. It is frequently very severe and often described by women as 'worse than childbirth'. The popular term 'biliary colic' is a misnomer since the pain is constant and unrelenting and not colicky in nature. It is therefore more accurately referred to as biliary pain. Similarly, use of the term 'chronic cholecystitis' should be avoided since it implies the presence of a chronic inflammatory infiltrate that may or may not be present. The number of stones, their size and the thickness of the gallbladder wall do not correlate well with the presence or absence, or severity of biliary symptoms. In many patients with significant biliary pain the gallbladder looks quite normal at the time of surgery.

The importance of clarifying what constitutes true biliary pain is to better predict relief following surgery (Table 11.1).[12] Cholecystectomy fails to relieve 'biliary pain' in 10–30% of patients with documented gallstones.[13,14] It is observed that patients who have had cholecystectomy for biliary pain often have improvement in other symptoms,

Table 11.1 • Typical features of biliary pain

Location	Epigastric/right upper quadrant
Duration	>30 minutes
Radiation	Round or through to back (band-like)
Severity	Severe (inhibits daily activity)
Periodicity	Intermittent
Less strongly associated	Nocturnal onset
	Post fatty meal

such as belching and low-grade epigastric discomfort ('biliary dyspepsia'). Some patients may be offered surgery for these symptoms alone. However, these more vague symptoms are probably vagal nerve-mediated and also frequently associated with other functional gut disorders such as irritable bowel syndrome or gastro-oesophageal reflux disease. Thus, results for cholecystectomy in patients with 'biliary dyspepsia' alone have worse outcomes than in patients who have more classic bouts of acute biliary pain, and should only be undertaken after appropriate exclusion of other causes where possible and with clear counselling that benefits are less likely.

Once patients have started to develop symptoms from their gallstones their likelihood of having further episodes is approximately 38–50% per annum.[15,16] Overall, approximately 30% of patients will never have further symptoms. The risk of developing complications of gallstones is higher in patients with symptomatic gallstones than in asymptomatic patients and is approximately 1–2% per annum.[17]

Acute cholecystitis

When biliary pain persists for more than a few hours and is accompanied by localised right upper quadrant (RUQ) discomfort, it is termed acute cholecystitis.

Pathophysiologically, prolonged obstruction of the cystic duct causes release of prostaglandins within the gallbladder mucosa resulting in fluid secretion producing a cycle of increased distension and further mucosal damage and inflammation. The inflammatory process results in irritation of the parietal peritoneum. Palpation of the RUQ is tender, and inspiration with the examiner's hand in this region results in pain as the inflamed gallbladder pushes against it (Murphy's sign), which can similarly be confirmed with the ultrasound probe. Inflammatory markers (WCC/ESR/CRP) may be elevated. Liver function tests are often deranged as a result of localised inflammation within the adjacent liver parenchyma or due to compression of the common bile duct from the inflamed gallbladder. Secondary infection can develop in this setting but is rarely the primary event.

The condition may, however, evolve and can result in a variety of complications (Fig. 11.6):

- Obstruction of the cystic duct, usually by a large stone in Hartmann's pouch, can cause a tense tender gallbladder due to mucus (mucocoele).
- If the obstructed gallbladder becomes infected, it may fill with pus (empyema), presenting classically with high swinging fevers, rising white cell count and a significantly elevated C-reactive protein (>50).

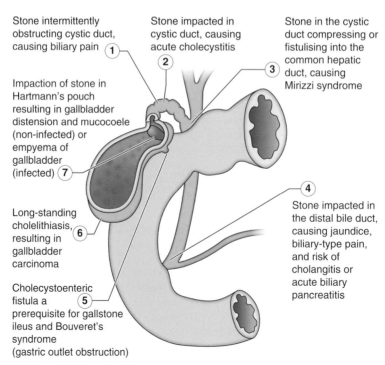

Figure 11.6 • Potential complications of gallstones.

- Emphysematous cholecystitis may develop when secondary infection in the gallbladder wall occurs with gas-forming bacteria, such as *Clostridium welchii*, *Escherichia coli* or anaerobic streptococci. Imaging may reveal the presence of gas within the gallbladder wall. It is most commonly seen in elderly diabetic men.

- The inflamed gallbladder may become adherent to an adjacent loop of bowel (duodenum, jejunum or colon) and eventually rupture into it, discharging its contents. Rarely a large stone passes through the gallbladder wall into the small bowel and causes obstruction (gallstone ileus) (**Fig. 11.7**). Gastric outlet obstruction due to impaction of a gallstone in the duodenum is known as Bouveret's syndrome. Discharge into the colon only rarely causes obstruction due to the larger diameter of the colon but can be encountered at cholecystectomy as a cholecysto-colic fistula.

- The gallbladder may rupture into the peritoneal cavity resulting in free pus and generalised peritonitis (1%), or may become walled off by adjacent bowel and omentum and form a localised pericholecystic abscess.

Common bile duct stones

Approximately 8–16% of patients with symptomatic gallbladder stones will have simultaneous common bile duct (CBD) stones and (with the exception of brown pigment stones) the vast majority (if not all) of these stones originate from the gallbladder and pass from there through the cystic duct into the CBD. The natural history of these CBD stones is

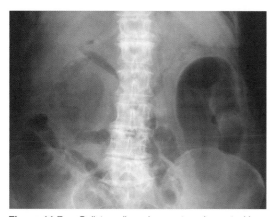

Figure 11.7 • Gallstone ileus. Large stone impacted in small bowel causing obstruction. Note pneumobilia from the cholecysto-jejunal fistula.

unknown, but there is evidence that many do not cause symptoms. Faecal sampling of patients with multiple gallbladder stones confirms that stones often pass freely into the gut without symptoms. Furthermore, studies of patients with known CBD stones awaiting or having had cholecystectomy and who are then re-imaged often show passage of the stones from the CBD.[18,19] Incidental (asymptomatic) CBD stones are also identified in patients undergoing imaging for unrelated non-biliary conditions. Thus, it would appear that many CBD stones may never cause any problems at all. However, because of the uncertainty in their natural history, once CBD stones are discovered, currently most clinicians would advise patients to have them removed, even if they are asymptomatic.

When stones enter the CBD and cause partial or complete obstruction, patients present with obstructive jaundice with an elevated bilirubin (conjugated), alkaline phosphatase (ALP) and gamma-glutamyl transferase (GGT). The transaminases (AST/ALT) may also be elevated ('a mixed pattern') as a result of secondary inflammation of the hepatocytes. Classically, obstructive jaundice is accompanied by pale stools due to lack of the brown pigment stercobilin (which requires the presence of bilirubin in the gut) and dark urine (due to increased bilirubin in the urine). These features are not always present, particularly in the early phases of obstruction or in incomplete biliary obstruction. Obstructive jaundice resulting from CBD stones is often associated with biliary pain, or with a history of biliary pain from previous attacks of gallbladder pain. This contrasts with jaundice associated with malignant obstruction which is usually painless, but the distinction is not absolute. As obstruction progresses, dilatation of the biliary tract occurs which is evident on ultrasound or cross-sectional imaging (e.g. magnetic resonance imaging [MRI], computed tomography [CT]).

CBD stones, when present, are only occasionally identified with ultrasound because the lower part of the bile duct lies behind the gas-filled duodenum preventing visualisation. The presence of a dilated CBD or intrahepatic ducts with elevated liver function tests (LFTs) raises the suspicion of CBD stones, which are best visualised by magnetic resonance cholangiopancreatography (MRCP) or endoscopic ultrasound (EUS). A recent meta-analysis has shown that EUS and MRCP are equally good at identifying CBD stones, with similar sensitivity and specificity.[20] However, EUS is more costly, less widely available and more invasive than MRCP. These techniques have replaced the use of endoscopic retrograde cholangiopancreatography (ERCP) (with its attendant risks) as a diagnostic tool.

If infection develops in an obstructed bile duct, jaundice is invariably accompanied by high temperatures and RUQ pain (Charcot's triad) and is termed cholangitis. Fevers are typically fluctuating, with high temperatures of 39–40°C punctuated by chills and shaking bouts (rigors). Cholangitis is caused by secondary infection within the biliary tract, usually caused by enteric bacteria from the duodenum (most commonly Gram-negative spp. – *E. coli* (25–50%), *Klebsiella* spp. (15–20%), *Enterobacter* spp. (5–10%) or less commonly, Gram-positive bacteria, *Enterococcus* spp. (10–20%)).[21] Early management with intravenous antibiotics (broad-spectrum cephalosporin or ciprofloxacin) followed by early decompression of the ducts by stone removal or stenting is essential. Failure to treat this condition frequently results in septicaemia, which can be fatal.

Acute pancreatitis

CBD stones (usually small) may pass out of the papilla at the bottom of the bile duct and in some cases result in acute pancreatitis. The most popular theory for the pathogenesis of gallstone pancreatitis is that an impacted gallstone in the distal bile duct obstructs the pancreatic duct, increasing pancreatic pressure, thereby damaging ductal and acinar cells (see Chapter 14).

Mirizzi syndrome

First described by Argentinian surgeon Pablo Mirizzi in 1948, the term is used to describe the situation where a stone impacted in Hartmann's pouch produces an inflammatory process that results in adherence of Hartmann's pouch to the CBD with loss of the space between the two structures (i.e. obliteration of Calot's triangle). The result is a partial obstruction of the common hepatic duct (CHD) with deranged LFTs. The most useful subclassification is into type I, where there is no fistula present, and type II, where the stone has eroded into the bile duct itself resulting in a cholecysto-choledochal fistula (Figs. 11.8).

Intrahepatic stone disease

In certain parts of the world primary bile duct stones (synonyms include intrahepatic stone disease (IHSD), oriental hepatolithiasis, cholangiohepatitis, recurrent pyogenic cholangitis, Hong Kong disease), form by a very different pathogenesis to cholesterol and black pigment stones, and present with a different clinical picture. The greatest frequency of this disease is seen in South-East Asia where it has been associated with the liver fluke *Clonorchis sinensis*. However, it also exists in other areas of the world, most notably South Africa, Pakistan and Colombia in the absence of *Clonorchis*, where the main linked epidemiological factor is severe poverty. In these communities, there may be an association with the round worm *Ascaris lumbricoides* infestation.

Stones formed in this disease are very different from cholesterol and bilirubin-rich stones and are brown, soft and friable. The stones form in any part of the biliary tract as a result of anaerobic-bacteria-secreting enzymes that hydrolyse ester and amide linkages in biliary lipids as insoluble anions or calcium salts. These precipitates deposit on obstructing elements such as small cholesterol crystals, black stones from the gallbladder, parasite eggs and dead worms or flukes.[22]

Patients with IHSD present with sepsis and RUQ pain, and initial management is with antibiotics. Symptoms are far more commonly related to ductal stones, and infective and inflammatory processes around the stones result in strictures and proximal dilatation of the ducts. Simple cases caught early can be managed by decompression of pus from the CBD with a plastic stent. Subsequent definitive surgical management aims to clear the biliary tract of stones, provide adequate biliary drainage and, where necessary, provide adequate access to the biliary duct. When there is an extrahepatic or hilar duct stricture, hepatico-jejunostomy is performed leaving the afferent loop long and fixing it to the abdominal wall as an 'access loop' which permits subsequent percutaneous or endoscopic management of recurrent stones and strictures.[23] A proportion of patients require resection of an atrophied portion of the liver containing multiple stones. The disease more frequently affects the left lobe than the right. Patients with intrahepatic stone disease have a 10% risk of developing cholangiocarcinoma.[24]

Management of gallstones

Conservative

> ✅ Asymptomatic gallstones in the gallbladder do not require further investigation or management. Patients with symptomatic gallbladder stones should be offered laparoscopic cholecystectomy unless medically unfit for surgery.

Patients with gallstones without symptoms do not require treatment. The risk of people with asymptomatic cholelithiasis developing symptoms (biliary pain) is low, averaging 2–3% per year, or approximately 10% by 5 years.[25] Major complications related to gallstones are very rare in asymptomatic patients.[26] Expectant management is therefore an appropriate choice for silent gallstones in the general population.

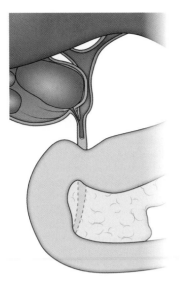

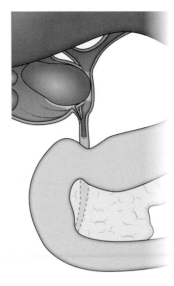

Type 1 Mirizzi
(pressure from stone in gallbladder
on common bile duct)

Type 2 Mirizzi
(stone eroded through gallbladder
wall into common bile duct—
a cholecysto-choledochal fistula)

Type 1

Type 2

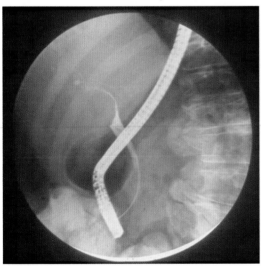

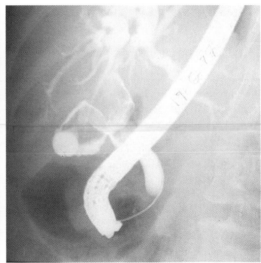

Figure 11.8 • Mirizzi syndrome.

Non-operative management

Even in the laboratory gallstones are difficult to dissolve and most chemicals that successfully dissolve gallstones are too toxic to ingest or inject into the gallbladder (e.g. methyl tetra butyl ether (MTBE), mono-octonoin, carbon tetrachloride). During the 1970–80s there were many attempts to develop strategies to achieve non-medical management of gallstones by oral dissolution, injection of solvents into the biliary tract and extracorporeal shock wave lithotripsy (ESWL). However, none achieved significant reliable dissolution of the stones, even in highly selected study groups, and all required long-term bile salt therapy (with a high incidence of abdominal cramps and diarrhoea) to prevent recurrent stone formation.[27] With the development of laparoscopic cholecystectomy in the late 1980s with its low morbidity and ability to definitively remove the 'stone factory', research in this area has dwindled.

Alternative treatments such as the 'gallbladder flush' (essentially consisting of giving purgative agents such as Epsom salts, olive oil and lemon juice) have been popularised by the Internet, but there is no evidence of any efficacy, although they do result in the production of small pellet-like faeces which can be mistaken by enthusiasts of the procedures as stones![28]

Cholecystectomy

Patients with biliary pain should be offered cholecystectomy as definitive treatment for their disease. Up until the early 1990s, the operation was usually performed through an incision in the right upper quadrant (Kocher's incision). The cholecystectomy procedure consists of detaching the gallbladder from the biliary tract by division of the cystic duct, division of the cystic artery and subsequent removal of the gallbladder from its attachments to the gallbladder fossa of segments 4 and 5 of the liver.

The first laparoscopic cholecystectomy (LC) was performed on 12 September 1985 by Erich Muhe in Boblingen, Germany.[29] Within a few years the 'open' procedure was superseded by the laparoscopic procedure, and in 2016 >98% of cholecystectomies were performed laparoscopically in England (HES data). Although never subjected to large-scale randomised trial, improved clinical outcomes led to rapid adoption. Smaller incisions result in less tissue damage, less pain and a faster recovery. The average length of stay following cholecystectomy reduced from approximately 5 days to 1 day. This has progressed further to widespread realisation that the procedure can be carried out as a day case procedure. In 2016, over 70% of laparoscopic cholecystectomies in England were performed as day case procedures (HES data). Patients are now routinely discharged within a few hours of their operation.

The major disadvantage following the widespread introduction of LC has been cited as a rise in the incidence of bile duct injury. The true incidence of major bile duct injury (defined as injury affecting >25% circumference of the CBD) in the open cholecystectomy era was poorly documented, but was in the order of 0.1–0.5%.[30,31] Initial results from small series of LC demonstrated an increase in these rates,[32,33] but subsequent large multicentre and single-centre prospective studies show that bile duct injury rates are similar to the open era at aproximately 0.2–0.3%.[34,35] A number of studies have shown that the incidence of bile duct injury is related to the surgeons inexperience with the technique,[36,37] but the risk is always present however experienced the surgeon. When bile duct injury does occur with laparoscopic cholecystectomy, it is frequently more proximal and more extensive than with open cholecystectomy (i.e. involving complete transection or excision of the bile duct).

The technique for a routine elective LC consists of gaining entry to the abdominal cavity under general anaesthesia, usually by an open 'Hasson' technique around the umbilical area, followed by insufflation of the cavity with carbon dioxide gas at a pressure of 12 mmHg. Following insertion classically of three additional ports in the right upper quadrant and epigastrium, the fundus of the gallbladder is grasped and pushed cephalad to expose the porta hepatis. Careful dissection of the peritoneum overlying the structures in Calot's triangle (Fig. 11.9) permits identification of the cystic artery and duct. Once clearly confirmed as such, these two structures are clipped and divided and the gallbladder is dissected free from its attachments to the undersurface of the liver. Following inspection of the gallbladder fossa to ensure no bleeding or bile leak, and that the clips on the cystic duct and artery remain intact, the gallbladder is removed, usually within a bag to reduce contamination of the port sites. The gas is emptied from the abdominal cavity and the port sites are closed. Antibiotics are not routinely given. The patient is fed within a few hours of the procedure and typically is discharged home the same day with an expectation of return to full normal function and activities over the following 2–4 weeks.

There are variations in the number and size of the ports (5 mm/12 mm) used to perform the laparoscopic procedure. Newer even less invasive techniques have been developed – SILS (Single Incision Laparoscopic Surgery) involves a single larger incision at the umbilicus to further reduce scarring;[38] NOTES (Natural Orifice Transluminal Endoscopic Surgery) allows scarless abdominal surgery using a flexible endoscope inserted via the mouth or vagina to remove the gallbladder.[39] Whilst feasibly possible, these techniques have failed to convince the majority of surgeons and patients that the elimination of three or four small incisions offers a significant benefit to patient recovery sufficient to justify the longer operative times, greater costs, greater technical challenges in more difficult cases, and increased additional potentially serious risks of these procedures. The standard four-port laparoscopic technique remains the gold standard allowing, as it does, better triangulation of Calot's triangle and reducing the potential error of excessive cephalad traction and misidentification of the CBD for the cystic duct.

There are very few true contraindications to the laparoscopic approach and most of the former contraindications, including acute cholecystitis, obesity, respiratory disease and pregnancy (middle trimester ideally when necessary), are now the preferred options compared to 'open' surgery. Multiple previous laparotomies and RUQ stomas remain a relative indication for open surgery.

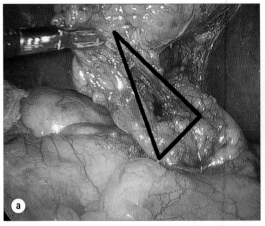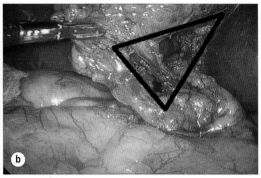

Figure 11.9 • Calot's triangle and the cystohepatic triangle. Calot's original description bounded by the cystic duct, cystic artery and common hepatic duct. (a) The cystohepatic triangle bounded by the gallbladder wall, cystic duct and common hepatic duct, with the cystic artery lying within the space. (b) Although technically incorrect, the term Calot's triangle is widely used in surgical texts to refer to the cystohepatic triangle.

✅✅ Laparoscopic cholecystectomy is the only recommended treatment for symptomatic gallbladder stones.

Intraoperative bile duct imaging and prevention of bile duct injury

Intraoperative cholangiography (IOC) is an essential skill for all surgeons performing cholecystectomy. It enables identification of CBD stones and the biliary tract anatomy. Routine use of IOC is held by some as reducing the incidence of bile duct injury;[40] however, there are many series that have shown no difference in incidence, nor in the number of bile duct injuries missed during surgery.[41] Other series have shown that more than 50% of injuries revealed on the cholangiograms were missed by the operating surgeon. In the UK, selective cholangiography appears to be the favoured approach, with IOC performed in <10% of LCs (HES data).

Laparoscopic ultrasound (LUS) is a fast and reliable technique to identify CBD stones and with the addition of colour Doppler can aid identification of anatomical structures (vessels and ducts) within the porta hepatis. It is not widely available but has been shown to be superior to IOC in identification of CBD stones.[42]

Recently indocyanine green (IGC) given intravenously 15 minutes before surgery has been shown to facilitate identification of the biliary anatomy in LC. ICG is concentrated in the liver and excreted from the biliary tract and with the aid of a near infrared (NIR) filter on the laparoscope, the ICG within the ducts fluoresces and can be clearly seen. The sensitivity of ICG in the recognition of the cystic duct and CBD was 100% irrespective of the presence of fat or inflammation in Calot's triangle.[43] It has also been shown to be useful in identifying the origin of bile leaks at surgery although the specialist equipment required is not widely available at present.

Safe cholecystectomy and prevention of bile duct injuries require clear visualisation of the anatomy which itself demands proper exposure of the critical structures. Avoiding these injuries requires use of caudal and lateral traction on Hartmann's pouch to counter-tract the cephalad retraction of the fundus, and always dissecting as close to the gallbladder wall as possible. No structure should be clipped or divided unless its identity is certain and an intraoperative cholangiogram should be performed if any uncertainty exists. Conversion to open surgery should not be seen as a failure and should be considered if doubts persist.

Several methods have been proposed to reduce the incidence of bile duct injury – e.g. identification of Rouviere's sulcus, the flag technique, the infundibular technique and the critical view of safety (CVS). The critical view (Fig. 11.10) has become the most widely used technique and is the method recommended and taught by SAGES (Society of American Gastroenterological and Endoscopic Surgeons). The CVS requires demonstration of three criteria – Calot's triangle is cleared of fat and fibrous tissue; the lower third of the gallbladder is separated from the liver to expose the cystic plate; demonstration of two (and only two) structures to be seen entering the gallbladder.[44] Its usage has been shown to reduce the incidence of bile duct injury in several large studies.[45,46]

When the anatomy in Calot's triangle is unclear as a result of inflammation and fibrosis, subtotal cholecystectomy is a safe technique avoiding the need to dissect in the hostile area of Calot's

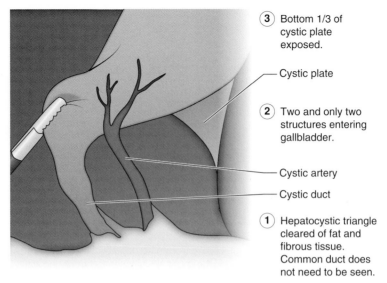

(3) Bottom 1/3 of cystic plate exposed.

Cystic plate

(2) Two and only two structures entering gallbladder.

Cystic artery

Cystic duct

(1) Hepatocystic triangle cleared of fat and fibrous tissue. Common duct does not need to be seen.

Figure 11.10 • The critical view of safety.

triangle. Subtotal cholecystectomy is with division of the gallbladder at the level of Hartmann's pouch, removal of the stone(s) with or without complete removal of the posterior wall of the gallbladder and securing Hartmann's pouch with endoloop, suture or stapler as appropriate. Occasionally the cystic duct cannot be secured at all due to friable tissues and a drain can be left, with the majority of leaks settling without further intervention. Further surgery is rarely required following subtotal cholecystectomy as long as all the stones are removed at the original procedure. In a review of over 1000 cases following subtotal cholecystectomy, further surgery was required in <2% of cases.[47] If the whole area is 'frozen' with dense adhesions, cholecystostomy (insertion of a drain directly into the gallbladder) offers a safe alternative allowing transfer to a specialist unit if required.

It is widely held that the majority of bile duct injuries are preventable and result from inadequate training, poor surgical technique or misidentification of the normal anatomy (Box 11.2). Perhaps surprisingly, unusual amounts of bleeding, severe inflammation and emergency operations are typically involved in <25% of injuries,[48] and it is noteworthy that in this extensive Swedish review, the patients most at risk of bile duct injury were young, slim females who had

Box 11.2 • Bile duct injuries – risk factors

Dangerous anatomy	7%
Dangerous pathology	9%
Dangerous surgery	84%

Adapted from Johnson GW. Iatrogenic bile duct injury: an avoidable surgical hazard. Br J Surg 1986;73:246–7.

not undergone previous surgery. Similar studies have suggested that 84% of injuries were in non-complicated LCs and 97% were due to perceptual errors.[49]

Acute cholecystitis

Patients with acute cholecystitis generally require admission for analgesia and intravenous fluid rehydration. Non-steroidal anti-inflammatory agents such as diclofenac or indomethacin have been shown to reduce inflammation and speed recovery.[50] Broad-spectrum antibiotics, such as a second-generation cephalosporin, are recommended to prevent secondary bacterial infection.

The approach to the management of acute cholecystitis has changed radically over the last 20 years. Optimal management has shifted from leaving the cholecystectomy for 6 weeks in an effort to reduce inflammation and facilitate easier dissection following a realisation that this practice resulted in a 20% need for urgent surgery, 20% readmission rates, as well as prolonged and unnecessary pain, discomfort and inactivity. It is now recognised that surgery should ideally be undertaken within 48 hours of the onset of symptoms when the inflammatory process is still acute and before the development of more difficult fibrosis sets in. Benefits are still evident up to 10 days from onset of symptoms.[51,52] These cholecystectomy procedures can be challenging and there remains a significant conversion to open surgery (10–30%). Surgeons operating on this group of patients must have the full repertoire of techniques and equipment (e.g. cholangiography and choledochoscopy) and be prepared to perform a subtotal cholecystectomy or cholecystostomy.

✅✅ Patients with acute presentation of cholecystitis or gallstone pancreatitis should undergo early cholecystectomy, preferably on the same admission unless there are contraindications to surgery.

Prophylactic cholecystectomy

There have been arguments made for certain patient groups to undergo prophylactic cholecystectomy – patients with diabetes mellitus (falsely assumed to have a higher incidence of acute cholecystitis and infective gallbladder complications); patients undergoing weight loss surgery (high incidence of postoperative gallstones); patients with hereditary spherocytosis undergoing splenectomy for their disease (high incidence of black pigment stones); patients awaiting heart transplant (higher incidence of post-transplant gallbladder problems) – however, the evidence in all these groups seems to suggest that complications of gallstones are not sufficiently frequent to warrant prophylactic cholecystectomy and that patients can be safely managed if symptoms develop.

Bile duct stones

There are two main approaches to the removal of CBD stones – endoscopic retrograde cholangiopancreatograpy (ERCP) or surgical bile duct exploration.

ERCP

The most common approach to the management of CBD stones is by ERCP (Fig. 11.11). This procedure involves insertion of a side-viewing endoscope

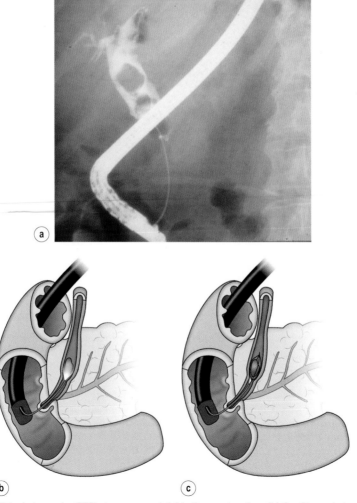

Figure 11.11 • ERCP techniques for CBD stone removal: **(a)** balloon extraction; **(b)** SpyGlass cholangioscopy with contact lithotripsy; **(c)** basket removal.

(a duodenoscope) through the mouth into the duodenum. The papilla is cannulated with a fine cannula to enter the bile duct. The papilla can be cut using a sphincterotome, which uses diathermy to divide the sphincter of Oddi, and stones can be extracted with baskets or balloons. Larger stones can be crushed with a mechanical lithotripter. Large, impacted or multiple stones that cannot be removed can be managed by insertion of a plastic stent left within the bile duct to prevent the stone obstructing. These stones might be suitable for extraction using an ultrathin endoscope that passes down the working channel of the duodenoscope (e.g. SpyGlass endoscope). This ultrathin scope can pass up the CBD and enables direct visualisation of the stone to permit piezoelectric or laser contact lithotripsy. ERCP is performed under sedation and carries a risk of acute pancreatitis due to manipulation of the papilla (approximately 5%), bleeding or perforation (approximately 1%) and death (0.1%).

Surgical bile duct exploration

Bile duct exploration was originally performed via laparotomy but increasingly the procedure is performed laparoscopically. At open surgery, the bile duct is opened longitudinally in the mid part of the anterior wall (choledochotomy) and stones are removed with Des Jardin's forceps, flushing and the use of a flexible choledochoscope. Prior to the development of flexible choledochoscopes, retention of CBD stones was high (10–15%) and a T-tube was inserted into the choledochotomy to prevent inadvertent leakage, potential stone impaction or swelling due to the traumatic stone extraction. With optical magnification, direct visualisation and more delicate instrumentation, trauma to the bile duct was reduced, missed CBD stones were rarer and primary duct closure became more common.

Laparoscopic bile duct exploration (LBDE) can be performed either via the cystic duct (transcystic) or directly through a choledochotomy (transductal). Small stones (<5 mm) can be removed by a transcystic approach with a 3-mm choledochoscope or caught in a basket under fluoroscopy and retrieved via the cystic duct, or can be pushed through the papilla. A balloon to occlude the proximal duct whilst giving a smooth muscle relaxant, such as buscopan or glucagon, and then flushing through the balloon catheter can also be used to clear small distal duct stones. The transcystic approach is limited to stones small enough to be retrieved through the cystic duct (typically stones <5 mm) and it is not usually possible to access the proximal hepatic duct due to inability to retroflex the choledochoscope and other instruments.

Larger stones can be managed by a transductal approach by making a choledochotomy (a longitudinal incision in the anterior surface of the bile duct) and extracting stones by a combination of manipulation of the duct, Dormia basket and balloon extraction with a 5-mm flexible choledochoscope. Large and impacted stones can be removed by shattering under direct vision with a piezoelectric or laser lithotripsy. Most bile ducts are primarily closed with an absorbable suture. Bile can leak through the choledochotomy suture line and a drain is usually left for 24 hours or so post procedure. Where the duct is inflamed and friable (e.g. after recent cholangitis), in the presence of pus or multiple small stones a T-tube can be left within the choledochotomy to be removed after a period of at least 2 weeks, to permit safe drainage and reduce the risk of peritoneal bile leakage. Post-procedural acute pancreatitis is rare unless there has been traumatisation of the papilla.[53] Regardless of exact technique, the high rates of duct clearance reported with LBDE[54,55] can be increased to near 100% with the availability of intraductal lithotripsy.[56] Long-term results also appear favourable.[57,58]

Approaches to the management of simultaneous CBD and gallbladder stones

Preoperative identification of CBD stones in the presence of gallbladder stones offers two principal management options – a two-stage preoperative clearance of the CBD followed by LC, or a single-stage LBDE and cholecystectomy. Several trials have shown that there is no significant difference in clinical outcomes between the two approaches.[59–61] However, most studies show that single-stage LBDE is associated with a reduction in overall hospital stay when compared to the two-stage approach and has a lower overall cost.[59,62] Furthermore, the complications of surgical duct exploration are predominantly related to choledochotomy (bile leak) and T-tube use (bile leakage, tube displacement) that has largely been replaced with primary bile duct closure, resulting in shorter operative time, reduced hospital length of stay, and faster return to work of approximately 8 days.[61] UK national guidelines currently recommend that both approaches are considered equally valid treatment options and that training of surgeons in LBDE is to be encouraged.[63]

LBDE is largely replacing open BDE, with approximately 80% of BDE now performed laparoscopically in England (HES data). However, for preoperatively identified stones, a US survey reported that 86% of surgeons would choose preoperative ERCP over BDE, and for intraoperatively discovered CBD stones, only 30% would choose LBDE, citing availability of ERCP, lack of equipment and lack of skill performing LBDE.[64]

A third option that has been used in a few centres is the use of intraoperative ERCP at the time of

LC.[65] Although feasible and with low morbidity, its use is not widespread due to the logistic difficulties of requiring ERCP equipment and staffing.

> ✓✓ Bile duct stones should be removed either by simultaneous bile duct exploration or perioperative ERCP depending on local resources and skills.

Approaches to abnormal LFTs prior to LC

The decision and desire of surgeons to identify the presence of stones in the CBD prior to LC is highly variable. There are now several different preoperative diagnostic techniques (MRCP and EUS) and intraoperative techniques for imaging (IOC and LUS), and several options to manage any common bile duct stones identified (pre-, intra-, or postoperative ERCP, open or laparosocpic BDE). At present, there are no studies to support one or other approach and it is therefore important to develop an individual strategy for the preoperative and operative management of patients with gallstones dependent upon the local availability of techniques and skills.

The financial and logistic implications of preoperative imaging of all patients undergoing LC would inflict a significant cost and strain on resources with currently around 100 000 procedures performed per annum in the UK and 60 000 in the USA, and would be of questionable benefit. Most clinicians will therefore attempt to stratify their patients in some way according to the probability of bile duct stones being present. Patients with normal LFTs, non-dilated bile ducts on ultrasound and no history of jaundice will have a <1.5% chance of having a common bile duct stone.[66] This low-risk group can undergo LC without the need for further preoperative imaging or intraoperative cholangiography, with an incidence of retained CBD stones of <1% and a very low risk of significant problems from retained stones.[67,68]

Patients who are at highest risk of bile duct stones are those with jaundice at the time of surgery and those with preoperative US visualisation of a stone in the CBD (positive predictive value [PPV] of 0.86 and 0.74 at subsequent IOC). Another study found that patients with persistently abnormal LFTs, tested prior to MRCP with the presence of at least two of bilirubin >110 μmol/L, ALP >400 IU/L or ALT >750 IU/L together with a dilated CBD (>8 mm) or dilated IHDs, had a PPV of 87% for stones (compared to only 32% if the bile ducts were not dilated), and even less correlation with the presence of subsequently confirmed CBD stones when only the incident LFTs were used for prediction.[69]

The combination of US duct dilatation and abnormal LFTs yields the next highest incidence of CBD stones preoperatively, e.g. the presence of two or more of: presentation with jaundice/bilirubin >20 mmol (2 g/dL), alkaline phosphatase 150 mmol, CBD >10 mm and/or a CBD stone seen on US, yielded a PPV for CBD stones of 56%. Similar findings were reported in patients with a history of jaundice and dilated ducts on preoperative US, with a PPV of 56%.[67] Thus, these criteria might be used to identify patients at intermediate risk of CBD stones to select for preoperative MRCP prior to preoperative ERCP, or for selection of patients for referral to a surgeon who performs single-stage LBDE. However, in a significant number of patients identifed preoperatively with definite stones, at least 25% had passed stones spontaneously without problems by the time of surgery.[67]

Less marked or singly elevated LFTs, particularly with non-dilated biliary ducts, have very poor sensitivity and specificity for predicting CBD stones, with an incidence in these groups of approximately 15–16% (Table 11.2).[70] This is only slightly higher than the incidence of CBD stones in the overall population of patients with symptomatic gallstones (9–13%).[71] The choice between the various strategies in this low-risk group of patients at present depends largely upon the quality of the surgical and endoscopic therapies available, but ERCP should not be performed without prior demonstration of stones in this group.

Table 11.2 • Risk stratification for likelihood of CBD stones

	Criteria	Relative risk of CBD stones
High risk	Preoperative US showing CBD stone	0.74–0.86
	Jaundice at time of procedure	
Intermediate risk	At presentation, two of: Bilirubin >20 mmol/L ALP or AST/ALT >2–3 × normal Dilated CBD (>8 mm)	0.56
	History of jaundice + dilated ducts	
Low risk	Single elevated ALP or AST/ALT	0.15
	History of acute gallstone pancreatitis	
Minimal risk	Normal LFTs	0.01

CBD, common bile duct; LFTs, liver function tests; US, ultrasound.

There are three possible approaches to management of patients undergoing cholecystectomy with regard to the dilemma of the CBD and possible CBD stones:

1. Identification of CBD stones prior to LC in order to remove them by ERCP prior to surgery. This approach sets a threshold at which to perform MRCP based on abnormalities of LFTs ± - ultrasound findings. If stones are found at MRCP then ERCP can be performed and CBD stones removed. Most would then avoid intraoperative IOC. The disadvantage of this approach is a very high level of unnecessary MRCPs (around 85% depending on the threshold) and exposure to the risks of ERCP in the positive MRCP group.

2. Using preoperative stratification to perform selective IOC (or LUS) or alternatively simply performing routine IOC (or LUS) on all patients. If CBD stones are identified then the options are:

   (a) Exploration of the bile duct with removal of the CBD stones intraoperatively by transcystic removal or choledochotomy.

   (b) Secure closure of the cystic duct and perform postoperative ERCP.

   The potential disadvantage of this approach is the risk of failure of ERCP to remove the CBD stones, although in practical terms this is <5%. Some surgeons place an antegrade stent at LC to further reduce this risk.

3. Not performing any pre- or intraoperative imaging and assessing patients on symptoms, or persistence of abnormal LFTs to select for postoperative CBD imaging.

It is clear that a small proportion of patients undergoing LC regardless of pre- or intraoperative investigations will thus have 'missed' CBD stones. The *potential* risks posed by these CBD stones are of subsequent acute gallstone pancreatitis, and postoperative bile leak due to CBD stone impaction and raised intrabiliary pressure causing clip failure in the first few days before the cystic duct has sealed. A study of 10 000 LC procedures in Switzerland identified that the immediate risk of acute postoperative pancreatitis was 0.34% and was due to CBD stones in only four patients (0.0004%).[72] The incidence of CBD stones in patients with cystic duct stump leaks is only 3–5%,[73,74] and thus neither of these concerns is significant.

Furthermore, several studies have shown that the incidence of symptoms relating to retained CBD stones is itself low and in fact not significantly different to the incidence of symptoms in patients who had undergone IOC with supposedly clear ducts.[75,76] The complication rate in these groups of patients with retained stones was very low.[72,73]

The author's favoured approach is the use of preoperative imaging (MRCP) in the small group of patients presenting with gallbladder stones and obstructive jaundice (where the presence of CBD stones is >50%) and selective IOC in patients with acute gallstone pancreatitis or deranged LFTs. If stones are found on IOC, the favoured approach would be to proceed with LBDE for large stones if the CBD is >8 mm, or post-LC ERCP for small stones/small ducts (Fig. 11.12).

With so many options available, and with differences in availability of resources, this area requires further research to establish the best and most cost-effective approach. A large multicentre study in the UK is in progress (the Sunflower study).

☑ Patients with mild or moderately elevated LFTs can safely undergo laparoscopic cholecystectomy with intraoperative bile duct imaging or postoperative investigation of ongoing biliary symptoms, reducing the high number of unnecessary preoperative MRCPs.

Management of specific scenarios

Gallstone ileus

Gallstone ileus (another misnomer) is not a dysfunction of motility but is a mechanical obstruction of the bowel caused by an impacted gallstone. It occurs as the result of an acutely inflamed gallbladder becoming adherent to a segment of bowel with subsequent inflammation and erosion of the stone through the bowel wall. The median age of affected patients is 70 years. It represents 1% of small bowel obstructions in patients <70 years, but 5% aged >70 years.[77] Presentation is with vomiting and abdominal distension and only rarely with acute cholecystitis. Half will have a preceding history of symptomatic gallstone disease. The stones are invariably large (>2.5 cm) and obstruction is most frequently at the level of the terminal ileum. Management following resuscitation is to remove the stone via a small enterotomy with primary closure of the bowel usually possible. Bowel resection is only necessary in the presence of perforation or ischaemia. Removal of the gallbladder is fraught with hazard due to the presence of the inflammation and cholecysto-enteric fistula. In most cases the stones have passed and the fistula closes spontaneously. Elective cholecystectomy and closure of the fistula is rarely necessary.[78]

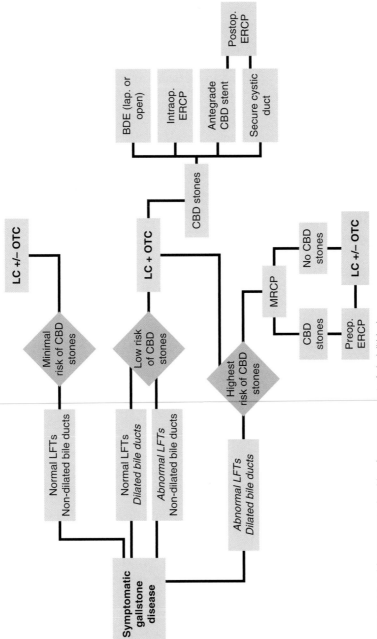

Figure 11.12 • Management algorithm for management of cholelithiasis.

Mirizzi syndrome

Type I Mirizzi syndrome can be managed by subtotal cholecystectomy with removal of the majority of the gallbladder leaving the posterior wall where it is adherent to the bile duct, and ligation of the cystic duct if identified and still patent. Sometimes no cystic duct is found and a drain is simply left in the gallbladder fossa in case a later leak does occur. Type II Mirizzi is defined by the presence of a fistula between the gallbladder and the bile duct due to erosion of the impacted gallbladder stone in Hartmann's pouch. There is usually a large amount of chronic inflammation present and primary closure and T-tube insertion rarely works. Typically, the CBD will need to be reconstructed with a Roux-en-Y hepatico-jejunostomy (see Chapter 12).

Postcholecystectomy complications – identification and management

Early presentation

With the majority of LCs performed as day case procedures surgeons need to have a high index of suspicion for complications, and patients deviating from the normal pathway of early and rapid return to normal function within the first few hours or days of an elective cholecystectomy should be reviewed by an experienced surgeon.

Excessive pain in the early postoperative period may be an indicator of intraperitoneal leakage of bile or bowel contents. Significant hypotension and pain may be an indicator of bleeding. Early re-laparoscopy, to identify and correct these problems, is preferred to diagnostic imaging, which is likely to add delay and may be inconclusive.

Common sites of bleeding are from a slipped cystic artery clip or missed cystic artery, damage to the middle hepatic vein within the gallbladder bed of the liver, or damage to the superior epigastric vessels from port insertion. Bile leaks may be from slipped cystic duct clips, damage to the cystic duct during IOC, a duct of Luschka injury or injury to the main bile duct.

The duct of Luschka is a subvesical duct which lies within the gallbladder bed of the liver close to the surface and can be damaged during removal of the posterior gallbladder wall. These ducts are small and away from the porta hepatis. When a leak is identified it should be clipped or sutured to seal it and prevent ongoing leakage (Fig. 11.13). Failure to identify the exact source of a small bile leak should be managed by insertion of a drain. Most low volume leaks from a duct of Luschka will resolve with simple drainage. In prolonged drainage (>5 days), resolution may be expedited by ERCP and stent insertion. Persistent leakage requires formal identification of the damaged duct and suturing, or rarely, resection of a segment of liver and should be dealt with in a specialist hepatopancreaticobiliary (HPB) unit.

Cystic duct stump leak requires further clip application or suturing. Clips used to hold a

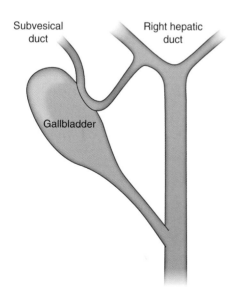
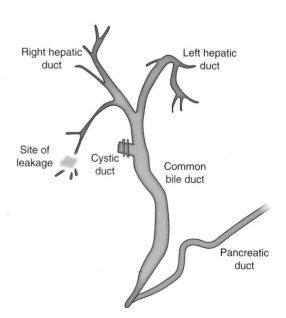

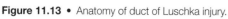
Figure 11.13 • Anatomy of duct of Luschka injury.

cholangiogram catheter in place can cause a small hole when removed and caution should be used to ensure that the lower most definitive clip is placed below the IOC cannula clip to prevent this.

Identification of a bile leak from the porta hepatis should be managed by insertion of a drain to the gallbladder fossa area, with discussion and early transfer to an HPB unit for investigation. The algorithm for investigation of a potential bile duct injury will depend on the timing post cholecystectomy, the presence or absence of sepsis and physiological well-being of the patient (see below).

> ✅ Patients who do not follow the normal pattern of straightforward recovery within the first 48 hours following cholecystectomy should be suspected of having a biliary leak until proven otherwise.

Delayed presentation

Patients who have been discharged home and re-present with ongoing or new onset of abdominal pain following LC should be investigated with assessment of full blood count and LFTs and consideration of CT. Ultrasound is rarely helpful in this setting due to the presence of RUQ tenderness and intra-abdominal gas. A small amount of gas and fluid in the gallbladder bed may be normal but collections of fluid or gas elsewhere may represent a bile leak. If haemostatic agents (e.g. Surgicel) have been used to control bleeding in the gallbladder bed there may be gas containing foreign material seen on US or CT. Elevated abnormal LFTs also raise suspicion of a bile leak or retained CBD stone. MRCP or ERCP will be diagnostic and the exact approach is dictated by the initial findings and clinical suspicion, the patient's condition and clinical urgency, and local availability and expertise. Concerns over MRI and dislodgement of cystic duct or artery clips in the immediate postoperative period are unfounded since virtually all metallic clips in current usage are non-ferrous.[79] The presence of bile collections or dilated intrahepatic ducts raises the suspicion of a bile duct injury and warrants early discussion and transfer to a specialist HPB unit.

Visualisation of a fluid collection in the presence of excessive pain, sepsis and/or abnormal LFTs should be evaluated with a percutaneous radiologically sited drain (or alternatively returned to theatre for laparoscopy). If bile is drained, an MRCP should be arranged to look for bile leakage or CBD stones with progression to ERCP if either is identified. If neither is identified and the patient is not septic then it is likely that the leak is small and will settle without further intervention and the drain can be removed once dry.

Retained CBD stones identified by MRCP in the postoperative period are best dealt with by ERCP. Success rates in most centres exceed 95% and recent developments of ultra-thin cholangioscopy (e.g. SpyGlass) permitting break-up of stones under direct vision using either electrohydraulic or laser lithotripsy are likely to increase this rate further.[80] LBDE can be performed in those where ERCP is not possible, e.g. large duodenal diverticulum, previous gastric bypass surgery.

> ✅ Patients re-presenting following cholecystectomy should undergo CT to look for a collection. In the presence of sepsis or significant abdominal pain, needle aspiration and subsequent drainage is mandated to look for a bile leak.

Bile duct injury

It is widely held that the incidence of bile duct injuries increased twofold following the introduction of laparoscopic surgery to around 0.4%.[81] Increasing recognition and the development and promulgation of techniques to prevent bile duct injury have reduced the rates to approximately 0.2–0.3%; however, this disguises the fact that there has been a significant incidence in more severe injuries in the laparoscopic group and a recognition that injury to the right hepatic artery is also present in approximately 25% of patients with a major bile duct injury.[82]

Davidoff described the mechanisms and errors involved in the causation of a 'classical' bile duct injury in the laparoscopic era. In this injury there is misidentification of the common duct for the cystic duct with subsequent ligation and division of the CBD, often with ligation of the right hepatic artery. This injury results in complete excision of a segment of the bile duct (Fig. 11.14).[83] The classification of bile duct injuries and their management is further discussed in Chapter 12.

Postoperative problems (chronic)

Postoperative pain resolution following cholecystectomy is dependent upon case selection. Post-cholecystectomy pain is invariably the result of precholecystectomy symptoms/other diagnoses and there is no evidence that the procedure of LC in itself results in the development of abdominal pain.

A proportion of patients (approximately 5%) develop looser bowel habit or urgency of defaecation, although this is usually in patients who had some degree of symptoms (e.g. irritable bowel syndrome) pre-LC. Severe high volume diarrhoea

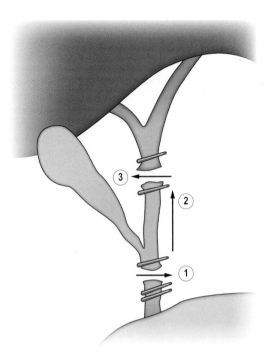

Figure 11.14 • The 'classical' bile duct injury. Excessive cephalad retraction of the gallbladder leads to dissection of the CBD low down (1). Subsequent mobilisation of the bile duct occurs (2). Removal of the gallbladder specimen requires further division of the bile duct (3) and, in around 25% of cases, division of the RHA as well.
Adapted from Davidoff AM, Pappas TN, Murray EA, et al. Mechanisms of major biliary injury during laparoscopic cholecystectomy. Ann Surg 1992;215(3):196–202.

is fortunately extremely rare.[84,85] Loose stools may be due to the more constant flow of bile entering a relatively empty bowel resulting in irritation of the bowel rather than a bolus of bile delivered by the contraction of the gallbladder in response to cholecystokinin into a small bowel containing fat. In half of these patients a degree of adaptation appears to occur with resolution of symptoms over a period of 3–6 months. Patients who continue to be troubled with diarrhoea may benefit from loperamide to control urgency and/or a bile-binding agent such as cholestyramine.[86]

Gallstones which are dropped at the time of cholecystectomy as a result of perforation of the gallbladder are quite commonly seen with an estimated incidence of spilled stones in approximately 7% of LCs, and of stones definitely left within the peritoneal cavity of approximately 2%.[87] Complications of dropped stones are, however, uncommon. The commonest complication of dropped stones is the development of an intra-abdominal abscess which occurs in 0.1–2.9% of patients with dropped stones at an average of 14 months after surgery.[88] Some of these present with subphrenic abscess formation requiring repeat laparoscopy or laparotomy to drain the pus and find the causative stone(s). The stones themselves may be very small but can usually be identified on CT. Attempts should therefore be made to remove all spilled stones where possible although conversion to laparotomy is not considered advisory to achieve complete clearance.

Gallstones and cancer

A number of studies purported to show both positive and negative associations between gallstones or cholecystectomy and various non-biliary tract cancers, in particular with the development of gastrointestinal tract cancers. A large population-based study in the USA suggests that there may be a slight increase in liver, pancreatic and gastro-oesophageal cancers but a decrease in colorectal cancers. Whether these increases are true or occur by chance, the risk ratios are small and insufficient to advise a change of practice either way.[89]

There is an association between gallstones and the development of gallbladder cancers, with a relative risk of 4.9.[90] The relative risk is further increased from 2.4 in patients with stones <3 cm, to 10 with stones >3 cm. However, there is no justification for removal of the gallbladder based solely on concerns over the risk of developing gallbladder cancer.

Porcelain gallbladder

Extensive calcium encrustation of the gallbladder wall is referred to as porcelain gallbladder. The incidence of porcelain gallbladder is reported to be 0.6–0.8%, with a male-to-female ratio of 1:5. Most porcelain gallbladders (90%) are associated with gallstones.[91,92] Patients with a porcelain gallbladder are asymptomatic, and the condition is usually found incidentally on plain abdominal radiographs, US or CT imaging. Surgical treatment of porcelain gallbladder is based on results from studies performed between1931 and 1973, which demonstrated a very high frequency (22–68%) of adenocarcinoma in porcelain gallbladder.[93]

However, the causal relationship between porcelain gallbladder and malignancy has not been established and the very high rates of carcinoma originally quoted seem, for whatever reason, to be less high than previously recorded in more recent case series (i.e. dating from 2001–11) that show incidences ranging from 2.3% to 7%.[94,95] Current guidance is that patients found to have porcelain gallbladder should undergo LC to prevent the risk of developing gallbladder cancer.

Other diseases of the gallbladder

Acute acalculous cholecystitis

Acute acalculous cholecystitis is a life-threatening condition that occurs in critically ill patients. It is an uncommon problem encountered largely in patients in intensive care or in cardiac patients as a result of poor perfusion. The cystic artery is an end-organ artery with no collateral circulation and poor perfusion can result in gallbladder ischaemia with resultant pain and tenderness. The diagnosis is often elusive and the condition is associated with significant mortality (up to 50%). Risk factors include severe trauma or burns, major surgery such as cardiopulmonary bypass, prolonged fasting, total parenteral nutrition, sepsis, diabetes mellitus, atherosclerotic disease, systemic vasculitis, acute renal failure and acquired immunodeficiency syndrome (AIDS). The condition is thought to be caused by microvascular occlusion of end arteries within the gallbladder wall resulting in ischaemia and, in up to 60% of cases, in gangrene.[96] Over 70% of patients have atherosclerotic disease, which might explain the higher prevalence of the condition in elderly men.[97]

The diagnosis of acute acalculous cholecystitis is often hindered by obtundation of the patient, the presence of pre-existing diseases or recent abdominal surgery, and requires a high index of suspicion. Ultrasound confirms the diagnosis within the intensive care unit and allows immediate percutaneous cholecystostomy which reduces the tension on the gallbladder wall and has become the preferred alternative to cholecystectomy in the treatment of the condition in severely ill patients.[98] Early cholecystectomy may still be appropriate depending on the patient's clinical condition and if cholecystostomy fails to improve the patient's conditions, as gangrene can develop with subsequent perforation of the gallbladder.

Primary infections of the gallbladder

Primary infective cholecystitis is rare and is more commonly seen in immunocompromised patients. Typical causative organisms include *Salmonella typhi*, *Campylobacter jejuni* and *Vibrio cholera*. The presentation is similar to patients with acute acalculous cholecystitis, but there is often an antecedent history of a gastroenteritis-like illness.

AIDS patients are susceptible to opportunistic gastrointestinal infections including acute cholecystitis and cholangitis, especially when the CD4 count falls below 200. In half the cases there are no associated gallstones within the biliary tract. The most common infecting agents are cytomegalovirus and cryptosporidium, and less commonly *Candida*, fungi and *Mycobacterium tuberculosis*. The 30-day mortality in AIDS patients with acute cholecystitis is 20%.

Treatment is by appropriate intravenous antibiotics followed by laparoscopic cholecystectomy.

Chronic acalculous cholecystitis

Chronic acalculous cholecystitis is a poorly understood condition. The term is used to describe patients with biliary pain but without cholelithiasis. In some cases biliary sludge may be responsible for a localised inflammatory response in the gallbladder with pain and tenderness typical of low-grade biliary pain. Occasionally a tiny stone within the spiral valve of the cystic duct is found at cholecystectomy which was missed preoperatively.

In patients with typical biliary pain, cholecystectomy may be justifiable in the absence of other disease processes and treatment options. Informed consent with an understanding of at best a 50% likelihood of pain resolution must be emphasised.

Isotope scans with HIDA or DISIDA (cholescintigraphy) have been used to improve outcomes in this group by selecting patients with a non-functioning gallbladder (failure to take up isotope within 4 hours of injection) or poorly functioning gallbladder. The gallbladder ejection fraction (GBEF) is used to calculate gallbladder function by giving a cholecystokinin (CCK) analogue or fatty meal following uptake of the isotope by the gallbladder. These stimulate emptying of the gallbladder, allowing an ejection fraction to be calculated. Administration of CCK may also recreate the pain. Normal GBEF is around 75% and LC in patients with low gallbladder ejection fractions (<40%) achieves long-term symptom relief in 65–80% of cases.[99,100]

Gallbladder disease in childhood

Underlying conditions are identified in 60% of children presenting with gallstones. These include haemolytic anaemias, congenital anomalies (choledochal cyst, prematurity, NEC), genetic disorders (Down syndrome, cystic fibrosis), Crohn's disease and ileal resection, liver disease and cirrhosis, cancer or leukaemia therapy.[101] Obesity is becoming an increasingly important risk factor in development of childhood cholelithiasis. Overall, the risk of gallstones in children is 0.13% (0.27% in females). Management is similar to that of adults, with LC.[102] CBD stones are the commonest cause of obstructive jaundice in children.

Acalculous cholecystitis in children may follow burns and trauma and may also be seen as a postoperative complication of abdominal surgery.

It occurs at any age from 1 month to 15 years[103] and is frequently misdiagnosed as appendicitis. Cholecystostomy is the treatment of choice.

Adenomyomatosis

Adenomyomatosis of the gallbladder is an acquired, hyperplastic lesion characterised by excessive proliferation of the gallbladder mucosa with invaginations into the muscle layer to produce deep clefts (Rokitansky–Aschoff sinuses). It may be generalised or localised to one area (adenomyoma). The involved gallbladder wall is thickened to 10 mm or greater. Gallstones are found in 60% of cases. It is usually an incidental radiological or pathological finding and simple adenomyomatosis is not considered a premalignant condition.

In the absence of biliary tract symptoms, adenomyomatosis requires no treatment. If the patient has biliary pain and evidence of adenomyomatosis with calculi, a cholecystectomy is indicated. The benefit of LC in patients with biliary pain and adenomyomatosis but no gallstones is more difficult to predict but the likelihood of benefit from surgery increases the more extensive or severe the adenomyomatosis.[104]

Key points

- Biliary pain is typically epigastric/right upper quadrant pain, radiating around or through to the back, lasting >20 minutes, often occurring at night or associated with eating fatty foods.
- People with gallstones but without symptoms do not require further management or follow-up.
- People with gallstones and biliary pain should be offered laparoscopic cholecystectomy as definitive treatment to prevent further episodes of pain and development of complications.
- Laparoscopic cholecystectomy is one of the commonest general surgical procedures in the UK, with around 100 000 procedure performed in England per annum.
- Current advice is to remove all CBD stones, which can be done most cost-effectively by simultaneous laparoscopic bile duct exploration but is still most frequently done by ERCP.
- Following cholecystectomy, patients presenting with abdominal pain in the first 48 hours should be investigated quickly to identify potential biliary leaks/bile duct injury.

🌐 Full references available at **http://expertconsult.inkling.com**

Key references

29. Reynolds W. The first laparoscopic cholecystectomy. J Soc Laparoend Surg 2001;5:89–94.
   Good review of the early history of laparoscopic cholecystectomy.

44. Strasberg SM, Brunt LM. Rationale and use of the critical view of safety in laparoscopic cholecystectomy. J Am Coll Surg 2010;211:132–8. PMID: 20610259.

Essential reading for rationale and technique of safe cholecystectomy avoiding bile duct injury.

63. Williams EJ, Green J, Beckingham I, et al. Updated guidelines on the management of common bile duct stones (CBDS). Gut 2017;66(5):765–82. PMID: 28122906.
   Definitive guidelines on current diagnosis and management of CBD stones.

83. Davidoff AM, Pappas TN, Murray EA, et al. Mechanisms of major biliary injury during laparoscopic cholecystectomy. Ann Surg 1992;215(3):196–202. PMID: 1531913.
   Analysis of causes of bile duct injury during laparoscopic cholecystectomy.

12

Benign biliary tract diseases

Benjamin N.J. Thomson
O. James Garden

Introduction

Apart from those disorders related to choledo-cholithiasis, benign diseases of the biliary tree are relatively uncommon (Box 12.1). The most challenging patients are those who present with symptoms associated with biliary strictures, which arise more commonly following iatrogenic injury during cholecystectomy. Congenital abnormalities such as choledochal cysts and biliary atresia are usually in the domain of the paediatric surgeon, although later presentation of cysts may occur after missed diagnosis or when revisional surgery is required. Most of the published literature regarding benign non-gallstone biliary disease is retrospective or at best prospectively gathered, non-randomised data, but clear guidelines can be followed based upon this experience.

Congenital anomalies

Biliary atresia

Biliary atresia occurs in approximately 1 per 10 000 live births but its aetiology remains unclear. There is experimental evidence for a primary perinatal infection as well as cellular and humoral autoimmunity. An inflammatory process before birth may result in failure of the biliary lumen to develop in all or part of the extrahepatic biliary tree. Two clinical variants are thought to originate during intrauterine development, biliary atresia malformation syndrome (BASM) and cystic biliary atresia (CBA).[1]

Presentation is usually in the early neonatal period with prolongation of neonatal jaundice. Most patients are treated in specialist neonatal surgical units; however, occasionally patients may be referred to adult units for assessment for liver transplantation following previous unsuccessful treatment. Management in the neonate is by porto-enterostomy (Kasai's operation), which involves anastomosis of a Roux limb of jejunum to the tissue of the hilum. Restoration of bile flow has been reported in 86% of infants treated before 8 weeks of age, but only 36% in older children.[2] Four-year survival is dependent on the timing of surgery. Of 349 North American children with biliary atresia, 210 (60%) required later liver transplantation, with a 4-year transplantation survival of 82%.[3] A properly performed Kasai porto-enterostomy can postpone the need for liver transplantation and improve outcome. Better outcomes are also seen following maternal living-related liver transplantation, potentially due to tolerance to non-inherited maternal antigens.[4]

Choledochal cysts

Presentation is usually in childhood, with jaundice, fever or an abdominal mass. Around 25% are diagnosed in the first year, although prenatal diagnosis is now possible with improvements in antenatal ultrasonography. Adult centres treat a small proportion of those presenting with late symptoms or complications from previous cyst surgery.

Strictures of the extrahepatic biliary tree
Iatrogenic biliary injury
Postcholecystectomy
Trauma
Other
Gallstone-related
Mirizzi's syndrome
Inflammatory
Recurrent pyogenic cholangitis
Parasitic infestation
   Clonorchis sinensis
   Opisthorchis viverrini
   Echinococcus
   Ascaris
HIV/AIDS cholangiopathy
Primary sclerosing cholangitis
Benign strictures imitating malignancy
Pancreatitis
IgG4-related disease
   Autoimmune pancreatitis
   IgG4-related cholangiopathy
   Inflammatory pseudotumour

The incidence of choledochal cysts in Western countries is around 1 in 200 000 live births but it is much higher in Asia. There is frequent association with other hepatobiliary disease such as hepatic fibrosis, as well as an aberrant pancreatico-biliary duct junction. Magnetic resonance cholangiopancreatography (MRCP) is the non-invasive imaging investigation of choice (**Fig. 12.1**).

Classification

The modified Todani classification is employed to describe the various forms of choledochal cyst[5] (**Fig. 12.2**). Type I, the most common, represents a solitary cyst characterised by fusiform dilatation of the common bile duct. Type II comprises a diverticulum of the common bile duct, whilst type III cysts are choledochocoeles. Type IV is the second most common, with extension of cysts into the intrahepatic ducts. Lastly, type V involves intrahepatic cystic disease with no choledochal cyst, which merges into the syndrome of Caroli's disease.

Risk of malignancy

In the Western literature, the incidence of cholangiocarcinoma (see Fig. 12.1) is reported to be approximately 12%,[6] but is higher in Japanese reports. Sastry et al. reported 434 cancers in 5780 patients with a choledochal cyst from 78 studies. Cholangiocarcinoma occurred in 70.4%, gallbladder cancer in 23.5% but cancer occurring before the age of 18 years was rare.[7] Cyst drainage without cyst excision does not prevent later malignant change, and there is continuing debate regarding the precise ongoing risk following cyst resection. In a report of 180 patients who underwent primary surgery, synchronous malignancy was found in 36 patients (20%), with only one of the remaining patients developing malignancy during follow-up.[8]

Management

Surgical resection is required to prevent recurrent episodes of sepsis and pain, to prevent the risk of pancreatitis from passage of debris and calculi, and because of the association with cholangiocarcinoma. Complete cyst excision with preservation of the pancreatic duct is required, with hepatico-jejunostomy for reconstruction. Some authors advocate liver resection for type IV cysts with intrahepatic extension for complete removal of the cyst, although the advantage is debatable. For those patients with Caroli's disease, resection may be feasible if the biliary involvement is localised to one part of the liver. For other patients, endoscopic or radiological techniques may be required to address biliary sepsis by improving biliary drainage, while others may need to be considered for hepatic replacement if liver failure develops.

Cyst-enterostomy, or drainage of the cyst into the duodenum, should no longer be performed

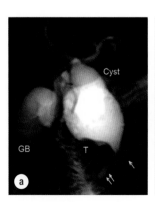
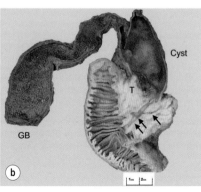

Figure 12.1 • MRCP **(a)** and macroscopic photograph **(b)** demonstrating a type I choledochal cyst with a distal cholangiocarcinoma in a 42-year-old Caucasian woman requiring a pancreatico-duodenectomy. Gallbladder (*GB*), tumour (*T*), pancreatic duct (*single arrow*) and aberrant common channel (*double arrow*) are shown.
Courtesy of Professor Prithi S. Bhathal, Pathology Department, University of Melbourne, Australia.

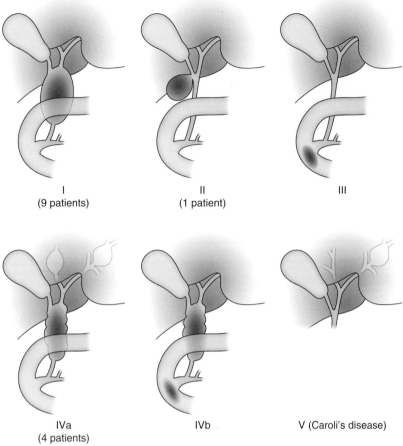

I
(9 patients)

II
(1 patient)

III

IVa
(4 patients)

IVb

V (Caroli's disease)

Figure 12.2 • Modified Todani classification for choledochal cysts.[9]
Reproduced from Todani T, Watanabe Y, Narusue M et al. Congenital bile duct cysts: classification, operative procedures, and review of thirty-seven cases including cancer arising from choledochal cyst. Am J Surg 1977;134:263–9. With permission from Elsevier.

for extrahepatic cysts as the cyst epithelium remains unstable and malignant potential exists. If previous drainage has been performed, symptoms of cholangitis generally persist and conversion to a Roux-en-Y hepatico-jejunostomy is advisable.

Special operative techniques

During operative exposure, intraoperative ultrasound is very useful to identify the biliary confluence, the intrahepatic extension of the cyst and the relationship to the right hepatic artery above and to the pancreatic duct below (**Fig. 12.3**). Small aberrant hepatic ducts may enter the cyst below the biliary confluence and these are missed frequently on preoperative imaging. Such aberrant ducts are usually identified once the cyst has been opened. The uncomplicated cyst is normally best excised in its entirety and this is facilitated by opening it along its anterior length. This aids identification of the vessels from which the cyst is freed. Early identification of

the biliary confluence aids the surgeon in planning the incorporation of any segmental duct into the eventual hepatico-jejunal Roux-en-Y anastomosis. Dissection into the head of the pancreas is made easier by use of bipolar scissors and the CUSA™ (ultrasonic surgical aspiration system, ValleyLab, Boulder, CO) if the plane of dissection is obscured by fibrosis or inflammation. It may be necessary to leave a small oversewn lower common bile duct stump to avoid compromise to the pancreatic duct lumen; however, recurrent pancreatitis and possible malignant transformation remain possible complications. Pancreatico-duodenectomy is difficult to justify in the uncomplicated case when dealing with the residual lower bile duct. Laparoscopic resection and reconstruction has been described; Senthinathan et al. reported 110 adults and children successfully managed, with three adults requiring conversion, a re-exploration rate of 1.8% and one death. Cholangitis occurred in

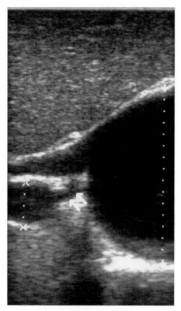

Figure 12.3 • Operative ultrasound scan of a type I choledochal cyst. The junction of the undilated proximal biliary tree with the cyst (*long dotted line*) is demonstrated. The right hepatic artery is posterior (*two arrows*), as is the right branch of the portal vein (*short dotted line*).

three patients, with three requiring intervention for anastomotic strictures on the short-term follow-up.[9] (See recommended video at end of chapter.)

> ✓✓ There is an accepted association between choledochal cyst and cholangiocarcinoma. The cyst should be excised and the biliary tree reconstructed by means of a Roux-en-Y hepatico-jejunostomy.

Iatrogenic biliary injury

The commonest cause of an injury to the extrahepatic biliary tree is as a result of an iatrogenic injury at the time of cholecystectomy. Although it is recognised that injury may also occur during other gastric or pancreatic procedures, this is much less common with the reduction in ulcer surgery and increasing specialisation in pancreatico-biliary surgery. Rarely, the injury may be related to abdominal trauma,[10] injection of scolicidal agents in the management of hydatid cyst, ablation of hepatic tumours or radiotherapy. The true incidence of biliary injury following laparoscopic cholecystectomy remains obscure but there has been a slight increase since its introduction, with a reported incidence of 0.3–0.7%.[11] Despite the expectation that the rate of injury would decrease with experience, the Swedish quality register reported a rate of 0.3% in 55 134 cholecystectomies performed from 2007 to 2011.[12]

Recent variations in technique such as single-incision laparoscopic surgery (SILS) cholecystectomy are not immune to biliary injury, with a rate of 0.72% reported in 2626 patients undergoing SILS.[13]

Aetiology

Previous reports of injury during laparoscopic cholecystectomy suggested that injury was more likely to occur when performed for pancreatitis, cholangitis or acute cholecystitis.[14] However, surgeons should remain vigilant regardless of the indication. In the majority of patients the problem is misinterpretation of the biliary anatomy, with the common bile duct being confused with the cystic duct. Associated injury to the right hepatic artery often occurs as it is mistaken for the cystic artery. Partial injury may occur to the common bile duct after a diathermy burn or due to rigorous traction on the cystic duct, leading to its avulsion from the bile duct.

Techniques to avoid injury

Many techniques have been described to decrease the risk of injury to the common bile duct during cholecystectomy. The main risk factors are thought to be inexperience, aberrant anatomy and inflammation.[14,15] However, in an analysis of 252 laparoscopic bile duct injuries, the authors suggested that the primary cause of error was a visual perceptual illusion in 97% of cases, whilst faults in technical skill were thought to have been present in only 3% of injuries.[16]

Correct identification of the biliary anatomy is essential in avoiding injury to the extrahepatic bile duct. Dissection of Hartmann's pouch should start at the junction of the gallbladder and cystic duct and continue lateral to the cystic lymph node, thus staying as close as possible to the gallbladder. The biliary tree and hepatic arterial anatomy is highly variable and therefore great care must be taken in identifying all structures within Calot's triangle before ligation. In Couinaud's published study of biliary anatomy, 25% had drainage of a right sectoral duct directly into the common hepatic duct.[17] Sometimes this structure may follow a prolonged extrahepatic course, where it can be at greater risk from cholecystectomy. The right hepatic artery may also course through this area. All structures should be traced into the gallbladder to minimise the risk of injury (**Figs 12.4 and 12.5**).

Calot's original description of gallbladder anatomy described a triangle formed by the cystic duct, common hepatic duct and superior border of the cystic artery. For satisfactory visualisation of the structures, dissection should also extend above

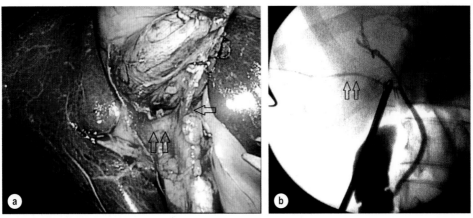

Figure 12.4 • Aberrant biliary anatomy. The normal biliary anatomy is a trifurcation of the right sectoral and left hepatic ducts forming the common hepatic duct which receives the cystic duct after a variable distance. Operative photograph **(a)** and a cholangiogram **(b)** of a short cystic duct (*single arrow*) draining into the right posterior sectoral duct (*double arrow*), which has a long extrahepatic course.

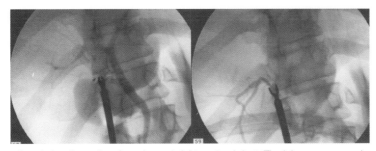

Figure 12.5 • Operative cholangiography of an aberrant right sectoral duct. The injury was recognised after division of the duct following cholangiography. The cholangiogram catheter was used to obtain a cholangiogram of the aberrant duct. The surgeon obtained advice by telephone and a decision was made to ligate the duct. The patient remains asymptomatic.

the cystic artery to the liver. Extensive dissection should be avoided in Calot's triangle as diathermy injury may occur to the lateral wall of the common hepatic duct. Furthermore, arterial bleeding in this area should not be cauterised or clipped blindly. Most bleeding can be controlled with several minutes of direct pressure with a laparoscopic forceps compressing Hartmann's pouch on to the bleed point. During the era of open cholecystectomy many advocated complete excision of the cystic duct to its insertion into the common bile duct to avoid a cystic duct stump syndrome. However, extensive dissection around the common bile duct with or without diathermy may cause an ischaemic stricture due to damage to the intricate blood supply of the common hepatic duct.

Strasberg described the 'critical view of safety' with complete dissection of Calot's triangle by mobilisation of the gallbladder neck from the gallbladder bed of the liver before transecting the cystic artery and duct.[15] More recently, Connor et al. suggested a five-point checklist to limit

the occurrence of biliary injury at laparoscopic cholecystectomy. The five steps are: '(i) confirm the gallbladder lies in the hepatic principal plane and is retracted to the 10 o'clock position; (ii) confirm Hartmann's pouch is lifted up and toward the segment IV pedicle; (iii) identify Rouvière's sulcus; (iv) confirm the release of the posterior leaf of the peritoneum covering the hepatobiliary triangle; and (v) confirm the critical view with or without intraoperative cholangiography'.[18]

Many authors argue that operative cholangiography is essential to avoid biliary injury.[11,14] Fletcher et al. reported an overall twofold reduction in biliary injuries with the use of operative cholangiography, with an eightfold decrease in complex cases.[14] Flum et al. analysed retrospectively the Medicare database in the USA and identified 7911 common bile duct injuries following cholecystectomy. After adjusting for patient-level factors and surgeon-level factors, the relative risk was 1.49 when intraoperative cholangiography was not used.[11] When the use of intraoperative cholangiography has undergone cost analysis, routine cholangiography has been found to be most cost-effective during high-risk operations when employed by less experienced surgeons.[19]

Unfortunately, many operative cholangiograms are interpreted incorrectly and injuries are missed. Although this event should be less frequent with the use of modern C-arm imaging, in reported series of biliary injuries only 6–33% of operative cholangiograms are interpreted correctly. For correct anatomical interpretation of the proximal biliary tree, both right sectoral/sectional ducts and the left hepatic duct should be visualised. In the presence of an endoscopic sphincterotomy, contrast will preferentially flow into the duodenum and the patient may need to be placed in a head-down position to fill the intrahepatic ducts. If the anatomy is unclear no proximal clip should be placed on what is presumed to be the cystic duct, to avoid a crush injury to what may be the common hepatic duct.

Retrograde cholecystectomy has been described previously as a safe technique when inflammation around Calot's triangle makes identification of the anatomy difficult. Nonetheless, care still needs to be exercised during dissection to avoid injury to the right hepatic artery and common hepatic duct, which may be adherent to an inflamed gallbladder. Eight such vasculobiliary injuries were described by Strasberg and Gouma.[20] If identification remains impossible then the gallbladder can be opened to facilitate identification of the cystic duct. A subtotal cholecystectomy should be considered if a safe plane of dissection cannot be established, thus avoiding injury to the common hepatic or left hepatic ducts. Originally described for open cholecystectomy, these techniques have now also been performed laparoscopically.

✔✔ Bile duct injury can be avoided by careful identification of the biliary anatomy, dissection close to the gallbladder and avoidance of diathermy in Calot's triangle. The use of operative cholangiography and its correct interpretation is associated with a reduced incidence of bile duct injury.

Classification

Injury to the distal biliary tree is less technically demanding to repair than involvement of the biliary confluence. The success of reconstruction depends on the type of injury and the anatomical location.[21] Bismuth first described a classification system for biliary strictures reflecting the relationship of the injury to the biliary confluence (Table 12.1).[22] Strasberg et al. further proposed a broader classification to include a number of biliary complications, including cystic stump leaks, biliary leaks and partial injuries

Table 12.1 • Bismuth classification of biliary strictures

Bismuth classification	Definition
Bismuth 1	Low common hepatic duct stricture – hepatic duct stump >2 cm
Bismuth 2	Proximal common hepatic duct stricture – hepatic duct stump <2 cm
Bismuth 3	Hilar stricture with no residual common hepatic duct – hepatic duct confluence intact
Bismuth 4	Destruction of hepatic duct confluence – right and left hepatic ducts separated
Bismuth 5	Involvement of aberrant right sectoral hepatic duct alone or with concomitant stricture of the common hepatic duct

to the biliary tree (**Fig. 12.6**).[23] Recently the European Association for Endoscopic Surgery (EAES) has proposed the ATOM (anatomic, time of detection, mechanism) classification to facilitate epidemiologic and comparative studies.[24]

Presentation

It is preferable that injuries are recognised at the time of surgery to allow the best chance of repair, but this occurs in less than a third of patients. An unrecognised injury may present early with a postoperative biliary fistula, symptoms of biliary peritonitis or jaundice. Early symptoms or signs may be lacking but ductal injury should be suspected in the patient whose recovery is not immediate or is complicated by symptoms of peritoneal or diaphragmatic irritation and/or associated with deranged liver function tests in the first 24–48 hours of surgery. Signs may range from localised abdominal tenderness through to generalised peritonitis with overwhelming sepsis. Ligation of the bile duct will present early with jaundice; however, later presentation may occur as a result of stricture formation from a partial injury, localised inflammation or ischaemic insult.

Ligation of sectoral ducts may cause subsequent or late atrophy of the drained liver segments, which may become infected secondarily. Occasionally liver resection or transplantation may be required for unilobar hepatic necrosis or fulminant hepatic failure secondary to combined biliary and vascular injuries.[25] More commonly, liver failure presents late with liver failure due to secondary biliary cirrhosis as a result of the injury, and may require liver transplantation.[25]

In many patients there is a delay in referral, despite suspicion or evidence of a biliary injury. In a report

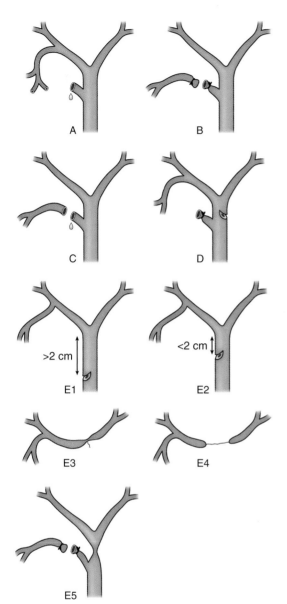

Management

Intraoperative recognition

In a review by Carroll et al., only 27% of patients underwent a successful repair by the primary surgeon responsible for the injury, whilst 79% of repairs performed following referral had a successful outcome.[27] If experienced help is not at hand, an attempt should not be made to remedy the situation since this may compromise subsequent successful management. Advice should be sought immediately and a T-tube or similar drain should be placed to the biliary injury and drains left in the subhepatic space, followed by referral to a specialist centre. Some specialist units may offer a specialist surgeon who can travel to the site of referral to expedite immediate repair. No attempt should be made to repair a transection or excision of the bile duct.

A partial injury to the bile duct may sometimes be managed by direct closure with placement of a T-tube through a separate choledochotomy. Primary repair with or without a T-tube for complete transection of the common bile duct is nearly always unsuccessful. This may result from unappreciated loss of common duct, an associated arterial injury, or result from local diathermy injury or devascularisation of the duct from overzealous dissection of the common bile duct (**Fig. 12.7a,b**). Successful endoscopic treatment is possible for failed primary repair; however, as many as 32% will require subsequent hepatico-jejunostomy.[28]

> ✔✔ If an injury to the biliary tree is suspected during cholecystectomy, help must be sought from an experienced hepatobiliary surgeon. A successful repair by the surgeon who has caused the injury is far less likely than one performed by a surgeon experienced in performing a biliary reconstruction.

Postoperative recognition: biliary fistula

Any patient who is not fit for discharge at 24 hours due to ongoing abdominal pain, vomiting, fever or bile in an abdominal drain should be considered to have a biliary leak. The lack of bile in an abdominal drain does not exclude the possibility of a biliary leak, particularly if there is liver function test derangement. Symptoms and signs vary widely, and widespread soiling of the abdominal cavity may be present with few signs in the early period following cholecystectomy.

Initial investigation should include full blood examination and determination of serum levels of urea, electrolytes, creatinine and liver function tests. Ultrasound is usually the initial investigation but it cannot readily differentiate bile and blood from

Figure 12.6 • Strasberg classification. Type A injuries include leakage from the cystic duct or subvesical ducts. Type B involves occlusion of part of the biliary tree, most usually an aberrant right hepatic duct. If the former injury involves transection without ligation this is termed a type C injury. A lateral injury to the biliary tree is a type D injury. Type E injuries are those described by Bismuth and subdivided into his classification (Table 12.1).
Adapted from Strasberg SM, Hertl M, Soper NJ, et al. An analysis of the problem of biliary injury during laparoscopic chole cystectomy. J Am Coll Surg 1995;180:102–25. With permission from the American College of Surgeons.

by Mirza et al., the median interval until referral was 26 days.[26] This delay is not inconsequential as the opportunity for an early repair is lost and may result in the liver sustaining further damage.

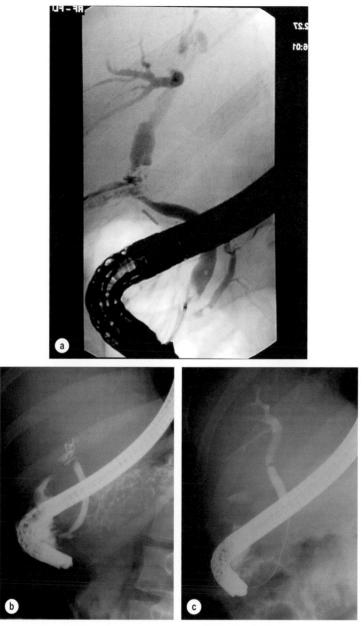

Figure 12.7 • (a) Failure of primary repair with T-tube. Primary repair was performed for an injury to the common bile duct presenting with biliary peritonitis. A T-tube was inserted through the anastomosis and this was removed at 4 weeks. An anastomotic stricture developed and the patient required a hepatico-jejunostomy 2 months later. **(b)** Failure of primary repair for ligation of the common bile duct. A complete transection of the common bile duct identified at postoperative endoscopic retrograde cholangiopancreatography (ERCP). Immediate repair was performed with a direct duct-to-duct repair. **(c)** A tight anastomotic stricture is demonstrated at a later ERCP.

a residual fluid collection following uneventful cholecystectomy. It may provide important information about the presence of intra-abdominal or pelvic fluid, biliary dilatation or retained stones within the bile duct. CT is normally preferred since it provides more objective information and allows assessment of the liver vasculature.

If there is evidence of significant peritoneal irritation from widespread biliary peritonitis, laparoscopy allows confirmation of this and provides an opportunity for abdominal lavage. The porta hepatis can be inspected to determine the cause of the bile leak. Whilst dislodged clips from the cystic duct can be managed by application of further clips or suture, any other form of bile leak should lead to specialist referral. Drains can be placed to the subhepatic space as well as the subdiaphragmatic space and pelvis if required. No attempt should be made to repair an injury at laparoscopy. If laparotomy is required, this should be considered in conjunction with specialist assistance if bile duct injury is suspected.

Further assessment depends on the clinical situation. The majority of biliary fistulas are due to leaks from the cystic duct stump or subvesicle ducts, and endoscopic retrograde cholangiopancreatography (ERCP) allows anatomical definition, endoscopic sphincterotomy or stent placement when abdominal contamination has been controlled. As complete transection of the bile duct precludes ERCP, computed tomography intravenous cholangiography (CT-IVC) or MRCP can determine continuity of the biliary tree prior to endoscopy. Occasionally, persistent bile drainage is associated with choledocholithiasis requiring endoscopic sphincterotomy and stone extraction. Most simple cystic duct stump leaks are resolved by endoscopic stenting if cannulation is possible at ERCP and occasionally side injury to the biliary tree can be controlled with endoscopic stent placement.

If ERCP is unsuccessful or the bile duct is ligated or occluded by clips, percutaneous transhepatic cholangiography (PTC) may facilitate biliary decompression but it is less frequently employed for diagnosis or delineation of the biliary anatomy. Occasionally, both sides of the liver may need to be externally drained to gain control of a biliary fistula, especially with Strasberg E4 injuries (Fig. 12.6) to the biliary confluence. However, injury to the biliary tree detected in this way may allow surgical repair to be considered within the first week of injury in the stable non-septic patient, and again such further investigation or management decisions should only be considered following specialist referral.

Where the diagnosis of bile duct injury has been delayed, the aim should be to control the biliary fistula with external drainage using surgical or radiologically placed drains. Further control may be required with endoscopic stenting or external biliary drainage. Delayed repair can be considered subsequently once sepsis and intra-abdominal soiling have resolved, as a planned elective procedure in a specialist unit, usually 2–3 months following injury. Such an initial conservative approach renders a potentially difficult operation into a repair that will be considerably easier.

✅✅ Diagnosis of a bile duct injury in the postoperative period should lead to immediate referral to a specialist centre since inappropriate attempts to manage this outside a specialist centre will compromise the outcome.

Postoperative recognition: biliary obstruction

Ligation or inadvertent clipping of the biliary tree presents early in the postoperative period with jaundice. Later, stricture formation may occur as a result of direct trauma during dissection, clips placed inadvertently on the cystic duct but compromising the bile duct, or from damage to the intricate vascular supply of the bile duct by extensive mobilisation or diathermy. Initial investigation should include haematology, assessment of coagulation by estimation of prothrombin time, and liver function tests. Ultrasound may indicate the level of obstruction or exclude the presence of a correctable cause of obstructive jaundice, such as a retained stone in the common bile duct.

ERCP will identify a stricture or complete transection of the bile duct; however, identification of complete transection with MRCP will avoid the risks of an unnecessary ERCP. CT IVC is not indicated as the contrast agent (Biliscopin) will not be excreted. Overzealous instillation of contrast at ERCP should be avoided due to the potential to introduce infection above the stricture. Placement of an endoscopic stent should be considered only after consultation with a specialist unit since this may introduce sepsis into the biliary tree and compromise further management. Furthermore, an undrained biliary tree may allow proximal biliary dilatation, thereby facilitating later reconstruction.

Although some have reported satisfactory resolution of biliary strictures with endoscopic stenting alone, the follow-up has usually been short and almost all patients require later surgery in our experience. Partial occlusion of the duct by a clip may be remedied by balloon dilatation with or without placement of a stent; however, delay in diagnosis may result in subsequent recurrent stricture formation. Nonetheless, de Reuver et al. reported 110 patients with bile duct strictures following cholecystectomy that were treated with endoscopic stenting, 48 (44%) of which had already undergone attempted surgical repair. At a mean follow-up of 7.6 years, 74% of patients had a successful outcome.[29] Parlak et al. recently reported 156 partial biliary strictures following cholecystectomy with only 11% requiring further intervention at 7.5 years median follow-up post stent removal.[30] The technique of placing multiple, increasing numbers of stents every 3–4 months was associated with a better outcome than stent replacement. The development of removable endoscopic expandable metal stents has recently been described,[31] although long-term results and large series are not yet available. Furthermore, stent migration can complicate treatment.

✅ If the diagnosis of ductal obstruction is made early within the first week after surgery, the bilirubin level is only moderately elevated and there is no coexisting coagulopathy or sepsis, immediate repair offers the best chance of a successful outcome.

✅ If repair needs to be delayed, stent placement may still be avoidable and a decision will generally be made based on the individual patient circumstances. Suspicion or evidence of arterial injury may influence the management decision.

✅ For strictures that declare late, appropriate indications for stent placement are the presence of sepsis, severe itch resistant to medical therapy, or significant hepatic dysfunction.

The timing of repair

Early repair

When an injury is recognised in the early postoperative period and there is minimal peritoneal contamination or sepsis, a definitive repair by an experienced surgeon can be successful (**Fig. 12.8**). In our series of 123 patients referred with injury to the biliary tree, 22 patients underwent primary biliary repair in the first 2 weeks following injury and three had revision of a failed biliary repair. Between 2 weeks and 6 months, a further 22 injuries were repaired selectively. Successful repair was possible in 22 of 25 early repairs compared with 20 of 22 delayed repairs.[32] Kirks et al. compared immediate repair (<48 hours) to delayed repair (>48 hours) and found equivalent outcomes in 61 patients when managed by an experienced team.[33] Dominguez-Rosado et al. reviewed 614 bile duct injuries and found that the intermediate group (repair between 8 days and 6 weeks) had a higher risk of complications when compared to early or delayed repair.[34]

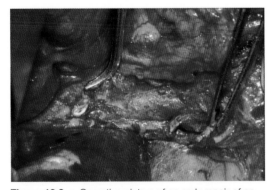

Figure 12.8 • Operative picture of an early repair of an E4 injury. A right-angle forceps is placed in the opening of the left hepatic duct whilst the open right hepatic duct is visible below. The portal vein is skeletonised with ligation and excision of both the extrahepatic biliary tree and right hepatic artery (held by forceps).

Delayed repair

Many injuries continue to be unrecognised or referral delayed, including patients with generalised peritonitis. Controlling the biliary injury and associated sepsis is the first treatment aim, which may require endoscopic or percutaneous biliary decompression, allowing jaundice to settle or biliary sepsis to be drained. Intra-abdominal collections may be drained percutaneously, or in the early postoperative period this may be better achieved by laparoscopic means. It is accepted, however, that bile collections are frequently loculated and difficult to eradicate in patients with intra-abdominal sepsis or widespread biliary contamination or peritonitis. The most effective treatment may be laparotomy with extensive lavage and the placement of large intra-abdominal drains. Definitive repair should not be contemplated if there is severe peritoneal soiling since injudicious attempts to repair the injury may aggravate the injury and result in a poor outcome.

Once these objectives have been met, the patient should be allowed to recover from the combined insult of surgery and sepsis. A period of rehabilitation at home is generally required before repair is contemplated in these compromised patients. Abdominal and biliary drainage can be managed on an outpatient basis with community nursing support. Nutritional supplementation may be required, particularly in those who have required a prolonged admission to the intensive care unit and hospital. Attention should be paid to the consequences of prolonged external biliary drainage and consideration given to recycling of bile.

Associated vascular injury

In patients with a delayed diagnosis, abdominal CT is required to ensure resolution of intra-abdominal collections and before repair to exclude the presence of liver atrophy. Atrophy can occur from prolonged obstruction to the segmental, sectional or hepatic ducts, but is generally associated with the presence of a vascular injury, most usually of the right hepatic artery. Liver resection may occasionally be needed at the time of definitive repair to remove a source of ongoing sepsis, or if satisfactory reconstruction to the left or right duct is not possible.

Buell et al. identified associated vascular injury as an independent predictor of mortality, with 38% of patients dying compared to 3% ($P < 0.001$) where no arterial injury was present.[35] Some authors advocate arteriography before repair to identify such associated vascular injury as a repair is less likely to be successful, or for consideration of hepatic arterial reconstruction at the time of hepatico-jejunostomy.[36] However, a recent review was unable to demonstrate any difference in outcome between patients with and without hepatic arterial injury.[37] Alves et al. described 55 patients with post-cholecystectomy strictures who underwent surgical reconstruction with a left duct approach and preoperative coeliac axis and superior mesenteric artery angiography.[38] Twenty-six patients (47%) had an associated vascular injury, of which 20 (36%) were of the right hepatic artery. In this series, only one patient in each group (vascular injury vs no injury) developed a recurrent stricture after repair.[38] A proximal anastomosis may offer a better blood supply, minimising the risk of anastomotic stricturing (**Fig. 12.9**). In support of this theory, Mercado et al. demonstrated that an anastomosis fashioned below the biliary confluence was more likely to require revisional surgery (16%) compared to an anastomosis performed at the biliary confluence (0%; $P < 0.05$).[39] Recent improvements in magnetic resonance imaging (MRI) and spiral CT provide impressive arterial and venous anatomical reconstructions, which should negate the need for invasive arteriography.

Injury to the hepatic arterial supply (usually the right hepatic artery) may present with haemobilia or intra-abdominal haemorrhage from a false aneurysm, usually associated with ongoing subhepatic sepsis. If suspected, urgent angiography is required (**Fig. 12.10**). Haemorrhage may be controlled by embolisation of the feeding vessel, although re-bleeding can occur and necessitate further embolisation. However, in our experience, further bleeding in the presence of ongoing sepsis usually requires laparotomy for control of bleeding and drainage of any subhepatic collection.

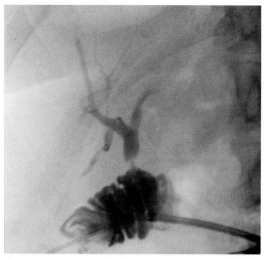

Figure 12.9 • Anastomotic stricture following repair of biliary injury. Percutaneous transjejunal cholangiogram (PTJC) of a Bismuth 1 injury repaired by hepatico-jejunostomy at the level of the transection of the common bile duct (not to the left hepatic duct). Three months later the patient required reconstruction of the anastomotic stricture.

Rarely, combined injury to the hepatic artery and portal vein can occur with resultant infarction of the affected hepatic parenchyma, usually the right liver. Such injuries may require urgent hepatic resection or transplantation.[25]

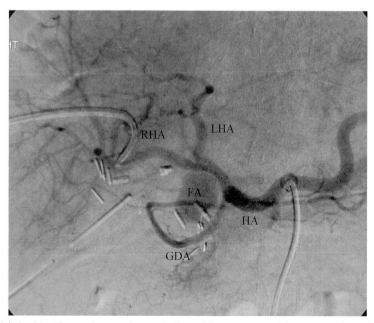

Figure 12.10 • Digital subtraction angiogram demonstrating a false aneurysm of the common hepatic artery. Embolisation was required for control. The patient has undergone a primary repair for a complete transection of the common bile duct. *FA*, false aneurysm; *GDA*, gastroduodenal artery; *HA*, common hepatic artery; *LHA*, left hepatic artery; *RHA*, right hepatic artery.

Further imaging

For patients with injury to the biliary confluence (E3 and E4), preoperative imaging will help in the planning of future repair. In the presence of a biliary stricture, invasive cholangiography by ERCP or PTC risks introducing sepsis. However, if PTC is required for external biliary drainage, an adequate cholangiogram may be obtained at this time. The quality of MRCP continues to improve, and detailed biliary anatomical reconstructions can be produced, thereby negating the need for more invasive imaging.

Operative techniques

Biliary reconstruction should be performed under optimal circumstances at the time of injury or soon thereafter. Once this opportunity has been lost, repair should only be considered when the patient has been optimised, in the absence of intra-abdominal sepsis, and when sufficient time has elapsed to allow for maturation of adhesions and the tissues at the porta hepatis.

A right subcostal incision is used for access, which can be extended across the midline if required. Retraction is provided with an upper abdominal (Omni-tract®, Omni-tract surgical, St Paul, MN) mechanical retractor. Laparotomy is undertaken to assess the liver and to allow adhesiolysis, thereby freeing the small bowel for reconstruction. Frequently the omentum, hepatic flexure, duodenum and hepatoduodenal ligament are involved in a dense inflammatory mass, and occasionally an unsuspected fistula between bile duct and duodenum or colon is identified. Dissection is often easier if commenced laterally and then directed towards the biliary structures. The common bile duct can be difficult to identify, particularly in the presence of extensive fibrosis, and intraoperative ultrasound is a useful tool in allowing its location and relationship to vessels to be determined.

For injuries that involve the biliary confluence, lowering of the hilar plate allows easier identification of the left and right hepatic ducts. This may be aided by the use of an ultrasonic dissector (CUSA), which is also employed to break down the contracted fibrotic tissue in the gallbladder bed and to facilitate the division of any bridge of liver tissue between segments III and IV. Opening these two planes on the right and left sides facilitates identification of and access to the biliary confluence.

Since the blood supply to the bile duct is often damaged at the time of injury, the common hepatic duct should be opened as proximally as possible, although frequently there has been retraction of the fibrotic remnant superiorly. Extension of the incision into the left hepatic duct allows a wide anastomosis to be fashioned with adequate views of the left- and right-sided ducts. Care should be taken since there may be a small superficial arterial branch crossing the left duct anteriorly and running above

to segment IV. For injuries involving separation of the confluence, the right and left hepatic ducts can be anastomosed together before formation of a hepatico-jejunostomy, allowing a single biliary anastomosis. If possible, injuries to an isolated right sectoral duct are best repaired or drained into a Roux limb of jejunum (Fig. 12.5). Simple ligation will lead to atrophy of the drained segments, which may become a nidus for sepsis. However, enteric drainage of a small sectoral duct may also lead to sepsis if an anastomotic stricture occurs.

Repair should be effected by a hepatico-jejunostomy with a 70-cm Roux limb of jejunum, thereby minimising the risk of enteric reflux and chronic damage to the biliary tree. Moraca et al. advocate hepatico-duodenostomy for biliary injury on the basis that it is more physiological, quicker to perform and allows later ERCP for imaging and intervention.[40] They found no difference in outcome following hepatico-duodenostomy when compared with hepatico-jejunostomy, although median follow-up was only 54 months. Hepatico-duodenostomy has largely been abandoned in the treatment of other benign biliary disease due to ongoing enteric reflux. There have been anecdotal reports of the late development of cholangiocarcinoma,[41] as well as the need to undertake liver transplantation in patients so managed when secondary biliary cirrhosis due to enteric reflux has resulted. Our own view is that hepatico-duodenostomy has no role in the management of bile duct injury.

Fine absorbable interrupted sutures of 4/0 or 5/0 polydioxanone sulphate (PDS II) should be used to fashion an end-to-side hepatico-jejunostomy, with care being taken to produce good mucosal apposition. Some authors advocate the use of an access limb, particularly for E3 and E4 injuries, to allow subsequent radiological intervention for dilatation of recurrent strictures. However, others believe that advances in percutaneous transhepatic techniques have made this unnecessary and have achieved satisfactory results without using this surgical approach.

Rarely, there may be no recognisable bile ducts visible in the porta hepatis. In such cases a variation of porto-enterostomy (Kasai procedure) can be considered with the Roux limb sutured to the fibrous structure of the hilar plate (S.W. Banting, personal communication).

Partial injury to the biliary tree can be repaired with fine interrupted sutures, although when resulting from diathermy dissection, formal hepatico-jejunostomy may be necessary as conduction of the thermal injury may cause later stricture formation. If a T-tube is placed to protect a primary duct repair, this should be placed through a separate choledochotomy. Laparoscopic repair has also been described with a recent report of 29 cases. The majority were managed with a primary repair with eight hepatico-jejunostomies and the longest follow-up only 36 months.[42] Our view is that laparoscopic repair offers little benefit over open biliary reconstruction and that primary repair is an inferior treatment modality.

Management of complications related to repair

Revisional surgery

Many patients with biliary injury continue to suffer from complications despite reconstruction. Factors such as the experience of the initial surgeon, the level of injury, the associated sepsis and liver atrophy all increase the chance of an unsuccessful repair. Following primary repair of a ductal tear or laceration, further stricture formation may result if there has been extensive dissection around the common hepatic duct. In such instances, surgical revision with the formation of a Roux-en-Y hepatico-jejunostomy is indicated.

The majority of patients requiring revisional surgery will have undergone a previous biliary enteric drainage procedure. Anastomotic stricturing will require revision of the anastomosis, with extension of the choledochotomy into the left hepatic duct (Fig. 12.9). There is very little literature to guide decisions about the management of anastomotic stricture formation following reconstruction of the bile duct with a Roux-en-Y hepatico-jejunostomy but surgical revision remains the gold standard.

Liver resection and transplantation

In the acute setting of bile duct injury, long-term damage to the hepatic parenchyma is difficult to predict. Major vascular injury or unrecognised segmental biliary obstruction may lead to atrophy of the liver, chronic intrahepatic infection, abscess formation or secondary biliary cirrhosis. In such patients, careful operative assessment is required; CT should be performed to identify areas of associated liver atrophy and to exclude portal vein thrombosis.

In our experience, the majority of patients requiring liver resection are those with ongoing sepsis in an obstructed segment or those where drainage of the extrahepatic biliary tree is not possible due to sectoral duct damage or fibrosis.[25] Truant et al. identified 99 patients (5.6%) requiring hepatectomy among 1756 post-cholecystectomy bile duct injury patients, with combined arterial and Strasberg E4 and E5 injuries more likely to require hepatic resection.[43] Occasionally, early hepatic resection is required for combined arterial, portal venous and biliary injury, although results are poor.[20] Very rarely, resection may be needed to gain access to the biliary tree, especially when the injury involves the biliary confluence (E4), although some authors routinely advocate resection of segments IVb and V for access to the right hepatic ducts.[44] The right lobe is most commonly affected by sepsis and atrophy as the right-sided sectoral ducts

and arterial supply are more likely to be damaged during cholecystectomy, although both left- and right-sided hepatic resections have been reported in patients with severe biliary injury. Resection of the right liver can be performed, for example at the time of delayed reconstruction if there is any doubt regarding the integrity of the anastomosis to the right sectoral or hepatic duct and when a satisfactory anastomosis can be achieved to the long extrahepatic left duct.

Failed reconstruction and persistent cholangitis may lead to end-stage liver failure within a few years and this may require liver transplantation (**Fig. 12.11**).[25] A long interval between injury and referral is known to be associated with end-stage liver disease. Rarely, liver transplantation may be needed when the combined biliary and vascular injury is so severe as to preclude attempted reconstruction, although the results are universally poor.[25]

Prognosis

Success of repair

Successful repair has been well described and can be achieved in 90% of patients in a specialised unit.[32,45] As for laparoscopic cholecystectomy, a learning curve for biliary repair has also been described for tertiary centres managing bile duct injury. Over a 20-year period, Mercado et al. reported an improvement with experience and a reduction of post-repair strictures from 13% to 5%.[46] Stilling et al. recently reported 139

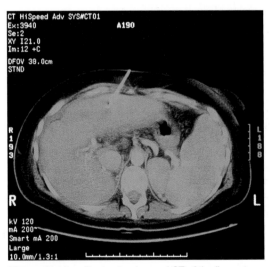

Figure 12.11 • Contrast-enhanced CT of the liver after unsuccessful revisional hepatico-jejunostomy. The surgeon who performed the laparoscopic cholecystectomy performed the hepatico-jejunostomy for an E4 injury. A revisional hepatico-jejunostomy was performed before referral, which was complicated by an anastomotic stricture and portal vein thrombosis. The CT shows evidence of right lobe atrophy and splenomegaly as well as a percutaneous biliary drain.

bile duct injuries repaired with a hepatico-jejunostomy in one of the five Danish HPB centres with only a 70% successful primary repair.[47] Forty-two patients (30%) developed an anastomotic stricture, with 19 managed with redo-hepatico-jejunostomy and the remainder with percutaneous transhepatic dilatation. As well as anastomotic strictures, liver atrophy and cirrhosis may also occur many years following repair. Predictors of a poor outcome include involvement of the biliary confluence,[21] repair by the injuring surgeon,[27,48,49] three or more previous attempted repairs[21] and recent active inflammation.[49]

Survival

Mortality following injury to the biliary tree is significant. Death may follow the acute injury itself, following the biliary repair, or occur later as a result of biliary sepsis or cirrhosis. In a report of a nationwide analysis of survival following biliary injury after cholecystectomy, Flum et al. identified 7911 (0.5%) injuries from 1 570 361 cholecystectomies.[48] Within the first year after cholecystectomy the mortality rate was 6.6% in the uninjured group and 26.1% in those with injury to the common bile duct. The adjusted hazard ratio for death during follow-up was higher for those with an injury (2.79; 95% CI 2.71–2.88). The risk of death increased significantly with advancing age and comorbidities. If the initial repair was performed by the injuring surgeon then the adjusted hazard of death increased by 11%.

Quality of life

Boerma et al. first undertook an assessment of quality of life in patients who had sustained biliary injury or leak that required additional intervention.[50] Five years after injury, quality of life in the physical and mental domains was significantly worse than controls, despite a successful outcome in 84% of treated patients and regardless of the type of treatment or severity of injury. However, the length of treatment was an independent predictor of a poor mental quality of life. Melton et al. report that quality of life in 89 patients who had undergone biliary repair following laparoscopic cholecystectomy showed no difference in the physical or social domains when compared to controls.[51] However, in the psychological domain, patients were significantly worse, particularly in the 31% of patients who sought legal recourse for their injury.

Associated malignancy

A small number of reports exist about the development of cholangiocarcinoma at the site of anastomosis 20–30 years following repair.[41] It is possible that enteric reflux into the biliary tree with sepsis and the production of mutagenic secondary bile salts may be responsible. Furthermore, hepatocellular carcinoma may develop due to secondary biliary cirrhosis (**Fig. 12.12**).[52]

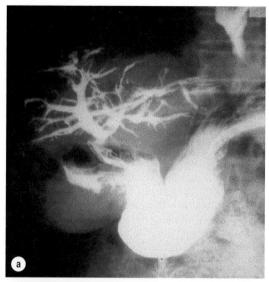

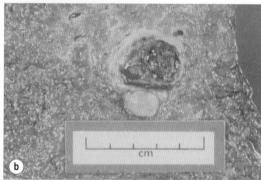

Figure 12.12 • Hepatocellular carcinoma as a consequence of biliary injury. This patient required a liver transplant for secondary biliary cirrhosis, which developed following hepatico-duodenostomy for a biliary injury **(a)**. At pathological examination a hepatocellular carcinoma was detected in the explanted liver **(b)**.

Benign biliary strictures

Mirizzi's syndrome – see Chapter 11

Hepatolithiasis – see Chapter 11

Parasitic infestation causing jaundice

Liver flukes (trematodes)

Infestation with liver flukes is caused through consuming inadequately cooked, pickled or salted infected fish. The immature fluke passes into the biliary tree, where it grows to maturity.

Ova are passed into the gastrointestinal tract and subsequently to water supplies, infecting molluscs and fish. Infection with *Clonorchis sinensis* occurs in China, Japan and south-east Asia, whilst *Opisthorchis viverrini* is found in parts of Eastern Europe and Siberia. Infection may be asymptomatic or the patient may present with an acute febrile illness or chronic symptoms. Chronic infestation results in hepatolithiasis (see Chapter 11).

Diagnosis is possible by the detection of ova within the stool or in duodenal aspirates, and an eosinophilia may also be present on blood film. ERCP may demonstrate slender filling defects within the bile duct as well as associated changes of fibrosis and calculus formation.

Echinococcus

Hydatid cysts involving the liver remain endemic in parts of the Mediterranean and Far East, as well as sheep farming areas of Australia, New Zealand, South America and South Africa. Infection is from *Echinococcus granulosus*, and less commonly *Echinococcus multilocularis* in central Europe.

Biliary obstruction can occur due to local compression of the common hepatic duct by the expanding cyst, or when daughter cysts pass down the common hepatic duct following rupture of the cyst into intrahepatic radicles. Erosion into the biliary tree is usually associated with death of the cyst contents due to toxicity of the bile. Secondary sclerosing cholangitis has been described following inappropriate injection of scolicidal agents into the hepatic cyst when there is communication with the biliary tree.[53]

Treatment

Preoperative endoscopic cholangiography may identify debris within the biliary tree, and endoscopic sphincterotomy may prevent further episodes of biliary obstruction. Endoscopic stenting may also allow resolution of obstruction secondary to a large intrahepatic cyst.

The secondary sclerosing cholangitis produced by inappropriate instillation of a scolicidal agent into the biliary tree will often only be amenable to hepatic replacement. Surgical bypass may be possible for localised strictures or Roux-en-Y hepaticojejunostomy and access loop formation for ongoing percutaneous radiological procedures (Fig 12.13).

Ascaris lumbricoides

The roundworm *Ascaris lumbricoides* is the commonest worm to infect humans. Rarely, an infected patient can present with obstructive jaundice due to migration of the worm into the biliary tree and this is difficult to distinguish from stone disease. The more frequent presentation is from cholangitis due to the worm traversing the

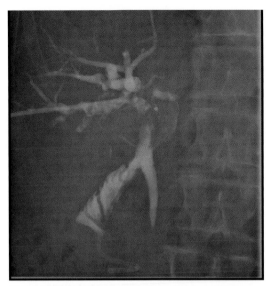

Figure 12.13 • Complicated hilar stricture secondary to a central hydatid cyst previously ruptured into the left hepatic duct. The patient required a hepatico-jejunostomy with access loop and percutanoues biliary drain when intrahepatic stones were unable to be removed endoscopically.

ampulla. *Ascaris* has also been associated with recurrent pyogenic cholangitis.

Ultrasound sometimes identifies a long, linear filling defect within the biliary tree. Identification may occur at the time of ERCP where endoscopic extraction may be possible. Medical treatment exists with the anthelmintics mebendazole or albendazole, which are often curative. The late complication of papillary stenosis can be treated with endoscopic sphincterotomy.

HIV/AIDS-associated cholangiopathy

HIV- or AIDS-associated cholangiopathy is thought to be secondary to opportunistic infection of the biliary tree by cytomegalovirus, *Cryptosporidium* and other organisms. The usual presentation is with right upper quadrant pain and abnormal liver function tests although jaundice is unusual. Magnetic resonance cholangiopancreaticography (MRCP) demonstrates the characteristic ductal abnormalities of multiple intrahepatic strictures, papillary stenosis and long segmental extrahepatic strictures.[54] Endoscopic retrograde cholangiography is the gold standard for diagnosis and provides symptomatic relief following endoscopic sphincterotomy for papillary stenosis.[55] Antiretroviral therapy has been associated with regression of cholangiographic abnormalities[56] but endoscopic interventions have not been associated with improvements in prognosis.[55]

Biliary strictures imitating malignancy

It is not unusual for benign biliary pathology to be found in resected specimens of the pancreatic head that had been thought to be malignant. Approximately 10% of Whipple resections for malignancy will be found to have benign pathology. Most commonly the pathology is chronic pancreatitis related to alcohol or gallstone disease. However, other confounding pathologies include IgG4-related disease, primary sclerosing cholangitis and choledocholithiasis.

Up to 14% of patients undergoing surgery for presumed malignant hilar obstruction are found to have a benign fibrotic stricture of the bile duct.[57] It is usually impossible to differentiate them from malignancy preoperatively and thus resection is often attempted and nearly always feasible. Successful treatment has been described with the use of steroids.

Primary sclerosing cholangitis

Aetiology
Primary sclerosing cholangitis is a rare condition, and although the precise cause has yet to be determined there is increasing evidence of an immunological basis as well as an overall increase in the incidence.[58] Between 60% and 80% of patients will have ulcerative colitis, or more rarely Crohn's disease. There is a strong association with a number of human leucocyte antigens.[59]

Presentation
Primary sclerosing cholangitis is a progressive obliterative fibrosis of the intrahepatic and extrahepatic biliary tree with a wide clinical spectrum and frequent remissions and relapses. In the early stages of disease most patients are asymptomatic but later in the disease process patients may have pruritus, ill-defined pain, fever, jaundice and weight loss. Many asymptomatic patients are diagnosed by detection of abnormal liver function tests during the investigation of inflammatory bowel disease. Although some patients may present at an advanced stage, signs of liver failure develop over a period of time. Sudden deterioration may suggest the development of cholangiocarcinoma, with which there is a strong association.

Investigation
Liver biochemistry demonstrates a cholestatic picture. Although antineutrophil cytoplasmic antibodies are present in the majority of patients, testing for autoantibodies is usually performed to exclude primary biliary cirrhosis, a condition from which it can be difficult to differentiate.

The mainstay of investigation is cholangiography, which usually demonstrates a diffuse picture of stricturing and attenuated intrahepatic bile ducts. As well as providing anatomical details of the biliary tree, ERCP enables endoscopic therapy and the opportunity for brush cytology if malignancy is suspected. MRCP is highly sensitive, with a diagnostic accuracy comparable to ERCP, and is now preferred as a means of both diagnosing and assessing the extent of disease to avoid the introduction of bacteria and causing severe biliary sepsis. CT intravenous cholangiography also provides a good alternative when MRCP is contraindicated.

Management
The prognosis of primary sclerosing cholangitis is poor, with a median survival of only 9.6 years from diagnosis to death or liver transplantation.[60] Survival may improve with earlier diagnosis and liver transplantation; however, subsequent development of cholangiocarcinoma and colorectal cancer has now become the leading cause of death.[61] The use of ursodeoxycholic acid has not been demonstrated to be of benefit following randomised studies[62] and there is little benefit from immunosuppression or antibiotics.[63] Episodes of cholangitis can be treated with antibiotics covering biliary pathogens. There is no evidence that colectomy for inflammatory bowel disease alters disease progression.

Endoscopic or transhepatic dilatation of short dominant strictures with or without endoscopic stenting has been described as effective, safe and well tolerated, although no randomised trials have been performed. Dilatation achieves palliation at 1 and 3 years in 80% and 60% of patients, respectively.[64] In those patients without cirrhosis but with jaundice secondary to a dominant stricture, surgical drainage with an access limb has been described.

Liver transplantation is necessary to treat end-stage liver disease and is the fifth commonest reason for liver transplantation in the USA.[65] However, it is now more usual for patients to be considered if there is persistent jaundice, intractable pruritus, recurrent cholangitis, malnutrition or fatigue. Many patients undergo transplantation before liver failure supervenes or when cholangiocarcinoma is suspected, with survival rates of 80–92% at 5 years.[66,67] Recurrence rates of 15–25% in the transplanted liver have been reported.[68]

Exclusion of associated malignant stricture
Cholangiocarcinoma and gallbladder cancer complicate 10–36% of patients with primary sclerosing cholangitis[60] and need to be excluded before liver transplantation.

In the majority of patients, concern regarding occult cholangiocarcinoma is small, and liver transplantation is undertaken in the absence of a dominant stricture. Serum carbohydrate antigen (CA) 19-9 has been used in an attempt to identify cases with an occult biliary malignancy. Patients with a sudden rapid deterioration in their clinical state or with a dominant stricture must be considered to have a cholangiocarcinoma and be investigated extensively. Brush cytology at ERCP may provide the diagnosis if a malignant smear is obtained but ERCP-based cholangioscopy with targeted biopsies appears to be the most accurate.[69] CT or MRI may demonstrate a mass lesion in association with the biliary tree, although the usual appearance is of a stricture indistinguishable from a benign disease. Positron emission tomography (PET) is superior to conventional radiological investigations to differentiate primary sclerosing cholangitis and cholangiocarcinoma.[70]

Laparoscopy identifies the majority of patients with unresectable biliary tract cancer,[71] and may be of use in assessing those considered for transplantation in whom a cholangiocarcinoma is suspected since tumour dissemination often occurs early. Laparoscopic ultrasound may further aid assessment, and occasionally laparotomy may be required if there is diagnostic doubt regarding cholangiocarcinoma.

Immunoglobulin G4 (IgG4)-related disease

IgG4-related disease has only been recognised in the last 11 years. It is an immune-mediated condition that mimics many malignant, infectious and inflammatory disorders but the aetiology remains obscure. Autoimmune pancreatitis was the first condition to be associated with high serum IgG4.[72] It is also known as lymphoplasmacytic sclerosing pancreatitis.

Other IgG4 diseases include IgG4 sclerosing cholangitis, retroperitoneal fibrosis, periaortitis, sclerosing mesenteritis, inflammatory pseudotumour and multifocal fibrosclerosis as well as other extra-abdominal diseases such as Riedel's thyroiditis.[73] Tissue is the gold standard for diagnosis, with demonstration of a high number of IgG4-positive plasma cells.[73] Several clinical entities can cause biliary strictures, which include autoimmune pancreatitis, IgG4-related sclerosing cholangitis and inflammatory pseudotumours. Adequate biopsy material from these disorders can be difficult to obtain at endoscopic ultrasound and biopsy.

Autoimmune pancreatitis

Two types of autoimmune pancreatitis are reported, with type I associated with IgG4 disease. Although only accounting for about 2.4% of pancreatic resections, the condition is important since a proportion of patients will develop either biliary anastomotic strictures or intrahepatic strictures following resection. In a series of 31 patients, eight (28%) went on to develop recurrent jaundice after resection.[74] Often the diagnosis is radiological, with an enlarged pancreatic head mass with delayed enhancement without pancreatic duct dilatation. Endoscopic ultrasound and fine-needle aspirate cytology may be helpful if plasma cells are detected but usually the diagnosis remains indeterminate.

IgG4-related sclerosing cholangitis

IgG4-related sclerosing cholangitis is commonly associated with type I autoimmune pancreatitis and can be difficult to differentiate from cholangiocarcinoma.

Treatment

Glucocorticoids are the mainstay of treatment,[75] but no randomised studies have been performed. In patients with jaundice, treatment with steroids should lead to resolution within 1–2 weeks so avoidance of endoscopic stenting may be beneficial to aid in the diagnostic process (**Fig. 12.14**). FDG PET CT response can also be useful in the assessment of treatment response.[76]

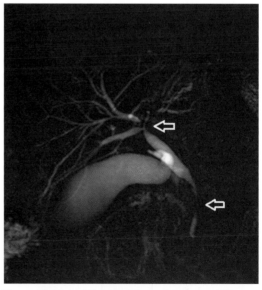

Figure 12.14 • IgG4-related cholangiopathy in a 70-year-old man presenting with jaundice and a recent history of retroperitoneal fibrosis. His jaundice resolved within 2 weeks after treatment with prednisolone without endoscopic stenting. The arrows point to benign biliary strictures at the hilum of the liver and intrapancreatic bile duct.

Functional biliary disorders

Most patients who present for investigation of sphincter of Oddi dysfunction have already undergone cholecystectomy for presumed gallbladder pain. However, 39–90% of patients with idiopathic recurrent pancreatitis may also have sphincter of Oddi dysfunction.[77] In those patients with post-cholecystectomy pain, the presentation and investigation identifies three types:[78]

- Type 1 – Abdominal pain, obstructive liver function tests, biliary dilatation and delayed emptying of contrast at ERCP.
- Type 2 – Pain with only one or two of the above-mentioned criteria.
- Type 3 – Recurrent biliary pain only.

Between 65% and 95% of group 1 patients will be found on biliary manometry to have sphincter of Oddi dysfunction compared to only 12–28% of type 3.[77] Diagnosis is usually by exclusion of other causes of abdominal pain such as peptic ulcer disease and irritable bowel syndrome. Liver function tests, abdominal ultrasonography, CT, endoscopy and MRCP have often already been performed. Morphine–neostigmine and secretin provocation MRCP studies may also be of diagnostic value.

At ERCP, biliary manometry is not required if there is delayed drainage of contrast in type 1 or 2 patients. This investigation should be reserved for those patients in whom the diagnosis remains unclear.

Medical therapy with calcium channel blockers, nitrates and botulinum toxin is available but long-term results are unknown. Avoidance of opiate analgesia, particularly over-the-counter preparations containing codeine, may prevent the onset of pain in the majority. The development of severe abdominal pain with codeine is almost diagnostic. Endoscopic sphincterotomy is a potential treatment; however, 5–16% of patients will develop postprocedural pancreatitis[79] and good or excellent responses are reported in only 69% of patients at long-term follow-up.[80] Surgical sphincterotomy is now indicated rarely due to the lower cost and lower morbidity of endoscopic sphincterotomy but it may be required if the endoscopic approach has been unsuccessful. Avoidance of codeine and reassurance about the benign nature of the condition is the safest path.

Key points

- Choledochal cysts should be treated with complete cyst excision and hepatico-jejunostomy due to the risk of malignancy in the remaining biliary epithelium.
- Identification of the biliary anatomy and minimisation of diathermy near the common bile duct are essential during laparoscopic cholecystectomy to avoid biliary injury.
- Operative cholangiography is useful for delineating the biliary anatomy during cholecystectomy; however, many cholangiograms are not interpreted correctly at the time of biliary injury.
- Following laparoscopic cholecystectomy, any patient who is not fit for discharge at 24 hours due to ongoing abdominal pain, vomiting, fever or bile in an abdominal drain should be considered to have a biliary leak.
- Diagnosis of a bile duct injury in the postoperative period should lead to immediate referral to a specialist centre since inappropriate attempts to manage this outwith a specialist centre will compromise the outcome.
- In the absence of sepsis, repair of injuries to the biliary tree can be performed successfully within the first week.

▶ **Excision of a choledochal cyst**

Although not the authors' recommended technique, this video offers excellent vision of the dissection:
- Laparoscopic excision of a choledochal cyst from SAGES 2015 – https://www.youtube.com/watch?v=gZRw8rf3l2Y
  [Comment: Decision not to excise the upper hepatic/common bile duct may increase risk of stricture formation given consideration of blood supply to the bile duct.]

🌐 Full references available at **http://expertconsult.inkling.com**

Key references

11. Flum DR, Dellinger EP, Cheadle A, et al. Intraoperative cholangiography and risk of common bile duct injury during cholecystectomy. JAMA 2003;289(13):1639–44. PMID: 12672731.

A retrospective analysis of more than 1.5 million cholecystectomies detailing the risk of injury and the decreased risk if operative cholangiography is used.

14. Fletcher DR, Hobbs MS, Tan P, et al. Complications of cholecystectomy: risks of the laparoscopic approach and protective effects of operative cholangiography: a population-based study. Ann Surg 1999; 229(4):449–57. PMID: 10203075.

A retrospective audit of biliary injury in Western Australia that identified the increased risk of biliary injury after laparoscopic cholecystectomy compared to open cholecystectomy. This study also identified a significantly reduced risk of injury if operative cholangiography was performed.

16. Way LW, Stewart L, Gantert W, et al. Causes and prevention of laparoscopic bile duct injuries: analysis of 252 cases from a human factors and cognitive psychology perspective. Ann Surg 2003;237(4):460–9. PMID: 12677139.

Analysis of 252 bile duct injuries according to the principles of the cognitive science of visual perception judgment and human error showing that the majority of errors result from misperception, not errors of skill, knowledge or judgement.

23. Strasberg SM, Hertl M, Soper NJ. An analysis of the problem of biliary injury during laparoscopic cholecystectomy. J Am Coll Surg 1995;180(1):101–25. PMID: 8000648.

This paper describes a very useful classification system for biliary injury that includes the Bismuth classification as well as other less major injuries.

48. Flum DR, Cheadle A, Prela C, et al. Bile duct injury during cholecystectomy and survival in medicare beneficiaries. JAMA 2003;290(16): 2168–73. PMID: 14570952.

A retrospective analysis of survival following bile duct injury among Medicare beneficiaries in the USA. This study demonstrates the increased hazard ratio of death following injury in comparison to a control group of routine cholecystectomy patients.

50. Boerma D, Rauws EA, Keulemans YC, et al. Impaired quality of life 5 years after bile duct injury during laparoscopic cholecystectomy: a prospective analysis. Ann Surg 2001;234(6):750–7. PMID: 11729381.

A prospective analysis of quality of life that demonstrated a poor outcome at 5 years, despite successful repair.

51. Melton GB, Lillemoe KD, Cameron JL, et al. Major bile duct injuries associated with laparoscopic cholecystectomy: effect of surgical repair on quality of life. Ann Surg 2002;235(6):888–95. PMID: 12035047.

A study of the impact of biliary injury on quality of life that demonstrated a significantly worse psychological domain, especially in those pursuing legal action.

75. Kamisawa T, Shimosegawa T, Okazaki K, et al. Standard steroid treatment for autoimmune pancreatitis. Gut 2009;58(11):1504–7. PMID: 19398440.

An excellent and comprehensive review article for IgG4 disease.

13

Malignant lesions of the biliary tract

Russell C. Langan
Shishir K. Maithel
William R. Jarnagin

Introduction

Malignant lesions of the biliary tract can present a formidable diagnostic and treatment challenge. These malignancies are rare and account for only approximately 15% of hepatobiliary neoplasms and 3% of all gastrointestinal (GI) malignancies. Specifically, it has been estimated that there will be 11 420 new cases and 3710 deaths from a biliary malignancy within the United States in 2016.[1] The gallbladder is the most common site of biliary tract malignancy (60%) and the fifth most common GI malignancy. The remaining 40% are distributed throughout the extrahepatic and intrahepatic biliary tree.

Currently, surgery remains the mainstay of multidisciplinary care, the only chance at cure and the best option to increase long-term survival. Unfortunately, the majority of patients present with locally advanced, unresectable or metastatic disease. Additionally, due to the rarity of these tumours and their frequently advanced stage at presentation, randomised prospective trials assessing different treatment regimens have not been performed. However, there is a plethora of data to guide the algorithm of care.

The diagnosis of a biliary malignancy requires the thoughtful integration of clinical experience, radiological evaluation and objective diagnostic data. Herein, we discuss the entity, work-up, management, outcomes and address controversies in patients with biliary adenocarcinoma, including cholangiocarcinoma (hilar, intrahepatic and extrahepatic) and gallbladder carcinoma.

Cholangiocarcinoma

Epidemiology

Cholangiocarcinoma is an uncommon cancer with an incidence of 1–2 per 100 000 in the USA and accounts for 3% of all GI malignancies.[2] In the United States, cholangiocarcinoma will prove fatal in approximately 5000 individuals per year.[3] Interestingly, recent data have suggested that the incidence of intrahepatic cholangiocarcinoma has dramatically risen within the USA and over the last two decades there has been an increase in the ratio of intrahepatic to extrahepatic cholangiocarcinoma.[3–5] In fact, over the past 20 years, intrahepatic cholangiocarcinoma has become the leading cause of primary liver tumour-related death. Moreover, this observation is most likely not due to reclassification, better detection or a rise in primary sclerosing cholangitis (PSC), but rather a true increase in this tumour; however, the aetiology to this change remains poorly understood.[3,6] That being said, some have postulated that there may be a direct correlation to the rising incidence of obesity-related, non-alcoholic fatty liver disease and also chronic hepatitis C infection.[7] Separately, the true incidence of extrahepatic cholangiocarcinoma remains uncertain, since traditionally these malignancies were grouped with gallbladder adenocarcinoma and current data suggest that the incidence and mortality rates are declining for both pathologies.[3,4,6]

Overall, men are affected 1.5 times as often as women and the majority of patients are greater than 65 years of age. In fact, the peak incidence is within the eighth decade of life.[2] With respect to race, cholangiocarcinoma has a higher prevalence in Hispanics and Asians as compared to their white and black counterparts.[3]

Risk factors

The majority of patients with cholangiocarcinoma do not have any of the known or suspected risk factors and present with sporadic disease. However, there are several well-known entities that increase risk for developing cholangiocarcinoma.

Primary sclerosing cholangitis
The most common and best-known risk factor is primary sclerosing cholangitis (PSC). The majority of patients (70–80%) with PSC have associated inflammatory bowel disease; however, only a minority of patients with inflammatory bowel disease develop PSC.[8] Unlike sporadic cases, the age at presentation is younger and typically occurs between 30 and 50 years. The natural history of PSC is variable, and the true incidence of cholangiocarcinoma is unknown. In a Swedish series of 305 patients followed over several years, 8% of patients eventually developed cancer. On the other hand, occult cholangiocarcinoma has been reported in up to 40% of autopsy specimens and in up to 36% of liver explants from patients with PSC.[8] Unfortunately, patients with cholangiocarcinoma associated with PSC are often not candidates for resection because of multifocal disease or severe underlying hepatic dysfunction.

Congenital cysts
Congenital biliary tree abnormalities (choledochal cysts, Caroli disease) are associated with an increased risk in the development of cholangiocarcinoma, with the estimated risk ranging from 7% to 28%.[3,9,10] Although the cause is unknown, it has been hypothesised that the abnormal pancreatico-biliary duct junction found in this patient population predisposes the patients to reflux of pancreatic secretions into the biliary tree, leading to chronic inflammation and bacterial contamination.[11] Over time, this insult leads to malignant transformation. In a series of 119 patients subjected to this procedure for benign conditions, Hakamada et al. found a 7.4% incidence of cholangiocarcinoma over a period of 18 years.[12]

Hepatolithiasis
Additionally, hepatolithiasis has been documented as a well-known risk factor for the development of cholangiocarcinoma in Japan and parts of South-East Asia, as up to 10% of those affected will develop cholangiocarcinoma. Chronic portal bacteraemia and portal phlebitis lead to intrahepatic pigment stone formation, obstruction of intrahepatic ducts and recurrent episodes of cholangitis and stricture formation.[13,14] This recurrent inflammatory state is likely the main contributing factor to cholangiocarcinogenesis.

Parasitic infection
The literature has suggested a pathogenic association between liver fluke infestation (*Opisthorcis viverrini*, *Clonorchis sinensis*) and the development of cholangiocarcinoma.[15] Although exceedingly rare in the USA, these organisms are endemic in South-East Asia.

Viral hepatitis and cirrhosis
Extrapolating data from population-based studies, viral hepatitis and cirrhosis have been linked to the development of cholangiocarcinoma. In a prospective study from Japan, the risk of developing cholangiocarcinoma in patients infected with hepatitis C virus was 3.5% at 10 years, compared to their non-infected counterparts who harboured a rate 1000 times less.[16] Moreover, the fact that cholangiocytes and hepatocytes arise from the same progenitor cell and that the hepatitis C virus has been found within cholangiocarcinoma tumour specimens allude to a strong probable pathogenic association.[3]

Chemical exposure
Several chemical agents have been implicated in the development of cholangiocarcinoma. In particular, exposure to Thorotrast (a radiological agent used in the 1960s) is associated with a 300-fold increase in the development of biliary malignancy.[6] Moreover, environmental toxins, such as dioxin and vinyl chloride, may directly increase the chance of developing cholangiocarcinoma.[6]

Classification/histopathology

Cholangiocarcinoma is classified according to the site of origin within the biliary tree. Malignancies arising from the biliary confluence are classified as hilar cholangiocarcinoma and are the most common type of cholangiocarcinoma (60% of all cases).[17] The remainder of cholangiocarcinomas comprise those originating within the extrahepatic bile duct (20–30%) and from the intrahepatic biliary tree (10%).[18] Of note, patients can present with multifocal or diffuse involvement of the biliary tree, although this is quite rare.[19] Cholangiocarcinoma can be classified further by the Bismuth–Corlette classification system: type I tumours involve the common hepatic duct below the biliary confluence, type II involve the biliary confluence, type IIIa involve the biliary confluence extending into the right hepatic duct, type IIIb involve the biliary confluence extending into the left hepatic duct and type IV involve the confluence and extend into both the left and right hepatic ducts.

The vast majority of cholangiocarcinomas are adenocarcinoma, whereas other histologic variants comprise 5%.[3] A small number show different patterns with focal areas of papillary carcinoma with mucous production, signet-ring cells, squamous cell, mucoepidermoid and spindle cell variants.[20,21] The Liver Cancer Study group of Japan established a subclassification of these tumours based on morphology: (1) mass-forming type; (2) periductal-infiltrating type; (3) intraductal growth type.[20] Periductal infiltrating is the most common, and as the name suggests, is associated with infiltrative characteristics while also causing fibrosis of periductal tissues and annular bile duct thickening.[3,20,21] As a consequence, a non-diagnostic preoperative biopsy is not uncommon.[21] Although outside the scope of this review, tumours with both hepatocellular and cholangiocellular differentiation (combined tumours) are rare but well described. Their clinical behaviour more closely resembles that of cholangiocarcinoma than hepatocellular carcinoma, and they tend to display aggressive biology.[22]

Three macroscopic subtypes of extrahepatic cholangiocarcinoma are described: sclerosing, nodular and papillary, of which the first two are often combined into one (i.e. nodular-sclerosing) since features of both types are often seen together.[23] Papillary tumours represent a less common morphological variant, accounting for approximately 10% of tumours arising from the extrahepatic biliary tree.[23] Papillary tumours are soft and friable, may be associated with little transmural invasion, and are characterised by a mass that expands rather than contracts the duct (**Fig. 13.1**). Although papillary tumours may grow to significant size, they often arise from a well-defined stalk, with the bulk of the tumour mobile within the ductal lumen. Despite this histological variant being the minority of cases, recognition of this entity is important since they are more often resectable and have a more favourable prognosis than their histological counterparts.[24]

Tumours of the lower bile duct, namely mid- and distal bile duct, are classified according to their anatomical location, although there may be considerable overlap. Mid-bile duct tumours arise between the upper border of the duodenum and the cystic duct, while distal bile duct tumours arise from the duodenum to the ampulla of Vater. Tumours of the distal bile duct represent approximately 5–10% of all periampullary tumours.[17] True mid-duct tumours are distinctly uncommon, and thus Nakeeb et al. have proposed an alternative classification scheme that divides cholangiocarcinomas into intrahepatic, perihilar and distal subgroups, thereby eliminating the mid-duct group, which is often difficult to classify accurately.[17] As is true throughout the biliary tree, adenocarcinoma is the principal histological type in the lower bile duct, and it has previously been suggested that the papillary variant is more common at this location compared to the biliary confluence.[24]

Clinical presentation

The clinical presentation of cholangiocarcinoma is directly determined by the location/level of biliary involvement. Patients with extrahepatic cholangiocarcinoma may present earlier due to outflow obstruction of the biliary tree. Therefore, these patients can present with the classic signs and symptoms of hyperbilirubinaemia (painless jaundice, pruritus, pale stool and dark urine). The clinical presentation of distal bile duct cancer is generally indistinguishable from that of hilar cholangiocarcinoma or other periampullary malignancies. Progressive jaundice is seen in 75–90% of patients, with serum bilirubin levels often exceeding 10 mg/dL.[25] Distal bile duct tumours are frequently mistaken for adenocarcinoma of the pancreas, the most common periampullary malignancy. Of note, patients with papillary tumours may give a history of intermittent jaundice, perhaps due to the ball-valve effect of a pedunculated mass within the lumen or, more likely, small fragments of tumour having passed into the common bile duct.

In stark contrast, intrahepatic cholangiocarcinoma patients are typically asymptomatic. In the majority of cases, early symptoms are nebulous (weight loss, abdominal discomfort) and many are identified incidentally on cross-sectional imaging or following the discovery of abnormal liver function tests. In patients with no previous biliary intervention, cholangitis is rare at initial presentation. Occasionally, patients with long-standing biliary obstruction and/or portal vein involvement may present with symptoms related to portal hypertension. Additionally, in those with PSC, distal ductal or periductal lesions can be difficult to differentiate from benign biliary strictures.[3]

Diagnostic assessment

Radiological investigation

Preoperative staging should be aimed not only at the exclusion of distant metastases but

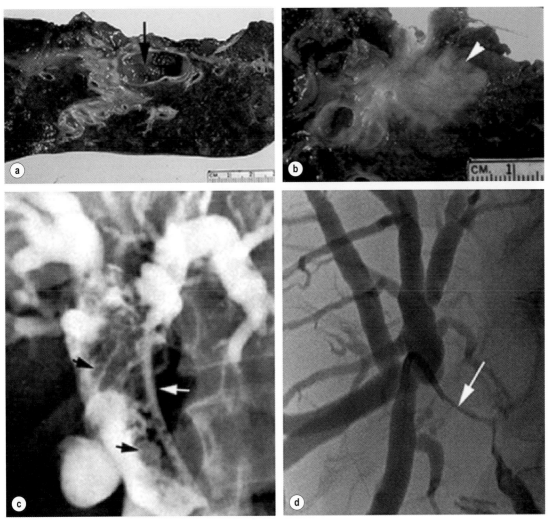

Figure 13.1 • Gross and cholangiographic appearance of a papillary cholangiocarcinoma **(a, c)** and a nodular-sclerosing tumour **(b, d)**. In **(a)** and **(c)**, note that the papillary tumour occupies the lumen and expands the duct (*black arrow*). A biliary stent is visualised (*white arrow*). In **(b)** and **(d)**, the nodular-sclerosing variant constricts the lumen, nearly obliterating it (*white arrow*).
Reproduced with permission from Blumgart LH, editor. Surgery of the liver, biliary tract, and pancreas. 4th ed. Elsevier Saunders; 2006.

also the assessment of local extent of disease. Cross-sectional, contrast-enhanced imaging is the mainstay of investigation. Multiphasic computed tomography (CT) of the chest, abdomen and pelvis to include portal venous and arterial phases should be used to assess the extent of disease in the liver and porta hepatis while also evaluating for metastatic disease. Imaging should include thin cuts to elucidate detailed relationships between the tumour and porta hepatis structures. It should be noted that initial imaging studies should be performed prior to biliary stenting (if it is to be performed), as stenting will cause local inflammation, making assessment of tumour extent difficult.

Computed tomography

Cross-sectional imaging provided by CT remains an important study for evaluating patients with biliary obstruction and can provide valuable information regarding the level of obstruction, vascular involvement and liver atrophy. As portal venous inflow and bile flow are important in the maintenance of liver cell size and mass, segmental or lobar atrophy may be evident on CT that would suggest portal venous occlusion or, alternatively, long-standing biliary obstruction in the absence of portal venous involvement.[26] Generally speaking, CT offers excellent assessment of the radial extent of soft-tissue involvement, direct liver invasion

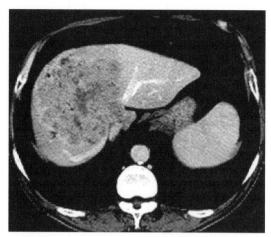

Figure 13.2 • Characteristic CT appearance of intrahepatic cholangiocarcinoma demonstrating heterogeneous enhancement.

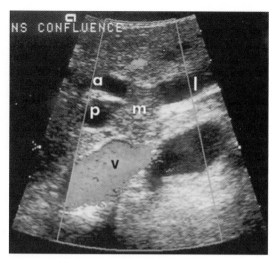

Figure 13.3 • Ultrasonographic view of a hilar cholangiocarcinoma showing a papillary tumour (*m*) extending into the right anterior (*a*) and posterior (*p*) sectoral ducts and the origin of the left duct (*l*). The adjacent portal vein (*v*) is not involved and has normal flow. Reproduced with permission from Blumgart LH, editor. Surgery of the liver, biliary tract, and pancreas., 4th ed. Elsevier Saunders; 2006.

of perihilar lesions and the relationship to portal structures. For instance, dilated intrahepatic ducts with a normal or collapsed gallbladder allude to a perihilar cholangiocarcinoma, particularly if there is any evidence of a soft-tissue mass. Whereas a distended gallbladder with normal intrahepatic ducts alludes to either stone disease or tumour obstructing the cystic duct, and a distended gallbladder with dilated intra- and extrahepatic ducts suggests either choledocholithiasis or a distal biliary malignancy.[3] On contrast-enhanced CT, variable rim-like enhancement can be observed, predominantly on the arterial phase images with gradual centripetal enhancement on delayed imaging (**Fig. 13.2**).

Current CT imaging has been found to identify cholangiocarcinoma in 94–100% of patients and the positive and negative predictive values for determining resectability are 92% and 85%, respectively.[27–29] However, CT imaging tends to underestimate the proximal extent of tumour within the bile duct and is thus not ideal as the primary determinant of resectability.[30] In fact, reported accuracy for detecting the longitudinal spread along bile ducts is 81% as compared to an accuracy of 100% for detecting radial spread into adjacent structures.[31] Another limitation is the detection of lymph node metastases, since CT has a documented sensitivity ranging from 35% to 65%.[31]

Duplex ultrasonography

Ultrasonography is a non-invasive, but operator-dependent, study that often precisely delineates the level of the tumour within the bile duct (**Fig. 13.3**). It can also provide information regarding tumour extension within the bile duct and in the periductal tissues.[32] In a series of 19 consecutive patients with malignant hilar obstruction, ultrasonography with colour spectral Doppler technique was equivalent

to angiography and CT portography in diagnosing lobar atrophy, level of biliary obstruction, hepatic parenchymal involvement and venous invasion.[32] Duplex ultrasonography is particularly useful for assessing portal venous invasion. In a series of 63 consecutive patients from the Memorial Sloan-Kettering Cancer Center (MSKCC), duplex ultrasonography predicted portal vein involvement in 93% of cases, with a specificity of 99% and a 97% positive predictive value. In the same series, angiography with CT angio-portography had 90% sensitivity, 99% specificity and a 95% positive predictive value.[33]

Magnetic resonance cholangiopancreatography (MRCP)

Several studies have demonstrated the utility of magnetic resonance cholangiopancreatography (MRCP) in evaluating patients with biliary obstruction, and it has now become the imaging modality of choice.[34,35] MRCP may not only identify the tumour and the level of biliary obstruction, but may also reveal obstructed and isolated ducts not appreciated at endoscopic or percutaneous study. By virtue of being an axial imaging modality, MRCP has further advantages over standard cholangiography by also providing information regarding the patency of hilar vascular structures, the presence of nodal or distant metastases, the presence of lobar atrophy and with its high tissue contrast helps to detect hepatic parenchymal involvement or metastatic

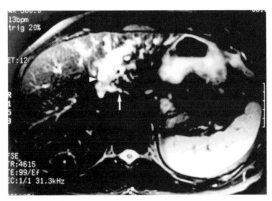

Figure 13.4 • Cross-sectional MRCP from a patient with hilar cholangiocarcinoma extending into the left hepatic duct and left lobe atrophy. The bile ducts appear white. The left lobe is small with dilated and crowded ducts (*arrowhead*). The principal caudate lobe duct, seen joining the left hepatic duct, is also dilated (*arrow*).
Reproduced with permission from Blumgart LH, editor. Surgery of the liver, biliary tract, and pancreas. 4th ed. Elsevier Saunders; 2006.

hepatic disease (**Fig. 13.4**). As compared to invasive cholangiopancreatography, MRCP has comparable rates of detecting the location and extent of tumour within the biliary tree.[27,36] Furthermore, because it does not require biliary intubation, it is not associated with the same incidence of bacterobilia and infectious complications that is frequently associated with standard cholangiography.[37]

In general, cholangiocarcinoma is hypointense on T1-weighted images and hyperintense on T2-weighted imaging.[3] These lesions demonstrate initial rim enhancement characterised by progressive and concentric enhancement post-administration of contrast material. Generally, the lesions do not completely enhance post-contrast. In the absence of a separate primary source of disease, a lesion in the liver with this morphology on magnetic resonance imaging (MRI) evaluation can be considered virtually diagnostic of cholangiocarcinoma without a tissue diagnosis. Intrahepatic cholangiocarcinomas may only enhance completely on delayed imaging obtained hours after contrast administration, a finding related to the desmoplastic nature of the tumour. Capsular retraction may also be seen.[38,39]

Additionally, magnetic resonance cholangiopancreaticography (MRCP) can more accurately evaluate biliary ducts proximal to a lesion that may not be adequately filled with contrast during endoscopic retrograde cholangiopancreatography (ERCP), since the MRI provides biliary imaging above and below the obstruction.[3] In fact, reported accuracy in determining the extent of bile duct involvement is 71–96%.[40,41] That being said, MRCP has limitations, in that it will understage up to 20% of perihilar cases, can overstage patients with indwelling biliary stents and is overly sensitive to motion.[3]

Positron emission tomography

Traditional fluorodeoxyglucose positron emission tomography (FDG-PET) imaging may have benefit in the assessment of cholangiocarcinoma. In one prospective series comparing patients with cholangiocarcinoma to those with benign biliary disease, PET imaging diagnosed cholangiocarcinoma with a sensitivity of 92% and a specificity of 93%.[42] Additionally, with respect to the assessment of metastatic nodal disease, PET was found to have a specificity of 100%, compared to CT which had a specificity of 59%.[43] Moreover, it has been reported that FDG-PET imaging has altered surgical treatment plans in up to 30% of patients by identifying occult distant metastatic disease and also proving findings suspicious on CT to be negative.[44,45] In the authors' experience with FDG-PET for all biliary tract cancer, the information provided influenced management in 24% of patients.[46] However, false-positive findings are common, specifically in patients with indwelling biliary stents. Although the evidence is limited to small reviews, PET imaging should be considered when evaluating newly diagnosed biliary malignancies, not only to evaluate for distant metastatic disease but also to confirm/refute questionable findings on cross-sectional imaging.

Invasive modalities
Direct cholangiography

Although ERCP may provide helpful information, percutaneous transhepatic cholangiography (PTC) displays the intrahepatic bile ducts more reliably. Moreover, PTC may be required in patients with an obstructive perihilar lesion. Unlike diagnostic radiographic imaging modalities, PTC offers the ability to obtain tissue for sampling (brushing, biopsy) and also to place a biliary stent to relieve symptoms of obstructive jaundice.

Endoscopy

In cases of biliary dilatation without an obvious mass lesion seen on cross-sectional imaging, endoscopic modalities (endoscopic ultrasound [EUS] and ERCP) offer the ability to further characterise indeterminate biliary strictures, assess for the presence of a biliary ductal mass, assist with staging by identifying lymphadenopathy or liver lesions and perform biliary stenting.

Cytology

Pathology results obtained through brushings during PTC or endoscopy must be interpreted with great caution since sensitivities for brush cytology for diagnosing cholangiocarcinoma range from 30% to 60%.[47,48] A postulation for this low yield is the dense fibroplastic reaction observed with cholangiocarcinoma. This relatively low yield, in combination with the lack of standardised criteria for cytologic evaluation and reporting, continue to limit the usefulness of this modality.[3]

In an attempt to improve these results, advanced cytology techniques to detect aneuploidy (fluorescence in situ hybridisation [FISH] using fluorescent probes to detect chromosomal amplification and digital image analysis that quantifies nuclear DNA as a ratio of normal ploidy) have been studied.[49,50] Preliminary results have found that when used in combination with routine cytology, the sensitivity may increase without compromising the specificity for diagnosing cholangiocarcinoma.[50]

Choledochoscopy

Endoscopic choledochoscopy utilises a narrow-calibre fibreoptic choledochoscope passed through the working channel of a standard duodenoscope. It can be used to directly observe luminal filling abnormalities noted on MRCP or direct cholangiography. Malignant biliary strictures can be identified by the presence of dilated or tortuous vessels, mucosal ulceration, polypoid or nodular masses, or villous mucosal morphology.[51,52] Endoscopic choledochoscopy allows for passage across strictures to second-order and third-order bile ducts, making it particularly useful in patients with PSC, when it can be used to locate and directly biopsy a dominant stricture.[3] With respect to diagnosis, the combination of endoscopic choledochoscopy with ERCP and tissue sampling has been reported to increase the sensitivity for the detection of malignancy in patients with indeterminate biliary strictures from 58% to 100%.[53]

SpyGlass endoscopy

SpyGlass may overcome some limitations of conventional cholangioscopy. A recent prospective analysis of a cohort of patients with indeterminate biliary lesions following ERCP was performed. Fifty-two patients underwent SpyGlass and targeted biopsies and a definite diagnosis was made in 94% of cases. A concordance rate of 90% was found between SpyGlass biopsy results and surgical pathology specimens. The sensitivity, specificity, and positive and negative predictive values were 88%, 94%, 96% and 85%, respectively. Overall, SpyGlass allowed adequate biopsy sampling and definite diagnosis in the vast majority of patients with indeterminate biliary lesions.[54] Although a paucity of data remains, this technology may prove beneficial.

Serum markers

CA 19-9 and carcinoembryonic antigen (CEA) levels may be elevated. Unfortunately, these markers can also be elevated in patients with cholestasis, hepatic parenchymal injury, benign biliary obstruction and gastric, pancreatic, colorectal and gynaecological cancers. However, serum markers may prove beneficial in certain circumstances; for instance, CA 19-9 levels >100 U/mL in diagnosing cholangiocarcinoma in patients without PSC have a sensitivity of 53%.[55,56] In those with PSC, however, the sensitivity of CA 19-9 ranges from 38% to 89%, with a specificity of 50–98%.[55,56] Although the diagnostic accuracy of CA 19-9 in patients with cholangiocarcinoma is variable, an extremely elevated level may be indicative of unresectable or metastatic disease.[3]

Staging

Hilar cholangiocarcinoma

The staging systems currently used for hilar cholangiocarcinoma do not account fully for all of the tumour-related variables that influence resectability, namely biliary tumour extent, lobar atrophy and vascular involvement. The modified Bismuth–Corlette classification stratifies patients solely based on the extent of biliary duct involvement by tumour.[57] Although useful to some extent, it is not indicative of resectability or survival. Similarly, the earlier American Joint Committee on Cancer (AJCC) T-stage system (6th edition) was based largely on pathological criteria and had little applicability for preoperative staging. The ideal staging system should accurately predict resectability and the likelihood of associated metastatic disease, and also correlate with survival.

✔ The authors have proposed such a preoperative staging system (Blumgart Clinical Staging System).[58,59] This staging system places the finding of portal venous involvement and lobar atrophy into the proper context for determining resectability, especially when partial hepatectomy is an important component of the operative approach (Table 13.1).

Specifically, the MSKCC system stratifies the extent of disease based on four factors: (1) involvement of the biliary confluence; (2) second-order biliary radical involvement; (3) portal vein involvement; (4) hepatic lobar atrophy. Based upon these factors, a clinical T stage is determined.[59] For example, a tumour with unilateral extension into second-order bile ducts that is associated with ipsilateral portal vein involvement and/or lobar atrophy would still be considered potentially resectable, while such involvement on the contralateral side would preclude a resection. The authors initially found that this staging system correlated well with resectability,

Table 13.1 • Proposed T-stage criteria for hilar cholangiocarcinoma

Stage	Criteria
T1	Tumour involving biliary confluence ± unilateral extension to second-order biliary radicles
T2	Tumour involving biliary confluence ± unilateral extension to second-order biliary radicles AND *ipsilateral* portal vein involvement ± *ipsilateral* hepatic lobar atrophy
T3	Tumour involving biliary confluence + bilateral extension to second-order biliary radicles OR unilateral extension to second-order biliary radicles with *contralateral* portal vein involvement OR unilateral extension to second-order biliary radicles with *contralateral* hepatic lobar atrophy OR main or bilateral portal venous involvement

Reproduced with permission from Jarnagin WR, Fong Y, DeMatteo RP, et al. Staging, resectability, and outcome in 225 patients with hilar cholangiocarcinoma. Ann Surg 2001;234:507–19.

Box 13.1 • Criteria of unresectability

Patient factors

Medically unfit or otherwise unable to tolerate a major operation

Hepatic cirrhosis

Local tumour-related factors

Tumour extension to secondary biliary radicles bilaterally

Encasement or occlusion of the main portal vein proximal to its bifurcation

Atrophy of one hepatic lobe with contralateral portal vein branch encasement or occlusion

Atrophy of one hepatic lobe with contralateral tumour extension to secondary biliary radicles

Unilateral tumour extension to secondary biliary radicles with contralateral portal vein branch encasement or occlusion

Metastatic disease

Histologically proven metastases to distant lymph node basins*

Lung, liver or peritoneal metastases

*Includes peripancreatic, periduodenal, coeliac, superior mesenteric or posterior pancreatico-duodenal lymph nodes. Reproduced with permission from Jarnagin WR, Fong Y, DeMatteo RP, et al. Staging, resectability, and outcome in 225 patients with hilar cholangiocarcinoma. Ann Surg 2001;234:507–19.

the likelihood of associated distant metastatic disease, and median survival (Table 13.2).

✓✓ Independent confirmation of the utility of the Blumgart Clinical Staging System was recently reported in a series of 85 patients from China as well as 380 patients from MSKCC where the preoperative clinical T-staging system predicted resectability (*P* < 0.001), metastatic disease (*P* < 0.001) and R0 resection (*P* = 0.007).[59,60]

The authors' criteria for unresectability are detailed in Box 13.1. This staging scheme is now incorporated in the 7th edition (2009) of the AJCC staging system for hilar cholangiocarcinoma.

Extrahepatic cholangiocarcinoma

Carcinomas of the distal common bile duct are staged according to the AJCC system (7th edition) for tumours of the extrahepatic bile ducts. This system is of limited clinical use, as it is based on pathological information and does not provide any information pertaining to factors that define resectability. The most important of these is the presence of tumour involvement of the portal vein, superior mesenteric artery or common hepatic artery. Tumours involving a short segment of the portal vein (<2 cm) may be resected with reconstruction of the vein. Metastatic disease to distant sites, such as the liver or peritoneum, represents an absolute contraindication to proceeding with resection; however, involvement of regional lymph nodes should perhaps be viewed as a relative contraindication, given the poor survival in patients with node-positive disease.

Table 13.2 • Resectability, incidence of metastatic disease and survival stratified by T stage

T stage	n	Explored with curative intent	Resected	Negative margins	Hepatic resection	Portal vein resection	Metastatic disease	Median survival (mth)
1	87	73 (84%)	51 (59%)	38	33	2	18 (21%)	20
2	95	79 (83%)	29 (31%)	24	29	7	40 (43%)	13
3	37	8 (22%)	0	0	0	0	15 (41%)	8
Total	219	160 (71%)	80 (37%)	62	62	9	73 (33%)	16

Reproduced with permission from Jarnagin WR, Fong Y, DeMatteo RP et al. Staging, resectability, and outcome in 225 patients with hilar cholangiocarcinoma. Ann Surg 2001234:507–19.

Intrahepatic cholangiocarcinoma

Currently, there is no useful consensus regarding a clinical staging system for intrahepatic cholangiocarcinoma. The AJCC TNM classification for primary liver cancers is applied both to hepatocellular carcinoma and intrahepatic cholangiocarcinoma, but is of little clinical value. Because intrahepatic cholangiocarcinomas tend to be relatively silent lesions, they are often large at presentation. Thirty per cent of patients will have peritoneal or hepatic metastases at presentation and many of these will not be detected until staging laparoscopy or exploratory laparotomy is performed.

Management

Preoperative tissue diagnosis

In the authors' view, histological confirmation of malignancy is not mandatory prior to exploration. With no prior suggestive history (i.e. prior biliary tract operation, PSC, hepatolithiasis), the finding of a focal stenotic lesion combined with the appropriate clinical presentation is sufficient for a presumptive diagnosis of intrahepatic or hilar cholangiocarcinoma.[61] It is dangerous to rely entirely on a negative result from a needle biopsy or biliary brush cytology, since they are often misleading, particularly in the face of compelling radiographic evidence of malignant disease.[62] In patients with a stricture of the distal bile duct and a clinical presentation consistent with cholangiocarcinoma (or any other periampullary malignancy), histological confirmation of malignancy is also generally unnecessary, unless non-operative therapy is planned. Benign strictures do occur in the lower bile duct, but these are difficult to differentiate definitively from malignant strictures without resection.

Preoperative biliary drainage

Although patients with lesions suspicious for cholangiocarcinoma who meet resection criteria should be taken for an upfront resection, there are certain situations in which biliary stenting is necessary.

While the use of routine preoperative drainage remains controversial, several studies have reported that the treatment of hyperbilirubinaemia is associated with decreased postoperative complications; there has not, however, been a documented improvement in mortality or survival. Proponents argue that stenting improves hepatic function and nutritional status, and reduces the risk of cholangitis and postoperative liver failure.

Specifically, Kennedy et al. found preoperative biliary drainage to be associated with improved perioperative outcomes in patients with a predicted future liver remnant (FLR) <30%.[63] Similarly, on an assessment of 287 consecutive patients undergoing major liver resection for perihilar cholangiocarcinoma, incomplete drainage of the future liver remnant in patients with FLR volume <50% predicted postoperative mortality.[64] However, in a multicentre, retrospective study, preoperative biliary drainage did not result in improved postoperative outcomes in patients undergoing major surgical resection for perihilar cholangiocarcinoma. That being said, on a subset analysis in patients requiring right hepatectomy, there was an association with decreased mortality due to liver failure.[65] On the other hand, opponents believe preoperative drainage increases the risk of tumour seeding, cholangitis, perioperative infectious complications and lengthens overall and postoperative stay.[3]

Of note, the median patency of metallic endoprostheses placed at the biliary confluence is approximately 6 months, which is significantly lower than that reported for similar stents placed in the distal bile duct.[66] Becker et al. reported 1-year patency rates of 46% and 89% for Wallstents placed at the biliary confluence and the distal bile duct, respectively.[67] Due to this higher occlusion rate, 25% of patients will require re-intervention. This concurs with our findings of a mean patency of 6.1 months in 35 patients palliated for malignant high biliary obstruction by placement of expandable metallic endoprostheses. The periprocedural mortality was 14% at 30 days, and seven patients (24%) had documented stent occlusion requiring repeated intervention.[66]

Additionally, hilar tumours frequently involve all three major hilar ducts (left hepatic, right anterior sectoral hepatic and right posterior sectoral hepatic), and thus may require two or more stents for adequate drainage. That being said, a randomised clinical trial assessed bilateral and unilateral stent placement and found unilateral stenting to be associated with higher rates of successful drainage (87% vs 77%, $P = 0.041$), lower complications (19% vs 27%, $P = 0.026$) and lower rates of cholangitis (9% vs 17%, $P = 0.013$). There was no significant difference between the two groups with regard to procedure-related mortality, 30-day mortality, complications and median survival.[68]

✔ Biliary decompression of an atrophic lobe does not typically provide much benefit in terms of lowering serum bilirubin or improving hepatic function, and should only be performed if necessary to treat cholangitis.

As alluded to above, endoscopic or percutaneous instrumentation significantly increases the incidence of bacterial contamination and the subsequent risk of clinical infection. In fact, the incidence of bacterobilia approaches 100% after endoscopic biliary intubation, thus making cholangitis more common.[37] The presence of overt or subclinical infection at the time of surgery is a major source of postoperative morbidity and mortality. Thus, endoscopic and percutaneous intubations are both associated with greater morbidity and mortality following surgical resection or palliative bypass for hilar cholangiocarcinoma. In an analysis of 71 patients who underwent either resection or palliative biliary bypass for proximal cholangiocarcinoma, all patients stented endoscopically and 62% of those stented percutaneously had bacterobilia. Moreover, postoperative infectious complications were doubled in those patients stented before operation compared to their non-stented counterparts. Of note, non-infectious complications were equal in both groups.[37] *Enterococcus*, *Klebsiella*, *Escherichia coli*, *Streptococcus viridans* and *Enterobacter aerogenes* are the most common organisms, and this spectrum of bacteria must be considered when administering perioperative antibiotics. It is imperative to take intraoperative bile specimens for culture in order to guide selection of postoperative antibiotic therapy.

Neoadjuvant therapy

To date, there remains a paucity of data on the efficacy of neoadjuvant therapy in patients with resectable disease. However, questions have been raised regarding potential benefits in down-staging locally advanced hilar disease, although its utility remains unproven. One meta-analysis has suggested that systemic therapy, in properly selected patients, may help achieve an R0 resection and improve survival.[69] However, adequate prospective data on using chemotherapy alone for down-staging locally advanced hilar tumours prior to surgical resection are scarce. The likelihood of achieving meaningful local tumour response with systemic chemotherapy alone is low and most neoadjuvant therapy regimens are combinations of chemotherapy along with radiation.[70]

Furthermore, there are even fewer data regarding neoadjuvant therapy in resectable disease. However, one small series encompassing 40 patients who underwent resection for extrahepatic cholangiocarcinoma retrospectively evaluated the use of neoadjuvant chemoradiotherapy. A pathological complete response was observed in 3/9 (33%) patients. On an assessment of margins, 100% of the preoperative chemoradiotherapy group had a margin-negative resection compared to 54% for the group who did not receive preoperative chemoradiotherapy (P <0.01).[71] Moreover, in a series of 45 patients with extrahepatic cholangiocarcinoma, 12 received neoadjuvant chemoradiotherapy and were compared to an adjuvant chemoradiotherapy group. In the neoadjuvant setting, three had a

complete pathological response and 11 were able to undergo a complete (R0) resection. Despite having more advanced disease at presentation, patients who received neoadjuvant chemoradiotherapy had longer 5-year survival rates compared to their adjuvant counterparts (53 vs 23 months, respectively).[72]

Lastly, one retrospective review recently assessed neoadjuvant and adjuvant therapy in resectable biliary tract malignancies. Of 94 patients who underwent resection for cholangiocarcinoma, 18% received neoadjuvant chemotherapy. Neoadjuvant therapy was found to delay resection by an average of 7 months (P <0.0001) and was associated with inferior median overall survival outcomes compared to those who underwent upfront resection (42 months vs 54 months; P = 0.01).[73] These trials are presented as hypothesis-generating and allude to the need for randomised trials testing this strategy.

Portal vein embolisation

Currently, it remains common practice to consider portal vein embolisation (PVE) in patients who have an estimated/anticipated FLR <20–30% of the total liver volume. Additionally, in patients with underlying liver dysfunction, or those who have been heavily pre-treated with systemic therapy, a FLR <40% may be used as the cutoff to consider PVE.[3] Traditionally, it has been used more often in the setting of an extended right hepatectomy, since the left lateral sector may not encompass enough future volume. On average, up to a 15% increase in the total volume of the future liver remnant can be expected.[3]

> ✅✅ PVE can theoretically reduce the risk of postoperative hepatic dysfunction by inducing preoperative compensatory hypertrophy of the non-embolised lobe.

As previously identified by our group, a FLR <30% in patients undergoing liver resection for hilar cholangiocarcinoma was associated with increased risk for hepatic insufficiency and death.[63] Moreover, in a series of 287 consecutive perihilar cholangiocarcinoma patients who underwent resection, postoperative mortality at 90 days was independently associated with a FLR <30%.[64] Therefore, the authors recommend PVE in patients at risk of a FLR of <30%. To date, numerous studies have reported the safety and efficacy of PVE in increasing the remnant liver volume before extended hepatectomy.[74–76]

General operative principles

Cholangiocarcinoma remains an aggressive malignancy, and complete tumour extirpation remains the definitive management and only chance in achieving long-term survival. Unfortunately, unresectable or systemic spread of disease is common at initial presentation. In the setting of hilar cholangiocarcinoma, only 50–75% of patients meet resection criteria at diagnosis.[77] At the authors' institution, 23% of all patients presenting with hilar cholangiocarcinoma had advanced or unresectable disease.[58] Additionally, in a review of 53 peripheral intrahepatic cholangiocarcinomas treated at MSKCC over an 8-year period, the median tumour diameter was 7.1 cm at presentation.[78] Twenty patients were found to be unresectable at exploration (overall resectability rate was 62%). Operative findings precluding resection were intrahepatic metastases (35%), peritoneal metastases (30%), coeliac lymph node metastases (25%) and portal vein involvement (10%).[78] Additionally, in a more recent review, a total of 270 patients with intrahepatic cholangiocarcinoma were seen over a 16-year period. Of these, 54% had unresectable disease at presentation and ultimately only 34% of the entire cohort underwent a potentially curative resection (70% of those explored with curative intent).[79]

✅ In general, irresectability is defined by bilateral spread to secondary biliary radicals, bilateral portal vein involvement, bilateral hepatic arterial involvement or unilateral hepatic artery involvement with contralateral ductal spread.[70] Moreover, even when deemed resectable by modern imaging, 30–40% of patients will be deemed unresectable at the time of exploration. Therefore, diagnostic laparoscopy has become a prudent step at the time of operation.

Diagnostic laparoscopy

Despite improvements in preoperative imaging, a considerable number of patients are still found to have unresectable disease at the time of exploration. In a recent report from MSKCC, this number approached 50% of patients with cholangiocarcinoma explored with curative intent.[24] In an effort to minimise the number of non-curative laparotomies performed, staging laparoscopy should therefore be utilised. Two recent studies specifically analysing patients with biliary cancer have shown that laparoscopy can identify a large proportion of patients with unresectable disease primarily in the form of radiographically occult metastases, the yield of which is greatest in locally advanced tumours.[80,81] Weber et al. evaluated 56 patients with potentially resectable hilar cholangiocarcinoma; 33 were ultimately determined to have unresectable disease, of which 14 (42%) were identified at laparoscopy and spared an unnecessary laparotomy.[81] With respect to intrahepatic cholangiocarcinoma, staging

laparoscopy spared 27% of patients at MSKCC undergoing a laparotomy due to findings of peritoneal and intrahepatic metastases.[78]

Margin-negative resection

✅✅ Whether intrahepatic, hilar or extrahepatic in origin, the achievement of pathologically negative margins (R0 resection) is the most predictive factor of oncologic outcome. This concept has been shown in previous studies, which found survival for patients with incomplete (R1 or R2) resections to be equivalent to those with unresectable tumours **(Fig. 13.5).**[58]

The extent of resection should be dictated by what is necessary to achieve a negative margin and this may require an extended resection. For instance, Bismuth IIIb lesions typically require a left hepatectomy, while Bismuth I, II, IIIa lesions usually require an extended right hepatectomy. Simple excisions of the extrahepatic biliary tree should be avoided, as this approach is associated with a high probability of R1/R2 resections and inferior overall survival.[82] Over time, the increased utilisation of hepatic resection has been responsible for the increased percentage of R0 resections and the observed improvement

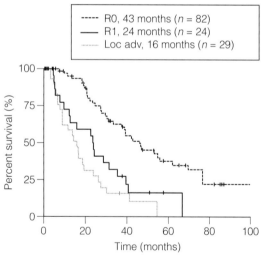

----- R0, 43 months (n = 82)
—— R1, 24 months (n = 24)
········ Loc adv, 16 months (n = 29)

Figure 13.5 • Survival curves after resection of hilar cholangiocarcinoma. R0 indicates complete resection with histologically negative resection margins (median survival 43 months). R1 indicates histologically involved resection margins (median survival 24 months; P <0.001, R0 vs R1). Loc Adv indicates patients explored, but found to have unresectable tumours owing to local invasion (no metastatic disease) (median survival 16 months; P <0.19, R1 vs Loc Adv).
Reproduced with permission from Blumgart LH, editor. Surgery of the liver, biliary tract, and pancreas. 4th ed. Elsevier Saunders; 2006.

in postoperative survival. This point is emphasised by a reported series of 269 patients accumulated over a 20-year period demonstrating a progressive increase in the proportion of patients subjected to partial hepatectomy, with a corresponding increase in the incidence of negative histological margins and in turn, survival.[83] Moreover, a more recent study from MSKCC reported results of resection in 106 consecutive patients and showed a median survival of 43 months in patients who had an R0 resection compared to 24 months in those with involved resection margins.[24] On multivariate analysis, R0 resection, concomitant hepatectomy, well-differentiated histology and papillary tumour phenotype were all independent predictors of long-term survival.

Intraoperative frozen section should be obtained and, if positive, extended resections should be undertaken to obtain pathologically negative margins. This technique is dictated by the location of the tumour. For extrahepatic cholangiocarcinoma frozen section should be obtained on the proximal and distal bile duct margins and, if positive, hepatectomy or pancreaticoduodenectomy should ensue. For perihilar cholangiocarcinoma, distal and proximal margins should be assessed and, if positive, extended hepatectomy and/or pancreatico-duodenectomy should ensue. In an MSKCC analysis of extrahepatic cholangiocarcinoma, 82% of proximal lesions required a combined hepatectomy whereas 92% of distal lesions required a pancreatico-duodenectomy.[84] That being said, there remains doubt as to the true efficacy of intraoperative frozen section. In an analysis of 90 patients found to have a negative intraoperative frozen section of the proximal bile duct, 9% were confirmed positive at final pathology. Therefore, frozen section analysis of the proximal bile duct margin was misleading in a substantial subset of patients. Additionally, in those patients who were determined to have negative duct margins intraoperatively, only 60% had margins adequately wide enough to be associated with an improvement in disease-specific survival.[85]

✔ If the portal vein is involved with tumour, portal vein resection should not be considered a contraindication to resection. Although series have reported potentially higher postoperative morbidity and mortality rates, hepatic resection combined with portal vein resection has been demonstrated to be associated with superior survival.

In an assessment of 95 patients resected for hilar cholangiocarcinoma, 42 required resection of the portal vein. Patients who underwent portal vein resection had perioperative mortality and morbidity

similar to those who did not. Median survival was 38 months (95% CI 29–51 months), with a 5-year survival rate of 43%. Similar to the studies reported above, negative margins were achieved in 84% of cases and were associated with improved survival ($P <0.01$). More impressive, the 5-year survival rate in patients with an R0 resection was 50%, and on multivariate analysis the only predictor of survival was negative margin status.[86]

In contrast, the role of arterial resection and reconstruction is more controversial since the majority of studies have shown arterial resection and reconstruction to be associated with significantly increased morbidity and mortality without long-term survival benefit.[87]

Portal lymphadenectomy

In addition to resection margin status (i.e. an R0 resection), metastatic disease to regional lymph nodes is a critical determinant of outcome. An international study group for intrahepatic cholangiocarcinoma has recently advocated routine portal lymph node dissection at the time of resection, as approximately 30% of patients who underwent evaluation were found to have lymph node involvement.[88]

✔✔ Although the survival benefits of node dissection are unproven and unlikely, the diagnostic information gained regarding node positivity is important and may inform decisions about adjuvant therapy.

Fong et al. found that lymph node status was the only independent predictor of long-term survival after complete resection, with positive nodes conferring a 6.7 times greater likelihood of recurrence and death.[89] Similarly, Allen et al. reported lymph node positivity to be an independent predictor of 5-year disease-specific survival (node-negative 42% vs node-positive 22%) in both proximal and distal resected cholangiocarcinoma.[84] Lastly, the authors' group also assessed the prognostic significance of the highest peripancreatic lymph node. In a series of 85 patients who underwent curative resection, 30% had a positive peripancreatic lymph node. This highest peripancreatic lymph node positivity correlated to statistically lower recurrence-free (24 vs 10 months) and disease-specific survival (62 vs 21 months). Further, on multivariate analysis, positivity within the highest peripancreatic lymph node was an independent predictor of recurrence-free survival (HR 3.73, 95% CI 1.86–7.45; $P <0.01$) and disease-specific survival (HR 3.98, 95% CI 1.89–8.38; $P <0.01$).[90]

The extent of lymphadenectomy that should be performed remains an area of controversy. Some surgeons advocate an extended nodal dissection as

Table 13.3 • Summary of selected series showing proportion of number of patients surviving 5 years after resection of hilar cholangiocarcinoma with metastatic disease to regional lymph nodes

Author	Resections (n)	Node-positive (%)	Five-year survivors with positive nodes (n)
Sugiura (1994)	83	51	3
Klempnauer (1997)	151	29	2
Nakeeb (1996)	109	–	0
Ogura (1998)	66	52	0
Iwatsuki (1998)	72	35	0
Kosuge (1999)	65	46	4
Jarnagin (2001)	80	24	3
Kitagawa (2001)	110	53	5
Total	**802**	–	17 (2.1%)

some studies have demonstrated measurable 5-year actuarial survival in the presence of metastatic disease to distant lymph nodes (e.g. para-aortic).[91] However, an analysis of studies specifically reporting 5-year survival suggests that distal nodal involvement is a marker of advanced/systemic disease and very few patients benefit from an aggressive surgical approach (Table 13.3). Thus, while a complete porta hepatis lymphadenectomy should be routinely performed at the time of resection, the authors do not advocate an extended lymph node dissection.

With respect to the number of lymph nodes needed, the clinical implication of negative lymph nodes on histopathological analysis is likely dependent on the total number of lymph nodes sampled. A study from MSKCC reported that seven lymph nodes appear to be the target sampling number in order to accurately stage hilar cholangiocarcinoma.[92] This must be weighed against the reality that, in most series, the median number of nodes sampled from a porta hepatis lymphadenectomy is usually approximately three.

In brief, given the low yield of lymph nodes from a portal lymphadenectomy, the accuracy of lymph node evaluation is questionable, and thus its use as a selection criterion for adjuvant therapy is controversial. Perhaps pathological criteria from evaluation of the primary tumour, such as lymphovascular invasion and perineural invasion, should be used instead as selection criteria for adjuvant therapy, as the presence of these factors has been associated with poor survival that is similar to lymph node-positive disease.[93]

Caudate lobectomy

✓✓ Although initially controversial, resection of the caudate lobe en bloc for hilar or intrahepatic cholangiocarcinoma is now widely accepted as standard of care.

In an assessment of 171 patients with resected hilar cholangiocarcinoma, total caudate lobectomy was significantly associated with more opportunity to achieve curative resection ($P < 0.01$), without an accompanying increase in morbidity ($P = 0.39$) or mortality ($P = 0.67$).[94] Additionally, results of a 15-year experience with 127 resected hilar cholangiocarcinoma patients found those who underwent caudate lobectomy ($n = 70$) had significantly improved overall survival compared to those who did not (64 vs 35 months, $P = 0.010$). Also, multivariate analysis found caudate lobectomy to statistically improve disease-free survival ($P = 0.016$).[95] Moreover, in a recent analysis of 243 resected hilar cholangiocarcinoma patients, caudate lobectomy was identified as an independent predictor of long-term survival (>5 years) ($P = 0.006$).[96] In general, a surgical approach that includes resection of the extrahepatic biliary tree along with hepatic resection including the caudate lobe should yield negative pathological margins in up to 80% of patients.[70]

No touch technique

This concept of 'no-touch' was initially proposed by Neuhaus et al. in 1999 and combines an extended right hepatectomy with portal vein resection and caudate lobectomy in order to avoid hilar dissection and the possible intraoperative microscopic dissemination of malignant cells.[97] This technique places vascular clamps on the left portal vein branch within the umbilical fissure as well as on the main portal vein (directly above the head of the pancreas). These vessels are then divided without dissecting the portal vein within the hilar region. A retrospective review of this technique found improved 5-year survival rates (58% vs 29%, $P = 0.02$) compared to those who underwent a conventional surgical approach.[98] Although the authors reported no increase in morbidity or mortality, this technique may not be applicable to all surgeons or centres. Of note, this technique has not been widely adopted partially due to the fact that morbidity and mortality rates are already high in this patient population and the above data are based on a small cohort of patients. As such, more data are certainly needed before the 'no touch technique' becomes the standard of care for all hilar tumours. This is clearly an aggressive surgical approach that is likely best applied only to a highly selected population.

Postoperative oncological outcomes

Generally, 5-year survival rates are in the range 20–40% for intrahepatic cholangiocarcinoma and 30–40% for perihilar cholangiocarcinoma.[99] Five-year survival rates have been reported to be higher for distal/extrahepatic cholangiocarcinoma, and may be as high as 54%.[89] Interestingly, Neuhaus et al. compared outcomes following lobar and extended hepatic resections for hilar cholangiocarcinoma and found 5-year survival rates to increase from 18–23% in the lobar hepatectomy group to 52–72% in the extended resection cohort.[100]

Technical aspects of resection

Technical aspects of intraoperative tumour assessment, exposure and resection are outside the scope of this chapter and the reader is referred to speciality texts for a detailed description of surgical techniques.[101] However, video links are provided at the end of the chapter.

Adjuvant therapy

The rarity of cholangiocarcinoma has, until recently, prevented any meaningful clinical trials evaluating the use of adjuvant therapy. Several small, single-centre studies have attempted to investigate the benefit of postoperative adjuvant chemoradiotherapy in patients with hilar cholangiocarcinoma. Traditionally, data suggested no benefit of adjuvant external beam or intraluminal radiation therapy. However, in contrast, Kamada et al. suggested that radiation may improve survival in patients with histologically positive hepatic duct margins.[102] It must be noted, however, that none of these studies was randomised and most consisted of small, heterogeneous groups of patients. The only phase III trial investigating adjuvant chemotherapy, which used mitomycin/5-fluorouracil (5FU), included 508 patients with

resected bile duct tumours ($n=139$), gallbladder cancers ($n=140$), pancreatic cancers ($n=173$) and ampullary tumours ($n=56$).[103] On subset analysis, there were no significant differences in overall or disease-free survival for bile duct tumours.

Given the lack of randomised data to guide management of adjuvant therapy for resected biliary malignancies, a meta-analysis of 20 studies encompassing 6712 patients is worth considering. Compared to surgery alone, there was a non-significant improvement in overall survival with the use of adjuvant therapy (OR 0.74; 95% CI 0.55–1.01 [$P=0.06$]). In particular, patients who received chemotherapy or chemoradiotherapy derived statistically greater benefit than those who received radiation alone (OR 0.39, 0.61 and 0.98, respectively; $P=0.02$). Moreover, patients who benefited the most from adjuvant therapy included those with lymph node-positive disease (OR 0.49; $P=0.004$) and those with positive margins disease (OR 0.36; $P=0.002$).[104] On the basis of this meta-analysis, adjuvant therapy with either chemotherapy or chemoradiotherapy may be an appropriate treatment option after surgical resection. With respect to therapy, the positive results found for those with unresectable disease in the ABC-02 trial (Cisplatin plus Gemcitabine vs Gemcitabine for Biliary Tract Cancer) are generally extrapolated to the adjuvant setting in patients with resected disease.

The recently reported BILCAP (multi-institution phase III randomised) trial randomised patients with biliary tract cancer to 6 months of adjuvant capecitabine ($n=223$) or observation ($n=224$) after resection. Of note, the trial included all sites of biliary tract cancers (intrahepatic, hilar, distal and gallbladder) and both R0 and R1 resections. Given the known heterogeneity of these diseases, the grouping of all types of biliary tract cancer into one trial can be criticised, but does represent a clinical and practical reality, given the rarity of these cancers and the feasibility of performing a clinical trial. Although on an intent-to-treat analysis, the P-value did not reach significance ($P=0.97$), the difference in median overall survival between the treatment arm (51 months) and the observation arm (36 months) cannot be ignored. On per-protocol analysis, which only excluded 27 patients since the adjuvant capecitabine regimen was so well tolerated, the results were statistically significant (treatment arm 53 months vs control arm 36 months; $P=0.028$). Adjuvant capecitabine also significantly extended the median recurrence-free survival (treatment arm 25 months vs control arm 18 months; $P=0.036$). Given these data, adjuvant capecitabine will likely become the new standard of care for patients undergoing upfront resection of biliary tract malignancies. Further trials evaluating site-specific biliary tract cancers, which will necessitate international collaboration, are now needed to better define the optimal treatment regimen for these patients.[70,105]

Additionally, radiation therapy (external beam radiation therapy [EBRT] along with intraluminal brachytherapy) following R1 resection for hilar cholangiocarcinoma has been studied. In an analysis of 91 patients, overall median survival after treatment with adjuvant radiotherapy was longer than after resection without additional radiation (24 vs 8 months, P <0.01). No significant benefit from the use of intraluminal brachytherapy was identified. Therefore, additional radiotherapy after resection of hilar cholangiocarcinoma may improve survival following an R1 resection and should be discussed in a multidisciplinary setting.[106]

More recently, the SWOG S0809 study – a single-arm prospective phase II trial of adjuvant capecitabine/gemcitabine chemotherapy followed by concurrent capecitabine and radiotherapy in extrahepatic cholangiocarcinomas and gallbladder cancer – assessed 79 patients to estimate 2-year survival and patterns of relapse. The 2-year survival was 65% (95% CI 53–74%) in all-comers and 67% and 60% in R0 and R1 patients, respectively. Additionally, the median overall survival was 35 months (R0, 34 months; R1, 35 months).[107] Overall, although double-arm or phase III trials are lacking, there is mounting evidence to support consideration of adjuvant chemotherapy.

Transplantation

Orthotopic liver transplantation has been investigated for unresectable hilar tumours. Klempnauer et al. reported four long-term survivors of 32 patients who underwent transplantation for hilar cholangiocarcinoma.[108] The same group also reported a 17.1% 5-year survival for their transplant group.[109] Comparable results were reported by Iwatsuki et al.[110] The results of transplantation have previously not been sufficiently adequate to justify its use, and most centres now do not perform liver transplantation for cholangiocarcinoma. More recently, however, data from the Mayo Clinic have emerged suggesting good results with transplantation in highly selected patients with low-volume unresectable disease with an intensive pre-transplant treatment regimen.[111,112] Although the data are compelling, routine use of vascular resection, even when there is no obvious tumour infiltration, will likely lead to higher perioperative morbidity. Therefore, this approach would seem applicable to only a very small proportion of patients.

Orthotopic liver transplantation has been utilised in the management of some patients with intrahepatic cholangiocarcinoma.[113] However, many of these lesions are suitable for resection, which would likely produce similar results. Given the critical shortage of liver grafts, transplantation for intrahepatic cholangiocarcinoma is not performed in most centres, unless it is done in the context of a clinical trial.

Palliative therapy

Intrahepatic biliary-enteric bypass

Patients with hilar cholangiocarcinoma with unresectable disease identified at operation, particularly after the bile duct has been divided, may be candidates for intrahepatic biliary-enteric bypass. The segment III duct is usually the most accessible and is the preferred approach of the authors, but the right anterior or posterior sectoral hepatic ducts can also be used.[114] Segment III bypass provides excellent biliary drainage and is less prone to occlusion since the anastomosis can be placed remote from the tumour. The 1-year bypass patency rates approach 80%.[114] Decompression of only one-third of the functioning hepatic parenchyma is usually sufficient to relieve jaundice. Furthermore, provided that the undrained lobe has not been percutaneously drained or otherwise contaminated, communication between the right and left hepatic ducts is not necessary.[115] As discussed above for stenting, bypass to an atrophic lobe or a lobe heavily involved with tumour is generally not effective.

Systemic therapy

Data remain scarce on the true effectiveness of chemotherapy for cholangiocarcinoma since trials have been limited by small sample sizes and heterogeneous accrual of various biliary and gallbladder malignancies.

In cases of advanced biliary tract cancers where curative surgical resection is not an option, palliative chemotherapy has been used to potentially improve quality of life, reduce symptoms and increase survival. One randomised study assessed the role of chemotherapy in 37 patients with advanced biliary tract cancers who were randomised to receive chemotherapy (5FU/leucovorin with or without etoposide) or best supportive care.[116] Short-term improvements in survival (6.5 vs 2.5 months) were noted in the chemotherapy group. In addition, the treatment group also demonstrated improvement in quality of life as measured by the EORTC QLQ-C30 instrument.

Generally speaking, chemotherapy is reserved for patients with systemic spread of disease, unresectable disease or locally advanced disease.

As compared to historical 5FU-based therapy, gemcitabine regimens, used in multiple phase II trials as a single agent, found response rates of 18–36%.[117,118] Moreover, when gemcitabine was combined with capecitabine, response rates were 25% and overall survival was 12–14 months.[119,120] Additional survival improvements were seen with the addition of oxaliplatin to gemcitabine. Response rates increased to 50% and in treatment-naïve patients, median overall survival was as high as 18 months.[121,122]

✔✔ Currently, gemcitabine in addition to cisplatin remains the standard of care for patients with advanced biliary cancer.

In a randomised prospective trial in patients with metastatic biliary cancers, Valle et al. found that cisplatin plus gemcitabine was associated with a significant advantage in overall survival compared to gemcitabine alone (11.7 vs 8.1 months, $P <0.001$), along with an improvement in median progression-free survival (8 vs 5 months, $P <0.001$). The use of gemcitabine with a platinum agent, barring any contraindications, has now become the treatment regimen of choice for patients with advanced disease. This finding now raises the question of whether appropriately selected patients might benefit from this regimen in the adjuvant setting as well.[123]

Novel agents

Recently, interest has shifted to targeted-based therapy for advanced biliary malignancy, the first of which was the epidermal growth factor receptor (EGFR), expressed in both cholangiocarcinoma and gallbladder carcinoma. However, data have not found this target to be efficacious. In a randomised phase III trial of gemcitabine and oxaliplatin with and without the anti-EGFR agent erlotinib, there was no difference noted in progression-free or overall survival.[124] Additionally, smaller phase II trials combining other anti-EGFR agents (cetuximab or panitumumab) to gemcitabine/oxaliplatin found overall survival to be 7–15 months, which is synonymous to historical chemotherapy controls.[125,126] Another recent target has been the inhibition of the vascular endothelial growth factor pathway. The addition of bevacizumab to gemcitabine/oxaliplatin was associated with an objective response rate of 40% and a median overall survival of 13 months.[127] A recent randomised phase II trial assessing gemcitabine/cisplatin with the addition of cediranib compared to chemotherapy alone reported an overall survival of 14 months and progression-free survival of 7.7 months, neither of which were statistically superior to chemotherapy

alone.[128] More recently, MEK inhibition utilising selumetinib in combination with a gemcitabine/cisplatin regimen has been studied in a phase 1b study. Median progression-free survival was 6.4 months, 25% of patients had a partial response and 42% had stable disease.[129] In essence, although novel, the addition of targeted agents in advanced biliary malignancy remains investigational.

Regional chemotherapy/hepatic arterial infusion

Two clinical trials assessing the role of regional hepatic chemotherapy utilising hepatic arterial infusion (HAI) with floxuridine (FUDR) with or without bevacizumab in unresectable intrahepatic cholangiocarcinoma have been performed at MSKCC. Forty-four patients were analysed (26 FUDR and 18 FUDR/bevacizumab). At a median follow-up of 29 months, partial response, as measured by RECIST criteria, was found in 48% and 50% had stable disease. Median survival was 29 months and compared favourably to historical controls.[130,131] The disease control rate was 98% (median 8 months; range 1.4–37.9), 23% of patients survived more than 3 years and 11% survived beyond 5 years. Of note, the addition of bevacizumab increased the incidence of biliary toxicity without any improvement in survival (31.1 vs 29.5 months; $P =$ NS). In summary, HAI therapy may result in prolonged survival for patients with unresectable intrahepatic cholangiocarcinoma and should be in the armamentarium of those caring for such patients.[130,131]

Y-90 radioembolisation

Radioembolisation with yttrium-90 microspheres is another treatment modality for those with unresectable intrahepatic cholangiocarcinoma. Although prospective data are lacking, a recent systemic review and meta-analysis of 12 studies (seven prospective case series and five retrospective reviews) identified 298 patients treated with Y90 radioembolisation. Overall median survival was 15.5 months, with 28% of patients obtaining a partial response and 54% of patients had stable disease at 3 months. Seven patients were able to be down-staged and taken for definitive resection.[132] Additionally, Ibrahim et al. reported a median survival of 31.8 months in patients with unresectable IHC treated with yttrium-90 (Y-90) who had a performance status of ECOG 0. This study included only 24 patients and a positive effect of Y-90 was not observed in patients with ECOG performance status of 1 or 2.[133] In brief, the use of yttrium-90 microspheres should be discussed in a multidisciplinary setting as a treatment option for those with advanced intrahepatic cholangiocarcinoma.

Gallbladder cancer

The gallbladder is the most common site of biliary tract malignancy and the fifth most common gastrointestinal malignancy and yet remains an uncommon malignancy with fewer than 10 000 new cases per year in the USA.[1] Historically, reported median survival ranged from 2 to 5 months for untreated gallbladder cancers; moreover, even those treated had a less than 5% chance of surviving beyond 5 years. However, improved understanding of the disease and its treatment has led to prolonged survival and cure in selected patients. To date, documented 5-year survival rates for resected gallbladder carcinoma range from 20% to 50%.[134–142] Specifically, in a review of 410 gallbladder carcinoma patients who presented to MSKCC between 1986 and 2000, the median and 5-year survivals for resected patients were 26 months and 38%, respectively. Currently, the only chance of cure is with complete surgical extirpation of the cancer.

Epidemiology/aetiology

Worldwide, the highest incidence of gallbladder cancer is found among people indigenous to the Andes Mountains of South America. In North America, the incidence is approximately 1.2 per 100 000, the highest being among native American Indians and Mexican Americans. It occurs in women almost three times more often than in men across all populations studied.[143] As with other biliary tract tumours, chronic inflammation leading to high cellular turnover is a common denominator of associated risk factors. The most common risk factor is cholelithiasis; other factors include the presence of a cholecystoenteric fistula, typhoid bacillus infection and an anomalous pancreatico-biliary junction.[143] As with other gastrointestinal malignancies, the adenoma to carcinoma sequence has been demonstrated within adenomatous polyps of the gallbladder as well. Gallbladder polyps are noted in 3–6% of the population undergoing ultrasonography, although the vast majority are cholesterol polyps or adenomyomatosis, both of which are benign and have no malignant potential.[144] However, about 1% of cholecystectomy specimens contain adenomatous polyps, which do have malignant potential.[144] Conditions that increase the risk of malignancy include polyp size >1 cm, patient age >50 years and the presence of multiple lesions.[144] The conservative recommendation is to perform a prophylactic cholecystectomy for polypoid lesions >0.5 cm in size, although the likelihood of malignancy in polyps even up to 1 cm appears to be extremely low. This is in contrast to gallbladder polyps arising in the setting of primary sclerosing cholangitis, which are more often neoplastic.[144] The authors' practice is to recommend cholecystectomy for polyps >1 cm, although carcinoma in such lesions appears to be much lower than previously thought. Polypoid lesions <0.5 cm have an extremely low likelihood of harbouring malignancy and are safe to follow with serial ultrasounds for evidence of growth or change in character.[144]

A gallbladder with a calcified wall, also known as a 'porcelain gallbladder', is also associated with an increased risk of developing cancer (**Fig. 13.6**). The deposition of calcium most likely reflects a state of chronic inflammation. Although the risk of malignancy in a porcelain gallbladder previously was considered to be extremely high (10–50%), recent studies demonstrate a much lower incidence (P <10%), with stippled calcification actually

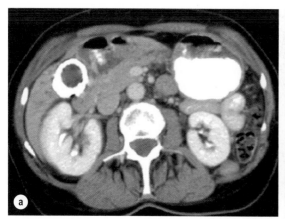
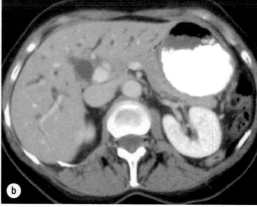

Figure 13.6 • Axial CT images of a porcelain gallbladder. Note the marked circumferential calcification of the gallbladder wall **(a)** and the intrahepatic biliary ductal dilatation **(b)**. This patient had a gallbladder cancer arising in the setting of a porcelain gallbladder, which had progressed to involve the common hepatic duct.

carrying a higher risk than diffuse intramural calcification.[145] Nevertheless, the current recommendation for patients with a porcelain gallbladder is to perform a cholecystectomy, which in most cases can be safely done laparoscopically.

Clinical presentation and diagnosis

Many patients present late in the course of their disease, and 75% of patients present with unresectable disease. Two-thirds of patients present with abdominal pain/biliary colic. Approximately one-third will present with jaundice and 10% will have significant weight loss. For early-stage cancers, the diagnosis is usually made on pathological examination of a cholecystectomy specimen resected for symptoms presumed to be benign biliary colic. Preoperative diagnosis should be suspected for any mass or irregularity of the gallbladder wall noted on radiological investigation.

Histopathology and staging

The overwhelming majority of gallbladder cancers are adenocarcinomas, with a papillary subtype being associated with a relatively better prognosis compared to others.[146] Other histological subtypes, such as adenosquamous carcinoma or pure squamous cell carcinoma, are seen in the gallbladder more commonly than at any other site within the biliary tree. The AJCC staging system was updated in 2002 (6th edition) and was based on the standard TNM classification, of which the T stage has the greatest clinical impact on the extent of surgery performed, because it is dependent on the depth of invasion into the gallbladder wall and adjacent organs. The wall of the gallbladder consists of a mucosa and lamina propria, a thin muscular layer, perimuscular connective tissue and a serosa. However, it should be noted that the gallbladder wall lacks a serosal covering along its border with the liver and the perimuscular connective tissue is continuous with the liver connective tissue. T1 tumours are divided into T1a and T1b lesions, where the former are limited to the lamina propria and the latter have invaded the muscle layer. T2 tumours have invaded through the muscle layer into the perimuscular connective tissue. T3 tumours have penetrated the serosa and directly invade either the liver or another single extrahepatic organ. T4 tumours reflect locally advanced tumours into the main portal vein, hepatic artery or multiple extrahepatic organs. Previously, the N stage was divided into locoregional and distant lymph node involvement, but due to the powerful adverse negative impact of any positive lymph node, the 6th edition staging system simply divided tumours into being either node-negative or node-positive, i.e. N0 or N1, respectively. Metastatic disease refers to distant metastasis. The AJCC 6th edition staging system is detailed in Table 13.4. The 7th edition of the AJCC staging system (2009) reverted back to stratifying nodal involvement based on location, thus creating an N1 and N2 designation, and considers T4 tumours as stage IV disease (Table 13.5).

Table 13.4 • AJCC staging system (6th edition) for gallbladder cancer (TNM classification)

Primary tumour (T)	
TX	Primary tumour cannot be assessed
T0	No evidence of primary tumour
Tis	Carcinoma in situ
T1	Tumour invades lamina propria or muscle layer
T1a	Tumour invades lamina propria
T1b	Tumour invades muscle layer
T2	Tumour invades perimuscular connective tissue: no extension beyond serosa or into liver
T3	Tumour perforates serosa (visceral peritoneum) or directly invades the liver and/or one other adjacent organ or structure, e.g. stomach, duodenum, colon pancreas, omentum, extrahepatic bile ducts
T4	Tumour invades main portal vein or hepatic artery, or invades two or more extrahepatic organs or structures
Regional lymph nodes (N)	
NX	Regional lymph nodes cannot be assessed
N0	No regional lymph node metastasis
N1	Regional lymph node metastasis
Distant metastasis (M)	
MX	Presence of distant metastasis cannot be assessed
M0	No distant metastasis
M1	Distant metastasis
Stage grouping	
Stage 0	Tis, N0, M0
Stage IA	T1, N0, M0
Stage IB	T2, N0, M0
Stage IIA	T3, N0, M0
Stage IIB	T1, N1, M0
	T2, N1, M0
	T3, N1, M0
Stage III	T4, any N, M0
Stage IV	Any T, any N, M1

Reproduced with permission from Sobin LH, Wittekind C, editors. TNM classification of malignant tumours, 6th ed. Wiley–Liss; 2002.

Table 13.5 • AJCC staging system (7th edition) for gallbladder cancer (TNM classification)

Primary tumour (T)

TX	Primary tumour cannot be assessed
T0	No evidence of primary tumour
Tis	Carcinoma in situ
T1	Tumour invades lamina propria or muscular layer
T1a	Tumour invades lamina propria
T1b	Tumour invades muscular layer
T2	Tumour invades perimuscular connective tissue; no extension beyond serosa or into liver
T3	Tumour perforates the serosa (visceral peritoneum) and/or directly invades the liver and/or one other adjacent organ or structure, such as the stomach, duodenum, colon, pancreas, omentum or extrahepatic bile ducts
T4	Tumour invades main portal vein or hepatic artery or invades two or more extrahepatic organs or structures

Regional lymph nodes (N)

NX	Regional lymph nodes cannot be assessed
N0	No regional lymph node metastasis
N1	Metastases to nodes along the cystic duct, common bile duct, hepatic artery and/or portal vein
N2	Metastases to periaortic, pericaval, superior mesenteric artery and/or coeliac artery lymph nodes

Distant metastasis (M)

M0	No distant metastasis
M1	Distant metastasis

Stage grouping

Stage 0	Tis, N0, M0
Stage I	T1, N0, M0
Stage II	T2, N0, M0
Stage IIIA	T3, N0, M0
Stage IIIB	T1, N1, M0
	T2, N1, M0
	T3, N1, M0
Stage IVA	T4, N0, M0
	T4, N1, M0
Stage IVB	Any T, N2, M0
	Any T, any N, M1

Reproduced with permission from Sobin LH, Gospodarowicz MK, Wittekind C, editors. TNM classification of malignant tumors. 7th edition. Wiley–Blackwell; 2010.

Radiological assessment

Preoperative staging should exclude distant metastases and assess the local extent of disease. It is therefore prudent to obtain cross-sectional, contrast-enhanced imaging (CT and/or MRCP). Multiphasic CT of the chest, abdomen and pelvis to include portal, venous and arterial phases should be used to assess the extent of disease in the liver and porta hepatis while also evaluating for metastatic disease. In order to elucidate relationships between the tumour and porta hepatis structures, imaging should include thin cuts through the liver and porta hepatis.

With respect to the local assessment of disease, a study of 118 patients with gallbladder carcinoma found CT to be 79% accurate for differentiating T1 and T2 tumours, 93% accurate for differentiating T2 and T3 tumours and 100% accurate for differentiating T3 and T4 tumours.[147] Additionally, MRCP with intravenous contrast is a valuable modality to assess the extent of gallbladder carcinoma. Specifically, analyses of MRI have found sensitivities of 70–100% for hepatic invasion, 100% for vascular involvement and 75% for lymph node metastases.[148,149] However, it remains unclear and relatively unstudied as to whether MRI has added benefit to that of CT. Therefore, these two imaging modalities should be considered complementary.

Along with cross-sectional imaging, hepatic duplex ultrasound imaging can add valuable information in patients with locally advanced tumours. Specifically, duplex ultrasonography has added benefit in the assessment of the extent of transmural tumoural invasion into hepatic parenchyma or biliary structures (87% accuracy). Also, duplex ultrasonography has the added benefit of simultaneously assessing for involvement of portal venous or hepatic arterial structures which can be challenging to assess on cross-sectional imaging.[150] Of note, and as is the case with cholangiocarcinoma, initial imaging studies should be performed prior to biliary stenting (if it is to be performed) as stenting will cause local inflammation making assessment of tumour extent difficult. Similar to cholangiocarcinoma, FDG-PET imaging is helpful in the identification of distant disease.

For the identification of distant metastases, a study of 61 patients with biliary tract malignancies found PET/CT to have a sensitivity of 100% compared to 25% for CT alone (P <0.001), and PET results changed surgical management in 17% of cases.[151] In an analysis of 41 patients with gallbladder carcinoma at MSKCC, preoperative PET results altered surgical management in 23% of patients (for either the initial operation or re-resection after an incidental finding following cholecystectomy).[46] Furthermore, in a recent analysis of the efficacy of PET imaging compared to CT and MRI, PET identified occult distant metastatic disease and also showed that some suspicious CT findings were negative, and altered surgical decision-making in 17% of patients.[152] Therefore, PET should be considered when evaluating patients with newly diagnosed gallbladder carcinoma, largely to evaluate for distant metastatic disease and to confirm/refute questionable findings on cross-sectional imaging.

Obstructive jaundice

Jaundice in the setting of a newly diagnosed gallbladder cancer is an ominous finding, usually representing a sign of advanced disease. Except for the uncommon patient with concomitant common bile duct stones, patients presenting with obstructive jaundice and a gallbladder malignancy have tumour involvement of the porta hepatis by either direct extension of the tumour, diffuse invasion of the porta hepatis or extensive nodal disease. Although theoretically, local extension should not necessarily affect oncologic outcome, studies have found jaundice to be an indicator of advanced malignancy with a direct survival relationship.

The authors' group has assessed 240 patients with gallbladder carcinoma and compared oncologic outcomes between those who presented with obstructive jaundice and those who did not.[153] Overall, 34% of patients within the cohort presented with obstructive jaundice. Of the jaundiced patients, 67% underwent operative exploration. Within this cohort, diagnostic laparoscopy was performed in 45% and found peritoneal metastases in 68%, precluding further exploration. Ultimately, exploratory laparotomy was undertaken in 37 patients. Among these 37 patients, distant peritoneal and liver metastases were found in 22% and locally unresectable disease in the porta hepatis was found in an additional 27% of patients. In summary, 52% of jaundiced patients who underwent exploratory laparotomy were resected with curative intent, however this represented only 7% of the entire population of jaundiced patients.[153]

With respect to oncologic outcomes, jaundiced patients compared to their non-jaundiced counterparts were more likely to have advanced-stage disease (stage III/IV) at the time of presentation (96% vs 60%, $P <0.001$) and a lower median disease-specific survival (6 vs 16 months, $P <0.0001$). Moreover, there were no disease-free survivors at 2 years in the jaundiced group, whereas 21% of the non-jaundiced patients were alive without disease at this time-point.[153]

As noted above, obstructive jaundice is a poor prognostic indicator and a marker of advanced disease in patients with gallbladder cancer. Although there is no proven correct approach to this patient population, a multidisciplinary discussion and consideration for systemic therapy, prior to undertaking surgical exploration, is warranted. As with cholangiocarcinoma, gemcitabine in combination with a platinum agent (cisplatin/ oxaliplatin) remains the standard of care.[123]

General operative principles

Contraindications to resection include distant spread (peritoneum, discontiguous liver lesions), tumour involvement of the hepatic vasculature or biliary tree that would preclude a complete resection, and presence of disease in distant lymph node groups (peripancreatic, periduodenal, periportal, coeliac and/or superior mesenteric). Although upfront resection is controversial in locally advanced disease, surgical intervention remains the mainstay of definitive therapy for gallbladder cancer.

As in patients with suspected cholangiocarcinoma, a suspicious gallbladder mass does not require a preoperative tissue diagnosis. Biopsies can result in false-negative findings and may spread tumour into the peritoneum. However, staging laparoscopy should be considered for all malignant-appearing gallbladder masses in an attempt to avoid non-therapeutic laparotomy.[154] If there is no evidence of peritoneal or hepatic metastases, laparotomy should be performed and resection undertaken with the paramount goal being to achieve a negative pathological margin.

Margin-negative resection

In an analysis of 135 patients subjected to definitive resection following an incidentally diagnosed gallbladder carcinoma, the presence of residual disease at any site was associated with significantly worse survival; specifically, the median disease-free survival (DFS) (11.2 vs 93.4 months, $P <0.0001$) and disease-specific survival (DSS) (25.2 months vs not reached, $P <0.0001$) were dramatically lower than patients without residual disease.[155] Moreover, residual disease identified at any particular site predicted DFS (HR 3.3, 95% CI 1.9–5.7, $P = 0.0003$) and DSS (HR 2.4, 95% CI 1.2–4.6, $P = 0.01$) and was independent of all other tumour-related variables.[155] The primary finding of this analysis was that survival among patients with residual disease at any site was not significantly different than those with stage IV disease.[155] Therefore, the recommended surgical approach for gallbladder carcinoma greater than T1a utilises an extended cholecystectomy to include resection of segments IVb and V of the liver along with a portal lymph node dissection. However, the reason to extend an operation beyond this (such as major hepatectomy or bile duct resection) would be an inability to obtain a negative margin.

Portal lymphadenectomy

Additionally, there are data to support portal lymphadenectomy for accurate staging.[90,156] Specifically, with locally advanced lesions it has been found that on progression of T stage from T2 to T4, nodal and distant metastases increased from 16% to 79% and from 33% to 69%, respectively.[134] Although the impact of node dissection on survival is controversial (rare 5-year survivors with N1 disease), the diagnostic information gained regarding node positivity may help in determining adjuvant therapies.[157–161]

Regional lymphadenectomy for gallbladder carcinoma should include removal of nodes in the porta hepatis, gastrohepatic ligament and retroduodenal space.[156,162,163] However, prior to proceeding with resection, the authors would recommend a complete search for metastatic disease that would preclude resection. Mobilisation of the duodenum and assessment for aortocaval, retropancreatic and/or coeliac lymphadenopathy should be performed. If the nodes in these areas are suspicious for metastatic disease, intraoperative frozen section should be obtained and the case aborted for positive results, as these nodes would be representative of distant metastatic disease.

T1/T2 tumours

T1a tumours, or those that are confined to the lamina propria, are most often discovered after, and adequately treated with, a simple cholecystectomy since the potential for nodal involvement is small and cure rates approach 85–100% if negative margins are achieved.[164] T1b tumours, i.e. those that have extended into, but not through, the muscle layer, in theory should be cured by a simple cholecystectomy as well. However, there have been reports in the literature documenting recurrence and death following a simple cholecystectomy for T1b tumours.[165] Given the limited data regarding T1b gallbladder cancers, the decision to perform a simple cholecystectomy versus a more radical procedure should be made on a case-by-case basis.

T2 lesions, or tumours that extend into the perimuscular connective tissues, should be treated with an aggressive resection, including removal of adjacent liver, lymphadenectomy of the hepatoduodenal ligament and a bile duct resection only if necessary to obtain a negative margin on the cystic duct. As discussed above, the extent of hepatic resection required depends on whether or not there is tumour involvement of the right portal pedicle (i.e. major inflow vascular structures or right hepatic duct). In the absence of such involvement, the authors prefer to perform a segmental resection of segments IVb and V, and most T2 tumours are amenable to such an approach. It should be noted that the normal plane of dissection of simple cholecystectomy, open or laparoscopic, is within the perimuscular connective tissue intimately associated with the liver. Thus, a simple cholecystectomy will not achieve tumour clearance with certainty. A lymphadenectomy is performed in the treatment of T2 tumours given that up to 50% of these lesions have associated lymph node metastases.[140] The benefit of an extended resection over simple cholecystectomy is supported by data that demonstrate improved survival. This is underscored by the fact that liver involvement can be found after radical resection in up to a quarter of patients with presumed T2 disease after cholecystectomy alone, a finding that is associated with markedly reduced recurrence-free and disease-specific survival.[162] De Aretxabala et al. reported 5-year survival rates of 70% compared with only 20% after simple cholecystectomy alone.[166]

Extended resections

In the setting of locally advanced disease (T3/T4), many cases will require division of the left hepatic duct and excision of the biliary confluence along with an extended right hepatectomy. If the right hepatic duct and/or biliary confluence is involved, an extended right hepatectomy is mandatory for complete resection of the tumour. In most cases, it is the involvement of major hepatic vascular structures rather than parenchyma involvement that dictates the extent of hepatic resection required.

> ✔✔ With respect to the extent of resection, an analysis at MSKCC in 104 patients with gallbladder cancer found tumour biology and stage, rather than the extent of resection to predict disease-specific survival. Major hepatic resections, including extended hepatectomy and CBD excision, were proven appropriate when necessary to achieve negative pathological margins and were associated with acceptable long-term survival.[135] Therefore, as in cholangiocarcinoma, the extent of resection should be dictated by what is necessary to achieve a negative margin.

Unsuspected malignancy at exploration

It should be routine to inspect the gallbladder mucosa after simple cholecystectomy. Suspicious lesions should be sent immediately for frozen section. If a carcinoma is diagnosed, the need to perform additional surgery is dictated by the T stage on frozen section, although the information will be limited since a full histopathological evaluation is not available at the time of operation. The authors prefer to perform an oncologically correct resection, suitable for an invasive lesion, at the time it is discovered, unless there are extenuating circumstances that mandate otherwise. However, if the surgeon is not comfortable with performing a radical cholecystectomy/hepatic resection, the patient is best served by transferring them to a centre/surgeon with experience in performing the appropriate operation. A delayed radical and appropriate resection does not negatively influence the patient's outcome.[134]

Malignancy diagnosed post-cholecystectomy

When the cancer is diagnosed by postoperative histology, the need for a more radical resection will be based on T stage, as outlined above. Fong et al. demonstrated a much improved 5-year survival rate in patients undergoing a second operation compared to those who did not. Five-year survival rates of 61% were achieved in patients who were re-resected compared to 19% for patients who did not undergo a radical second operation.[134] However, prior to undertaking a second operation, high-quality cross-sectional imaging (CT/MRI) should be obtained to appropriately stage the disease. Postoperative inflammatory changes may be indistinguishable from tumour and thus may necessitate bile duct resection or a more aggressive hepatic resection to ensure complete tumour eradication.

✅ Given that inadvertent cholecystotomy during cholecystectomy is rarely documented, it is difficult to predict who is at increased risk for peritoneal dissemination and, specifically, port site recurrence. In the past, routine resection of laparoscopic port sites was recommended, in an effort to ensure clearance of microscopic disease that may have implanted during the laparoscopic procedure. However, there is little evidence to support the efficacy of routine resection of all port sites at re-operation. In the authors' experience, recurrence at the port sites is a harbinger of generalised peritoneal recurrence that will not be prevented with resection of these limited areas.

Adjuvant therapy

In order to provide a rational framework upon which to develop adjuvant therapies for patients having undergone resection, Jarnagin et al. investigated the initial pattern of recurrence after resection of biliary tract cancers. Sixty-six per cent of patients with gallbladder cancers who underwent a potentially curative resection recurred within a median follow-up of 24 months. Only 15% of patients developed a locoregional recurrence as the first site of failure, while the majority of patients (85%) had recurrence that involved a distant site.[167] Thus, local therapies targeted at locoregional disease, such as radiotherapy, are unlikely to significantly impact the course of this disease, further emphasising the importance of developing effective systemic adjuvant therapies.

Most data for the use of adjuvant therapy are derived from phase II trials in which treated patients are compared with historical controls. Most of these trials are limited by small numbers, combine chemotherapy with radiation treatment, and are confounded by inclusion of patients with an R1 resection.[168] Thus, minimal conclusions can be drawn regarding the use of external beam radiation/chemotherapy in the adjuvant setting. In cases of incomplete resection, there remains a theoretical benefit to adding an additional locoregional therapy such as external beam radiation therapy for disease control.

✅✅ One phase III multi-institutional trial of adjuvant chemotherapy was performed in Japan as reported by Takada et al.[103] It should be noted that this trial included 508 patients with biliary and pancreatic cancers. However, on subset analysis, this study included 140 patients with gallbladder cancer who were randomised to undergo surgical resection alone or resection plus adjuvant mitomycin and 5FU. In considering only the patients with gallbladder cancer, the actuarial 5-year disease-free survival favoured the adjuvant chemotherapy group in comparison to the surgery-alone group (20.3% vs 11.6%). From these data, it is reasonable to offer adjuvant chemotherapy with 5FU and mitomycin; however, no consensus has been reached regarding routine use of adjuvant chemotherapy.

Key points

- In hilar cholangiocarcinoma preoperative assessment is mainly a decision of resectability. Attention should be paid to the extent of bile duct involvement, portal vein involvement and to the presence or absence of hepatic atrophy.
- Complete resection for hilar cholangiocarcinoma necessitates a hepatectomy; achievement of a negative pathological margin (R0) is of paramount importance (in terms of survival, residual disease is synonymous with stage IV disease).

- Chemotherapy and radiotherapy may have benefit in the adjuvant setting but currently remain investigational.
- The clinical presentation in distal cholangiocarcinoma is very similar to that of other periampullary tumours.
- Similar to hilar disease, a preoperative tissue diagnosis is not necessary to proceed with surgical resection.
- When possible, endoscopic palliation is the preferred method to relieve symptomatic jaundice in the setting of unresectable disease.
- Hepatocellular carcinoma must be excluded in patients with an intrahepatic mass.
- Metastatic adenocarcinoma to the liver from a remote primary, such as lung, breast or gastrointestinal, must be excluded.
- Similar to all other locations of cholangiocarcinoma, complete surgical resection of an intrahepatic cholangiocarcinoma is the optimal treatment and only chance for cure.
- In gallbladder cancer, a cholecystectomy should be performed for adenomatous polyps >1 cm, or those that are smaller but growing and changing in character. Cholesterol polyps and adenomyomatosis are not premalignant conditions.
- Complete surgical resection is the goal, whether the diagnosis is made preoperatively, intraoperatively or after a non-curative laparoscopic cholecystectomy.
- In patients with invasion into the common bile duct, consideration should be given to neoadjuvant chemotherapy prior to surgical exploration in an attempt to best select patients for potentially curative resection.
- Obstructive jaundice in the setting of gallbladder carcinoma portends poor survival and systemic therapy should be considered prior to entertaining surgical resection.

⬤ Recommended videos:

- Extended right hepatectomy – https://tinyurl.com/ybkfl6dp
- Extended left hepatectomy – https://tinyurl.com/yaseqppf
- Hepatectomy with portal vein resection – https://tinyurl.com/ya9np7s9

🌐 Full references available at **http://expertconsult.inkling.com**

Key references

3. Esnaola NF, Meyer JE, Karachristos A, et al. Evaluation and management of intrahepatic and extrahepatic cholangiocarcinoma. Cancer 2016;122(9):1349–69. PMID: 26799932.
This current review focuses on recent advances in the diagnosis and treatment of patients with cholangiocarcinoma and, in particular, on the role of endoscopy, surgery, transplantation, radiotherapy, systemic therapy and liver-directed therapies in the curative or palliative treatment of these individuals.

57. Bismuth H, Nakache R, Diamond T. Management strategies in resection for hilar cholangiocarcinoma. Ann Surg 1992;215(1):31–8. PMID: 1309988.
Seminal paper where results indicate that improved survival in hilar cholangiocarcinoma can be achieved by resection, with minimal morbidity and zero mortality rates, if histologically free resection margins are obtained.

58. Jarnagin WR, Fong Y, DeMatteo RP, et al. Staging, resectability, and outcome in 225 patients with hilar cholangiocarcinoma. Ann Surg 2001;234(4):507–17; discussion 517–9. PMID: 11573044.
By taking full account of local tumour extent, the proposed staging system for hilar cholangiocarcinoma accurately predicts resectability, the likelihood of metastatic disease, and survival. Complete resection remains the only therapy that offers the possibility of long-term survival, and hepatic resection is a critical component of the surgical approach.

59. Matsuo K, Rocha FG, Ito K, et al. The Blumgart preoperative staging system for hilar cholangiocarcinoma: analysis of resectability and outcomes in 380 patients. J Am Coll Surg 2012;215(3):343–55. PMID: 22749003.
The preoperative clinical T-staging system of Blumgart, defined by the radial and longitudinal tumour extent, accurately predicts resectability of

hilar cholangiocarcinoma. The full outcomes benefit of resection is realised only if a concomitant partial hepatectomy is performed.

64. Wiggers JK, Groot Koerkamp B, Cieslak KP, et al. Postoperative mortality after liver resection for perihilar cholangiocarcinoma: development of a risk score and importance of biliary drainage of the future liver remnant. J Am Coll Surg 2016;223(2):321–31. e1. PMID: 27063572.
The mortality risk score for patients with resectable hilar cholangiocarcinoma can be used for patient counselling and identification of modifiable risk factors, which include FLR volume, FLR drainage status, and preoperative cholangitis. No evidence to support preoperative biliary drainage in patients with an FLR volume >50% was identified.

76. Ribero D, Abdalla EK, Madoff DC, et al. Portal vein embolization before major hepatectomy and its effects on regeneration, resectability and outcome. Br J Surg 2007;94(11):1386–94. PMID: 17583900.
This study evaluated the safety of portal vein embolisation (PVE), its impact on future liver remnant (FLR) volume and regeneration, and subsequent effects on outcome after liver resection.

94. Cheng QB, Yi B, Wang JH, et al. Resection with total caudate lobectomy confers survival benefit in hilar cholangiocarcinoma of Bismuth type III and IV. Eur J Surg Oncol 2012;38(12):1197–203. PMID: 22992326.
Study to identify prognostic predictors for overall survival of patients with hilar cholangiocarcinoma of Bismuth type III and IV, and to determine survival benefit and safety of total caudate lobectomy. Resection with total caudate lobectomy offers a long-term survival opportunity for patients with hilar cholangiocarcinoma, with high curative resectability rates and an acceptable safety profile.

97. Neuhaus P, Jonas S, Bechstein WO, et al. Extended resections for hilar cholangiocarcinoma. Ann Surg 1999;230(6): 808–18; discussion 819. PMID: 10615936.
Extended resections, especially right trisegmentectomy resulted in the highest rate of R0 resection. Right trisegmentectomy together with portal vein resection best represents the principles of surgical oncology and may be regarded as the surgical procedure of choice.

105. Primrose JN, Fox R, Palmer DH, et al. Adjuvant Capecitabine for biliary tract cancer: The BILCAP randomized study. Journal of Clinical Oncology 2017;35(15_suppl):4006.
The results of the BILCAP trial will shape the practice of adjuvant therapy after resection of biliary tract malignancies. Given these data, adjuvant capecitabine will likely become the new standard of care for patients undergoing upfront resection of biliary tract malignancy.

123. Valle J, Wasan H, Palmer DH, et al. Cisplatin plus gemcitabine versus gemcitabine for biliary tract cancer. N Engl J Med 2010;362(14):1273–81. PMID: 20375404.
This study shows a significant survival advantage for cisplatin plus gemcitabine over gemcitabine alone in patients with advanced biliary cancer. Cisplatin plus gemcitabine is an appropriate option for treatment of these patients.

131. Konstantinidis IT, Groot Koerkamp B, Do RK, et al. Unresectable intrahepatic cholangiocarcinoma: systemic plus hepatic arterial infusion chemotherapy is associated with longer survival in comparison with systemic chemotherapy alone. Cancer 2016;122(5):758–65. PMID: 26695839.
In patients with unresectable intrahepatic cholangiocarcinoma confined to the liver or with limited regional nodal disease, a combination of systemic therapy and hepatic arterial infusion chemotherapy is associated with greater survival than systemic alone.

135. D'Angelica M, Dalal KM, DeMatteo RP, et al. Analysis of the extent of resection for adenocarcinoma of the gallbladder. Ann Surg Oncol 2009;16(4):806–16. PMID: 18985272.
Tumour biology and stage, rather than extent of resection, predict outcome after resection for gallbladder cancer. Major hepatic resections, including bile duct excision, are appropriate when necessary to clear disease but are not mandatory in all cases.

14

Complicated acute pancreatitis

Euan J. Dickson
C. Ross Carter
Colin J. McKay

Introduction

Complications following acute pancreatitis occur on a spectrum of severity, complexity and chronology. The majority of patients with acute pancreatitis (AP) recover with simple supportive management including intravenous fluids and analgesia. Approximately 20%, however, develop severe acute pancreatitis with local and/or systemic complications. Of this subgroup, up to half will die as a result of complications of their disease.

Successful management of the patient with complications following AP is challenging and best undertaken by a multidisciplinary team. Decision-making is complex, multimodal therapy is often required and the hospital stay is likely to be protracted. Increasingly, these patients are managed, at least initially, in the base hospital. Early and regular discussion with a specialist unit is recommended and those patients who exceed local institutional capability should be considered for transfer.

Initial management

The initial management of acute pancreatitis is covered in the relevant chapter of the Core Topics in General and Emergency Surgery volume of this series and is addressed in several guidelines and consensus statements. The most recent and relevant of these is the International Association of Pancreatology/American Pancreatic Association Guidelines of 2013 (IAP/APA Working Group 2013).[1] This chapter will therefore focus on the management of complications of acute pancreatitis.

Key concepts

There are three key concepts in the current management of complications of acute pancreatitis (Box 14.1).

Definitions and terminology in acute pancreatitis

The original Atlanta Classification of acute pancreatitis was published in 1993[2] in an effort to define the disease and clarify the terminology. Over the subsequent two decades, understanding of the correlation between clinical, radiological and pathological features has improved. This is largely as a result of advances in medical imaging technology and, in particular, contrast enhanced computed tomography (CECT).

The revised Atlanta Classification was published in 2013[3] and sought to address the recognised deficiencies and confusion inherent in the previous definitions. Two phases of the disease process are identified: early and late, arbitrarily defined as less than/more than 4 weeks from presentation. A third category has been added to disease severity, which is now classified as mild, moderate or severe (Box 14.2).

The ability to interpret fluid collections and necrosis is critical to decision-making regarding management, particularly intervention. The revised Atlanta Classification of these local complications is a significant improvement over the original definitions. Local fluid collections are now defined based on time from presentation and content,

1. Patient pathophysiology, rather than anatomy of disease, determines the need for intervention. Serial clinical review identifies global trends in patient trajectory and guides management.
2. If intervention is considered necessary it should in general be delayed for as long as possible (unless immediately life-saving) and is best avoided in the first 2 weeks following the index episode.
3. Each intervention carries risk and benefit – therapeutic gain is maximised when the intervention is limited to that which is absolutely necessary (the 'step-up approach'). Radiological, endoscopic and other minimally invasive techniques are replacing major open surgical intervention.

Box 14.2 • Revised Atlanta Classification (2012)

Mild acute pancreatitis
– no organ failure, local or systemic complications and usually resolves within a week

Moderately severe acute pancreatitis
– transient organ failure, local complications or exacerbation of comorbid disease

Severe acute pancreatitis
– persistent organ failure (duration >48 hours)

as acute peripancreatic fluid collections (APFC), pseudocyst, acute necrotic collection (ANC) and walled-off necrosis (WON). Collections may be sterile or infected. The management of each of these differs and is outlined below with the updated definitions.

Acute peripancreatic fluid collection (APFC)

In the early stages of acute pancreatitis, up to 25% of patients will develop a fluid collection in the peripancreatic region. On contrast-enhanced computed tomography (CECT), APFCs are ill-defined, homogeneous and may be multiple. Pancreatic vascular perfusion on CECT is normal, and there should be no necrotic material (e.g. peripancreatic fat) within the collection. Most acute fluid collections remain sterile, usually resolve without intervention and are of little clinical significance. There are, however, significant risks associated with aspiration and especially external drainage. These unnecessary interventions may introduce infection. Whilst most APFCs resolve spontaneously, a small number may persist beyond 4 weeks and develop into a pancreatic pseudocyst.

Pancreatic pseudocyst

A pancreatic pseudocyst refers specifically to a fluid collection with no solid component persisting beyond 4 weeks of presentation. It is predominantly in the peripancreatic tissues, although it may be partially or wholly within the pancreatic parenchyma. With time a well-defined wall will develop. Most post-acute collections described as pseudocysts are actually walled-off necrotic collections with a relatively minor volume of necrosis. Persistence of an acute fluid collection beyond 4 weeks is thought to result from disruption of the main pancreatic duct or its side branches, and the fluid within has a very high amylase content. Disruption of the duct will only occur following necrosis of either the duct or parenchyma and pancreatic necrosis must be present by definition. Therefore, a pancreatic pseudocyst is extremely rare in acute pancreatitis and most persistent collections should be thought of and managed as walled-off necrotic collections. CECT often underestimates the degree of solid material and MRI or EUS may be required to determine the volume of necrosis.

Asymptomatic or small pseudocysts do not require treatment, and many will eventually resolve spontaneously. Acute pseudocysts are most commonly retrogastric, and may or may not communicate with a disrupted pancreatic duct. Three-quarters will be associated with a mild to moderate hyperamylasaemia.

Necrosis

The revised Atlanta Classification dichotomises necrosis according to the phase of the disease process, with an arbitrary cut-point at 4 weeks.

Acute necrotic collection

Acute necrotic collection (ANC) is the terminology used to describe a fluid collection with a solid necrotic component within the first 4 weeks following presentation. The fluid and solid components occur in variable proportions. It is therefore distinct from an APFC, which contains fluid only. The necrotic process may involve both the pancreas and peripancreatic tissues. On CECT these collections may be multiple, ill-defined and loculated.

Walled-off necrosis

Walled-off necrosis (WON) also contains necrosis but occurs later in the disease process (after 4 weeks). On CECT it has a well-defined, mature, enhancing wall of reactive tissue and contains fluid and solid necrotic material. The nomenclature of this entity has perhaps undergone the greatest number of revisions over the last few decades and these are not revisited here in an effort to minimise confusion. WON can also occur at multiple sites, which may or may not communicate with each other, and can extend to more distant areas including the mesentery, making access challenging.

Sterile and infected collections

As will be discussed later, the development of infection within a collection has a profound effect on the clinical course and the need for intervention. All collections can become infected but this is unusual in the absence of necrosis, and infected acute fluid collections or pseudocysts are rare. Sepsis almost universally presents as an infected ANC or infected WON, the management of which will be discussed in a subsequent section. Infection may occur at any stage but is most frequent in the second and third weeks following presentation, and may be suspected through clinical deterioration, usually associated with a rising inflammatory response, and should prompt urgent CT.

> ✔ Local complications of acute pancreatitis are defined by time (< / > 4 weeks) and by necrosis (present or absent).

Clinical patterns and complications

Complications of acute pancreatitis may be broadly considered as systemic or local. These are inextricably linked and both may be present to varying degrees.

The clinical progress of a patient with pancreatitis, including the development of systemic or local complications is not a binary process but rather a dynamic continuum with the potential for rapid deterioration. Within this continuum, patterns of clinical behaviour are apparent.

Early phase complications (<4 weeks)

Systemic complications

Organ failure

The majority of patients with clinically mild acute pancreatitis may be managed in a ward environment. Patients with evidence of clinical deterioration, and in particular those with persistent organ dysfunction, should be managed in a critical care environment. Early indication for critical care support is usually as a result of an uncontrolled systemic inflammatory response resulting in organ failure. Late deterioration requiring critical care support is often the consequence of inadequately controlled sepsis, which is a risk factor for life-threatening haemorrhage, and often precedes terminal decline.

Severe acute pancreatitis is frequently associated with organ failure. Respiratory, cardiovascular, renal and gastrointestinal dysfunction are the most commonly involved systems. Deteriorating organ function mandates critical care support in the high dependency unit (HDU) or intensive care unit (ICU).

Respiratory failure should prompt early discussion with the critical care team. Whilst non-invasive respiratory support may be sufficient for some patients, others require early mechanical ventilation and the transition from one level of support to the other can be rapid.

Cardiovascular collapse is treated with aggressive volume resuscitation directed towards optimising tissue perfusion. This should include addressing both haemodynamic targets and parameters of cellular respiration. Acid–base balance, lactate and mixed venous oxygen saturation are helpful in assessing adequacy of volume restoration. Vasoactive support is often required as a bridge whilst restoring circulating volume.

Renal failure as a consequence of cardiovascular compromise and reduced perfusion is common. Management again involves prompt volume resuscitation and close attention to fluid balance. Dialysis may be required for fluid overload, hyperkalaemia or acidosis. Recovering renal function in this context is a helpful marker of global improvement in physiology.

Reduced visceral perfusion may also result in gastrointestinal dysfunction. Gastrointestinal blood flow is further compromised by splanchnic vasoconstriction, either as a consequence of shock physiology or secondary to exogenous vasoconstrictor support. This manifests as abdominal bloating, nausea and vomiting and has two significant clinical sequelae. Firstly, patients may be unable to tolerate enteral nutrition including nasojejunal feeding. Secondly, inadequate mucosal perfusion leads to breakdown of the intestinal barrier function and is associated with bacterial translocation and infection of pre-existing necrosis.

> ✔ Deteriorating physiology should prompt early critical care input regardless of 'predicted severity'.

Intra-abdominal hypertension (IAH)

IAH is recognised as a contributing factor to organ dysfunction in the context of a variety of acute abdominal processes. Most of the literature to date focuses on trauma patients, but there is increasing interest in its role in patients with severe acute pancreatitis. There are data to suggest that raised intra-abdominal pressure (IAP) may be associated with disease severity, organ failure and mortality in severe acute pancreatitis.

There are, however, no data to suggest improved outcome following surgical decompression for raised IAP in acute pancreatitis, and indeed this may be harmful. Abdominal compartment syndrome (raised IAP with associated organ failure) should initially be managed medically according to existing guidelines.[4] A decision to proceed to decompressive laparostomy may be made on an individual case basis within a multidisciplinary team setting, but there is currently no evidence base for this approach.

> ✔ There is currently no evidence base for the role of decompressive laparostomy in acute pancreatitis.

The role of ERCP in acute pancreatitis

There has been long-standing controversy over the role and timing of endoscopic retrograde cholangiopancreatography (ERCP) in gallstone pancreatitis, with conflicting results from randomised trials. However, there are now several meta-analyses of the randomised evidence clarifying the position.[5,6]

There is no role for early ERCP in mild pancreatitis. Following complete resolution of mild gallstone pancreatitis there may be a role for ERCP and sphincterotomy as definitive management where cholecystectomy is precluded by comorbidity.[7]

In patients with severe disease, there is a subgroup that present with hyperamylasaemia, pain, jaundice and fever within 12 hours of presentation. Early recognition that these patients have organ dysfunction secondary to biliary sepsis rather than pancreatitis, the hyperamylasaemia being incidental, should prompt an ERCP and biliary decompression.

A management dilemma, however, exists in the subgroup of patients with acute pancreatitis and jaundice as it may be difficult to differentiate between the systemic inflammatory response syndrome (SIRS) driven by acute pancreatitis and 'true' cholangitis. There is a lack of clear evidence regarding the role of early ERCP in patients with pancreatitis and jaundice but without evidence of cholangitis. In addition, unnecessary ERCP carries risk and may be technically challenging in the context of duodenal and periampullary oedema. The majority of duct stones causing acute pancreatitis are expected to pass spontaneously, and it may therefore be helpful to observe these patients for 24–48 hours and then divide them into one of three groups to determine if there is a need for ERCP (Box 14.3).

Box 14.3 • ERCP algorithm for acute pancreatitis

1. Patients with resolving jaundice
   – **observe**
2. Patients with persistent jaundice but clinically improving
   – biliary **imaging** with MRCP or EUS
3. Patients with persistent jaundice and clinical deterioration
   – **ERCP** and biliary decompression

ERCP, endoscopic retrograde cholangiopancreatography; EUS, endoscopy-guided ultrasound; MRCP, magnetic resonance cholangiopancreatography.

Early haemorrhage

In the era of early surgical debridement, the term haemorrhagic pancreatitis[8] was often used to describe the presence of blood within the necrotic pancreatic and peripancreatic tissue found at laparotomy. Active haemorrhage is, however, extremely rare in the acute phase in the absence of intervention.

Colonic ischaemia

Mesenteric vascular compromise is extremely common in severe acute pancreatitis, usually as part of global systemic hypoperfusion. Mucosal hypoperfusion has been postulated as a potential source of secondary infection of acute necrotic collections.[9] This is believed to be modulated through bacterial translocation as a result of a breakdown in the mucosal barrier. At laparotomy and debridement, the vascular integrity of the colon often appears questionable, leading to a relatively high incidence of colectomy. Full-thickness intestinal ischaemia is fortunately relatively rare, and is seen much less frequently in the minimally invasive era. Patchy full-thickness ischaemia may lead to fistulation with secondary sepsis (Fig. 14.1). Defunctioning ileostomy may be required for sepsis control.

Late complications (>4 weeks)
Management of collections associated with acute pancreatitis
Management of necrosis

As previously stated, intervention is usually required only for ANC or WON, the majority of acute fluid collections resolving spontaneously. The management algorithm for pancreatic necrosis has altered radically in the last 20 years in response to evolving concepts, improved understanding of the disease process and the development of minimally invasive techniques. These techniques include percutaneous,[10–12] laparoscopic[13] and endoscopic drainage[14,15] procedures as an alternative to conventional open debridement.

The necrotic process associated with pancreatitis tends to involve both the pancreatic parenchyma and surrounding adipose tissue. Significant quantities of necrotic peripancreatic tissue can be present with an essentially viable gland. Complications relate to the extent of the necrotic process, and in particular the extent of parenchymal necrosis.

It is key to recognise that the presence of necrosis in itself is not an indication for intervention. The previously held concept that recovery would not occur until almost complete removal of necrosis had been achieved[16] has been progressively challenged and the focus of intervention is now on the 'adequate and maintained control of sepsis'. The PANTER trial[17] demonstrated that 35% of patients will resolve completely without necrosectomy in the absence of

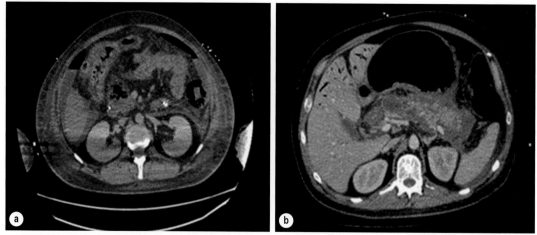

Figure 14.1 • Colonic ischaemia with fistulation. **(a)** Gas within acute necrotic collection in the head of pancreas, oedematous colon and free intraperitoneal gas and fluid levels laterally. **(b)** Portal pyaemia with gas within the peripheral intrahepatic portal venous radicals.

sepsis. Given sufficient time, 'organisation' occurs – solid components within a collection are gradually broken down through enzymatic and phagocytic activity, and pancreatic necrosis may resolve completely with resultant fibrosis and atrophy.

Successful management involves individualised multimodal care, selecting the appropriate intervention and technique for each stage of the patient pathway. A multidisciplinary approach has evolved, and it is now common for several different techniques to be utilised in an individual patient. The choice of intervention is dictated by physiology, anatomy and timing of disease and is underpinned by an understanding of the dynamic evolution of post-acute, necrosis-associated collections in pancreatitis. The success of various approaches will be dependent on the anatomical position of the collection and particularly the ratio of solid to fluid components.

The proess of maturation or 'organisation' takes in excess of 12 weeks to complete, during which four stages can be recognised (Box 14.4).

Historically, early aggressive debridement in the absence of infection was advocated. However, mortality

Box 14.4 • Evolution of pancreatic necrosis/collections

1. True pancreatic necrosis – minimal separation of devitalised tissue with a high solid/fluid ratio.
2. Transitional pancreatic necrosis with partial but incomplete separation.
3. Walled-off necrosis (WON) – good separation of devitalised tissue within a fluid-filled cavity and formation of a fibrous wall lined with granulation tissue.
4. Pseudocyst – almost complete resolution of any solid component and a well-formed fibrous wall lined with granulation tissue.

in this setting was high, and the only randomised study of early versus late (>12 days) necrosectomy[18] was discontinued as a result of the mortality rate in the early treatment group (56% vs 27%). The general principle is now to withhold surgery in the early phase of disease, operating for complications ideally once the acute inflammatory insult has subsided.

Indications for intervention

There are three main indications for intervention: sepsis, symptoms or persistence of the collection over several months. Early drainage (<6 weeks) may be potentially harmful by introducing infection into a poorly defined collection. Minimally invasive techniques often require sequential procedures within an established management protocol and should not be undertaken in isolation.

There is no role for the early drainage of acute collections in the absence of suspected sepsis. Clinical deterioration usually manifests through an escalation in the Early Warning Score,[19] along with a rise in biochemical or haematological markers of sepsis. Suspected sepsis mandates urgent CT confirmation of the diagnosis, resuscitation, antimicrobial therapy and prompt drainage for control. Of note, in the deteriorating patient with clinical evidence of sepsis, the absence of gas in a collection does not exclude infected necrosis. Although fine-needle aspiration of the collection to confirm or refute infection has been advocated,[20] the authors do not recommend it. In the patient with escalating SIRS or multiple organ dysfunction syndrome (MODS) and a drainable collection, percutaneous or endoscopic drainage should be performed within a step-up context, and positive culture of the aspirate is almost universally present.

A caveat exists where there is a clinical radiological mismatch on CECT (i.e. the patient is well but there

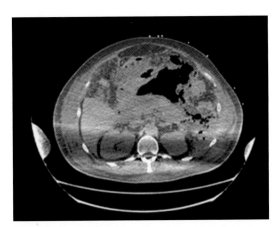

Figure 14.2 • Radiological mismatch – extensive gas within an acute necrotic collection following foregut fistulation in an otherwise clinically well patient.

is gas present in the collection, see Fig. 14.2), and the possibility of spontaneous discharge of the collection into an adjacent hollow viscus should be considered. In this scenario, whilst bacterial colonisation of the collection will have occurred, spontaneous discharge may result in resolution without intervention.

Symptoms requiring intervention include pain, early satiety and gastric outlet obstruction, the latter two arising from the local mass effect of the WON in relation to the stomach. Intervention for symptoms is not required with the same degree of urgency and there is often a place for nutritional optimisation with enteral feeding to allow the WON to 'mature' or even resolve.

Persistence of WON over several months is a relative indication for intervention and should be balanced against the individualised risks of the proposed procedure. Once the decision has been made to intervene, the options include percutaneous, endoscopic, laparoscopic or surgical drainage. This choice is largely determined by institutional capabilities, patient physiology and the position of the WON relative to other structures, particularly the stomach.

☑ There are three indications for intervention on collections: sepsis, symptoms and failure of resolution.

Sepsis control in an infected acute necrotic or walled-off collection (early phase, 2–6 weeks)

Infected pancreatic necrosis has previously been described as the most feared surgical complication of acute pancreatitis. This led to the development of protocol-driven management in the 1990s, aimed at the early identification of secondary infection within necrosis. The authors' approach has progressed from one based on the presence or absence of infection to one based on time from onset, organ dysfunction and anatomical position of the collection.

Methods of sepsis control

The traditional approach to infected necrosis was open laparotomy/debridement. These approaches are falling from favour with increasing evidence that minimally invasive intervention may reduce morbidity/mortality;[21] however, open debridement remains the method of choice in some countries.

Minimally invasive approaches to infected necrosis

Minimally invasive surgery provokes a reduced inflammatory response when compared to equivalent open surgery, and there is experimental evidence suggesting that local sepsis and the inflammatory response may be lessened by a minimally invasive rather than an open technique.

☑☑ The PANTER trial and several prospective cohort series have suggested that by avoiding the massive inflammatory 'hit' of open pancreatic necrosectomy, a minimally invasive approach to infected pancreatic necrosis may reduce the risk of post-procedural organ failure and wound morbidity.[17,21]

However, there is as yet no evidence that one minimally invasive approach is superior to another,[22] and the choice of modality is dependent on the anatomical position of the collection and the available local skills and resources.

Percutaneous drainage

Freeny et al.,[10] combining aggressive CT-guided percutaneous drainage (PCD) with continuous post-drainage lavage, demonstrated resolution of pancreatic abscesses in nearly 50% of patients. The remaining patients required subsequent surgical intervention for residual sepsis. Drain occlusion is common due to necrotic debris and repeated drains may be necessary. Simple drainage, even with small-diameter drains, may be associated with complete resolution and within the PANTER trial[17] 'step-up' arm, 35% of patients were successfully managed by small-bore (4-mm) percutaneous drainage alone.

Minimally invasive surgery

Control and prevention of recurrent sepsis is core to recovery. Inadequate control leads to failure to progress and an increased rate of secondary complications (e.g. bleeding). Enhanced percutaneous drainage (+/– percutaneous necrosectomy) aims to optimise sepsis control. Sequential drain tract dilatation allowing insertion of a large bore (30-Fr) double-lumen lavage system is the simplest 'step-up' approach over PCD. Formal debridement using a urological rigid-rod lens system can remove devitalised tissue and prevent drain blockage. In other centres as well as within our own patient cohort, this technique has significantly reduced mortality.

The Dutch Pancreatitis Study Group have popularised a video-assisted retroperitoneal debridement technique[23] (VARD) using a variation of the Fagniez technique[24] through a small, 5-cm incision in the left flank. Their management approach has evolved from being initially performed on all patients with infected necrosis, to now being used as a 'step-up' approach should initial PCD fail to control sepsis. The Dutch group has completed a randomised trial comparing this minimally invasive two-stage 'step-up' approach with open necrosectomy[17] and has shown a reduction in early organ failure (respiratory) and late morbidity, but the study was underpowered to address mortality.

Endoscopic necrosectomy

The principle of tract dilatation and minimally invasive necrosectomy has also been used with the endoscopic approach. Seifert et al.[25] have reported the dilatation of an endocyst-gastrostomy tract, allowing insertion of the endoscope into the retroperitoneum and subsequent piecemeal debridement. More recently, the use of multiple transgastric cystgastrostomy puncture sites has been reported, allowing nasocystic lavage and stent-assisted drainage through alternative drainage sites with good sepsis control. Lumen-opposing stents (Hot AXIOS) allow rapid decompression of necrosis-associated WON, and are often the treatment of choice in a critically ill patient as this can be performed at the bedside in the ICU. It is essential that a post-drainage protocol is followed to prevent blockage of the cystgastrostomy with recurrent sepsis. Although extremely effective as an initial intervention, increased use has seen a relatively high incidence of stent-associated morbidity, with recurrent sepsis, haemorrhage and stent migration being described (Fig. 14.3).

> ✔ There is currently no evidence that one minimally invasive technique has any advantage over another and choice is often determined by institutional capability.

Open laparotomy/debridement

Although the method of choice in the 1980s, open surgery and debridement is now relatively uncommon in most UK specialist centres. As originally described, the complete exposure of the retroperitoneum, with mobilisation of both colonic flexures originally arose through the unavailability of adequate axial scanning. A more limited laparotomy focused on adequate drainage of acute necrotic or walled-off collections identified on CECT has been suggested by some as a superior alternative in a fit patient with no organ compromise (Fig. 14.4). This may allow rapid recovery and avoid the repeated interventions and prolonged hospital stay associated with minimally invasive procedures. This approach is most appropriate where the collection has matured and complete separation of the necrosis has occurred. Fig. 14.4 illustrates the exposed SMA following open evacuation of haematoma following a bleed into a walled off necrotic cavity. Adequate and definitive drainage can

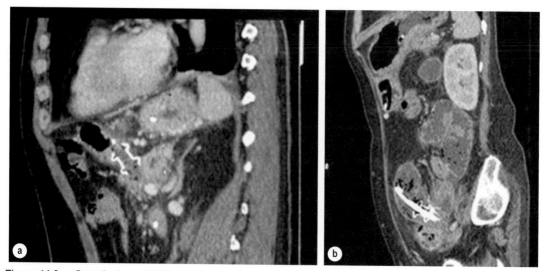

Figure 14.3 • Complications of EUS-guided cystgastrostomy. **(a)** Internal migration of SEMS; **(b)** intraluminal migration with small bowel obstruction.

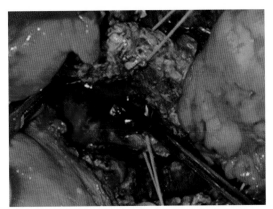

Figure 14.4 • Open necrosectomy following acute haemorrhage managed by interventional radiological embolisation of a branch of the superior mesenteric artery, with loss of the head and uncinate process.

then be achieved through a single intervention, often draining a collection through the posterior wall of the stomach (cystgastrostomy). This can be performed at open surgery or by laparoscopy.

Where organisation is incomplete, usually as a result of early intervention being mandated for sepsis, incomplete debridement carries a high incidence of recurrent sepsis, and several methods of maintaining sepsis control following debridement have been described. The commonest approach is closed lavage, popularised by Beger,[26] but open laparostomy[27] or closed packing[28] approaches are equally effective, and the method of choice often reflects local experience.

Retrocolic/perineal/mesenteric necrosis

Peripancreatic extension of the necrotic process commonly follows fat planes into the small bowel or colonic mesentery. It may also extend extraperitoneally behind the colon and abdominal wall, occasionally reaching the perineum. Adequate drainage of mesenteric extension without compromising the vasculature can be challenging, and patience is often rewarded. Retrocolic extensions often require multimodal, minimally invasive access drainage at several sites and, particularly with horseshoe collections, the VARD approach can be particularly useful (Fig. 14.5).

> ✓ Open surgery has largely been replaced by minimally invasive alternatives, but may occasionally be required to achieve control of sepsis and/or bleeding.

Nutritional support

Acute pancreatitis, particularly in the context of complications, is often a prolonged and profoundly catabolic illness. Nutritional insufficiency should

be anticipated and managed proactively. There are two important but distinct considerations: (1) the mode of nutritional delivery, and (2) the potential to impact the disease process through the use of immunomodulating feeds.

Nutritional delivery in the patient with acute pancreatitis

The traditional management of acute pancreatitis was to promote gut rest and address nutritional requirements parenterally, yet there is no evidence to support this. The early randomised studies of total parenteral nutrition (TPN) versus fasting,[29] or enteral feeding[30] demonstrated a negative effect of TPN, as a result of TPN-associated side-effects.

> ✓✓ A Cochrane review including eight randomised trials, demonstrated a reduction in mortality, systemic complications and surgical intervention in patients given enteral nutrition.[31]

Most experience to date has been with enteral feeding distal to the duodenojejunal flexure. More recently, nasogastric (NG)[31a] feeding has been shown to be a practical alternative to jejunal feeding. All studies in this area are underpowered but in the absence of definitive evidence it is reasonable to attempt this route prior to considering nasojejunal (NJ) tube support.

It is important to recognise that there are situations where parenteral nutrition must be considered. These include failure to meet nutritional requirements with enteral feeding, complex gastrointestinal fistulas and high output losses such as intractable diarrhoea. Occasionally, a combination of enteral and parenteral support is required, for example when enteral feed is not adequately absorbed. A multidisciplinary approach with nutrition team input is imperative, regardless of the route of feeding.

In summary, oral or enteric nutrition is the preferred route in acute pancreatitis. There is no requirement to fast patients with acute pancreatitis, assuming diet is tolerated. Normal diet may be augmented with commercially available nutritional supplements. If this is inadequate, NG feeding may be attempted followed by NJ support if this also fails. Finally, TPN should only be used when enteral options are exhausted or contraindicated for the reasons outlined above (Box 14.5).

Disease modulation through content or mode of delivery

There has been interest in the role of the intestine in the pathophysiology of multiple organ failure in critical illness, with loss of gut barrier function potentially leading to endotoxaemia and SIRS. These are largely non-clinical data but a small study from the authors reported a reduction in the

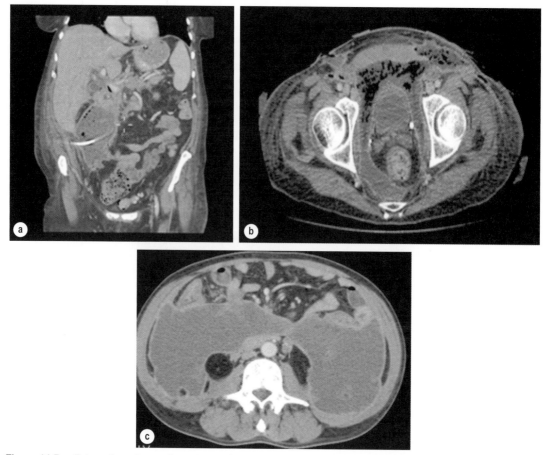

Figure 14.5 • Retrocolic and preperitoneal extension of peripancreatic necrosis. **(a)** Paraduodenal abscess managed by percutaneous drainage. **(b)** Preperitoneal extension pointing in the perineum via the inguinal canal. **(c)** Horseshoe collection extending down right and left paracolic gutters.

Box 14.5 • Escalating nutritional support algorithm for acute pancreatitis

| Diet with oral supplements |
| Nasogastric (NG) feeding |
| Nasojejunal (NJ) feeding |
| Total parenteral nutrition (TPN) |

inflammatory response and organ failure in those receiving enteral support.[32] Unfortunately there were only 13 patients with severe disease, limiting the validity of the conclusions. There have been several trials comparing so-called 'immunonutrition' with standard enteral feeding in critically ill patients, but so far no evidence of benefit has been demonstrated in acute pancreatitis.[33] Similarly, there has been interest in the role of 'probiotics', but a randomised trial from the Netherlands found an increase in fatal complications in the probiotic group, with an unexpectedly high incidence of intestinal necrosis.[34]

Delayed gastric emptying/gastric outlet obstruction

Gastric outlet obstruction resulting in persistent vomiting or high-volume gastric aspirates from NG suction may complicate up to 10% of patients with severe acute pancreatitis. The recent trend towards NJ intubation has rendered this complication less troublesome and the majority of patients can be treated by nasoenteric feeding until the local oedema/ileus settles. Occasionally, a gastroenterostomy is required for long-standing gastric stasis.

Management of acute phase complications

Haemorrhage

Haemorrhage into a walled-off collection or following necrosectomy is a relatively common problem. This is a consequence of a combination of factors: a large raw surface, partly controlled sepsis and exposed major vessels leading to primary or reactionary haemorrhage. Fresh blood in a drain, even of modest volume, requires attention as this will often represent a 'herald bleed' of imminent catastrophic haemorrhage. Urgent CT angiography (CTA) to identify a target, followed by embolisation with endovascular metal coils, is the treatment of choice. Fig. 14.6 illustrates active bleeding from a gastro-duodenal artery pseudoaneurysm. The increase in intracavity pressure associated with bleeding into an infected necrotic collection often results in a simultaneous episode of sepsis with bacteraemia and organ dysfunction, the hypotension being multifactorial.

A normal CTA suggests a venous source and bleeding in this context is usually associated with venous congestion, often secondary to portal venous thrombosis. Where percutaneous access to the cavity is possible, local packing will often arrest the bleeding, either with balloon tamponade (Fig. 14.7) or gauze strips, but surgical intervention and suture ligation of the bleeding point may be required. The challenges of gaining surgical access and achieving haemostasis in a patient with active haemorrhage, escalating organ dysfunction, coagulopathy and venous hypertension within a hostile abdomen should not be underestimated. The combination of haemorrhage and subsequent laparotomy frequently precipitates escalating organ failure and death.

Venous thrombosis

All patients with severe acute pancreatitis should be considered high risk for venous thromboembolic disease and receive prophylactic low molecular weight heparin (LMWH) and compression stockings. Splenic vein thrombosis is frequently identified on serial CT and is the result of a combination of local inflammation, extrinsic compression from collections and a low flow state. Splenic vein thrombosis does not require active treatment with therapeutic LMWH.[35] Superior mesenteric or portal vein thrombosis should be managed by therapeutic LMWH for 6 months in an attempt to maintain patency and avoid cavernous transformation of the portal vein. Despite active treatment, recanalisation rarely occurs in practice, and collateralisation will ensue. LMWH is preferred to warfarin, heparin, or one of the oral Factor Xa inhibitors, as it does not require monitoring and avoids compromising timing of interval intervention should it be required.

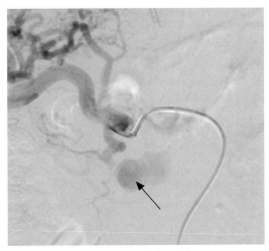

Figure 14.6 • Selective cannulation of the common hepatic artery showing filling of a pseudoaneurysm (marked with an arrow) arising from the gastroduodenal artery in a patient with haemorrhage into central pancreatic necrosis.

Enteric fistula

Abscess formation in conjunction with focal enteric ischaemia can lead to fistulation between the acute necrotic or walled off collection and the lumen of the bowel. This is almost universally associated with the presence of gas and sometimes a fluid level within the cavity. Historically this was seen as an indication for intervention, but the physiological impact and clinical course are dependent upon the site of fistulation into the gastrointestinal tract.

Spontaneous discharge of a post-acute collection into the upper gastrointestinal tract is not uncommon, effectively mimicking what happens when an EUS-guided cystgastrostomy is performed. This may decompress the collection and result in clinical improvement. Fluid levels are common and the radiological appearance does not correlate with the clinical condition of the patient. Immediate intervention is not usually required but care must be taken to observe for inadequate resolution which can lead to late recurrent sepsis.

In contrast, fistulation into the lower gastrointestinal tract more often results in a poorly drained collection, bacterial contamination and persistent sepsis. These rarely settle without intervention. Colectomy was formally proposed as part of a debridement procedure, but adequate

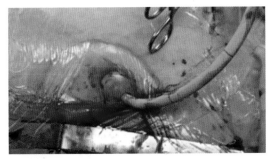

Figure 14.7 • Balloon tamponade (using the oesophageal balloon of a Sengstaken–Blakemore tube) for venous haemorrhage following a percutaneous necrosectomy – resolved without further intervention.

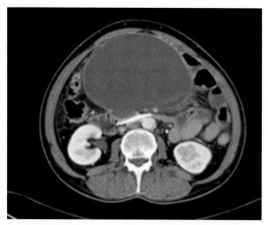

Figure 14.8 • Large pseudocyst resulting in gastric and extrahepatic biliary obstruction with jaundice. Both resolved following decompression by EUS-guided cystgastrostomy.

control can often be achieved by formation of a trephine defunctioning ileostomy minimising the surgical hit in a compromised patient.

Biliary obstruction

Extrahepatic biliary obstruction may complicate the management of severe acute pancreatitis due to extrinsic compression of the common bile duct by a large acute necrotic collection. ERCP in this situation is extremely difficult as the duodenum is usually oedematous and visualisation of the ampulla often impossible. In the acute phase it is unusual to have a true stricture and biliary decompression will often result from endoscopic or percutaneous drainage of the acute collection to relieve the pressure (see Fig. 14.8).

> ✅ Foregut fistulas often lead to clinical improvement; hindgut fistulas usually result in marked clinical deterioration.

Long-term complications

Pancreatic duct fistula

This complication most commonly follows prior intervention for an acute post-inflammatory collection or infected necrosis, and manifests as persistent drainage of amylase-rich opalescent fluid, in the absence of significant sepsis. Simple removal of the drain may facilitate closure of small volume leaks, but if persistent, the management is similar to that of a communicating pseudocyst, initially by transpapillary stenting where possible. Central gland necrosis may result in stricture formation and duct occlusion at the level of the pancreatic neck, with preferential drainage of pancreatic juice arising from viable pancreatic tissue in the pancreatic tail along the drain tract. A significant

advantage of the endoscopic drainage approach is that any residual fistula from the pancreatic tail is at least initially clinically silent as the fistula drains into the gastric lumen.

Intraperitoneal rupture of a pseudocyst can result in pancreatic ascites or pleural effusion (Fig. 14.9). These patients are usually profoundly catabolic. More invasive management of a persistent fistula, either inaccessible or failing to respond to ductal stenting, should be delayed by percutaneous or endoscopic control, until the patient has made a full recovery, and again often requires surgical resection (distal pancreatectomy and splenectomy).

Pancreatic duct stricture

Pancreatic duct stricture can occur following resolution of an attack of acute pancreatitis as a result of local tissue damage and fibrotic repair. A pancreatic duct stricture may be present on its own, or in association with a duct disruption causing a pseudocyst or pancreatic fistula. Isolated pancreatic duct stricture can result in recurrent attacks of abdominal pain, hyperamylasaemia and dilatation of the distal duct system. Management of the stricture may be by simple dilatation and temporary stenting at ERCP, by surgical resection of the stricture along with the pancreatic tail, or by surgical drainage of the pancreatic duct system into a Roux loop.

After significant central necrosis complete occlusion occurs, resulting in 'disconnected duct syndrome' should a remnant of viable tail remain. The treatment of this is described below.

Disconnected duct syndrome

Cutaneous or gastric mucosal closure of a pancreatic fistula may be followed by the development of a pseudocyst lying in the former pancreatic bed. This is preceded by necrosis, fibrosis and atrophy of the middle of the gland. It leads eventually to 'disconnected duct syndrome', with a pseudocyst forming between the proximal pancreas and a viable distal parenchymal remnant. Endoscopic transgastric drainage under endoscopic ultrasound may be a useful option. The presence of a fibrotic pancreatic ductal occlusion often at the pancreatic neck usually precludes transpapillary options. Surgical resection or drainage procedures are often required if resolution is not achieved. Surgery in this context is challenging, particularly if there are large venous collaterals secondary to splenic vein occlusion. A 'salvage' distal pancreatectomy and splenectomy is frequently required.

Late extrahepatic biliary stricture

In contrast to biliary obstruction in the acute phase, jaundice developing months after resolution is usually a result of focal fibrosis and scarring within the pancreatic head. Debris and stones may form

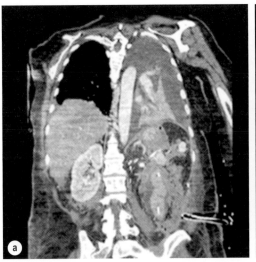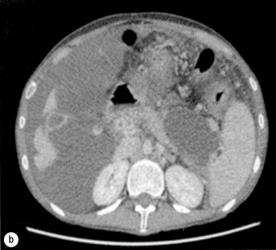

Figure 14.9 • Post acute pancreatitis: **(a)** pancreatico-pleural fistula and **(b)** pancreatic ascites.

above the stricture leading to episodes of cholangitis. Endoscopic stenting at ERCP can alleviate an acute attack but does not address the underlying pathology.

Remodelling of the fibrotic segment using a fully covered self-expanding metal stent (SEMS) will often result in prolonged relief but recurrence is common on stent removal. Failure of endoscopic remodelling is an indication for a formal hepatico-jejunostomy where fitness allows.

Portal and splenic vein thrombosis and cavernous transformation

Splenic and portal vein thrombosis is associated with up to 15% of patients dying with acute pancreatitis. In those patients with established thrombosis who survive the acute attack, the venous drainage is diverted through the short gastric, gastroepiploic and cardinal veins resulting in large venous collaterals. Segmental portal hypertension limited to the drainage territory of the splenic vein may result in a concerning endoscopic or radiological appearance. Despite the frequency of venous collaterals on follow-up CT, late gastrointestinal haemorrhage due to gastric varices is rare. Surgical intervention is more commonly required for a disconnected duct syndrome than for bleeding, and if there is significant concern regarding segmental venous collateralisation prior to surgery, preoperative embolisation of the splenic artery may decompress the system to facilitate resection.

Right-sided, or global superior mesenteric and portal venous occlusion with cavernous transformation of the pancreatic head, duodenum and hepatico-duodenal ligament is a more significant problem as it may preclude even intermediate surgical intervention (e.g. hepatico-jejunostomy for extrahepatic biliary obstruction). Recurrent low-grade sepsis in the presence of cavernous transformation is one of the most challenging complications of acute pancreatitis. On rare occasions, consideration of a multivisceral transplant may be the only option.

Key points

- Approximately 20% of patients with acute pancreatitis develop severe AP, with local and/or systemic complications, of whom half will die.
- The Revised Atlanta Classification defines local complications according to timing and presence of necrosis, and adds a new category (moderately severe pancreatitis).
- Necrosis *per se* is not an indication for intervention, but infected necrosis is the most feared complication of AP.
- Intervention for complications of AP should be delayed for as long as possible and is guided by patient physiology.
- Efforts should be made to minimise the negative impact of each intervention – 'the step-up approach'.
- There is no role for ERCP in the management of AP in the absence of biliary sepsis.

- The nutritional support algorithm starts with oral intake and ends with TPN.
- The key to successful management of infected necrosis is control of sepsis.
- Endoscopic and other minimally invasive techniques have largely replaced open surgery in the management of both early and late complications of AP.
- A key principle in managing the complications of AP is 'do as little as you can, as late as you can'.

🌐 Full references available at **http:// expertconsult.inkling.com**

Key references

1. Working Group IAPAPAAPG. IAP/APA evidence-based guidelines for the management of acute pancreatitis. Pancreatology 2013;13(4 Suppl. 2):e1–15. PMID: 24054878.
   These international guidelines provide 38 evidence-based recommendations relating to the clinical management of acute pancreatitis. They offer a comprehensive summary of the existing literature for all those involved in the care of this patient group from referring clinician to hospital specialist.

3. Banks PA, Bollen TL, Dervenis C, et al. Classification of acute pancreatitis – 2012: revision of the Atlanta classification and definitions by international consensus. Gut 2013;62(1):102–11. PMID: 23100216.
   International Consensus revision of the original Atlanta classification of acute pancreatitis. It uses clinical and radiological criteria to provide clear definitions of severity and associated complications.

6. Uy MC, Daez ML, Sy PP, et al. Early ERCP in acute gallstone pancreatitis without cholangitis: a meta-analysis. JOP 2009;10(3):299–305. PMID: 19454823.
   Previous data suggested that early ERCP in the context of acute pancreatitis improved outcome. This meta-analysis only included two RCTs but demonstrated a trend towards increasing mortality when ERCP was used in AP *in the absence of* cholangitis.

11. Carter CR, McKay CJ, Imrie CW. Percutaneous necrosectomy and sinus tract endoscopy in the management of infected pancreatic necrosis: an initial experience. Ann Surg 2000;232(2):175–80. PMID: 10903593.
   This paper reported the initial experience of the minimally invasive approach to infected pancreatic necrosis including technique and outcome. It demonstrated that sepsis resolution can be achieved with an apparent reduction in postoperative organ dysfunction and critical care support.

14. Seifert H, Biermer M, Schmitt W, et al. Transluminal endoscopic necrosectomy after acute pancreatitis:

a multicentre study with long-term follow-up (the GEPARD Study). Gut 2009;58(9):1260–6. PMID: 19282306.
   This key paper demonstrated good clinical outcomes with an endoscopic transluminal approach to infected necrosis. Of significance, this is a large series (*n*=93) with excellent long-term follow-up (mean period of 43 months).

17. van Santvoort HC, Besselink MG, Bakker OJ, et al. A step-up approach or open necrosectomy for necrotizing pancreatitis. N Engl J Med 2010;362(16):1491–502. PMID: 20410514.
   Landmark, multicentre randomised trial demonstrating a reduction in the composite endpoint of major complications or death with the 'step-up' approach when compared to open necrosectomy. Of note, 35% of patients were managed with percutaneous drainage alone.

30. Kalfarentzos F, Kehagias J, Mead N, et al. Enteral nutrition is superior to parenteral nutrition in severe acute pancreatitis: results of a randomized prospective trial. Br J Surg 1997;84(12):1665–9.
   Although a relatively small study (*n*=38), this randomised trial provided data to challenge the previously held dogma that patients with acute pancreatitis required parenteral nutrition. Feeding was both safer and cheaper in the enteral nutrition cohort.

31. Al-Omran N, AlBalawi ZH, Tashkandi MF, et al. Enteral versus parenteral nutrition for acute pancreatitis. Cochrane Rev 2010;. (1):CD002837. PMID: 20091534.
   A review of eight RCTs in patients with acute pancreatitis showing that enteral nutrition significantly reduced mortality, multi-organ failure, systemic infections and the need for operative interventions compared to parenteral nutrition.

34. Besselink MG, Timmerman HM, Buskens E, et al. Probiotic prophylaxis in patients with predicted severe acute pancreatitis (PROPATRIA): design and rationale of a double-blind, placebo-controlled randomised multicenter trial [ISRCTN38327949]. BMC Surg 2004;4:12. PMID: 15456517.
   This randomised, placebo-controlled multicentre trial addressed the question of probiotic prophylaxis in patients with *predicted* SAP. One of the key outcomes was a reduction in bacterial translocation overall, but an increase in bacterial translocation and enterocyte damage in patients with organ failure.

15

Chronic pancreatitis

Ajith K. Siriwardena
C. Ross Carter

Introduction

Chronic pancreatitis is defined as a benign inflammatory disease, characterised by chronic pancreatic inflammation and scarring, irreversibly damaging the gland and resulting in loss of pancreatic exocrine and endocrine function.[1] The most common aetiological factor is long-term excessive consumption of alcohol.[2] There is also an association with cigarette smoking.[2,3] Chronic pancreatitis is associated with mutations in trypsin activation genes and also cystic fibrosis genes.[4,5] Abdominal pain is typically the dominant symptom. Baseline assessment, in addition to careful clinical examination, must include cross-sectional imaging (typically CT). Treatment planning should ideally take place on a multidisciplinary basis. Pancreatic exocrine and endocrine function should be assessed and insufficiency treated. Pain control should follow the World Health Organisation's analgesic ladder originally developed for cancer pain.[6] Co-analgesics such as gabapentin may be used in conjunction with conventional analgesics.[7] Specialist interventions take the form of endoscopic and surgical treatment. Endoscopic interventions are directed at improving pancreatic duct drainage, managing pancreatic duct disruption, treatment of extrahepatic biliary obstruction, and/or pain control through coeliac plexus nerve block. Surgical interventions depend on the morphology of the diseased pancreas. In patients with a pancreatic head mass and concomitant chronic pancreatitis, pancreatic cancer must be considered in the differential diagnosis. Endoscopic ultrasound with fine-needle aspiration (EUS-FNA) should be considered. If concern over cancer cannot be excluded, a resectional treatment such as pancreatico-duodenectomy is appropriate. In patients without a pancreatic mass but with a dilated duct, pancreatic ductal drainage procedures such as lateral pancreatico-jejunostomy can be considered. In patients with small duct chronic pancreatitis, management is more difficult but can include the V-shaped excision. In selected patients, total pancreatectomy with islet autotransplantation can be considered.[8] The long-term complications of chronic pancreatitis all relate to recurrent or persistent episodes of inflammation with subsequent healing with fibrosis. These include biliary stricture, duodenal stenosis, pseudocyst, false aneurysms of visceral vessels and portal or splenic vein occlusion leading to extrahepatic portal hypertension.[9] Important long-term risks to monitor during follow-up include development of diabetes mellitus, malnutrition and the increased risk of cancer.[10]

Definition

✓✓ Chronic pancreatitis is defined as a benign inflammatory disease, characterised by chronic pancreatic inflammation and scarring, irreversibly damaging the pancreas and resulting in loss of exocrine and endocrine function.[1]

Classification of chronic pancreatitis

Classifications of chronic pancreatitis have been based on the aetiology of the disease, such as alcohol-related, genetic or idiopathic.[1] Alternatively, the disease can be classified according to morphology – large-duct disease, small-duct disease and minimal-change pancreatitis.[11] Classifications incorporating the temporal changes along the time course of chronic pancreatitis have also been used (early-stage, late-stage disease).[12] The availability of better diagnostic tests such as endoscopic pancreatography were the stimulus for morphologically based categorisations, and the Cambridge classification based on pancreatogram appearance is still used today.[11] Contrast-enhanced magnetic resonance scanning has replaced diagnostic pancreatography.[13] Morphologically based classifications have the practical advantage that treatment can potentially be tailored to the disease variant. In addition to these systems of classification, there have since been national classifications from (amongst others) Japan, Switzerland and the USA.[14-16] The most contemporary classification system is that described in the American Pancreatic Association's practice guideline on chronic pancreatitis in 2014.[16] This provides criteria for the diagnosis of chronic pancreatitis based on computed tomography (CT), magnetic resonance imaging (MRI) and endoscopic ultrasonography (EUS).

Incidence

✅✅ Data from the North American National Pancreas Foundation suggest an incidence of approximately 4 new patients per 100 000 population per year in the USA.[17] As this is a chronic disease, the prevalence is 40–50 per 100 000 people.[17] There is substantial worldwide geographic variation in the clinical profile of the disease.[18]

Aetiology

The TIGAR-O risk factor list is a modern, comprehensive list of the aetiological causes of chronic pancreatitis (see Table 15.1).[19] TIGAR-O considers toxic-metabolic causes, idiopathic, genetic, autoimmune, recurrent and obstructive factors. The M-ANNHEIM aetiology list is similar but adds the important option to consider multiple coexistent aetiological factors.[20] Excessive alcohol consumption is the single most common aetiologic factor.[19,20] Cigarette smoking is a common cofactor to alcohol, and as a modifiable risk factor, smoking cessation should be prioritised from the outset.[3] High caloric intake of protein and fat, and deficiency of fat-soluble vitamins in the diet, are associated with chronic pancreatitis but without proof of a causal link.[21,22]

There have been substantial important advances in understanding the genetic basis of chronic pancreatitis.[4] Mutations in the cationic trypsinogen gene *PRSS1* lead to premature intra-acinar activation of trypsin.[4] Similarly, mutations in the pancreatic secretory trypsin inhibitor also termed serine protease inhibitor Kazal Type 1 (*SPINK1*) compromise intracellular inactivation of trypsin and are associated with chronic pancreatitis.[23] Cystic fibrosis gene mutations, especially the $\Delta 508$ mutation are associated with chronic pancreatitis and are thought to be due to abnormalities in mucin production and secretion.[24] Alcohol susceptibility genes are also associated with alcohol-related chronic pancreatitis.[23]

Pathogenesis of pain in chronic pancreatitis

Pain in clinical chronic pancreatitis is complex and multifactorial. Logically, pain in chronic

Table 15.1 • The TIGAR-O classification system of risk factors for chronic pancreatitis

Toxic–metabolic	Alcohol, tobacco smoking, hypercalcaemia, hyperlipidaemia, chronic renal failure, medications, toxins
Idiopathic	Associated with early-onset CP and also with late-onset CP Tropical CP
Genetic mutations	*PRSS1*, *CFTR*, *SPINK1*, others
Autoimmune	Isolated or as part of a syndrome
Recurrent and severe AP-associated CP	Post-necrotic severe AP, vascular disease/ischaemic, post-irradiation
Obstructive	Pancreas divisum, sphincter of Oddi disorders, duct obstruction (e.g., tumour), post-traumatic pancreatic duct scars

AP, acute pancreatitis; CP, chronic pancreatitis.
The TIGAR-O classification is a comprehensive classification system of the risk factors for chronic pancreatitis.[19] It is worthwhile remembering that in clinical practice, there may be more than one coexistent aetiological factor.
Modified from Etemad B, Whitcomb DC. Chronic pancreatitis: diagnosis, classification, and new genetic developments. Gastroenterology 2001;120:682–707.

pancreatitis can be considered as having both a 'pancreatic' component and an 'extra-pancreatic' component. Pancreatic pain relates to inflammation of the gland and obstruction of the main pancreatic duct. Extra-pancreatic components relate to abnormal neural pathways and aberrant central nervous system perception of pain.[25,26] Objective evidence of the 'extra-pancreatic' component comes from studies which show that the number and diameter of non-myelinated type C pain fibres are significantly increased in patients with chronic pancreatitis.[27,28] In addition, central nervous system processing of pain may be altered with long-standing chronic pancreatitis.[29] These 'extra-pancreatic' factors may account for some of the treatment failures of pancreas-directed surgery or endoscopy. It should also be remembered that there may be treatment related side-effects such as opiate-induced gut dysmotility. In practical terms, patients should be counselled before undergoing surgical or endoscopic intervention and should understand that no individual intervention is associated with a guarantee of symptom relief in chronic pancreatitis.

> ✓✓ Pain in chronic pancreatitis is multifactorial and can include a pancreatic parenchymal component, an extra-pancreatic neural component and components due to treatment-related side-effects such as opiate-induced gut dysmotility.

Clinical presentations

Acute presentation of chronic pancreatitis

There is a substantial overlap between acute and chronic pancreatitis in their modes of presentation. To address this practically, if patients present with acute abdominal pain, hyperamylasaemia or meet the diagnostic criteria for acute pancreatitis defined in the Atlanta 2012 consensus[30] (see chapter on acute pancreatitis) they should be diagnosed as acute pancreatitis and receive treatment according to the current International Association of Pancreatology/American Pancreatic Association (IAP/APA) guidelines for the treatment of acute pancreatitis.[31] The practical importance of this is to ensure adequate initial resuscitation and also to detect and treat avoidable causes of recurrent pancreatitis. Principally, gallstones should be sought by transabdominal ultrasound and treated by cholecystectomy. The presence of parenchymal calcification on CT and/or a dilated main pancreatic duct are pointers toward an underlying diagnosis of chronic pancreatitis.

Chronic presentation of chronic pancreatitis

The majority of admissions secondary to established chronic pancreatitis are as a result of abdominal pain with normal or marginal hyperamylasaemia. Unlike severe acute pancreatitis, these episodes usually require little more than a temporary escalation of analgesia and maintenance fluids, but to avoid recurrent admissions an effective interim strategy is required. An important component of care is provision of counselling to help avoid continued alcohol overuse and there is good randomised trial evidence that professional counselling on the harms of alcohol consumption is associated with a reduction in future admissions with pancreatitis.[32,33] These patients may also be considered for endoscopic and/or surgical management (see below).

Index presentation with complications of chronic pancreatitis

Occasionally the index presentation will be as a result of a complication of chronic pancreatitis such as a pseudocyst, bleed from false aneurysm or biliary or duodenal obstruction from chronic fibrosis. The management of these is discussed in the section on complications.

Asymptomatic incidental finding

The widespread availability and use of CT occasionally results in the detection of patients with pancreatic parenchymal calcification without associated symptoms. In this setting, it is worthwhile assessing and excluding diabetes mellitus and malnutrition, but there is no role for intervention in the absence of symptoms.

Practical differential diagnoses in chronic pancreatitis

Three important differential diagnoses must be considered.

Pancreatic cancer

Initial assessment of a patient presenting with a focal pancreatic mass, on a background of known or newly diagnosed chronic pancreatitis, should consider the possibility of pancreatic cancer in the differential diagnosis. Biomarkers such as carbohydrate antigen 19-9 (CA 19-9) are insufficiently accurate to allow for reliable distinction between chronic pancreatitis and cancer, especially in the setting of biliary obstruction.[34] Chronic pancreatitis is itself an independent risk factor for the development of pancreatic ductal adenocarcinoma.[35] Sonographic artifact from fibrosis and calcification compromises the accuracy of endoscopic ultrasound, and whilst a diagnosis of cancer may be confirmed by EUS/FNA, it cannot exclude neoplasia despite negative cytology, and in patients in whom there is a suspicion of cancer, surgical resection should be considered.

Autoimmune pancreatitis

Autoimmune pancreatitis (AIP) is a chronic inflammatory condition in which patients may present with a pancreatic mass, pain and jaundice that can closely resemble chronic pancreatitis.[36,37] AIP is associated with extra-pancreatic stricture of the upper and intra-hepatic bile ducts and not typically with pancreatic calcification, and these pointers may help differentiation from chronic pancreatitis.[38] AIP is also associated with elevation of the immunoglobulin IgG4 subtype.[39] The diffuse nature of the inflammatory process leads to a classical 'sausage-shaped' swollen pancreas which can be distinguished from chronic pancreatitis.[40] Ideally a tissue diagnosis of AIP should be established, usually by pancreatic biopsy.

Intraductal papillary mucinous neoplasm (IPMN)

Main-duct IPMN presents with dilatation of the main pancreatic duct and can closely resemble chronic pancreatitis.[41] Main-duct IPMN typically has intraductal mucin which may be seen extruding from the ampulla whereas the duct dilatation associated with chronic pancreatitis is associated with stricture formation and parenchymal calcification. It is important to distinguish between the two as main-duct IPMNs are regarded as pre-malignant lesions and require resectional surgery.[41]

Clinical course

Typically the disease has a relapsing course characterised by intermittent abdominal pain.[42] At the onset, patients will have conserved exocrine and endocrine function but both are compromised during the clinical course. Diabetes mellitus is more frequent in long-standing chronic pancreatitis.[43] Historical series proposed a 'burnout' hypothesis, suggesting pain may

spontaneously decrease over time, coinciding with the occurrence of exocrine insufficiency.[44] However, two large prospective cohort studies[43,45] showed no association between the duration of chronic pancreatitis and pain.

Baseline assessment of a patient with suspected chronic pancreatitis

Clinical history is central to management and must focus on the nature and duration of symptoms, age of first onset of abdominal pain and associated factors such as jaundice and/or vomiting. An accurate history of alcohol consumption is important and must include information on type of alcohol, years of consumption and current intake in units. Smoking history and counselling on the significance of smoking on disease progression, and an accurate family history, may identify hereditary kindreds. Clinical examination should record body mass index, abdominal examination findings and urinalysis.

Baseline laboratory tests include blood count, urea/electrolytes, biochemical liver function tests, blood glucose (and glycosylated haemoglobin), C-reactive protein and CA 19-9. Transabdominal ultrasonography will provide information on the presence or absence of gallstones and also on common coexistent liver diseases such as steatohepatosis. CT, and to a lesser extent MRI, are the mainstay of detailed assessment in chronic pancreatitis.[16]

☑ APA Practice Guidelines key points on diagnosis of chronic pancreatitis (CP):[16]
- Intraductal pancreatic calcifications are the most specific and reliable sonographic and CT signs of CP.
- Compared with ultrasound and CT, MRI is a more sensitive imaging tool for the diagnosis of CP.
- Computed tomography is helpful for the diagnosis of complications of CP.
- Computed tomography is helpful for diagnosis of other conditions that can mimic CP.
- Endoscopic retrograde pancreatogram (ERP) is rarely used for diagnostic purposes.
- The ideal threshold number of EUS criteria necessary to diagnose CP has not been firmly established, but the presence of 5 or more and 2 or less strongly suggests or refutes the diagnosis of CP. The relatively poor inter-observer agreement for EUS features of chronic pancreatitis limits the diagnostic accuracy and overall utility of EUS for diagnosis.[46]

CT features of chronic pancreatitis include dilatation of the pancreatic duct, pancreatic calcification and parenchymal atrophy (**Fig. 15.1**). These features are usually present late in the course of the disease and thus may not be evident at an early stage. MRI is reportedly more specific for the diagnosis of CP because ductal abnormalities are very reliably detected. The addition of intravenous secretin may improve the accuracy of MRI, and may provide indirect evidence of residual exocrine function.[47]

EUS complements cross-sectional imaging and is more sensitive than CT in diagnosing the early stages of chronic pancreatitis. The Rosemont criteria,[46] derived from a consensus conference, combine the detection of parenchymal abnormalities with ductal irregularity or dilatation to produce a score for the prediction of chronic pancreatitis.

Although endoscopic retrograde cholangiopancreatography (ERCP) was a mainstay of diagnosis in the 1980s and was used in the Cambridge classification, purely diagnostic ERCP should no longer be undertaken as accurate information on ductal abnormalities can be obtained by cross-sectional imaging.

In addition to morphological assessment of the gland, functional assessment of the endocrine component of pancreatic function involves testing for diabetes mellitus. Baseline measurement of glycosylated haemoglobin (HbA1C) may be of value in non-diabetics at time of index presentation.

The exocrine component of pancreatic function can be assessed indirectly by measurement of faecal elastase, serum trysinogen or chymotrypsin and does not require direct hormonal stimulation of the pancreas.[48] These tests are of practical value only in the late stages of the disease, when clinical features such as steatorrhoea are already present. Direct assessment of pancreatic exocrine function by intubation of the duodenum, provision of a secretory stimulus and collection of pancreatic juice is not widespread and seems to be most widely utilised in North America.[49] In many units a clinical diagnosis of chronic pancreatitis serves as an indication for commencement of pancreatic exocrine replacement therapy given the high prevalence of subclinical malnutrition and vitamin deficiency in this disease.[48]

Medical management of chronic pancreatitis

The treatment of chronic pancreatitis and its complications remains a major challenge. A holistic approach is based on accurate assessment of symptoms, nutritional status, pancreatic endocrine and exocrine function and morphological assessment of the integrity and patency of the duct and the nature of the pancreatic parenchyma.

Analgesia

This is a key component of the non-operative treatment of chronic pancreatitis. Pain control should follow the World Health Organisation's analgesic ladder, starting with a non-opioid, progressing to weak opioid and then a strong opiod.[6] Typically, patients will already be on regular analgesic medication by the time of referral to specialist care. Co-analgesics such as gabapentin may be used in conjunction with these medications.[7]

Alcohol avoidance

There is good randomised trial evidence that professional alcohol avoidance counselling results in reduced hospital admission.[33] If alcohol consumption can be stopped at an early stage in the disease, progression may also be ameliorated.[32]

Smoking cessation

Formal guidance on cessation of smoking is useful. Cessation of smoking may modify disease progression.[3] If smoking cessation clinics are available, these should be utilised.

Exocrine replacement therapy

Exocrine replacement therapy should be considered in all patients with chronic pancreatitis. Treatment

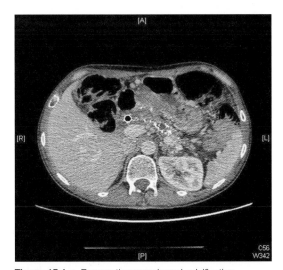

Figure 15.1 • Pancreatic parenchymal calcification. Venous contrast phase of a CT showing typical pancreatic parenchymal calcification and segmental dilatation of the main pancreatic duct. An indwelling metallic endobiliary stent is also seen.

does not need to be dictated by complex pancreatic intubation tests or by measurement of faecal elastase but can be based on pragmatic clinical assessment.[48]

Medications of unproven benefit

The search for effective treatment in chronic pancreatitis has resulted in the assessment of a wide range of therapies of unproven benefit. Antioxidant therapy was evaluated on the assumption that orally administered cocktails of vitamin C, selenium and methionine would be absorbed into the pancreas in sufficient concentration to quench oxidative stress. Antioxidant therapy has been evaluated by two reasonably large and well conducted randomised trials. An Indian trial reported a reduction in 'painful days' but showed a substantial placebo response and treated a population with striking dietary deprivation.[50] The European ANTICIPATE trial randomised patients with painful chronic pancreatitis to a 6-month period of antioxidant therapy or placebo.[51] The principal findings were of no intervention-related reduction in pain or improvement in quality of life. Although there is one further study whose results are awaited, it seems unlikely that antioxidant therapy is of any benefit in chronic pancreatitis. Medications of unproven benefit should be avoided in this population of vulnerable patients.

✔ Key points in medical management of chronic pancreatitis:
- Treatment decision-making should be in a multidisciplinary forum.
- Counselling on avoidance of alcohol consumption and cigarette smoking.
- Treatment of malnutrition, pancreatic exocrine and endocrine insufficiency.
- Analgesic use following the WHO ladder combined with co-analgesics such as gabapentin.

Endoscopic management of chronic pancreatitis

Surgery and endoscopy should be seen as complementary rather than competitive treatments. Hence treatment planning is best undertaken on a multidisciplinary basis.

Endoscopic drainage compared to surgical drainage of the main pancreatic duct

There have been two relatively small randomised trials comparing surgical drainage to endoscopic therapy for painful chronic pancreatitis. The first, in 2003, randomised 72 patients and reported the superiority of surgical resection or drainage over endoscopic duct stenting/duct clearance at 5 years in terms of pain relief and weight gain, with no difference in the rate of new onset diabetes.[52] In the second study from Holland, endoscopic decompression (with prior pancreatic lithotripsy in 80%) was compared to open surgical duct drainage in 39 patients.[53] At the end of follow-up (after 24 months) complete or partial pain relief was achieved in 32% assigned to endoscopic intervention and 75% treated surgically ($P=0.007$). Longer-term outcome in this cohort was reported in 2011, and again suggested a better outcome at 5 years in patients treated surgically.[54] Although complication rates, length of hospital stay and changes in pancreatic function were similar between the groups, endoscopically treated patients required more procedures than did patients in the surgery group (8 vs 3; $P <0.001$). The conclusion was that surgical drainage was more effective than endoscopic intervention. An important observation from the Dutch study was that whilst the response rate in terms of pain relief following endoscopy was inferior to surgery, those that did obtain relief did so within the first 3 months, suggesting persistence with endotherapy in the absence of a rapid response is unlikely to be beneficial.

An important limitation of the Dutch study is that the findings apply only to patients with large-duct disease without a pancreatic head mass as the surgical group were managed by lateral pancreatico-jejunostomy.[55]

Endoscopic drainage/stenting of the main pancreatic duct

Endoscopic drainage is best considered in patients with a dilated main pancreatic duct without a pancreatic head mass. The principles of endoscopic drainage are to access the pancreatic duct, typically by pancreatic duct sphincterotomy, to remove intraductal stones and to leave either a single endobiliary stent or multiple stents in situ to facilitate prolonged drainage.[56–59]

More recently, fully covered self-expanding metallic stents have been used within the pancreas.[56] A variable proportion of patients will be definitively treated by endoscopic decompression. Pancreatic ductal stones are different to common bile duct stones in that they may represent focal parenchymal calcifications with intraductal projections. Where large ductal calculi are evident on CT, extracorporeal shockwave lithotripsy (ESWL) should be used in combination with endoscopic attempts at clearance.[57,59]

Endoscopic coeliac plexus block

Endoscopic ultrasonography allows for good visualisation of the coeliac plexus around the coeliac trifurcation. Injection of local anaesthesia at

EUS can be used as a practical means of assessing for symptom relief.[60] In those patients who achieve an improvement in pain control after EUS-guided injection of local anaesthetic, destruction of the coeliac plexus can be considered by injection of alcohol.

Some operators are reluctant to consider alcohol ablation of the coeliac plexus in benign conditions and in these, surgical ablation of the greater, lesser and least splanchnic nerves in the thorax by the thoracoscopic route remains an option in patients with good temporary relief, although long-term outcomes tend to be unsatisfactory.[61]

Endoscopic treatment of complications of chronic pancreatitis

Endoscopic treatment can be considered for the treatment of distal bile duct stricture,[62] pancreatic pseudocyst (**Fig. 15.2**) and short-term duodenal stenting can be considered in patients with duodenal obstruction due to inflammation. Long-term benign, symptomatic duodenal obstruction in chronic pancreatitis is more typically treated by laparoscopic gastro-jejunostomy.

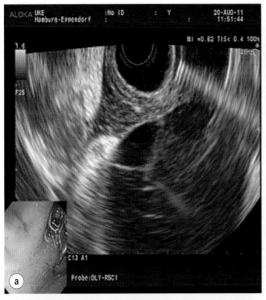

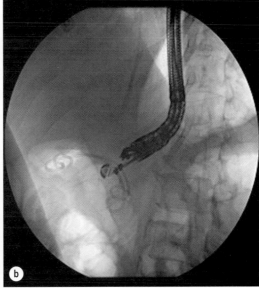

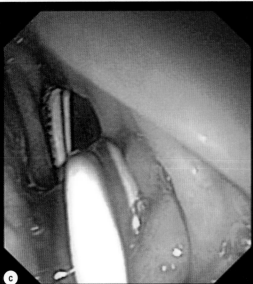

Figure 15.2 • Endoscopic drainage of pancreatic pseudocyst: **(a)** shows the pseudocyst on endoscopic ultrasound, **(b)** shows the endoscopic approach to the pseudocyst and **(c)** shows a pigtail stent in situ protruding into the duodenal lumen.

Surgical management of chronic pancreatitis

Indications for surgery

Surgery can be undertaken on an elective basis for pain control in patients with chronic pancreatitis. Surgery can also be indicated for management of the complications of chronic pancreatitis. Complications that can be effectively managed by surgery include distal bile duct stricture in younger patients where long-term biliary stenting is not optimal; gastric outlet obstruction secondary to duodenal stricture and occasionally patients with pseudocysts in the tail of the gland may require distal pancreatectomy.

Case selection for surgery in chronic pancreatitis

In terms of elective surgery, there is evidence of substantial variation in the thresholds for intervention[63] and thus, where possible, the decision to offer surgery should be taken in a multidisciplinary setting. Pain is the typical symptom which drives patients to seek surgery and for which operation is considered. Although there is little evidence to support the view that patients who continue to drink alcohol must have a period of abstention (including avoidance of cigarette smoking), patients being selected for elective surgery for chronic pancreatitis should ideally have avoided alcohol consumption for at least 6 months and preferably longer. The selection of the specific intervention is determined by the morphology of the gland, age and comorbidity.

Timing of surgery

There is no clear consensus on the optimal timing of surgery. Earlier surgical intervention in the disease course of chronic pancreatitis may avoid long-term sequelae such as habituation to pain and opioids. However, earlier intervention may also result in patients having surgery when this could potentially have been avoided.

Preparation for surgery

Patients with long-standing chronic pancreatitis being considered for surgery are often on high-dose opiates, may be insulin-dependent diabetics and are likely to have varying degrees of malnutrition. Cardiopulmonary exercise testing (CPET) provides a very reliable assessment of dynamic, functional reserve and modifiable risk factors. Although it has been evaluated prior to elective pancreatic cancer surgery it has not been formally evaluated as an assessment tool before surgery for chronic pancreatitis.[64] Dietitian and physiotherapy review before surgery should be considered and thought given to management of postoperative pain with either epidural or patient-controlled analgesia (PCA).

Selection of surgical procedure

For practical purposes, patients with chronic pancreatitis being prepared for surgery can be categorised into those with and without a pancreatic head mass and also those with and without main pancreatic duct dilatation. A guide to the selection of procedures is seen in Table 15.2.

Surgery for chronic pancreatitis in patients with a pancreatic head mass

In this setting there is often a concern about underlying malignancy. Preoperative assessment should include EUS with fine-needle aspiration. Intraoperatively, frozen section may be considered but Trucut-type biopsy of the pancreatic head may yield false-negative results. Differentiation of adenocarcinoma arising in the typical fibrous stroma of pancreatic cancer from the fibrous inflammatory infiltrate of chronic pancreatitis can be very difficult on frozen section and therefore it is preferable to have an operative strategy in place prior to commencing surgery rather than be exclusively reliant on frozen section histology.

A high index of suspicion may persist in patients with a hypodense mass in the head of the gland in the setting of chronic pancreatitis and in this scenario, resection in the form of pancreatico-duodenectomy should be considered. Appropriate counselling is required to explain that major resection may be undertaken, with all its attendant risks, for a final diagnosis of benign disease.

Table 15.2 • Matching the type of endoscopic or surgical procedure to the disease variant in chronic pancreatitis

Indications	Treatment options
Isolated pancreatic pseudocyst	Endoscopic pseudocyst-jejunostomy.
Pain + dilated duct without a pancreatic mass	Partington–Rochelle modification of lateral pancreatico-jejunostomy
Pain + dilated duct with a pancreatic mass	Frey pancreatico-jejunostomy
	Beger 'duodenum-preserving pancreatic head resection'
	Pancreatico-duodenectomy
Pain + pancreatic head mass + suspicion of malignancy	Pancreatico-duodenectomy
Pain + small duct disease (main duct <3 mm)	'V-shaped' resection + pancreatico-jejunostomy
Disconnected duct syndrome	Endoscopic stent
	Distal pancreatectomy

In those patients with a pancreatic head mass but where there is a low risk of cancer, the main surgical treatment options are between duodenum-preserving pancreatic head resection (DPPHR) and pancreatico-duodenectomy. Beger et al. introduced the duodenum-preserving resection of the pancreatic head as an organ-sparing procedure[65,66] (**Fig. 15.3**). The operation is a subtotal resection of the pancreatic head after transection of the pancreas above the portal vein. The pancreas is drained by pancreatico-jejunostomy. A systematic review and meta-analysis of four randomised trials comparing DPPHR to pancreatico-duodenectomy for pain relief in chronic pancreatitis reported that both procedures are equally effective in terms of postoperative pain relief, overall morbidity and incidence of postoperative endocrine insufficiency.[67] DPPHR is associated with better preservation of quality of life and lower long-term malnutrition.

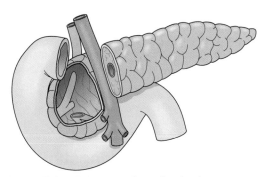

Figure 15.3 • Beger procedure – the duodenum-preserving pancreatic head resection. The pancreas is divided at its neck over the portal vein. The pancreatic head has been cored out and the bile duct is exposed within the head. Note that the duodenum has been preserved. Reconstruction is by a Roux pancreatico-jejunostomy.

Surgery for chronic pancreatitis in patients with a dilated main pancreatic duct without pancreatic head mass

Puestow and Gillesby described decompression of the main pancreatic duct with resection of the pancreatic tail, splenectomy and longitudinal lateral pancreatico-jejunostomy.[68] In a classic paper, Partington and Rochelle of the Cleveland Clinic reported a modification of this operation, preserving the spleen to avoid postsplenectomy complications and also avoiding distal pancreatectomy in order to preserve islet function.[69] Their modification of the operation of lateral pancreatico-jejunostomy with drainage of the opened pancreatic duct into a retrocolic Roux loop is frequently incorrectly termed a 'Puestow' procedure and is an effective and relatively simple surgical treatment for large-duct chronic pancreatitis without a pancreatic mass. The operation has been undertaken laparoscopically although this is not a standard method.[70] An important practical consideration is to exclude main-duct IPMN before undertaking duct drainage. Frey and Amikura reported a combined longitudinal pancreatico-jejunostomy of the body and tail of the pancreas (Partington–Rochelle procedure) with a limited duodenum-preserving resection or 'coring' of the pancreatic head.[71] In contrast to the Beger procedure, the pancreas is not divided over the superior mesenteric/portal vein (**Fig. 15.4**). The head of the pancreas is cored out in this procedure. Drainage of the cavity of the pancreatic head and the opened main duct of the body and tail is performed with a longitudinal pancreatico-jejunostomy using a Roux-en-Y loop.[71] Main-duct decompression may delay the progressive loss of pancreatic function.[72]

Indications for total pancreatectomy for chronic pancreatitis

In current practice, total pancreatectomy is not a widely used option in chronic pancreatitis. Total

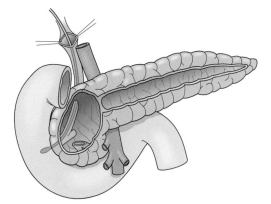

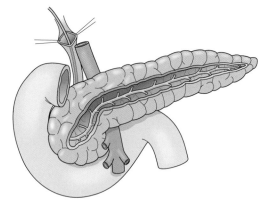

Figure 15.4 • The Frey procedure. Note the important similarities and differences from the Beger procedure. Frey describes a lateral pancreatico-jejunostomy, opening the main pancreatic duct out into the tail of the gland but making no attempt to undertake splenectomy. The head is then cored out. The key difference from the Beger operation is that the pancreas is not divided at its neck. In this illustration, the common bile duct is opened above the pancreas and a sound or dilator passed through into the duodenum. This is not usually necessary but can be done to ensure that there is no accidental injury to the intrapancreatic portion of the distal bile duct.

Figure 15.5 • V-shaped excision. The V-shaped excision is a variant of lateral pancreatico-jejunostomy undertaken for small-duct chronic pancreatitis. The main duct is opened out to the tail but a V-shaped core of tissue deep to the duct and from both above and below the duct is also excised. The term 'V' refers to the excision of a 'V-shaped' area of tissue which incorporates the main pancreatic duct. This core of tissue is removed from the head of the gland out to the tail taking care not to inadvertently damage the portal vein behind the gland. Reconstruction is by retrocolic Roux pancreatico-jejunostomy.

pancreatectomy with islet autotransplantation (TPIAT) does, however, have strong proponents.[73,74] In practical terms, this procedure can only be offered if there are facilities for islet isolation from the resected pancreas. Although tempting to consider TPIAT as a salvage procedure after failed drainage or subtotal resection, prior surgical treatments reduce the possibility of achieving a successful islet yield. The Mayo Clinic experience suggests that a tissue volume of 0.25 mL/kg be sought during islet manufacture and that intraportal infusion should be halted, at least temporarily, if the perfusion pressure exceeds 25 cm H_2O.[75] This procedure must be reserved for settings of established chronic pancreatitis with a low risk of cancer. In practice, the procedure is therefore optimal in younger patients with genetic chronic pancreatitis. It would be fair to say that as yet TPIAT for chronic pancreatitis is not a universally accepted procedure and further evidence is required before more widespread adoption can be recommended.

Surgical management of small-duct chronic pancreatitis

The V-shaped resection operation was developed for use in small-duct chronic pancreatitis. Izbicki suggests a longitudinal V-shaped excision of the ventral aspect of the pancreas combined with a longitudinal pancreatico-jejunostomy[76] (**Fig. 15.5**). If this condition is accompanied by an enlarged pancreatic head, pancreatic head resection should be performed.

✔✔ Key points in the surgical management of chronic pancreatitis:
- Large-duct disease without a mass can be effectively treated by pancreatic duct drainage combined with 'coring' of the pancreatic head. The head and decompressed duct are then drained into a Roux loop by lateral pancreatico-jejunostomy.
- Where there is a mass, consider pancreatico-duodenectomy if there is a high index of suspicion of an underlying cancer.
- The Beger procedure (duodenum-preserving pancreatic head resection or DPPHR) is an effective alternative treatment for chronic pancreatitis with a mass but a low index of suspicion of cancer.
- Total pancreatectomy with islet autotransplantation may be considered in young patients where there is a low risk of cancer. The procedure is not as yet widely accepted.
- Surgical bypass provides definitive treatment for biliary and/or duodenal strictures complicating chronic pancreatitis.

Complications of longstanding chronic pancreatitis

Complications include distal bile duct stricture with jaundice,[77,78] gastric outlet obstruction secondary to duodenal stricture, pseudoaneurysm of one of the major peripancreatic visceral arteries,[79] duct disruption resulting in pseudocyst,[80] pancreatic ascites or fistula.[81]

Biliary stricture

Long-term pancreatic and peripancreatic fibrosis can lead to distal bile duct stricture. Patients may present with jaundice or pain, or following investigation of abnormal liver function tests.[77,78] Initial management will usually involve exclusion of neoplasia by combinations of cross-sectional imaging, EUS/FNA, and internal biliary drainage at ERCP whilst long-term options are evaluated. Jaundice secondary to extrahepatic biliary obstruction may be managed by multiple stents or a self-expanding metal stent. However, biliary bypass should be considered in patients who are stent dependent with minimal comorbidity, but have a persistent, symptomatic stricture. Roux-en-Y hepatico-jejunostomy is the preferred intervention of choice. Choledochoduodenostomy and cholecystoduodenostomy carry high rates of failure and are regarded as obsolete for the treatment of benign biliary stricture.

Duodenal stenosis

Duodenal obstruction from fibrosis can be managed by short-term placement of a removable duodenal stent but gastro-jejunostomy, ideally undertaken laparoscopically, is the preferred treatment.

Pancreatic ascites

This is a rare complication. It is defined as a massive accumulation of pancreatic fluid in the peritoneal cavity.[81] The amylase level in the ascitic fluid is typically elevated threefold above plasma levels although plasma amylase levels are also usually raised. Pancreatic fluid secondary to duct disruption may also track along tissue planes through the diaphragmatic hiatus to the mediastinum, occasionally reaching the pleura or bronchus. Initial management is usually by percutaneous drainage and nutritional support followed by ERCP to localise the site of leakage with insertion of a transpapillary pancreatic duct stent. Surgery is rarely required. Additional treatment with somatostatin or octreotide together with diuretics and repeated paracentesis may be beneficial for some patients.

Pseudocyst complicating chronic pancreatitis

The revised Atlanta Classification of acute pancreatitis retains the term pseudocyst when describing a persistent fluid collection lasting more than 4 weeks from an episode of acute pancreatitis but the definition also carries the cautionary advice that such a collection should contain little or no necrosis.[30] In practical terms, all persistent fluid collections following acute pancreatitis contain some necrosis and should not be termed pseudocysts – a term that should be reserved for an amylase-rich fluid collection lined by granulation tissue more typically seen in association with chronic pancreatitis. These are invariably associated with main pancreatic duct disruption, fibrosis and stricturing of the main pancreatic duct. Features that point to a pseudocyst complicating chronic pancreatitis include parenchymal calcification on CT, pancreatic duct irregularity with segmental dilatation and absence of acute post-inflammatory changes in the peripancreatic fat. Pseudocysts complicating chronic pancreatitis are not liable to resolve spontaneously and usually require intervention. Endoscopic drainage is the preferred modality. Transpapillary stenting may be effective if any duct stricture can be negotiated. Endoscopic ultrasound-guided transgastric drainage will often result in medium-term resolution and stents are often left in situ to prevent closure of the endoscopic cystgastrostomy. Disruption of the main pancreatic duct in its mid-body – typically a consequence of severe acute pancreatitis but also seen in chronic disease – produces the 'disconnected duct syndrome' where the distal gland continues to secrete into the cavity around the middle of the gland.[83] Disconnected duct syndrome can be managed by endoscopic drainage but is one of the rare indications for distal pancreatectomy in chronic pancreatitis.[83]

False aneurysm of visceral vessels

Rarely, patients with chronic pancreatitis can present with gastrointestinal haemorrhage due to false aneurysms of the visceral vessels (**Fig. 15.6**).[84] The splenic artery and gastroduodenal artery are the most frequently affected and optimal intervention is angiographic embolisation.[79]

Extrahepatic portal hypertension

Chronic peripancreatic inflammation and swelling involving the head of the gland can lead to portal vein occlusion resulting in the development of a collateral circulation and cavernous transformation (**Fig. 15.7**).[85] Often this is an asymptomatic late-stage finding in chronic pancreatitis. Although there is some evidence favouring anticoagulation in acute portal vein thrombosis, the evidence in chronic occlusion is less clear and the risks of anticoagulation are considerable. Occlusion of the

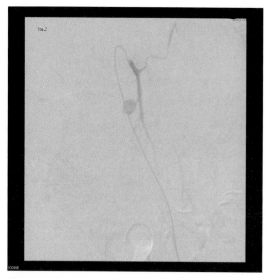

Figure 15.6 • False aneurysm in chronic pancreatitis. Selective mesenteric angiography with cannulation of the superior mesenteric artery (SMA) showing a 2-cm false aneurysm arising from the first jejunal branch.

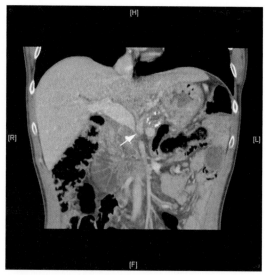

Figure 15.7 • Portal vein occlusion in chronic pancreatitis. Coronal view of a venous phase contrast CT showing a smooth post-inflammatory stenosis of the main portal vein at the level of the spleno-portal confluence (*white arrow*). There is post-stenotic dilatation of the portal vein. Parenchymal calcification is also seen.

splenic vein can lead to sinistral (or left-sided) portal hypertension with a variceal collateral circulation running through the wall of the stomach.[86] It should be noted that transjugular portosystemic stent shunt (TIPSS) is not effective in extrahepatic portal hypertension due to portal vein thrombosis, as the procedure creates a shunt between the intrahepatic portal circulation and the systemic circulation. Gastrointestinal bleeding is rare, and the significance of superior mesenteric vein/portal vein thrombosis, with formation of venous collaterals, is the restriction of subsequent surgical options and approaches.

Pancreatic cancer complicating chronic pancreatitis

There is an increased lifetime risk of cancer arising in long-standing chronic pancreatitis and this should be borne in mind in older patients. The relative risk is 13.3 for developing pancreatic cancer in those with chronic pancreatitis, with a 10–20-year lag between the incidences of pancreatitis and pancreatic malignancy.[87]

Key points

- Long-term alcohol overuse and cigarette smoking are the commonest aetiological factors for chronic pancreatitis.
- Abdominal pain is the most frequent presenting symptom.
- Baseline assessment must include, in addition to clinical history and physical examination, cross-sectional imaging (usually by CT), assessment of nutritional status, exocrine insufficiency and diabetes mellitus.
- Medical management is typically the first step, with analgesia following the WHO analgesic ladder.
- Endoscopic treatment is widely utilised as a second step in patients with chronic pancreatitis. Many patients may be effectively managed without surgery.
- Surgical duct decompression by lateral pancreatico-jejunostomy (the Partington–Rochelle procedure) has been shown to be superior to endoscopic treatment for patients with large duct chronic pancreatitis without a pancreatic head mass.
- In patients with a pancreatic head mass, coexistent pancreatic cancer must be excluded.

- If cancer cannot reliably be excluded, resectional surgery such as pancreatico-duodenectomy is appropriate.
- In patients with a pancreatic head mass and a low risk of cancer, surgical treatment can either utilise the Frey procedure or the Beger duodenum-preserving pancreatic head resection.
- In longstanding chronic pancreatitis, there is an increased risk of diabetes mellitus, malnutrition and pancreatic cancer.

⊕ Full references available at **http://expertconsult. inkling.com**

Key references

16. Conwell DL, Lee LS, Yadav D, et al. American Pancreatic Association practice guidelines in chronic pancreatitis: evidence-based report on diagnostic guidelines. Pancreas 2014;43:1143–62. PMID: 25333398.

This paper provides a concise but comprehensive overview of the diagnostic standards for chronic pancreatitis.

23. Aghdassi AA, Weiss FU, Mayerle J, et al. Genetic susceptibility factors for alcohol-induced chronic pancreatitis. Pancreatology 2015;15(Suppl):S23–31. PMID: 26149858.

This paper provides a good overview of the genetic susceptibility factors for alcohol-induced chronic pancreatitis.

33. Nordback I, Pelli H, Lappalainen-Lehto R, et al. The recurrence of acute alcohol-associated pancreatitis can be reduced: a randomized controlled trial. Gastroenterology 2009;136:848–55. PMID: 19162029.

This important randomised trial shows the effect of counselling in avoidance of repeat admission in alcohol-related pancreatitis.

53. Cahen DL, Gouma DJ, Nio Y, et al. Endoscopic versus surgical drainage of the pancreatic duct in chronic pancreatitis. New Engl J Med 2007;356:676–84. PMID: 17301298.

This important randomised trial compares surgery to endoscopic therapy in patients with large-duct chronic pancreatitis.

16

Pancreatic adenocarcinoma

Shaheel M. Sahebally
Kevin C. Conlon

Introduction

Whilst adenocarcinoma of the pancreas accounts for only 3% of new cancer cases annually, it represents the fourth leading cause for cancer-related mortality for both men and women.[1] The aggressive nature of the disease, coupled with its ambiguous presentation and lack of a diagnostic biomarker, frequently result in delayed diagnosis.[2,3] Surgery remains the only cure for pancreatic cancer, yet only 10–15% of newly diagnosed patients have surgically resectable disease at presentation.[4] For those patients who undergo a curative R0 resection, most will still recur within 2 years, leading to disappointing 5-year survival rates of 20–25%.[5,6]

The majority (~95%) of pancreatic tumours are adenocarcinomas, originating from the exocrine part of the pancreas. Nearly all of these are ductal adenocarcinomas, which is the focus of this chapter.

Epidemiology

It is estimated that there will be 53 070 new cases of pancreatic cancer diagnosed in the United States alone in 2016, with an estimated 41 780 cases expected to die from the disease.[1] Pancreatic cancer is the eleventh commonest cancer in males and eighth commonest cancer in females.[7] Its incidence varies with age, sex and ethnicity, and is highest is Northern Europe and North America,[8] being 3-4 times higher than rates observed in tropical countries.[9] The UK incidence of pancreatic adenocarcinoma is approximately 9 per 100 000 population.[10] Keane et al.[11] explored incidence trends in pancreatic adenocarcinoma in a large UK primary care cohort between 2000 and 2010 and noted increases in annual incidence by an average of 3% per year (95% CI 1–4%) but found no association between incidence and social deprivation. The peak incidence for the disease occurs between the seventh and eighth decades of life, and is rare under the age of 30.[12]

Risk factors (see Box 16.1)

Smoking

Tobacco smoking remains the most consistent modifiable risk factor associated with the development of pancreatic cancer.[13,14–16] A meta-analysis of 82 studies[17] found the overall risk of pancreatic cancer in current and former smokers to be 1.74 (95% CI 1.61–1.87) and 1.2 (95% CI 1.11–1.29), respectively. It is postulated that a dose-dependent relationship occurs, necessitating long-term exposure.[18] For ex-smokers, the risk persisted for a minimum of 10 years following cessation.[17] The exact mechanism through which cigarette smoking affects pancreatic carcinogenesis is still unknown, but it is hypothesised that N-nitroso compounds in tobacco are carried haematogenously to the pancreas where they have been shown to induce pancreatic cancer in animal models.[19]

Diet and alcohol

A meta-analysis of observational studies comprising 6643 patients found an overall statistically significant

Box 16.1 • Risk factors for pancreatic cancer

Age (above 60 years)
Smoking
Obesity
High fat diet
Alcohol abuse
Pancreatitis
    Chronic pancreatitis
    Hereditary pancreatitis
Diabetes mellitus
Family history of pancreatic cancer
Genetic predisposition
    Peutz–Jeghers syndrome
    Li–Fraumeni syndrome
    Fanconi syndrome
    Familial adenomatous polyposis
    Lynch syndrome
    Gardner syndrome
    Multiple endocrine neoplasia
    BRCA1
    Von Hippel–Lindau syndrome

association between processed meat consumption and pancreatic cancer risk, while red meat consumption significantly increased the risk only in men.[20] It has been suggested that fruit and vegetable intake may confer a protective effect against the development of pancreatic cancer;[21,22] however, a pooled analysis of 14 prospective studies from North America, Europe and Australia found no overall statistically significant association.[23] In regards to dairy products (including calcium and vitamin D) and risk of pancreatic cancer, a recent pooled meta-analysis showed no statistically significant overall association.[24] Finally, heavy alcohol consumption (i.e. ≥9 drinks/per day) significantly increased the risk of pancreatic cancer.[25]

Occupation

Occupational exposure to electromagnetic fields, asbestos, acrylamide and halogenated hydrocarbons is associated with a higher risk of developing pancreatic adenocarcinoma. There is evidence of an amplified risk in people exposed to chlorinated hydrocarbon solvents (metal degreasing workers and dry cleaners) and nickel compounds as well as people working in the paint/varnish and textile industries.[26]

Past medical history

Prior meta-analyses have shown an association between diabetes mellitus and pancreatic adeno-carcinoma.[27–29] Song et al.[30] examined the influence of long-term diabetes mellitus on incidence of

pancreatic adenocarcinoma and noted that diabetes duration of 2 or more years was associated with a 1.5–1.7-fold increased risk of cancer. However, this risk was inversely proportional to disease duration.

✔✔ Diabetes mellitus, especially for ≥2 years, is associated with an increased risk of pancreatic carcinogenesis. However, the risk is inversely proportional to the duration of disease.[30]

The mechanism linking diabetes mellitus to pancreatic tumourigenesis may be partly explained by pronounced reactive oxygen species (ROS) production secondary to persistent hyperglycaemia, which in turn enhances the migratory capacity of tumour cells.[31]

Histories of gallstone disease or cholecystectomy have also been shown to be independent risk factors for pancreatic carcinogenesis.[32]

✔✔ Both gallstones and prior cholecystectomy significantly increase the risk of pancreatic cancer in Asian as well as white populations. This positive association was independent of factors such as smoking, diabetes mellitus, obesity and number of years post cholecystectomy.[32]

Chronic pancreatitis is characterised by irreversible glandular damage and accumulating evidence points to an increased risk of pancreatic cancer, although the highest risk is in patients with early onset pancreatitis, such as hereditary and tropical pancreatitis.[33] However, over a 20-year period, only around 5% of patients with chronic pancreatitis will develop pancreatic cancer.[33] Other conditions linked to pancreatic adenocarcinoma include cystic fibrosis,[34] Gardner's syndrome and multiple endocrine neoplasia type 1 syndrome (MEN 1).

Hereditary pancreatic cancer

Epidemiological evidence[35,36] suggests that first-degree relatives with pancreatic cancer have at least a twofold increased risk of developing the disease. A meta-analysis of 6568 pancreatic cancer cases showed a significant increase in pancreatic cancer risk associated with having an affected relative, with an overall summary RR of 1.8 (95% CI 1.48–2.12).[37] Patients with familial pancreatic cancer make up 8–10% of all cases of pancreatic cancer.[38,39] Familial pancreatic cancer kindreds have two or more first-degree relatives diagnosed with pancreatic adenocarcinoma.

Although novel genes that predispose to familial pancreatic cancer remain to be fully elucidated, it is now well established that an increased risk is associated with familial conditions such as Peutz–Jeghers syndrome and germ-line mutations in *BRCA1/BRCA2* (hereditary breast–ovarian cancer syndrome),[40] *CDKN2A* (familial atypical mole and melanoma syndrome),[40] *PALB2* (familial breast cancer syndrome),[40] *ATM* (familial breast cancer syndrome),[41] mismatch repair genes (Hereditary Non Polyposis Colorectal Cancer or Lynch syndrome) and *PRSS1* and *SPINK1* of hereditary pancreatitis. Guidelines for family members at risk of hereditary pancreatic cancer are being developed, albeit based on expert opinion.[42]

Precursor lesions

Pancreatic carcinogenesis comprises histologically distinct precursor lesions. Preneoplastic lesions are usually asymptomatic and are small in size (usually <5 mm), making them radiographically occult and hence they are more commonly discovered at the time of resection. They appear to follow a multi-step progression to invasive carcinoma, analogous to that in colorectal cancer.[43] These precursor lesions include pancreatic intraepithelial neoplasia (PanIN), intraductal papillary mucinous neoplasm (IPMN) and mucinous cystic neoplasm (MCN).[44]

The commonest of these is Pan-IN, observed in approximately 82% of neoplastic pancreases.[45] They are traditionally subclassified into PanIN-1, PanIN-2 and PanIN-3, depending upon the degree of cytological and architectural atypia.[45] However, following the recent Baltimore Consensus Meeting for Neoplastic Pancreatic Precursor Lesions, a revised two-tiered classification system has been suggested such that all precursor lesions are either low-grade (PanIN-1, Pan-IN-2) or high-grade (PanIN-3, carcinoma in situ) dysplastic lesions.[46]

These lesions, first observed adjacent to resected adenocarcinoma, exhibit similar genetic alterations to the frankly invasive samples. In particular, the frequency of p16 and K-ras mutations increases with the severity of PanIN and this observation led to the development of a pancreatic tumourigenesis model involving a stepwise progression from PanIN to invasive carcinoma,[47] in turn characterised by diverse molecular changes (**Fig. 16.1**). Evidence suggests that pancreatic adenocarcinoma harbours approximately 63 genetic alterations, of which the majority are point mutations, including genes such as K-ras, p16/CDKN2A, TP53 and SMAD4.[48] The commonest observed mutation is K-ras, seen in >90% of pancreatic adenocarcinoma and also in about 45% of low-grade PanIN lesions.[49,50] K-ras is involved in various downstream signalling pathways, and mutations result in constitutive activation.[51]

P16/CDKN2A (cyclin-dependent kinase inhibitor 2A gene) is a tumour suppressor gene that is inactivated in up to 90% of pancreatic adenocarcinoma.[52] It functions to regulate the cell cycle. *TP53* and *SMAD4* are also tumour suppressor genes that are inactivated in 75% and 55% of pancreatic cancer, respectively.[53,54] Typically, these mutations are seen in

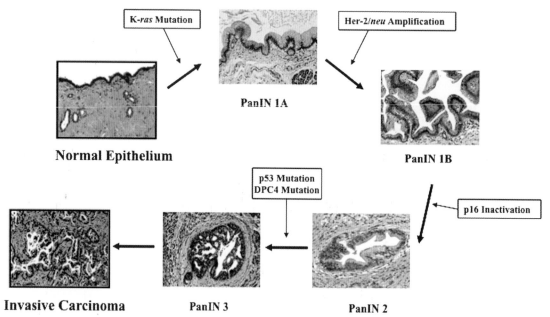

Figure 16.1 • Diagrammatic representation of the multi-step progression to invasive carcinoma from low-grade to high-grade neoplasm.
Images courtesy of Dr Paul Crotty.

late-stage precursor lesions, especially in high-grade PanIN.[55] Waddell et al.[56] performed whole-genome analysis of 100 pancreatic adenocarcinomas and implicated several other genes, including *KDM6A*, *PREX2*, *ERBB2*, *MET* etc. Similarly, whole-genome sequencing of 456 pancreatic ductal adenocarcinomas has recently identified 32 significantly mutated genes, which aggregated into 10 distinct molecular pathways.[57] Furthermore, work by the same group defined four independent pancreatic cancer subtypes (squamous, pancreatic progenitor, immunogenic and aberrantly differentiated endocrine exocrine), each of which is characterised by different transcriptional networks, histopathological features as well as survival. These data provide valuable insight into the mechanisms underlying pancreatic carcinogenesis and provide novel opportunities to target these molecular pathways. Unfortunately discussion about each of these genes and their associated transcription pathways is beyond the scope of this chapter.

Presentation

Most patients with pancreatic cancer present with non-specific symptoms such as weight loss, bloating and anorexia (Box 16.2). As a result, the disease is usually disseminated at diagnosis, and approximately 80% of patients have unresectable disease.[4]

Tumours in the body and tail of the pancreas usually present late. Painful jaundice is the commonest complaint (46%), followed by pain only (34%) or painless jaundice (13%). Weight loss and anorexia are seen in 7% of cases. Occasionally, haematemesis and malaena occur secondary to tumour invasion into stomach or duodenum. Late-onset diabetes mellitus or acute pancreatitis may also be the first sign of an underlying pancreatic neoplasm.[58] While widespread screening of asymptomatic cohorts does not appear cost-effective given the low incidence of the disease and the dearth of a cheap, sensitive and specific biomarker, targeted screening may be appropriate in high-risk individuals.[59] With regards to patients at increased risk for familial pancreatic cancer, experts at the recent International Cancer of the Pancreas Screening (CAPS) Consortium

Summit recommended screening with endoscopic ultrasound or magnetic resonance imaging for the following patients: first-degree relatives of patients with pancreatic cancer from a familial pancreatic cancer kindred with at least two affected first-degree relatives, patients with Peutz–Jeghers syndrome and *p16*, *BRCA2* and *HNPCC* mutation carriers with ≥1 affected first-degree relative.[60]

The classical Courvoisier's sign (palpable gallbladder with painless jaundice) occurs in less than 25% of patients. Jaundice may represent either primary disease causing biliary obstruction or external compression of the biliary system by metastatic nodal disease. Pain is a more common symptom than physicians typically appreciate, usually secondary to involvement of visceral afferent nerves or resultant local pancreatitis. Pain on initial presentation is suggestive of unresectability. Weight loss is common, often associated with early satiety, nausea or vomiting. The latter may be due to gastric outlet obstruction.

Virchow's node (left supraclavicular node associated with upper gastrointestinal malignancy), thrombophlebitis migrans (non-specific paraneoplastic sign named after Trousseau) and Sister Mary Joseph nodule (umbilical metastatic lesion via the falciform ligament) are well-recognised features of advanced disease. Hepatomegaly is seen in 65% of patients and may reflect hepatic metastases. Blumer's shelf (rectally palpable rectovesicle or rectovaginal mass) rarely occurs and is not usually sought as part of routine examination.

The most useful aid in making the diagnosis is a high index of suspicion. Vague epigastric symptoms and weight loss in the presence of normal endoscopy and preliminary radiology mandate further detailed investigation.

Investigation

Serology

Haematological and hepatic biochemical measurements are largely unhelpful in diagnosis. A mild normochromic anaemia may be present due to occult blood loss while thrombocytosis is also sometimes observed. Elevated serum bilirubin and alkaline phosphatase confirm obstructive jaundice; amylase and lipase may be elevated in those presenting with pancreatitis (5%). An elevated prothrombin time suggests hepatic dysfunction secondary to liver infiltration by metastases. Hyperglycaemia is non-specific and is seen in approximately 20% of patients and could be related to the fact that type 2 diabetes mellitus confers an increased risk of pancreatic cancer or may be the first presenting sign of the underlying cancer. Patients with malnutrition have hypoalbuminaemia and low cholesterol level.

Box 16.2 • Symptoms/signs suggestive of pancreatic neoplasm

Early satiety
Obstructive jaundice (± pain)
Unexplained weight loss
Endoscopy-negative epigastric/back pain
Late-onset diabetes
Signs of malabsorption without defined cause

Markers

As of yet, there remains no effective tumour marker for pancreatic adenocarcinoma. The most widely employed serum marker is sialylated Lewis blood group antigen on MUC-1 (Mucin 1, cell surface associated) carbohydrate antigen 19-9 (CA 19-9). It is a cell surface glycoprotein expressed by pancreatic neoplastic cells, as well as normal pancreatic and biliary duct cells, gastric, colonic, endometrial and salivary epithelia.[61] CA 19-9 has suboptimal sensitivity (41–86%) and specificity (33–100%) for detecting pancreatic cancer[62] and 4–15% of the general population do not express the antigen and hence do not have detectable serum CA 19-9 levels.[63] In addition, only 65% of resectable pancreatic adenocarcinoma demonstrated an elevated CA 19-9, while the marker was increased in 40% of patients with chronic pancreatitis.[64] Because of these limitations, CA 19-9 is mostly used as a prognostic marker to assess response to therapy in patients already diagnosed with pancreatic cancer.[65]

Other potential markers include CA494,[66] CEACAM1 (carcinoembryonic antigen-related cell adhesion molecule 1),[67] PTHrP (parathyroid hormone-related protein),[68] TuM2-PK (tumour M2-pyruvate kinase)[69] and serum β-HCG (beta-human chorionic gonadotropin).[70] However, further work is required before they can be translated into clinical practice. An in-depth discussion of each of these promising markers is beyond the scope of this chapter.

Diagnosis

Imaging studies

Transabdominal ultrasound (US) is the initial investigation in the jaundiced patient. It is superior to computed tomography (CT) to detect cholelithiasis. Common bile duct dilatation (>7 mm, >10 mm in post-cholecystectomy patients) is an indirect sign, together with pancreatic duct dilatation (>2 mm). The primary pancreatic lesion is often visible together with hepatic metastases and ascites if present. For lesions >3 cm, US is approximately 95% sensitive; however, sensitivity is considerably lower for smaller lesions.[71] The major drawback of US is machine quality difference and operator experience, making it user-dependent.[72] Colour Doppler US has been suggested to assess vascular involvement (portal or superior mesenteric vein/artery) by the tumour.

While US remains a useful imaging modality for the initial work-up of the jaundiced patient, additional imaging modalities are required to examine the pancreas and assess resectability status.

CT remains the commonest cross-sectional imaging modality. Conventional CT has been replaced by more sensitive and dynamic CT with thinner slice/cuts (1–3 mm) with multidetector and 3D reconstruction. For lesions >2 cm, the sensitivity is approximately 90%, decreasing to approximately 60% for smaller lesions.[73] CT not only allows assessment of the primary pancreatic lesion, but also its relationship to the remainder of the pancreas and peripancreatic vasculature, and determination of resectability (**Figs 16.2–16.5**). Direct evidence of a tumour is often seen as a hypodense mass, with other subtle signs such as pancreatic atrophy, deformity of the glandular contour or double duct dilatation (common bile duct and pancreatic duct; **Fig. 16.6**). Metastatic lesions can be detected as well as portal vein or superior mesenteric arterial involvement. However, despite these advances, CT-imaging is limited at detecting small liver or peritoneal metastatic deposits of occult disease.[74]

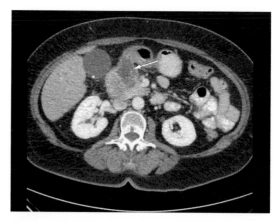

Figure 16.2 • Necrotic mass in the head of the pancreas (*arrow*).

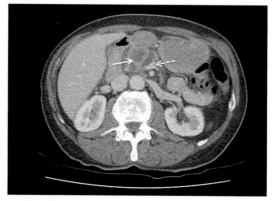

Figure 16.3 • Locally advanced borderline resectable tumour (*solid arrow*) with deformity of the superior mesenteric vein (*dashed arrow*).

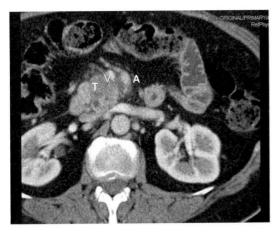

Figure 16.4 • Locally advanced unresectable tumour (*T*) with involvement of the superior mesenteric vein (*V*) and artery (*A*).

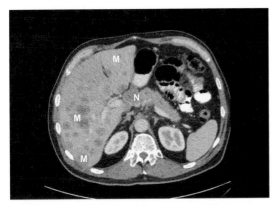

Figure 16.5 • Multiple hepatic metastases (*M*) from pancreatic neoplasm (*N*).

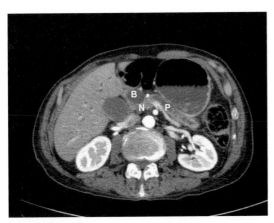

Figure 16.6 • Biliary duct (*B*) and pancreatic duct (*P*) obstruction by pancreatic neoplasm (*N*) denoting the double duct sign.

Magnetic resonance imaging (MRI) is mainly used as an adjunct to CT for planning treatment options. The combination of T1/T2-weighted imaging and magnetic resonance cholangiopancreatography (MRCP) is useful to visualise the primary tumour and its relationship to the biliary and pancreatic ducts, as well as peripancreatic vasculature. Kim et al. [75] suggested that MR imaging might be able to identify up to 79% of pancreatic tumours that appeared isodense on multiphasic CT.

Positron emission tomography (PET) shows accumulation of [^{18}F]2-fluoro-2-deoxy-D-glucose (FDG) by tumour cells, and has the advantage of combining metabolic activity with imaging characteristics while imaging the whole body. PET-CT scanners are able to detect small (up to 7 mm) pancreatic neoplasms and diagnose metastatic disease in about 40%.[76] PET is increasingly becoming a common method of assessing tumour response to treatment and may be prognostic. However, FDG-PET is not accurate in pancreatic disease due to its reliance on normal glucose homeostasis. The combination of PET-CT carries a sensivity of 92%, and is superior to either modality alone.[77]

Endoscopic retrograde cholangiopancreatography (ERCP) is reserved mainly to assess obstructive intraductal lesions and to relieve biliary obstruction in selected cases. MRCP has replaced ERCP as a diagnostic modality of choice.

Endoscopic ultrasound (EUS) is increasingly used to stage pancreatic adenocarcinoma. In addition to being more sensitive than CT in detecting small neoplastic lesions, it also provides tissue diagnoses through fine-needle aspiration (FNA) with higher sensitivity and specificity compared to CT-guided FNA, and without the need of administration of a contrast agent.[78] It may also help clarify benign conditions mimicking cancer, such as sclerosing pancreatitis or atypical choledocholithiasis. However, EUS is costly, invasive and operator-dependent.

Cytology/histology

Multidetector cross-sectional CT is the radiological modality of choice in the staging and diagnosis of pancreatic cancer. In selected cases, histological confirmation of malignancy may not be established prior to surgery. However, in patients selected for neoadjuvant therapy, histological confirmation is essential via FNA by EUS/ERCP or percutaneously by CT-guidance.

Advanced staging techniques

Laparoscopy

Despite advances in non-invasive imaging, laparoscopic staging and ultrasound have a role in selected cases. Laparoscopy can be performed immediately before conversion to laparotomy or as an interval staging measure. The routine use of diagnostic laparoscopy remains controversial and institution-dependent. However, laparoscopic ultrasonography can potentially identify radiographically occult metastatic disease and hence obviate the need for non-curative laparotomies. It enables direct visualisation of intra-abdominal organs and can detect metastatic deposits <3 mm on peritoneal and hepatic structures, thereby offering more accurate disease staging[79] (**Figs 16.7** and **16.8**).

✅ Staging laparoscopy (with a 30-degree lens) in patients diagnosed with pancreatic cancer should be used selectively. Hepatic and/or peritoneal deposits, if present, should be sampled. Laparoscopic ultrasound is reserved for patients with suspected vascular invasion and may help detect intrahepatic or lymph node metastases, and hence influence resectability status.

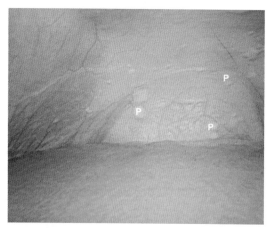

Figure 16.7 • Staging laparoscopy demonstrating peritoneal metastases (*P*).

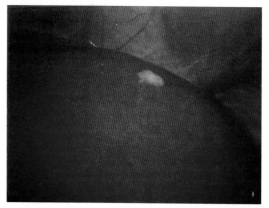

Figure 16.8 • Staging laparoscopy demonstrating a liver metastasis.

A recent meta-analysis concluded that diagnostic laparoscopy with biopsy of suspected lesions prior to definitive laparotomy avoided non-curative laparotomies in 21% of cases, all of which were deemed resectable by CT imaging.[80]

Detractors of laparoscopy argue that a significant proportion of patients require (open) surgical bypass and therefore laparoscopic staging should only be used if bypass would not be contemplated at open surgery.[81] Evidence from single-centre studies suggests that the need for subsequent operative palliation for established gastric outlet obstruction is less than 5%.[82] Moreover, less invasive options are now available for managing malignant gastric outlet obstruction such as endoscopic stenting and laparoscopic gastroenterostomy. A small (24 patients) randomised study comparing open versus laparoscopic gastroenterostomy concluded that the laparoscopic approach was associated with significantly less intraoperative blood loss, shorter time to oral solid food intake and less delayed gastric emptying.[83] Gurusamy et al. performed a meta-analysis to address the need for prophylactic gastrojejunostomy in patients with unresectable periampullary cancers (pancreatic cancer made up 92.1% of cases) and reported that prophylactic gastrojejunostomy was associated with a statistically significant lower risk of gastric outlet obstruction compared to controls.[84] However, there was no difference in quality of life between the two groups. The authors went on to recommend routine prophylactic gastroenterostomy in patients with unresectable disease (with or without hepatico-jejunostomy). However, it is important to mention that both trials included in this meta-analysis were associated with a high risk of bias and that all patients underwent exploratory laparotomy. Therefore, the results are not applicable to patients with unresectable disease diagnosed during staging laparoscopy.

General laparoscopy is performed with an angled (usually 30°) lens looking for small-volume peritoneal and liver metastases. The liver is examined systematically and usually all but segment 7 can be viewed. Biopsy of hepatic or peritoneal deposits for frozen-section histology is taken, and the procedure is terminated if positive. If metastases are not seen, the hepatico-duodenal ligament is inspected for nodal disease. The lesser sac is opened by incising the gastrocolic omentum to inspect for tumour, and biopsies of the primary may be undertaken. This is achievable in 80% of cases. In certain institutions, the duodenum is mobilised but this is unnecessary in the majority of cases. With more effective neoadjuvant regimens, it is important to use laparoscopic strategies to define patients who may be suitable for downstaging, similar to advanced rectal lesions.

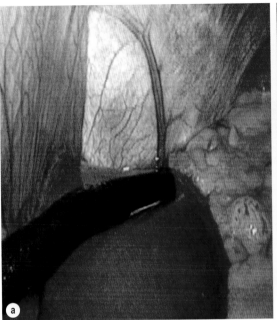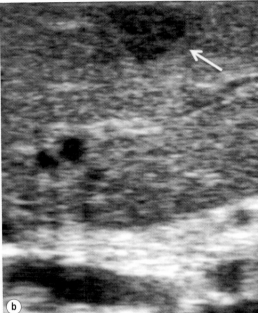

Figure 16.9 • **(a)** Laparoscopic ultrasonography, and **(b)** liver metastasis (*white arrow*).

Laparoscopic ultrasound (LUS) has been advocated as an additional aid to detect intrahepatic metastases, lymph node or vascular involvement to determine resectability (**Fig. 16.9**). However, the added value is <10% and therefore LUS should be reserved only for cases in which there is concern of vascular invasion.[85]

The role of peritoneal cytology taken during laparoscopic staging is less well defined, although it may improve staging accuracy. Recently, Oh et al. found that 14% of patients who would otherwise be classified as having potentially resectable disease had positive peritoneal cytology during routine staging laparoscopy and were subsequently upstaged to stage IV disease.[86] Moreover, most patients (86%) with positive cytology experienced disease progression after chemotherapy/chemoradiotherapy and their 5-year survival was zero.

Pathology

Ductal adenocarcinomas account for >85% of all pancreatic neoplasms. Other types of malignant tumours include the following:

- adenosquamous carcinoma
- mucinous non-cystic (colloid) carcinoma
- mucinous cystic neoplasms
- intraductal papillary mucinous neoplasm with an associated invasive carcinoma
- solid pseudopapillary neoplasm
- acinar cell carcinoma
- pancreatoblastoma
- serous cystadenocarcinoma
- undifferentiated (anaplastic) carcinoma
- signet-ring cell carcinoma
- giant cell carcinoma.

Treatment

Treatment strategies should be discussed at a multidisciplinary level, with emphasis on established guidelines. The American Joint Committee on Cancer TNM staging is outlined in Table 16.1.

Figure 16.10 outlines the authors' current treatment algorithm for patients with pancreatic cancer.

Resection

Surgical treatment remains the only potential cure for pancreatic cancer, yet patient selection remains paramount.

In patients with obstructive jaundice and surgically resectable disease, the use of preoperative biliary drainage is a topic of ongoing debate. Proponents of decompression argue that jaundiced patients undergoing surgery are at increased risk of perioperative sepsis, pancreatic fistula and wound infections[87] while detractors argue that routine biliary drainage is itself associated with an increased risk of procedure-specific complications such as cholangitis, pancreatitis and stent-related perforations.[88] A recent

Table 16.1 • American Joint Committee on Cancer TNM staging, 2013

Primary tumour (T)

TX	Primary tumour cannot be assessed
T0	No evidence of primary tumour
Tis	Carcinoma in situ
T1	Tumour limited to the pancreas, $\leq 2\,cm$ in greatest dimension
T2	Tumour limited to the pancreas, $>2\,cm$ in greatest dimension
T3	Tumour extends beyond the pancreas but without involvement of the coeliac axis or the superior mesenteric artery
T4	Tumour involves the coeliac axis or the superior mesenteric artery (unresectable primary tumour)

Regional lymph nodes (N)

NX	Regional lymph nodes cannot be assessed
N0	No regional lymph node metastasis
N1	Regional lymph node metastasis

Distant metastasis (M)

M0	No distant metastasis
M1	Distant metastasis

Stage	T	N	M
0	Tis	N0	M0
IA	T1	N0	M0
IB	T2	N0	M0
IIA	T3	N0	M0
IIB	T1	N1	M0
	T2	N1	M0
	T3	N1	M0
III	T4	Any N	M0
IV	Any T	Any N	M1

Courtesy of AJCC Cancer Staging Manual, Eighth Edition

meta-analysis reported that patients who underwent internal preoperative biliary drainage sustained statistically fewer major adverse events compared to those who had surgery only.[89] The authors' practice is not to decompress the bile duct preoperatively unless symptoms and signs of cholangitis or secondary signs of hyperbilirubinaemia are present. If a neoadjuvant approach is being considered, biliary stenting is required prior to commencing chemo/radiotherapy. Coagulopathy, if present, is treated with vitamin K, prior to resection.

Patient selection is key, including cardiovascular and respiratory evaluation. Curative surgery is associated with a median survival of 11–23 months, with approximately 10–27% alive at 5 years.[90] Previously, pancreatic resections were associated with significant mortality; however, with advances in perioperative supportive care, mortality rates are now <5% in high-volume centres.[91]

Pancreatico-duodenectomy

Pancreatico-duodenectomy was first described by Kausch in 1912, and later popularised by Whipple in 1935. The classical Whipple procedure (two-stage) was an en bloc resection of the pancreatic head, duodenum, common bile duct, with the distal stomach and surrounding lymph nodes. Later being performed as a one-stage operation, it still remains the surgical therapy for tumours of the pancreatic head and neck.

The right colon is mobilised, exposing the third and fourth parts of the duodenum, and an extended Kocherisation is performed. This allows a tumour in the head of the pancreas to be palpated and exposes the left renal vein. The aortocaval and portal vein (PV) nodal packages are dissected and the respective vessels are skeletonised. Resectability is finally assessed as extensive involvement of the confluence

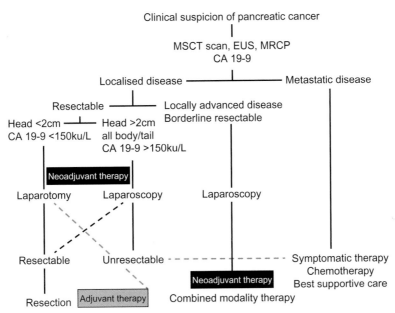

Figure 16.10 • Treatment algorithm for patients with pancreatic cancer.

of the PV/superior mesenteric vein (SMV) may herald termination of the procedure. It is important to remember that short segments of the PV can be resected if necessary, and therefore an involved PV does not necessarily denote unresectability.

> ✅ The relationship of the tumour to the first jejunal branch of the SMV is often the critical determinant of resectability. If this is involved by tumour, the likelihood of being able to reconstruct the SMV is low.

The remaining porta hepatis is dissected, and nodes are cleared. Cholecystectomy facilitates higher ligation of the bile duct, which is transected just proximal to the insertion of the cystic duct. It is the authors' practice to send a biliary aspirate for routine culture and sensitivity, as postoperative infective complications tend to involve enteric organisms.[92]

The common bile duct is mobilised distally and the hepatico-duodenal ligament is dissected along its length, taking care to identify and preserve the common hepatic artery and PV. The gastroduodenal artery is ligated while care is taken not to damage an aberrant right hepatic artery.

In a conventional Whipple, the distal stomach is resected. This is the authors' favoured approach as resection includes the nodes along the greater and lesser curves, reduces stomach-emptying dysfunction postoperatively, diminishes the density of parietal cells and theoretically reduces the risk of gastritis. The stomach is transected at the antrum along with the attached omentum. The proximal jejunum along

with its mesentery is transected and the mobilised duodenum and jejunum is delivered back under the ligament of Treitz.

The pancreas is transected between four stay sutures (to facilitate haemostasis in the marginal arteries) after the uncinate process has been dissected from the superior mesenteric vessels. Retroperitoneal dissection allows the tumour and nodal package to be delivered en bloc. If any doubt exists regarding the adequacy of tumour clearance, the pancreatic resection margin should be sent for frozen section histology. Verbeke and Menon had shown that a discrepancy between margin status and clinical outcome is due to frequent under-reporting of microscopic margin involvement.[93] The lack of a standardised pathological examination, with confusing nomenclature and controversy regarding the definition of microscopic margin involvement, results in the wide variation of reported R1 rates (between 18% and 85%).[94]

Reconstruction is undertaken with the biliary anastomosis followed by the pancreatic and finally the gastric. Pancreatico-jejunostomy and pancreatico-gastrostomy are the most commonly employed techniques for pancreatico-enteric reconstruction. A recent meta-analysis reported statistically significantly fewer rates of pancreatic fistula and intra-abdominal fluid collections after pancreatico-gastrostomy, with no significant differences in overall morbidity, mortality or length of hospital stay.[95]

The nature of the pancreatic reconstruction is subject to individual variation. The authors favour a two-layered pancreatico-jejunal anastomosis with mucosa-to-mucosa reconstruction. Choledocho-jejunostomy is performed in a similar end-to-side manner, leaving the gastrojejunostomy until the end. Abdominal drains are not routinely placed.[96]

Morbidity following resection varies, with the majority of complications being minor. The most significant cause of morbidity is development of a pancreatic fistula, observed in 7–18% of cases.[97,98]

> ✅✅ Octreotide administration in patients with a soft pancreas and non-dilated ducts did not significantly lower the rate of pancreatic fistula, overall morbidity or duration of hospital stay compared to patients who did not receive the medication although the trend favoured octreotide.[97]

Most complications can be dealt with either conservatively or using drains placed by interventional radiology. A minority (<5%) of cases requires re-laparotomy.

Pylorus-preserving pancreatico-duodenectomy (PPPDR)

Many centres recommend a PPPDR approach, first described by Watson in 1942. It is postulated to retain a functioning pylorus with an intact neurovascular supply, thereby ensuring good gastrointestinal function and diminishing nutritive, dumping and bile reflux sequelae.[99] A recent meta-analysis from Buchler's group showed no significant differences in overall survival, postoperative morbidity or mortality between PPPDR and a classical Whipple; however, the latter procedure was associated with significantly less delayed gastric emptying (DGE) whereas PPPDR resulted in significantly less operating time, intraoperative blood loss and red cell transfusions.[100]

> ✅✅ PPPDR and classical pancreatico-duodenectomy are similar with respect to morbidity, mortality and survival. However, rates of delayed gastric emptying are significantly lower with classical pancreatico-duodenectomy, whilst PPPDR results in significantly shorter operating time, less blood loss as well as fewer red cell transfusions.[100]

PPPDR dictates conventional mobilisation to the point where the stomach requires transection; the right gastric artery is preserved and the duodenum is transected at least 2 cm distal to the pylorus. Reconstruction is usually accomplished by duodenojejunostomy or gastrojejunostomy.

Subtotal stomach-preserving pancreatico-duodenectomy (SSPPD) is a relatively novel technique developed in an attempt to decrease the incidence of DGE.[101] It involves division of the stomach 2–3 cm proximal to the pyloric ring such that >90% of the stomach is preserved. In a meta-analysis comparing SSPPD and PPPDR, comprised of 650 patients, Huang et al. demonstrated that SSPPD was associated with a significantly lower rate of DGE but more intraoperative blood loss.[102] However, there were no differences in mortality, pancreatic fistula or intra-abdominal abscess rates between the two techniques. Nakamura et al. went one step further and compared rates of DGE between an antecolic side-to-side gastric greater curvature-to-jejunal anastomosis and a similar antecolic but end-to-side gastric stump-to-jejunal anastomosis in all patients undergoing SSPPD.[103] They showed that the former technique was associated with a significantly reduced rate of DGE, but similar overall morbidity compared to the end-to-side technique.

Extended lymph node and vascular dissection

It is the authors' practice to perform extended dissection including aortocaval nodal clearance in the majority of cases. At presentation, most tumours have involvement of lymph nodes beyond the gland and we believe that clearance of the left gastric and aortocaval nodes not only increases the specificity of staging and the resultant predicted prognosis but also the likelihood of a negative surgical margin. However, a recent meta-analysis examining previously published randomised trials failed to demonstrate improved overall survival with extended lymphadenectomy compared to standard dissection.[104] Moreover, extended dissection was associated with significantly worse postoperative morbidity.

> ✅✅ Whilst extended lymphadenectomy during pancreatico-duodenectomy increased the number of excised lymph nodes, it was associated with increased postoperative morbidity and failed to translate into improved overall survival, compared to standard lymph node dissection.[104]

The role of extensive vascular resection is very much an area of ongoing interest as the boundary of resectability for pancreatic cancer is continuously being pushed forward in an attempt to improve curability rates in patients who would otherwise be deemed unresectable. In a meta-analysis conducted by Zhou et al. comparing SMV/PV resection versus no resection in patients undergoing pancreatico-duodenectomy, there was no difference in postoperative morbidity or mortality between the two groups.[105] Furthermore, the 5-year overall survival rate was not significantly different between the two groups (12.3% in the vascular resection versus 17% in the no resection group); translating into better outcomes compared to strict palliative therapy. On the other hand, arterial resections may be indicated in selected cases, despite being associated with increased perioperative mortality compared to those without arterial resections.[106]

Distal pancreatectomy

Distal pancreatectomy is the procedure of choice for tumours of the body and tail of the pancreas. The pancreatic neck is dissected from the portal vein and the splenic flexure of the colon is taken down. In the majority of ductal cancers, the spleen is also resected to achieve an en bloc clearance. Splenic preservation is generally limited to patients with benign or borderline neoplasms. Patients undergoing distal pancreatectomy and splenic resection are vaccinated prophylactically preoperatively against encapsulated organisms such as *Haemophilus influenza* B, *Neisseria meningitidis* and *Streptococcus pneumoniae*.

Laparoscopic pancreatectomy

Laparoscopic pancreatectomy remains one of the most challenging minimally invasive abdominal operations to date. Accumulating evidence shows that laparoscopic pancreatico-duodenectomy is safe and feasible.[107] It has been shown to be associated with similar overall survival rates but significantly lower wound infection and pancreatic fistula rates, and reduced hospital stay, compared to the classic open approach.[108] Laparoscopic distal pancreatic resection is currently the most frequently performed minimally invasive pancreatic procedure, associated with decreased blood loss and reduced length of stay as well as lower rates of wound infections and similar oncological outcomes.[109,110] The Memorial Sloan-Kettering Cancer Center group published their experience of distal pancreatectomy using open, laparoscopic or robotic approaches.[111] There were no significant differences in 90-day morbidity and mortality or pancreatic fistula rates or oncologic outcomes between the three groups; however, the open group was associated with significantly more intraoperative blood loss. A recent review by Kocaay et al. concluded that laparoscopic pancreatic surgery remained a reasonable treatment modality for low-grade malignant tumours when performed by skilled surgeons in high-volume centres.[112] However, further research into its oncological safety and long-term outcomes is needed before it can be firmly established as first-line treatment.

Total pancreatectomy

Some suggest that pancreatic cancer is a multicentric disease and therefore advocate total pancreatectomy. It was initially proposed to avoid the risk of pancreatico-enteric leaks and to remove potential undetected synchronous disease in other parts of the gland. Although total pancreatectomy can be carried out safely, the survival benefit is so dismal it questions the indication for the operation.

Central pancreatectomy

The role of central pancreatectomy (CP) is rare and limited due to a narrow spectrum of indications. The procedure is historically reserved for patients with chronic pancreatitis and traumatic injuries. More recently, it has been advocated for use in lesions of the pancreatic neck. Opponents of this technique argue against higher rates of pancreatic anastomotic leakage whilst those in favour say it offers preserved functional elements (endocrine and exocrine) of the pancreas.[113]

Surgical palliation

Obstructive jaundice

In the majority of cases, biliary obstruction can be adequately relieved by endoscopic measures. However, in selected cases, surgical palliation may be required. Cholecysto-jejunostomy may be performed in cases where the cystic duct is patent and the tumour is not within 1 cm of the cystic duct. Alternatively, choledocho-jejunostomy may be used, which has equivalent outcomes.

Upper GI tract outflow obstruction

Gastric and duodenal outlet obstruction are said to occur in up to 20% of cases. Once jaundice has been addressed, persistent nausea and vomiting should raise the suspicion of underlying GI obstruction. If biliary obstruction is being dealt with at open operation, prophylactic duodenal bypass should be considered. Laparoscopic gastrojejunostomy has become the management of choice when warranted. Whilst endoluminal stenting is associated with more favourable short-term results, gastrojejunostomy may be a better treatment option in those with a predicted prolonged survival.

Adjuvant therapies

Despite surgery with curative intent, the 5-year survival rates remain disappointingly low. There is evidence to support the use of adjuvant chemotherapy after curative resection for pancreatic adenocarcinoma. Randomised controlled trials including ESPAC-3[114] and CONKO-001[6] show improved survival.

Gemcitabine is preferred to 5-fluorouracil (5FU) because its safety profile is better with similar efficacy.[115] The role of adjuvant chemoradiation is less well defined, with conflicting outcomes from the trials. While the Gastrointestinal Study Group (GISTG)[114] showed a survival benefit with 5FU and radiotherapy, albeit with a small sample size ($n=43$), the European Organisation of Research and Treatment of Cancer (EORTC) trial[116] failed to show a statistically significant survival benefit for those treated with adjuvant chemoradiation compared with an observation group. Finally, the Johns Hopkins–Mayo Clinic Collaborative Study[117] demonstrated improved survival associated with adjuvant chemoradiation following pancreatico-duodenectomy.

Two recent studies have shown promising results. In the first, Neoptolemos et al. presented the results of the European Study Group for Pancreatic Cancer 4 trial (ESPAC-4) which randomised 730 patients following surgery to either adjuvant gemcitabine ($n=366$) or gemcitabine plus capecitabine ($n=364$).[118] The latter regimen resulted in a statistically significant increase in median overall survival (28.0 vs 25.5 months, $P=0.032$).

✓✓ Dual adjuvant therapy with gemcitabine and oral capecitabine in patients undergoing surgical resection of pancreatic adenocarcinoma is associated with improved overall survival compared to gemcitabine monotherapy only.[118]

Also, the results of the Japan Adjuvant Study Group of Pancreatic Cancer (JASPAC) 01 trial comparing adjuvant gemcitabine to S-1, an oral fluropyrimidine, were recently published by Uesaka et al.[119] This multicentre, randomised, non-inferiority trial demonstrated an almost doubling of overall survival in the S-1 arm (44.1 vs 24.4 months, $P <0.0001$). Whether or not this intriguing result can be replicated in a non-Japanese population remains to be seen. Nonetheless, the results of both trials have shown promise and represent a new standard of care.

Despite the role of adjuvant therapy, survival remains poor, with a pressing need to discover more efficacious treatment and further studies to elucidate the optimal therapy protocol, with consideration of timing and the need for more tailored treatment regimens.

Neoadjuvant therapy

According to the National Cancer Control Network (NCCN) guidelines, indications for neoadjuvant chemoradiotherapy include locally advanced or borderline resectable disease, in an attempt to downstage the disease and allow for subsequent resection. Theoretical advantages include delivery of chemotherapy and/or radiotherapy to well-oxygenated tissue, and hence early treatment of micrometastatic disease. Detractors of neoadjuvant therapy argue that the resultant delay in surgery may result in disease progression; however, this is difficult to prove. In a recent retrospective study consisting of 575 patients, Hackert et al. showed that neoadjuvant therapy with folfirinox was associated with the highest resection rates (61%), compared to gemcitabine and radiation (46%) and other treatments (52%).[120] Several studies have evaluated the use of neoadjuvant therapy in resectable pancreatic adenocarcinoma. In the retrospective study by Mirkin et al. comprised of resectable (clinical stages I–III) pancreatic cancer patients from the National Cancer Database, more than 1700 patients who underwent neoadjuvant therapy were compared to 6706 patients who were treated with surgical resection alone, and nearly 10 000 patients treated with surgery followed by adjuvant therapy.[121] Within the neoadjuvant cohort, 22% received chemotherapy only, 8.5% radiotherapy only and the rest received both treatment modalities. While neoadjuvant therapy was associated with similar median survival to adjuvant therapy in stage I disease, it resulted in significantly improved survival compared to both surgery and adjuvant therapy in stage III disease. These findings are corroborated by Mokdad et al., who showed that neoadjuvant treatment followed by surgery in early stage, resectable pancreatic cancer is associated with improved survival, compared to surgery upfront.[122] Moreover, patients who underwent surgery alone had significantly higher T stages, number of positive lymph nodes and positive resection margins.

Future areas of interest

The last decade has seen considerable improvements in diagnosis, as well as advances in minimally invasive and endoscopic management strategies for pancreatic cancer. The boundaries for resectability of pancreatic cancer are constantly being expanded and biological agents such as erlotinib (epidermal growth factor receptor inhibitor), cetuximab, bevacizumab and axitinib are under investigation as potential therapies. The addition of erlotinib to gemcitabine has recently been shown to be superior to gemcitabine alone in patients with metastatic pancreatic cancer.[123]

Despite recent advances in imaging modalities, there remains a limited ability to detect pancreatic cancer at an early stage. Therefore, an emphasis on better understanding of cancer genomics as well as the role of tumour markers is crucial. Circulating tumour cells represent a promising research avenue and if they can be successfully isolated ex vivo,

they will provide an invaluable tool for biomarker development. Significant progress has been made recently in unravelling the molecular pathways underpinning pancreatic carcinogenesis and the identification of distinct mutated genes through whole-genome sequencing will undoubtedly provide novel therapeutic targets. Surgical techniques, especially oncological dissection methods, will need to be standardised to ensure stricter quality control and better data comparison.

Key points

- Prognosis remains poor since the majority of patients present with advanced, unresectable disease.
- Late onset diabetes mellitus may be the first presenting sign of an underlying pancreatic neoplasm.
- The classical Courvoisier's sign is seen in <25% of cases.
- Screening is recommended for the following: patients from a familial pancreatic cancer kindred with ≥2 affected first-degree relatives, patients with Peutz–Jeghers syndrome and *p16*, *BRCA2* and *HNPCC* mutation carriers with ≥1 affected first-degree relative.
- Multidetector row CT is the radiological staging modality of choice.
- Laparoscopic staging has a role in selected patients.
- Resectional surgery is associated with <5% mortality and 30–50% morbidity rates.
- Neoadjuvant therapy followed by surgery is associated with improved survival compared to surgery alone in early stage, resectable disease.
- The majority of patients re-occur with distal disease, hence the need for novel neoadjuvant and adjuvant therapies.

🌐 Full references available at **http://expertconsult. inkling.com**

Key references

6. Oettle H, Neuhaus P, Hochhaus A, et al. Adjuvant chemotherapy with gemcitabine and long-term outcomes among patients with resected pancreatic cancer: the CONKO-001 randomized trial. JAMA 2013;310(14):1473–81. PMID: 24104372.
   Patients receiving adjuvant gemcitabine for 6 months following curative pancreatic cancer resection had improved disease-free as well as overall survival, compared to observation alone.

20. Larsson SC, Wolk A. Red and processed meat consumption and risk of pancreatic cancer: meta-analysis of prospective studies. Br J Cancer 2012;106(3):603–7. PMID: 22240790.
    Red meat consumption was associated with an increased risk of pancreatic cancer in men but not in women. Consumption of processed meat also significantly increased the risk of pancreatic cancer.

24. Genkinger JM, Wang M, Li R, et al. Dairy products and pancreatic cancer risk: a pooled analysis of 14 cohort studies. Ann Oncol 2014;25(6):1106–15. PMID: 24631943.

Consumption of dairy foods, calcium or vitamin D did not result in an increased risk of pancreatic cancer.

30. Song S, Wang B, Zhang X, et al. Long-term diabetes mellitus is associated with an increased risk of pancreatic cancer: a meta-analysis. PLoS One 2015;10(7):e0134321. PMID: 26230263.
    Long-term diabetes mellitus increased the risk of pancreatic cancer development. However, the risk of cancer was inversely proportional to the duration of diabetes mellitus.

32. Fan Y, Hu J, Feng B, et al. Increased risk of pancreatic cancer related to gallstones and cholecystectomy: a systematic review and meta-analysis. Pancreas 2016;45(4):503–9. PMID: 26684857.
    Both gallstone disease and prior cholecystectomy are independent risk factors for pancreatic cancer development.

40. Zhen DB, Rabe KG, Gallinger S, et al. BRCA1, BRCA2, PALB2, and CDKN2A mutations in familial pancreatic cancer: a PACGENE study. Genet Med 2015;17(7):569–77. PMID: 25356972.
    BRCA2 and *CDKN2A* account for the majority of mutations in familial pancreatic cancer.

46. Basturk O, Hong SM, Wood LD, et al. A revised classification system and recommendations from the Baltimore consensus meeting for neoplastic

precursor lesions in the pancreas. Am J Surg Pathol 2015;39(12):1730–41. PMID: 26559377.
A two-tiered classification system (low versus high-grade dysplasia) was proposed for all pancreatic precursor lesions. Low-grade dysplastic lesions include PanIN-1 and PanIN-2, whereas high-grade lesions include PanIN-3 or carcinoma in situ.

60. Canto MI, Harinck F, Hruban RH, et al. International Cancer of the Pancreas Screening (CAPS) Consortium summit on the management of patients with increased risk for familial pancreatic cancer. Gut 2013;62(3):339–47. PMID: 23135763.
Screening with EUS or MRI is recommended for first-degree relatives of patients with pancreatic cancer from a familial pancreatic cancer kindred with at least two affected first-degree relatives, patients with Peutz–Jeghers syndrome and p16, BRCA2 and HNPCC mutation carriers with ≥1 affected first-degree relative.

80. Allen VB, Gurusamy KS, Takwoingi Y, et al. Diagnostic accuracy of laparoscopy following computed tomography (CT) scanning for assessing the resectability with curative intent in pancreatic and periampullary cancer. Cochrane Database Syst Rev 2016;7:CD009323. PMID: 27383694.
Diagnostic laparoscopy with biopsy of suspicious lesions would avoid 21 unnecessary laparotomies in 100 people who were deemed to have resectable disease by CT criteria.

84. Gurusamy KS, Kumar S, Davidson BR. Prophylactic gastrojejunostomy for unresectable periampullary carcinoma. Cochrane Database Syst Rev 2013(2):CD008533. PMID: 23450583.
Routine prophylactic gastrojejunostomy in patients with unresectable periampullary cancers significantly decreased the incidence of long-term gastric outlet obstruction. However, there were no differences in overall survival, perioperative mortality or morbidity, quality of life or hospital stay between the two groups. Only two trials encompassing 152 patients were examined and they were both at high risk of bias.

89. Moole H, Bechtold M, Puli SR. Efficacy of preoperative biliary drainage in malignant obstructive jaundice: a meta-analysis and systematic review. World J Surg Oncol 2016;14(1):182. PMID: 27400651.
Preoperative biliary drainage was associated with fewer major adverse events compared to direct surgery, in patients with malignant obstructive jaundice undergoing surgery. No significant differences were observed in mortality or length of hospital stay between the two groups.

95. Que W, Fang H, Yan B, et al. Pancreaticogastrostomy versus pancreaticojejunostomy after pancreaticoduodenectomy: a meta-analysis of randomized controlled trials. Am J Surg 2015;209(6):1074–82. PMID: 25743406.
Pancreatico-gastrostomy was associated with a significantly lower rate of postoperative pancreatic fistula and intra-abdominal fluid collection compared to pancreatico-jejunostomy. However, there were no significant differences in delayed gastric emptying, haemorrhage, wound infection, overall morbidity, mortality or length of hospital stay.

97. Kurumboor P, Palaniswami KN, Pramil K, et al. Octreotide does not prevent pancreatic fistula following pancreatoduodenectomy in patients with soft pancreas and non-dilated duct: a prospective randomized controlled trial. J Gastrointest Surg 2015;19(11):2038–44. PMID: 26302879.
Patients who received octreotide had a non-significantly lower rate of pancreatic fistula and morbidity compared to the control group.

100. Huttner FJ, Fitzmaurice C, Schwarzer G, et al. Pylorus-preserving pancreaticoduodenectomy (pp Whipple) versus pancreaticoduodenectomy (classic Whipple) for surgical treatment of periampullary and pancreatic carcinoma. Cochrane Database Syst Rev 2016;2:CD006053. PMID: 26905229.
There were no significant differences in postoperative morbidity, mortality or overall survival between the two techniques. However, pylorus-preserving pancreatico-duodenectomy was associated with significantly less operative time, less blood loss and less red cell transfusion but higher incidences of delayed gastric emptying.

102. Huang W, Xiong JJ, Wan MH, et al. Meta-analysis of subtotal stomach-preserving pancreaticoduodenectomy vs pylorus preserving pancreaticoduodenectomy. World J Gastroenterol 2015;21(20):6361–73. PMID: 26034372.
Subtotal stomach-preserving pancreatico-duodenectomy was associated with significantly less delayed gastric emptying but more intraoperative blood loss than pylorus-preserving pancreatico-duodenectomy. However, there were no significant differences in pancreatic fistula, intra-abdominal abscess, wound infection, haemorrhage or mortality between the two groups.

104. Dasari BV, Pasquali S, Vohra RS, et al. Extended versus standard lymphadenectomy for pancreatic head cancer: meta-analysis of randomized controlled trials. J Gastrointest Surg 2015;19(9):1725–32. PMID: 26055135.
Extended lymphadenectomy was associated with significantly worse postoperative morbidity compared to standard lymph node harvest. There were no significant differences in 30-day mortality, length of hospital stay or overall survival between the two groups.

108. Delitto D, Luckhurst CM, Black BS, et al. Oncologic and perioperative outcomes following selective application of laparoscopic pancreaticoduodenectomy for periampullary malignancies. J Gastrointest Surg 2016;20(7):1343–9. PMID: 27142633.
Laparoscopic pancreatico-duodenectomy was associated with significantly less pancreatic fistula, wound infections and shorter length of hospital stay.

Overall survival was similar for patients undergoing laparoscopic and open pancreatico-duodenectomy.

111. Lee SY, Allen PJ, Sadot E, et al. Distal pancreatectomy: a single institution's experience in open, laparoscopic, and robotic approaches. J Am Coll Surg 2015;220(1):18–27. PMID: 25456783.
     A series of 805 patients who underwent distal pancreatectomies (37 robotic, 131 laparoscopic and 637 open) during a 13-year period at Memorial Sloan Kettering Cancer Centre were analysed. Open surgery was associated with significantly more intraoperative blood loss. The robotic and laparoscopic approaches were comparable for most perioperative outcomes, with no clear superiority of one technique over the other.

118. Neoptolemos JP, Palmer DH, Ghaneh P, et al. Comparison of adjuvant gemcitabine and capecitabine with gemcitabine monotherapy in patients with resected pancreatic cancer (ESPAC-4): a multicentre, open-label, randomised, phase 3 trial. Lancet 2017;389(10073):1011–24. PMID: 28129987.
     Adjuvant gemcitabine combined with capecitabine was associated with significantly better overall survival compared to gemcitabine alone in patients who had R0 or R1 resection for pancreatic cancer.

119. Uesaka K, Boku N, Fukutomi A, et al. Adjuvant chemotherapy of S-1 versus gemcitabine for resected pancreatic cancer: a phase 3, open-label, randomised, non-inferiority trial (JASPAC 01). Lancet 2016;388(10041):248–57. PMID: 27265347.
     Adjuvant chemotherapy with S-1 was associated with significantly better 5-year survival rates compared to gemcitabine in Japanese patients with resected pancreatic cancer.

120. Hackert T, Sachsenmaier M, Hinz U, et al. Locally advanced pancreatic cancer: neoadjuvant therapy with folfirinox results in resectability in 60% of the patients. Ann Surg 2016;264(3):457–63. PMID: 27355262.
     Neoadjuvant therapy with folfirinox was associated with the highest resection rates compared to gemcitabine and radiotherapy, and other treatments. Multivariate analysis showed folfirinox to be an independent predictor of a favourable prognosis.

17

Cystic and neuroendocrine tumours of the pancreas

Saxon Connor

Introduction

Although pancreatic ductal adenocarcinoma accounts for the majority of patients with neoplastic disease of the pancreas, over the last three decades there has been an increasing recognition of cystic and neuroendocrine pancreatic neoplasms.[1] The aim of this chapter is to examine these tumours in more detail, with particular emphasis on intraductal papillary mucinous neoplasms (IPMNs) and pancreatic neuroendocrine tumours (PNETs). Where possible, evidence-based recommendations for the investigation and management of these tumours will be provided.

Intraductal papillary mucinous neoplasms

IPMNs are defined as a grossly visible, mucin-producing epithelial neoplasm of the pancreas, which arises from within the main pancreatic duct (main-duct IPMN) or one of its branches (branch-duct IPMN), and most often but not always has a papillary architecture. They are distinguished from mucinous cystic neoplasms (MCNs) by the absence of ovarian-type stroma.[2]

The incidence (95% confidence interval) is estimated at 2.04 (1.28–2.80) per 100 000 population; however, this increases significantly after the sixth decade.[3] The precise aetiology remains unknown, although an association with extrapancreatic primaries (10%), most commonly colorectal, breast and prostate, has been reported, but this is not significantly different to that seen with primary pancreatic adenocarcinoma.[4] IPMN has also been shown to be a predictor of

pancreatic cancer as compared to other intra-abdominal pathologies, with an odds ratio of 7.18.[5]

Clinical presentation

IPMNs most commonly present with symptoms related to pancreatic duct obstruction. The Johns Hopkins group reported their experience comparing the presentation and demographics to those patients presenting with pancreatic adenocarcinoma.[6,7] Although the mean age of presentation was similar to that of pancreatic adenocarcinoma (seventh decade), the clinical presentation was significantly different. Of the 60 patients with IPMNs, 59% presented with abdominal pain but only 16% presented with obstructive jaundice, compared to 38% and 74% of patients with pancreatic adenocarcinoma, respectively.[6] This is in spite of the fact that only five of the 60 patients with IPMNs had tumours within the body or tail.[6] In addition, those with IPMNs were more likely to have been smokers and 14% had suffered previous attacks of acute pancreatitis (compared to 3% of those with pancreatic ductal adenocarcinoma).[6] Weight loss was a prominent factor reported in 29% of patients with IPMNs.[7] Symptoms associated with invasive malignancy included the presence of jaundice, weight loss, vomiting[7] and diabetes.[8] Patients with invasive IPMNs were a mean of 5 years older (68 vs 63 years) compared to those with non-invasive IPMNs.[7] This led the authors to conclude that IPMN was a slow-growing tumour with a significant latency to develop invasive disease.[7] Increasingly, an important presentation is the incidental finding due to cross-sectional imaging for other medical indications. IPMN was the final diagnosis in 36% of pancreatic 'incidentalomas' that underwent pancreatico-duodenectomy.[9]

Investigation

Computed tomography (CT) and magnetic resonance imaging (MRI) form the mainstay of non-invasive radiological imaging of suspected IPMN. The classical features of main-duct IPMN are segmental or diffuse main pancreatic duct dilatation greater than 5 mm (**Fig. 17.1**), while branch-type IPMN can present with small cystic lesions (>5 mm^2) that may appear in a 'grape-like' configuration[2]. If both coexist then they are classified as mixed type. Although MRI and CT have been shown to identify accurately tumour location and communication with the pancreatic duct, the detection of invasive malignancy remains problematic.[10–12] Radiological features associated with malignancy have been grouped into high-risk stigmata or worrisome features.[2] High-risk stigmata include enhanced solid component and main pancreatic duct size >10 mm^2. Worrisome features have been defined as cyst size >3 cm, thickened enhanced walls, non-enhancing mural nodules, main pancreatic duct size 5–9 mm, abrupt change in main pancreatic duct calibre with distal pancreatic atrophy and lymphadenopathy.[2] In 2013 a systematic review of the use of ^{18}F-labelled fluorodeoxyglucose CT/positron emission tomography (PET) in patients with IPMN concluded, on the basis of a relatively small number of patients and studies, that it may be useful for separating benign from malignant tumours.[13] However, it should be noted that many of the included studies suffered from technical methodological heterogeneity and further research is required before it can become incorporated into routine practice. Differentiating IPMN from other cystic neoplasms (particularly branch-type IPMN from MCN) or pseudocysts can be difficult and the importance of considering the clinical picture cannot be underestimated, particularly the patient's age, gender and history of pancreatitis or genetic syndromes. Radiologically, localisation within the uncinate process, detection of non-gravity-dependent luminal filling defects (papillary projections) or grouped gravity-dependent luminal filling defects (mucin), and upstream dilatation of ducts (MCN ducts are normal) all favour the diagnosis of branch-type IPMN.[14] Differentiating diffuse main-duct IPMN from chronic obstructive pancreatitis can be

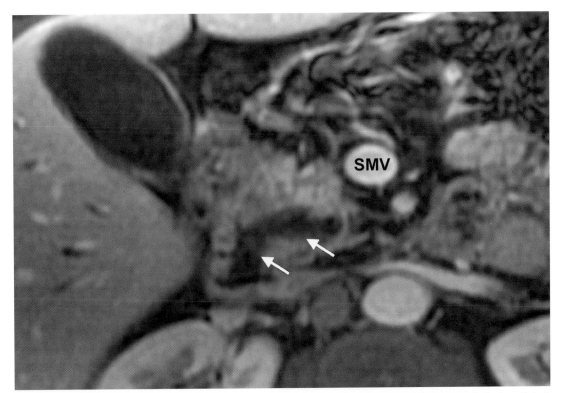

Figure 17.1 • MRI (post-gadolinium, T1-weighted, fat-saturated) image of the pancreas. *White arrows* indicate a dilated pancreatic duct with a widely open ampulla consistent with a main-duct intraductal papillary neoplasm. *SMV,* superior mesenteric vein. Histology is shown in Fig. 17.2.

challenging radiologically[14] (clinically, patients with IPMN tend to be 20 years older and lack a history of heavy alcohol use), but high-quality cross-sectional imaging looking for endoluminal filling defects (either mucin or papillary proliferations), cystic dilatation of collateral branches (particularly within the uncinate process), communication of dilated ducts with normal ducts without evidence of an obstructing lesion or a widely open papilla (**Fig. 17.1**) all favour IPMN.[14]

Endoscopic ultrasound (EUS) has the advantage of being able to sample cystic fluid and biopsy solid lesions at the time of assessment, although its utility over cross-sectional imaging has recently been questioned.[15] Features seen at EUS suggestive of malignancy include main duct >10 mm (for main-duct IPMN), while suspicious features for branch-type IPMN include tumour diameter >40 mm associated with thick irregular septa and mural nodules >10 mm.[16] In a systematic review and meta-analysis published in 2014 the sensitivity and specificity of EUS-FNA based cytology in detecting malignant IPMN was 65% and 91%, respectively.[17] Measuring tumour markers within cyst fluid has not proved to be accurate enough and in the future molecular analysis is likely to be more useful when combined with clinical presentation.[18] Although the absence of mucin does not exclude IPMN, the presence of necrosis is the only feature that is strongly suggestive of invasive carcinoma. Abundant background inflammation and parachromatin clearing are suspicious for carcinoma in situ.[19]

Endoscopic retrograde cholangiopancreatography (ERCP) can be used in the diagnosis of IPMN, although MRI (including the use of gadolinium) is increasingly replacing it (**Fig. 17.1**). The observation at ERCP of mucin protruding from a widely open papilla is diagnostic.[20] Biopsies and aspiration of ductal contents can be obtained; however, the yield is less than 50%.[20]

Although there are no tumour markers specific to IPMN, serum CA19-9, but not CEA, has been shown to be an independent predictor of malignancy.[8]

Given the increasing frequency of diagnosis and relatively low rate of malignancy within branch-duct IPMN, clinico-radiological scoring systems have been proposed.[8,21] In a large study by Hwang et al., 237 patients with branch-duct IPMN who underwent resection were studied.[21] Using multivariate analysis to identify independent predictors of either malignancy or invasiveness, formulae were created. However, the presence of a mural nodule, elevated serum CEA or cyst size >28 mm was sufficient to conclude that there was underlying malignant change or invasion and an indication for surgery.[21] An important point when considering the use of these scoring systems is that the radiological measurement varies by scan modality and may not correlate well with the final pathological measurement.[22]

> ✅ The American Gastroenterology Association (AGA) guidelines recommend that MRI is used as investigation of choice and EUS-FNA be restricted to those with two of three high-risk features, such as size >3 cm, dilated main pancreatic duct or presence of solid component (conditional recommendation, very low-quality evidence).[23]

Pathology

The importance of assessment by experienced pathologists cannot be overemphasised. There are now pathological guidelines for reporting of IPMN[24] but discussion of these is beyond the scope of this chapter. IPMNs involve the head of the gland in 70% of patients, while 5–10% are spread diffusely throughout the gland, and the rest are located within the body and tail.[25] On sectioning, the involvement can be diffuse or segmented, with projections of papillary epithelium (**Fig. 17.2**) and tenacious thick mucin within the involved dilated ducts. IPMNs are subclassified into main-duct,

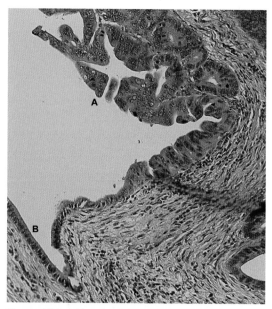

Figure 17.2 • Haematoxylin-and-eosin-stained section from the pancreatico-duodenectomy specimen of the patient in Fig. 17.1. Label *A* is in the lumen of the proximal pancreatic duct with adjacent proliferation of severely dysplastic glandular epithelium with intraluminal papillary growth, but no stromal invasion in this area. Elsewhere in the specimen focal stromal invasion was identified. Label *B* indicates remnant low columnar non-neoplastic epithelium of the duct.

branch-type or mixed, depending on site of origin. This is important as branch-type neoplasms are less likely to be associated with malignancy.[20] Surrounding pancreatic parenchyma may appear firm and hard due to scarring and atrophy from obstructive chronic pancreatitis secondary to the tumour. The presence of gelatinous or solid nodules should raise the suspicion of an invasive component. Microscopically, the most typical appearance is of mucin-secreting columnar epithelium with variable atypia (low-, moderate-, high-grade dysplasia or invasive carcinoma).[25] The growth pattern varies from flat ducts (ectasia) through to prominent papillae. The tumour tends to follow the pancreatic ducts and can be multifocal in 20–30% of patients.[25] IPMNs can contain intestinal, gastric or, less commonly, pancreatico-biliary type differentiation. The gastric type are more often associated with branch-type IPMN and would seem to be associated with a different (lower) malignant potential, growth pattern and type of mucin production compared to the intestinal type.[26,27] Invasive carcinoma occurs focally and is thought to result from a stepwise progression through increasingly dysplastic lesions.[25] The invasive growth pattern can be muconodular (colloid) or a conventional ductal pattern and would appear to be related to the underlying cellular differentiation (intestinal vs pancreatico-biliary, respectively).[25,27]

Pathologically, differentiating IPMN from other cystic neoplasms of the pancreas is important. The absence of ovarian stroma helps to separate IPMN from MCN.[2] For lesions between 0.5 and 1 cm, differentiating pancreatic intraepithelial neoplasia (PanIN) from IPMN is difficult. IPMNs tend to have taller and more complex papillae and are associated with abundant luminal mucin.[25] The presence of coarse and stippled chromatin with a smooth nuclear membrane will differentiate cystic pancreatic endocrine neoplasms from IPMNs.[25]

Management

In determining the most appropriate management of patients with IPMNs, the following should be considered. Given the preponderance for these to present in older patients and the fact that the majority will be located within the head of the pancreas, it is important to assess for comorbidities and general fitness for major pancreatic surgery. If the patient is deemed not fit enough for surgery, then simple medical management of symptoms is appropriate. Equally, in the event of an incidental diagnosis, intensive follow-up regimens are not indicated if tumour progression would not lead to surgical intervention. Presuming the patient is a suitable candidate for surgery (if required), then appropriate staging to determine surgical resectability (criteria equivalent to those for pancreatic adenocarcinoma) should be performed.

Despite over 250 publications per year being dedicated to IPMN, the level of evidence available to make clinical recommendations remains poor. There are more than 10 published sets of guidelines with little concordance and few using an evidence-based approach. For this reason much equipoise and controversy exists within the literature regarding this topic. Recently Falconi et al. reviewed the available guidelines as of 2014 in an attempt to answer several relevant clinical questions.[28] Universal agreement between the reviewing recognised experts could not be achieved.

> ✅ A summary of the key findings as interpreted by the current author with regard to indication for intervention and extent of intervention as recommended by Falconi et al.[28] is shown in Table 17.1 and **Fig. 17.3**.

Subsequent to this publication, the AGA commissioned a high-quality evidence-based review of the management of incidental pancreatic cysts.[23] Of the

Table 17.1 • Recommendation of management of IPMN as per current author's interpretation of an expert panel review of the guidelines for pancreatic cystic neoplasms by Falconi et al.[28]

Option	Must	May
Resect	Main-duct IPMN with duct size >10 mm Main-duct IPMN with duct size 5–9 mm and worrisome features* Branch-duct or main-duct IPMN with high-risk stigmata†	>2 cm branch-duct IPMN and <65 years Increase in size >2 mm/year for branch-duct IPMN Branch-duct IPMN with main duct >6 mm
Observe	Stable asymptomatic branch-duct IPMN with no worrisome features* and <4 cm	Family history of pancreatic cancer

*Worrisome features: size >3 cm, main duct 5–9 mm, thickened enhancing wall, non-enhancing mural nodule, pancreatitis, abrupt cut-off of pancreatic duct with atrophy, lymphadenopathy.

†High-risk stigmata: enhancing solid component, main duct >10 mm, jaundice.

Other high-risk factors to be considered: intraductal mucin, elevated serum CA19-9, cytological high-grade dysplasia.

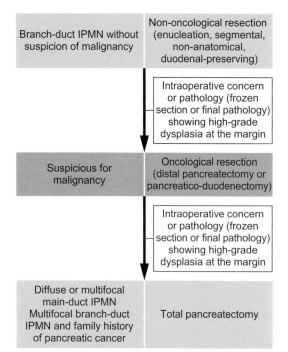

Branch-duct IPMN without suspicion of malignancy	Non-oncological resection (enucleation, segmental, non-anatomical, duodenal-preserving)
	Intraoperative concern or pathology (frozen section or final pathology) showing high-grade dysplasia at the margin
Suspicious for malignancy	Oncological resection (distal pancreatectomy or pancreatico-duodenectomy)
	Intraoperative concern or pathology (frozen section or final pathology) showing high-grade dysplasia at the margin
Diffuse or multifocal main-duct IPMN Multifocal branch-duct IPMN and family history of pancreatic cancer	Total pancreatectomy

Figure 17.3 • Extent of surgery for intraductal papillary mucinous neoplasm (IPMN) based on the current author's interpretation of an expert review of literature by Falconi et al.[28]

nine clinical questions the authors posed, all had very low-quality evidence and only one received a strong recommendation, with all others receiving a conditional recommendation.

✅ The AGA recommended that surgery was appropriate for asymptomatic patients with both a solid component and dilated pancreatic duct and/or concerning features on EUS and FNA (conditional recommendation, very low-quality evidence). Surgery should be performed in an expert centre (strong recommendation, very low-quality evidence).

Despite a robust methodological approach, it is important to recognise that these recommendations have not been met with universal acceptance and for those readers interested the author recommends reading the accompanying published correspondence.[23]

Given that branch-duct IPMN would appear to be a premalignant lesion, albeit a slow-growing one, it is important to know the outcome from long-term follow-up if conservative management is to be successful. In two large prospective contemporary studies of branch-duct IPMNs, in which indications for resection were based on IAP guidelines, patients

were allocated to a surgical or intensive follow-up arm.[29,30] In both studies, 18% of patients met the criteria for surgery at initial presentation. Of these patients, the final histology was malignant (in situ or invasive disease) in 3 of 20[29] and 8 of 34[30] patients. In those patients submitted to follow-up, intensive regimens (3–6-monthly for the first 2 years) were used in both studies, including combinations of CT, EUS and MRI. Between 5% and 12% of patients subsequently progressed to surgery during follow-up (median 12–18 months). Of these patients, 0 of 5[29] and 2 of 18[30] had malignant disease. All remaining patients ($n = 84$[29] and $n = 132$[30]) that were followed remained alive during median follow-up periods of 30 months, with no deaths attributable to their disease.

The methodology of the follow-up regimen of both these studies raises further questions. Both used state-of-the-art imaging at a frequency that many health systems may struggle to provide. Both studies showed that although the current recommendations for branch-duct IPMN are very sensitive in detecting malignancy, the specificity remains low and hence many patients are followed intensively and subjected to surgery without clear benefit. Unique to the AGA guidelines, consideration is given to such issues as potential harm, adverse outcomes and cost from intensive follow-up or subsequent interventions.[23] Thus, the AGA recommendations with regard to follow-up are perhaps the most controversial.

✅ The AGA suggests that patients without concerning EUS-FNA results should undergo MRI surveillance after 1 year and then every 2 years to ensure no change in risk of malignancy (conditional recommendation, very low-quality evidence). The AGA suggests that significant changes in the characteristics of the cyst, including the development of a solid component, increasing size of the pancreatic duct, and/or diameter >3 cm, are indications for EUS-FNA (conditional recommendation, very low-quality evidence). The AGA suggests against continued surveillance of pancreatic cysts if there has been no significant change in the characteristics of the cyst after 5 years of surveillance or if the patient is no longer a surgical candidate (conditional recommendation, very low-quality evidence).[3]

For those patients in whom surgery is indicated, the decision regarding the extent of pancreatic resection and nodal dissection needs to be decided. Falconi et al.[28] noted that there was lack of agreement amongst experts and some areas, such as use of duodenal sparing surgery, lacked evidence on which to make conclusive recommendations.

✓ Frozen section for margin assessment is currently recommended by two expert groups[2,28] although its true accuracy remains unclear.[31,32] Falconi et al. recommended frozen section with further resection until margins were without high-grade dysplasia or invasive malignancy.[28] Current recommendations from the IAP guidelines are that, in the presence of adenoma or borderline atypia, no further resection is required, but if in situ or invasive carcinoma is present, then further resection should be performed.[2] However, what has not yet been addressed in the literature is the effect of potentially spilling invasive carcinoma cells (i.e. cutting through invasive tumour) during surgery and the effect this has on long-term outcomes.

Fujino et al. reviewed the outcome in 57 patients who underwent surgical resection for IPMN.[31] Their approach was to perform a total pancreatectomy in patients with diffuse disease and a localised resection where preoperative imaging revealed localised disease, using intraoperative ultrasound (IOUS) to determine the point of pancreatic transection. Frozen section was undertaken and for patients with invasive carcinoma a radical resection was performed. Where non-invasive disease was detected, a tumour-free margin was sufficient. Of the 33 patients with main-duct IPMN, 14 met the pre-resection criteria for total pancreatectomy. All 24 patients with branch-duct tumours underwent partial resections, although two subsequently required completion pancreatectomy for complications. Correlating the IOUS findings with final pathological assessment indicated an accuracy of ductal spread of 74% for main-duct tumours and 96% for branch-duct tumours. Frozen section was performed in 30 of the patients who underwent partial resection and in 29 patients it correlated with the final result. Only one patient had invasive malignancy at the transected surface, while a further two patients who did not have frozen section assessment had invasive malignancy at the resection margin. In reviewing the final histology of the 16 patients undergoing total pancreatectomy, resection was found to be appropriate (frankly or potentially malignant tissue throughout all segments of the pancreas) in 12 patients. Importantly, six of these 16 patients had severe long-term problems with hypoglycaemia, two of whom died as a result of this complication. For those 41 patients undergoing partial pancreatectomy, five patients had an involved margin (three with invasive carcinoma, two with dysplasia). The three patients with invasive carcinoma all died from metastatic disease. Of the patients with clear margins, seven of 34 died from metastatic disease, while two developed metachronous pancreatic disease at 2 and 12 years. The authors of this study concluded that partial pancreatectomy should be performed if possible, and that the risk of severe long-term complications from total pancreatectomy outweighed the risk of patients developing recurrent malignancy in the remnant.

✓ For those undergoing resection, partial pancreatectomy is preferred to total pancreatectomy and intraoperative frozen section should be performed to ensure clear margins.[31]

Outcome

The main determinant of survival following resection is the presence of invasive disease. The AGA review process identified 37 studies evaluating 3842 patients.[33] For those with non-invasive disease 5-year survival was reported as between 80 and 100%, while for invasive disease it was between 3 and 68%. Factors associated with poor survival in those with invasive disease include the presence of jaundice,[4] tumour type (tubular worse than colloid), vascular invasion, perineural invasion, poorly differentiated tumours, percentage of tumour that was invasive and positive lymph node involvement, which has been reported in up to 41% of patients with invasive disease.[7,27,34-37] Invasive branch-type tumours have been shown to have similar survival to those with invasive main-duct disease.[34] Margin status has not been associated with worse long-term outcome.[7,34,35,37] In studies that have performed a multivariate analysis with adequate numbers of patients per variable, lymph node involvement,[35,37] invasive component >2 cm,[35] absence of weight loss,[35] morphological subtype[27] and tubular carcinoma[37] have been found to be independent predictors of poorer outcome. Invasive IPMN would still appear to have a better prognosis than pancreatic ductal adenocarcinoma,[36,37] although the tubular subtype may not.[37] The role of adjuvant therapy for those with invasive disease has not been addressed in formal trials. Outcomes from retrospective series have been analysed,[35,37] yet the role of either radiotherapy or chemotherapy remains unclear and currently cannot be recommended as the standard of care.

Recurrence following resection can be classified as disseminated arising from invasive disease or local (within the pancreatic remnant), which may or may not be invasive in nature. The AGA guidelines recommend that patients with invasive cancer or dysplasia in a cyst that has been surgically resected should undergo MRI surveillance of the remnant pancreas every 2 years (conditional recommendation, very low-quality evidence).[23] The authors acknowledge the lack of strong supporting evidence; however, the rationale is based on the concept that there may be a field change within the pancreatic remnant. Given the dismal survival for those with invasive disease and lack of subsequent curative therapies, it is questionable whether this type of follow-up should be limited to those with dysplasia or PANIN at the margin, or for patients with invasive disease >3 years from resection when the conditional survival is more favourable. In contrast, for those without high-grade dysplasia or malignancy at the margin, the AGA guidelines do not recommend ongoing surveillance (excluding mixed-type IPMN or family history of pancreatic cancer), again based on weak supporting evidence.[23]

✔ There is a lack of reliable evidence regarding recommended follow-up regimens. Both the IAP and AGA guidelines acknowledge this, but feel it is reasonable to perform cross-sectional imaging at a variable frequency (1–2 yearly).[2,23] The routine use of tumour markers is currently not supported.

Given that recurrence would seem to occur most commonly within the pancreatic remnant, Tomimaru et al. have proposed performing a pancreatico-gastrostomy to allow easy endoscopic follow-up of the duct.[38] Additionally, the association of IPMNs with other gastrointestinal malignancies should alert physicians to investigate new gastrointestinal symptoms promptly.

Pancreatic neuroendocrine tumours

Pancreatic neuroendocrine tumours (PNETs) are rare tumours with a reported incidence of 0.2–0.4 per 100 000, although post-mortem studies have reported PNETs in up to 10% of the population.[39] Eighty-five per cent of PNETs are non-syndromic (non-functional), with the rest comprised of syndromic tumours[40] of which carcinoid, insulinoma and gastrinoma are the most common.[41] The aetiology is poorly understood and although the majority of tumours are sporadic, there are associations with several hereditary syndromes, including Von Hippel–Lindau, multiple endocrine neoplasia-1 (MEN-1), neurofibromatosis type 1 and tubular sclerosis.[42]

Clinical presentation

The mode of presentation is dependent on the functional state of the tumour. Non-functioning tumours may present incidentally, whereas symptoms are usually related to mass effect or the presence of metastatic disease. For those tumours associated with a syndrome, this will be related to the specific hormone produced (Table 17.2).

Investigations

The order of investigations will be dependent on presentation. The general principle for functional tumours is to confirm the diagnosis (biochemically) prior to localisation (radiologically).

Biochemical

Specific fasting gut hormones can be measured for functional tumours but testing is complex and subject to change, therefore it is recommended that when faced with the need to investigate such a patient current guidelines are reviewed and the recommended tests are performed in centres with significant experience.[43] In the majority of patients with PNETs, including those with non-functional tumours, serum chromogranin A (protein produced from cells arising from the neural crest) will be elevated.[41] Although chromogranin A is sensitive, it is not highly specific and those interpreting the test must be aware of causes of false-positive results.[43] The degree of elevation of chromogranin A has been shown to correlate with burden of disease (although not with gastrinomas), response to treatment and recurrence.[43]

Other investigations, such as calcium, parathyroid hormone, calcitonin and thyroid function tests, should also be considered, particularly if there is a history that suggests MEN-1.[41] For those in whom a hereditary component is suspected, referral to an appropriate genetic service for further investigation should be initiated.

Radiology

For non-functioning tumours, where localisation is often not an issue, a high-quality arterial and portal venous phase CT will be sufficient to direct therapy, particularly in determining if surgery is indicated. Features suggestive of a PNET on CT include the presence of a hypervascular or hyperdense lesion within the pancreas; however, they can also appear cystic or contain calcifications.[44] The presence of a large incidental mass within the pancreas, particularly without vascular encasement or desmoplastic reaction, should also alert the clinician to the possibility of a PNET.[44]

Although somatostatinomas, VIPomas and glucagonomas tend to be large and easily identified and staged by contrast-enhanced CT, this is often not the case for insulinomas and gastrinomas, unless there is widespread metastatic disease. Most insulinomas are <2 cm and solitary. On CT they tend to be hypervascular (**Fig. 17.4**) with either uniform or target enhancement; however, given that they are often non-contour-conforming, detection of the vascular blush is essential to localise them (the chance of detection can be maximised by timing the images 25 seconds after contrast injection).[44] MRI features include low

Table 17.2 • Presentation, diagnosis and initial medical management of functional pancreatic neuroendocrine tumours

Tumour type	Syndrome	Symptoms	Diagnosis	Medical options for initial symptom control
Insulinoma	Whipple's triad	Neuroglycaemic or neurogenic symptoms relieved with eating	Insulin:glucose ratio >0.3 in presence of hypoglycaemia C-peptide suppression test	Overnight feeding Diazoxide titrated to symptom resolution Somatostatin analogue
Gastrinoma	Zollinger–Ellison	Complicated peptic ulceration or gastro-oesophageal reflux, diarrhoea, abdominal pain	Serum fasting gastrin >1000 pg/mL (if gastric pH <2.5) Secretin stimulation test	High-dose proton pump inhibition (may require up to 60 mg b.d.)
Glucagonoma	Glucagonoma syndrome	Necrolytic migratory erythema, weight loss, diabetes mellitus, stomatitis, diarrhoea, thromboembolism	Plasma glucagon >1000 pg/mL	Somatostatin analogue, hyperalimentation, thrombosis prophylaxis
VIPoma	Verner–Morrison syndrome	Profuse watery diarrhoea, hypokalaemia	Plasma VIP >1000 pg/mL	Somatostatin analogue
Somatostatinoma		Gallstones, steatorrhoea, hypochlorhydria, glucose intolerance	Raised plasma somatostatin	
Carcinoid	Carcinoid syndrome	Abdominal pain, if metastases then flushing, palpitations, rhinorrhoea, diarrhoea, bronchospasm, pellagra	24-hour urinary 5-HIAA	Somatostatin analogue

signal intensity on T1-weighted images and they are particularly well seen on fat-suppressed (T1- and T2-weighted) images.[44] In contrast to insulinoma, gastrinoma can be multiple and extrapancreatic (located within the gastrinoma triangle; the junction between neck and body of the pancreas medially, the junction of the second and third parts of the duodenum inferiorly and the junction of the common bile duct and cystic duct superiorly).[45] On radiological examination, they tend to be less vascular than insulinoma.[44] There is a high rate (70–80%) of lymph node and hepatic metastases.[44] The sensitivity of CT in the detection of gastrinoma is related to size and can be as low as 30–50%.[45] Although slightly better figures have been reported for insulinomas, this can be increased to 94% with the use of thin formats and, with the addition of endoscopic ultrasound, sensitivities of 100% have been reported.[45]

Endoscopic ultrasound is particularly useful for imaging the duodenal wall, regional lymph nodes and the pancreatic head, and has reported sensitivities of 79–100%, but is operator-dependent.[45] Equally, the use of intraoperative ultrasound has also been shown to be useful, particularly in gastrinomas, by identifying

occult multiple primaries or metastatic disease. The sensitivity for detecting small lesions in the pancreatic head is reported to be as high as 97%.[45]

PNET hepatic metastases often appear as low-attenuation lesions on pre-contrast CT and hyper-vascular lesions on post-contrast imaging.[45] It is, however, important to perform a hepatic arterial phase as they can be isointense with normal parenchyma on portal venous imaging. MRI appearances of hepatic metastases are usually of low signal intensity lesions on T1- and high signal intensity on T2-weighted images. Importantly, 15% of hepatic metastases were only seen on immediate post-gadolinium imaging.

In addition to standard radiological imaging, somatostatin receptor scintigraphy (SRS) is also very useful in the staging and treatment of PNETs (with the exception of insulinomas).[43] SRS works on the principle that PNETs express somatostatin receptors. The use of a somatostatin analogue labelled with a radioactive isotope (of which there are several) allows a functional image to be obtained but it requires somatostatin analogues to be stopped prior to the scan. As a single investigation, it is

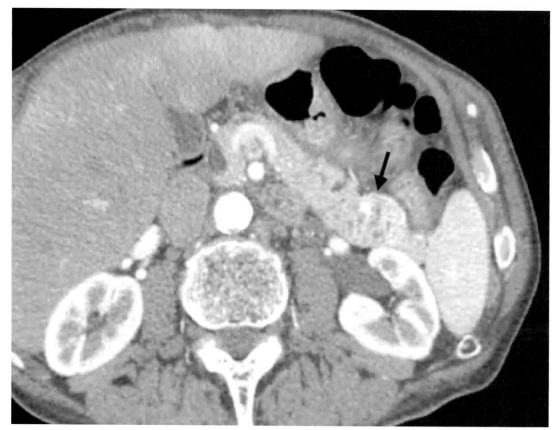

Figure 17.4 • A 78-year-old man presented with neuroglycaemic symptoms. Biochemical testing confirmed an insulinoma. Arterial phase computed tomography revealed a hypervascular lesion in the tail of the pancreas (*black arrow*). Laparoscopic spleen-preserving distal pancreatectomy was performed. Histology confirmed malignant, node-positive neuroendocrine tumour consistent with an insulinoma. After 4 years with no symptoms the patient re-presented with symptoms of hypoglycaemia. Further investigation revealed an isolated nodal recurrence adjacent to the superior mesenteric artery. The patient underwent a completion radical antegrade modular distal pancreatico-splenectomy with resolution of hypoglycaemic symptoms.

probably the most sensitive for the detection of PNETs; however, equivalence can be achieved with a combined approach of standard radiology (particularly MRI and EUS), which has the advantage of providing a detailed anatomical analysis.[46] SRS does, however, offer the advantage of reflecting functionality, which is important if treatment doses of radiolabelled somatostatin analogues or meta-iodobenzylguanidine (MIBG) are to be used. ^{18}F-labelled deoxyglucose PET has not been shown to be useful for the majority of PNETs; however, the development of newer alternatives to ^{18}F-labelled deoxyglucose would appear to be promising.[46] Invasive investigations such as selective arterial calcium (insulinoma) and secretin (gastrinoma) stimulation with hepatic/portal venous sampling are not used routinely and are undertaken only if there is a high suspicion but non-invasive imaging has failed to localise the tumour.[43]

Treatment

Once the diagnosis of a functioning tumour is established, control of the hormonal excess is the first priority in minimising symptoms and complications. Medications used for each individual tumour are shown in Table 17.2. Somatostatin analogue infusions are recommended pre- and intraoperatively for carcinoid tumours to prevent carcinoid crisis.[41] Surgery offers the only chance of cure for those with localised disease. The approach is dependent on tumour type and the presence or absence of an inherited syndrome.[43] The specific management of hereditary PNETs is beyond the remit of this chapter and readers are referred to more detailed reviews for an in-depth discussion.[42,47,48]

Over 80% of localised sporadic insulinomas are solitary, benign and <2 cm in size, making them ideal for consideration of enucleation and laparoscopic resection.[43] Enucleation is considered possible if the lesion can be clearly localised pre- or intraoperatively and if the relationship to the pancreatic duct has been clearly identified.[43] Intraoperative ultrasound has been shown to be particularly valuable in helping to assess these factors.[47] Postoperatively, histological confirmation of the benign nature must be established.[41] Resection is required for tumours where malignancy is suspected (hard, infiltrating tumour, duct obstruction or lymph node involvement), if there is major vascular involvement or the tumour is large.[47] Patients should be assessed for resection as for any pancreatic tumour. However, if a distal pancreatectomy is being performed, attempts to preserve the spleen should be made.[47] Blind pancreatic resection should be avoided.[47] Ablative therapies may also be appropriate in selected patients.[43]

✅✅ For localised sporadic gastrinoma, surgery has been shown to increase survival.[48]

Duodenotomy and intraoperative ultrasound combined with palpation (sensitivity 91–95%) are the key to successful intraoperative localisation.[49] For duodenal gastrinomas, small tumours (<5 mm) can be enucleated from the submucosa while larger tumours require full-thickness excision.[49] For pancreatic gastrinomas, intraoperative assessment regarding the suitability for enucleation (similar to that described above for insulinomas) should be performed. However, if the tumour is not suitable, a formal pancreatic resection (pancreatico-duodenectomy) should be performed. It is now recommend that formal oncological lymph node dissection be performed due to high rates of involvement and possible survival benefit.[43]

Most localised non-functioning tumours are detected at such a size that enucleation is not feasible, but given the increasing use of cross-sectional imaging and the earlier detection of smaller lesions, enucleation is likely to become a more frequent possibility. For asymptomatic suspected benign, non-functioning PNETs, it has been recommended that tumours <2 cm can be safely observed.[43] The risk of malignancy is related to size, and tumours between 1 cm and 3 cm can harbour malignant potential (**Fig. 17.5**).[50] Currently, patients should be assessed regarding fitness for surgery and an informed decision made with the patient regarding resection or observation. Central pancreatectomy has also been shown to be feasible for selected tumours and has the advantage of reducing the risk of postoperative diabetes.[51] A formal resection with lymphadenectomy should be performed for suspected malignant tumours as lymph node metastases are common (27–83%).[50]

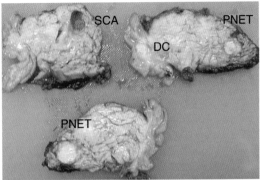

Figure 17.5 • A 30-year-old female with Von Hippel–Lindau disease underwent pancreatic screening. Radiological imaging revealed five neuroendocrine tumours within the pancreatic head. Pancreatico-duodenectomy was performed. Pathological sectioning of the pancreatic head revealed multiple neuroendocrine tumours (*PNET*), including at least one well-differentiated pancreatic endocrine carcinoma (node-positive) and a well-differentiated duodenal endocrine carcinoma (*DC*). All tumours were between 12 and 18 mm diameter. An incidental serous cyst adenoma (*SCA*) was also identified.

Resection is the treatment of choice for symptomatic patients with localised disease.[50] The median survival following resection was reported as significantly longer than for patients with metastatic or locally advanced unresectable disease (7.2 years vs 2.1 vs 5.2 years).[50] Importantly, however, 48% of patients who underwent resection for localised disease developed recurrence at a median follow-up of 2.7 years.[50] Because of the long natural history of these tumours and given that many are symptomatic and difficult to palliate without resection (e.g. tumour bleeding), the criteria for what determines unresectable disease may not be the same as those for adenocarcinoma of the pancreas. The MD Anderson experience would suggest that, in high-volume centres, major venous reconstruction can be performed safely, but only rarely should arterial reconstruction (isolated hepatic artery involvement) or upper abdominal exenteration be performed, due to the associated high long-term morbidity.[50] In addition, a recent report has also indicated that an incomplete resection (R2) is associated with a high perioperative mortality and may in fact be detrimental to the patient's survival.[52]

Metastatic disease

Only 10% of patients with hepatic metastases will be suitable for potentially curative resection.[41] However, it would appear that although recurrence rates are high, a survival advantage can be achieved, although randomised data are lacking.[53] Synchronous cholecystectomy should be performed to reduce complications from adjuvant therapy such as somatostatin analogues and hepatic artery embolisation.[53] For patients with non-functioning unresectable metastatic disease, there is no evidence to support palliative or 'debulking' resections, with possibly the only exceptions being those who have significant local symptoms from the primary and low-volume hepatic metastases.[50] For those with obstruction of the gastrointestinal or biliary tract, surgical bypass should be the first-line treatment in those with well-differentiated disease, given the indolent nature of the disease.[53]

☑ A cytoreductive approach (surgery or ablative therapies) has been advocated in patients with hormonal excess and hepatic metastases if 90% of tumour bulk can be removed, although randomised trials are lacking.[41,43] Other options assessed documented in the UK and European guidelines on the management of metastatic PNETs included somatostatin analogues (short- and long-acting), interferon-α, hepatic artery embolisation, radiolabelled analogues (MIBG and somatostatin), liver transplantation and radiofrequency ablation.[41,54]

Systemic chemotherapy for PNETs has been based around streptozocin and 5-fluorouracil after a randomised trial in 1979 showed a survival advantage for patients with metastatic carcinoid tumours receiving combination chemotherapy.[55] However, given the side-effects and variable behaviour of PNETs, it has not been widely accepted into clinical practice. More recently there is increased interest in the use of temozolomide-based chemotherapy.

☑☑ Two recent placebo-controlled randomised trials using the novel agents sunitinib[56] and everolimus[57] have shown an increase in overall and progression-free survival, respectively. In addition, a placebo-controlled trial of lanreotide in patients with enteropancreatic NETs has shown evidence of antiproliferative activity.[58] Thus, the results of these three trials would suggest these treatments should represent the standard of care.

The therapeutic options for patients with metastatic disease continue to evolve. It is clear that decision-making is complex and dependent on tumour and patient factors. It is strongly recommended that management decisions for these patients are made in a multidisciplinary forum.[54]

Pathology and outcome

PNETs are classified into four groups based on a combination of clinical, histological and molecular features.[41] Tumours confined to the pancreas are classified as well-differentiated endocrine tumours that can be subdivided into those of benign behaviour (<2 cm size, <2 mitoses per 10 high-power fields (HPFs), Ki67 index <2% and no vascular invasion) or uncertain behaviour (if the above criteria are not met). Tumours not confined to the pancreas (gross local invasion or metastases) or that exhibit evidence of small-cell carcinoma are considered endocrine carcinoma, which are further subdivided into well-differentiated (well to moderately differentiated (mitotic rate 2–10 per 10 HPFs, Ki67 index >5%) or poorly differentiated (small-cell carcinoma, necrosis, >10 mitoses per 10 HPFs, Ki67 index >15%, prominent vascular and perineural invasion). Importantly, the diagnosis of functional tumours is not made histologically but clinically, as immunohistochemical staining of specific hormones does not correlate with the clinical picture.[41] In 2010, the seventh edition of the American Joint Committee on Cancer (AJCC) published its first TNM staging classification for PNETs.[59] Using this, Strosberg et al. retrospectively applied the staging system to a dataset of 425 patients with PNETs.[60] Five-year overall survival for stages I–IV was 92%, 84%, 81% and 57%, respectively, thus indicating the proposed system is a useful adjunct for classifying PNETs.

Other tumours

The other two main types of cystic neoplasms are serous (SCA) and mucinous (MCN) cystic neoplasms. Because of the difference in malignant potential, the management of these two tumours differs, yet clinically and radiologically there is considerable overlap. It is therefore useful to contrast and compare them. The exact incidence of serous and mucinous cystic tumours is unknown; however, in a retrospective review of 24 039 patients undergoing radiological imaging, 0.7% had pancreatic cystic neoplasms. Of the 49 (0.2%) who underwent surgery, 10 and 16 patients had a final diagnosis of SCA and MCN, respectively.[61] A recent large multinational retrospective study reported on 2622 patients with SCA.[62] The median age at diagnosis was 58 years, with 74% occurring in women. Sixty-one percent of patients were asymptomatic. SCA were evenly distributed throughout the pancreas. In contrast, MCNs are almost exclusively found in women, with a peak incidence in the fifth decade, and are more likely to be located within the tail.[63] SCAs are also commonly associated with Von Hippel–Lindau syndrome[42] (**Fig. 17.5**), and young patients presenting with multiple cystic lesions involving the pancreas and kidneys should be genetically assessed.[64]

On cross-sectional imaging, the four typical appearances of SCA were microcystic (45%; multiple <2-cm cysts), macrocystic (32%; multiple >2-cm cysts), mixed type (18%; variable-sized cysts) and solid

(5%; no cysts visible on cross sectional imaging).[62] Central calcification (so-called sunburst calcification) occurred in 15%. When the classic features are present, differentiation from other tumours is not difficult; however, the presence of a uni- or oligolocular macrocystic (>2 cm) lesion is more difficult to diagnose and a wide differential exists. Both SCAs (oligocystic type) and MCNs can fall into this group, although MCNs are less likely to be multilocular and, if calcification occurs, it does so peripherally and may be a marker of underlying malignancy.[65] The presence of solid components within a cystic lesion indicates the presence of, or high risk of, malignancy and therefore surgical resection should be considered.[65] Included within this differential would be PNET, solid pseudopapillary neoplasm (young women) or mucinous cyst adenocarcinoma.[65] It is unusual for either SCAs or MCNs to communicate with the pancreatic duct, but it has been reported.[65]

The ability of non-interventional imaging to obtain an accurate diagnosis is limited. In a report of 100 SCAs from Bassi et al., the correct diagnosis was achieved in 53%, 54% and 76% by ultrasound (US), CT and MRI, respectively.[66] An incorrect diagnosis was made in 31%, 34% and 26%, and the investigation was non-diagnostic in 16%, 12% and 0% with US, CT and MRI, respectively.

In a study of solitary cystic (IPMNs were excluded) neoplasms, 71 patients underwent EUS and fluid aspiration (for mucin, viscosity, amylase, lipase, CEA, CA19-9, cytology) followed by surgery to assess its accuracy.[67] The authors concluded that an accurate algorithm using measurement of viscosity, lipase and CEA can be used to determine the diagnosis of cystic lesions. A viscosity of ≥ 1.6 indicates an MCN and the patient should be offered resection. If it is <1.6 and the lipase is <6000 U/mL, this indicates an SCA. If the viscosity is <1.6 and lipase is >6000 U/mL, then a CEA measurement should be performed, and if this value is less than 480 U/mL the diagnosis

is a pseudocyst. If it is >480 U/mL, a repeat EUS and fine-needle aspiration should be performed in 3–6 months. Using this algorithm, only 2 of 71 patients that underwent resection for suspected MCN had a final histology revealing a pseudocyst.

> ✅ The management of SCAs and MCNs differs based on their malignant potential. SCAs rarely undergo malignant transformation and if asymptomatic, no intervention is required.[62] Patients with significant symptoms may be offered resection.[62] Until recently it was recommended that all suspected MCNs undergo resection because of their malignant potential.[2] However, more recent series[68,69] have shown that it is safe to observe lesions less than 3 cm without mural nodules, thus aligning management with BD-IPMN.

Pathologically, SCAs demonstrate monomorphous cuboidal-shaped epithelium. The cells are glycogen-rich with cellular cytoplasm and small regular nuclei. There is a lack of mitotic activity. The cysts appear 'empty' on microscopy. In contrast, the cyst content of MCNs is turbid and tenacious,[64] and microscopically (unlike SCAs) the cyst lining can be highly variable. The cells are mucin-producing, which can be a single cell layer of flattened cuboidal epithelium or contain papillary tufting.[64] The tumours are classified as benign, borderline or malignant depending on the nuclear features of the cells.[64] It is important to examine the whole tumour as malignant invasion can occur without the presence of a mass.[64] The unique feature of MCNs, however, is the presence of ovarian stroma (highly cellular, densely packed, plump spindle cells). Current recommendations require the presence of this for a tumour to be classified as a MCN.[2] This is particularly important when the differential includes IPMN, in which this type of stroma is not seen.[2]

Key points

- As the use of cross-sectional imaging has become more frequent, there has been an increase in the diagnosis of cystic neoplasms within the pancreas.
- Main-duct IPMNs should be resected due to the high incidence of underlying malignancy; however, a selective approach to intervention for side-branch IPMNs should be taken (dependent on the presence of symptoms, tumour markers and tumour characteristics).
- Investigation and follow-up of cystic lesions of the pancreas requires a multimodal approach, of which endoscopic ultrasound with biopsy is becoming an increasingly important component.
- While asymptomatic SCAs do not require intervention, some MCNs should be resected due to their underlying malignant potential.
- The management of PNETs will be dependent on the presence or absence of an underlying genetic syndrome, whether the tumour is hormonally active, and stage of disease.
- New adjuvant therapies have been shown to increase progression-free survival in patients with advanced neuroendocrine tumours.

⏵ Recommended videos:

- Laparoscopic radical antegrade pancreatosplenectomy – https://tinyurl.com/yc3jgg9k (IHPBA members only)
- Laparoscopic pancreaticojejunostomy during laparoscopic pancreaticoduodenectomy –https://tinyurl.com/y9gtsmwn
- University of Toronto video atlas of pancreatic techniques and procedures – https://tinyurl.com/ya96srgv

🌐 Full references available at **http://expertconsult.inkling.com**

Key references

2. Tanaka M, Fernandez-del Castillo C, Adsay V, et al. International consensus guidelines for management of intraductal papillary mucinous neoplasms and mucinous cystic neoplasms of the pancreas. Pancreatology 2012;12:183–97. PMID: 22687371.
   This international guideline outlines a detailed management strategy for the IPMN and MCN of the pancreas. Importantly it differs in its recommendations from the AGA guidelines.

23. Vege SS, Ziring B, Jain R, et al. and Clinical Guidelines Committee. AGA Institute guideline on the diagnosis and management of asymptomatic neoplastic cysts. Gastroenterology 2015;148:819–22. PMID: 25805375.
   This highly controversial paper presents a sound methodological approach to the available evidence for the management of incidental pancreatic cystic neoplasms. It recommends a conservative approach to investigation and follow-up with stopping points due to the lack of supporting evidence and potential to do harm.

28. Falconi M, Crippa S, Chari S, et al. Quality and assessment of the guidelines on cystic neoplasms of the pancreas. Pancreatology 2015;15:463–9. PMID: 26100659.
   This paper examines the quality of the published guidelines on pancreatic cystic neoplasms. It highlights the deficits of the current literature and tries to achieve expert consensus on clinically important questions.

48. Norton JA, Fraker DL, Alexander HR, et al. Surgery increases survival in patients with gastrinoma. Ann Surg 2006;244:410–9. PMID: 16926567.
   In a study of 160 patients with gastrinomas, 35 patients (with similar staged localised disease) who did not undergo resection were compared to those who underwent resection. After 12 years' follow-up, 29% of those who did not undergo surgery had developed hepatic metastases compared to 5% in the resected group (P <0.001).

56. Raymond E, Dahan L, Raoul JL, et al. Sunitinib malate for the treatment of pancreatic neuroendocrine tumors. N Engl J Med 2011;364:501–13. PMID: 21306237.
   One hundred and seventy-one patients with advanced and progressive PNETs were randomised in double-blind fashion to placebo or sunitinib. The trial was stopped early due to increased complications and death in the placebo group. An improved progression-free survival (11.5 vs 5.5 months, P <0.001) and reduced risk of death (105 vs 255, P=0.02) were seen in the treatment group.

57. Yao JC, Shah MH, Ito T, et al. Everolimus for advanced pancreatic neuroendocrine tumours. N Engl J Med 2011;364:514–23. PMID: 21306238.
   In a placebo-controlled randomised crossover design trial, 410 patients with advanced and progressive PNETs were enrolled to placebo or everolimus. In those patients who received everolimus there was a 65% reduction in risk of progression (median progression-free survival was 11 months vs 4.6 months) as compared to placebo. In addition, tolerance was high.

62. Jais B, Rebours V, Malleo G, et al. SCN of the pancreas: a multinational study of 2622 patients. Gut 2016;65:305–12. PMID: 26045140.
   This large multinational study reported on 2622 patients with serous cystadenomas accumulated over three decades. The key points were: asymptomatic patients do not need resection and disease-specific mortality is extremely rare.

18

Hepatobiliary and pancreatic trauma

Adam Brooks

Alex P. Navarro

Introduction

Hepatobiliary and pancreatic trauma represents one of the most challenging scenarios faced by specialist surgeons. Equally, the non-specialist will find such situations daunting due to the anatomical complexity of the region. Despite this, with a modern approach excellent outcomes are achievable in nearly all grades of hepato-pancreato-biliary (HPB) organ injury. The key factors required are meticulously accurate assessment of injury through imaging or at initial laparotomy, basic damage control manoeuvres performed with anatomical respect and understanding, and finally, definitive surgery undertaken by specialist HPB surgeons in complex cases.

This chapter will address the presentation, initial assessment and management of patients with liver, biliary and pancreatic injuries. The selection criteria for non-operative management will be discussed together with the indications for operative intervention. The factors guiding surgical options and decision-making will be examined. The spectrum of complications and likely outcomes following trauma will also be reviewed. The American Association for the Surgery of Trauma Organ Injury Scale (OIS) provides a description of the injury categorised from minor injury (grade 1) to severe injury (grade 6). The primary concern of the surgical team managing a trauma patient is the patient's physiological status and this will determine surgical management; however, the OIS allows guidance based on available evidence for the management of liver, biliary and pancreas injuries.

Liver trauma

The liver is the most frequently injured organ in abdominal trauma.[1] The serious nature of liver injuries was noted by J. Hogarth Pringle in his seminal monograph published in 1908, where he commented 'Rupture of the liver is fortunately an accident not often met with, but one which may be associated with a condition of the patient as serious as any one can meet with in surgical practice'.[2] The capacity for torrential haemorrhage from the liver means that the patient can quickly enter a vicious cycle of physiological derangements consisting of coagulopathy, hypothermia and metabolic acidosis, rapidly leading to death.[3] A review of 7454 cases of severe hepatic injury by Asensio[4] in 1990 found that exsanguination accounted for 54% of deaths.[4]

Mechanisms of liver injury

The liver can be injured by two principal injury mechanisms: blunt and penetrating trauma. Motor vehicle crashes account for the majority of blunt injuries, whereas gunshot wounds and stabbings constitute the major cause of penetrating injuries. A 2017 review of 10 years of outcomes for hepatic trauma in the UK showed that, of 4368 cases of hepatic trauma, 81% were caused by blunt injuries with 19% due to penetrating trauma.[5] Whilst this is typical for other European centres,[6] it differs from the experience in South Africa, where penetrating injuries account for 66% of liver trauma,[7] and in North America, where up to 86% of liver injuries are penetrating wounds.[8,9]

Blunt liver trauma may be divided according to the mechansim of injury: deceleration (shearing) and crush injury. Deceleration injuries tend to occur in road traffic crashes and falls from a height where there is rapid forceful movement of the liver relative to its fixed diaphragmatic attachments.[10] Crush injuries are caused by direct trauma to the liver area. The two types of injury may coexist, but tend to produce somewhat different types of liver injury. Deceleration or shearing injuries create lacerations in the hepatic parenchyma, typically between the right posterior section (segments 6 and 7), the right anterior section (segments 5 and 8), and the right/left liver plane (segments 5/8 vs segment 4A/4B) which can extend to involve major vessels. In contrast, a direct blow to the abdomen may lead to a crush injury, with damage to the central portion of the liver (segments 4, 5 and 8). Compression between the right lower ribs and the spine may also cause bleeding from the caudate lobe (segment 1). Blunt trauma can rupture Glisson's capsule and can also lead to subcapsular or intraparenchymal haematoma formation.

Penetrating injuries are usually associated with gunshot or stab wounds, with the former usually resulting in more tissue damage due to the cavitation effect as the bullet traverses the liver substance.

Injury to the hepatic veins and juxtahepatic vena cava can occur as a result of shearing stress in blunt trauma. Typically such injuries are associated with rapid pre-hospital death. However, it is worth noting that there may not be initial exsanguinating haemorrhage if the weight of the liver provides sufficient compression against the retroperitoneum allowing tamponade.

Classification of liver injury

The severity of liver trauma ranges from a minor capsular tear, with or without parenchymal injury, to extensive disruption involving both lobes of the liver with associated hepatic vein or vena caval injury. The American Association for the Surgery of Trauma has adopted for general use the classification of liver injury described initially in 1989 by Moore and colleagues, and revised subsequently in 1994[11] (Table 18.1). The hepatic injury grade is calculated from assessment of the liver injury using information derived from radiological study, operative findings or autopsy report. Where there are multiple injuries to the liver, the grade is advanced by one stage. As stated previously, it is the physiological status of the patient rather than the anatomical grade of injury that dictates management. Grade I–III injuries are considered minor; they represent 80–90% of all cases and the majority can be managed non-operatively. Grade IV–V injuries are considered severe injuries and non-operative management or surgical intervention can be applied depending on the patient's physiology and clinical progression. Grade VI lesions are generally regarded as incompatible with survival.

The initial assessment of an injured patient should be performed according to Advanced Trauma Life Support (ATLS) protocols developed by the American College of Surgeons Committee on Trauma. A rapid primary survey should be completed to identify immediately life-threatening injuries that require emergency intervention. Simultaneously, adequate intravenous access should be established to allow resuscitation to begin.

Table 18.1 • Hepatic injury scale used by the American Association for the Surgery of Trauma

Grade*		Description
I	Haematoma	Subcapsular, <10% surface area
	Laceration	Capsular tear, <1 cm parenchymal depth
II	Haematoma	Subcapsular, 10–50% of surface area
	Laceration	Intraparenchymal <10 cm in diameter, 1–3 cm parenchymal depth, <10 cm in length
III	Haematoma	Subcapsular, >50% surface area or expanding; ruptured subcapsular or parenchymal haematoma; intraparenchymal haematoma >10 cm or expanding
	Laceration	>3 cm parenchymal depth
IV	Laceration	Parenchymal disruption involving 25–75% of hepatic lobe or 1–3 Couinaud segments within a single lobe
V	Laceration	Parenchymal disruption involving >75% of hepatic lobe or >3 Couinaud segments within a single lobe
	Vascular	Juxtahepatic venous injuries – retrohepatic cava, major hepatic veins
VI	Vascular	Hepatic avulsion

*Advance one grade for multiple injuries up to grade II.

Current resuscitation strategies advocate haemostatic resuscitation and the transfusion of 1:1:1 blood, fresh frozen plasma and platelets.[12] Techniques and protocols based on 'Damage control' principles are encouraged.[13]

Diagnosis of liver injury

In penetrating abdominal trauma, hepatic injury should be considered in any patient with a wound to the abdomen. Hepatic injury should also be considered in patients with penetrating low thoracic wounds (it is important to be aware that the liver anteriorly is situated at the level of the nipple) and also in posterior penetrating wounds below a coronal plane at the tips of the scapulae.

Patients with major hepatic injury may present with profound clinical shock and abdominal distension. Hypotension resistant to fluid resuscitation combined with gross abdominal distension remains an indication for immediate laparotomy. The operative management options for patients in this situation will be discussed in detail subsequently. Emergency room thoracotomy with cross-clamping of the descending thoracic aorta is a dramatic but sometimes necessary intervention for exsanguinating abdominal haemorrhage.

The Eastern Association for the Surgery of Trauma (EAST) published practice guidelines for Emergency Department thoracotomy in 2015,[14] based on a meta-analysis of 72 studies that included 10 238 patients. This EAST study showed that overall survival rate for patients with penetrating thoracic trauma and signs of life on arrival at hospital was 21.3%, with a neurological intact survival of 11.7%. In patients with penetrating thoracic trauma with no signs of life on arrival at hospital, the survival rate was 8.3%, with a lower neurologically intact survival rate of 3.9%.

The outcomes for blunt injuries are worse. The survival rate of blunt trauma patients with signs of life on arrival at hospital is 4.6% and a neurological intact survival rate of 2.4%. Blunt trauma patients with no signs of life on arrival have an extremely poor survival rate of 0.7%. In the EAST analysis, one patient survived neurologically intact to discharge after blunt injury traumatic arrest with no signs of life out of 825 patients who underwent resuscitative thoracotomy in the Emergency Department.[14]

REBOA (Resuscitative Endovascular Balloon Occlusion of the Aorta) is a technique where a balloon catheter is inserted into the femoral artery and the balloon inflated within the aorta to control distal bleeding. Relatively limited data exist to support its widespread deployment in the exsanguinating trauma patient; however, the technique is rapidly gaining interest.[15,16]

> ✅ Emergency room thoracotomy remains a potentially life-saving manoeuvre in patients with significant injury. However, these patients are better served by rapid transport to the operating theatre.

Patients who are haemodynamically stable or respond to resuscitation should undergo appropriate imaging to determine the nature and extent of their injuries. Collateral history from the emergency services is invaluable – photos of the scene give information regarding the mechanism and likely injury pattern. Conscious patients may complain of abdominal pain. Shoulder tip pain may arise from blood in the subdiaphragmatic space causing phrenic nerve irritation.

Clinical signs may be detected during the initial examination including anterior abdominal wall bruising, which may indicate compression from a seatbelt, and flank bruising, which may indicate retroperitoneal extravasation of blood. Signs of localised or generalised peritonitis are recorded in the conscious patient. Baseline investigations consist of a full blood count (for haemoglobin and haematocrit), serum urea and electrolytes, liver function tests, a coagulation screen, and blood for crossmatching. It will often be necessary to activate local Major Transfusion Protocols. Following initial assessment, patients who are conscious but have haemodynamic instability with clinical signs of peritonitis should undergo laparotomy. In patients who are haemodynamically stable and have suspected liver injury, further diagnostic tests may be undertaken at this stage to define the nature of the injuries. An ideal test will establish the presence and extent of any liver injury together with providing information on concomitant visceral injury.

Formerly, diagnostic peritoneal lavage (DPL) was the procedure of choice for the quick diagnosis of haemoperitoneum, particularly in patients with an impaired level of consciousness and equivocal physical signs. However, DPL is invasive and a positive result for blood provides no information regarding either the site or the nature of the injury, and in the context of liver injury may lead to patients undergoing surgery where they may be better treated non-operatively.

An alternative investigation advocated in initial trauma evaluation is Focused Assessment with Sonography for Trauma (FAST).[17] This involves ultrasonographic assessment of the pericardium, right upper quadrant including Morrison's pouch, left upper quadrant and pelvis. This evaluation is not designed to identify the degree of organ injury, but rather the presence of blood. A large meta-analysis of the use of emergency ultrasonography for blunt abdominal trauma reported sensitivity rates ranging from 28% to 97% and specificity rates close to 100%.[18]

Rozycki et al. demonstrated a significant correlation between haemoperitoneum in the right upper quadrant and injury to the liver, and suggested that adherence to a pre-agreed protocol increased the reliability of ultrasound assessment of abdominal trauma.[19] Other centres have also reported that ultrasound is a reliable 'first' test for the assessment of a patient with suspected liver trauma.[20] However, an important cautionary note comes from a study by Richards et al.[21] In a series of 1686 abdominal ultrasound scans for trauma, 71 patients had bowel or mesenteric injury and 30 patients had a negative ultrasound scan (43% false-negative rate). Limitations of FAST include operator dependence, poor assessment of the retroperitoneum, unreliable detection of pneumoperitoneum and difficulty in scanning obese patients or those with overlying wounds.

Computed tomography (CT) is the 'gold standard' investigation for the evaluation of a patient with suspected liver trauma (**Fig. 18.1**). Modern CT protocols provide simultaneous arterial and portovenous images. CT has high sensitivity and specificity for detecting liver injuries. Specific CT features of liver trauma have been reported by a number of authors. Fang et al. described intraparenchymal 'pooling' of intravenous contrast that correlated strongly to the presence of ongoing haemorrhage.[22] Yokota and Sugimoto documented 'periportal tracking' to consist of a circumferential area of low attenuation around the portal triad.[23] Periportal tracking is thought to represent blood or fluid within the condensation of the Glissonian sheath around the portal structures and indicates the presence of injury to structures in the portal triad. If the sign is present in the periphery of the liver it may alert the clinician to the presence of a peripheral bile duct injury that in turn may present as a bile leak. Addition of oral contrast does not add to the diagnostic yield of CT in the assessment of liver injury and simply delays the acquisition of images.[24]

In order to maintain a balanced perspective, it is worthwhile considering some of the limitations of CT in the assessment of liver trauma. The CT-defined grade of injury may differ from the grade of liver injury found at operation, with the predominant tendency being to overdiagnose the grade of injury on CT as compared with subsequent operative findings. Croce et al. concluded that CT should not be used in isolation to estimate blood loss and that CT may not provide an accurate assessment of the extent of a liver laceration in some areas of the liver – specifically in the vicinity of the falciform ligament.[25]

Bearing the above limitations in mind, CT will define the extent of the liver injury and will be of value in the detection of injury to other intra-abdominal viscera, in particular pancreatic injury. CT allows the liver injury to be graded and thus will provide objective information if non-operative treatment is to be contemplated. Further refinements now permit accurate three-dimensional image reconstruction, and demonstration of vascular anatomy (CT angiography).

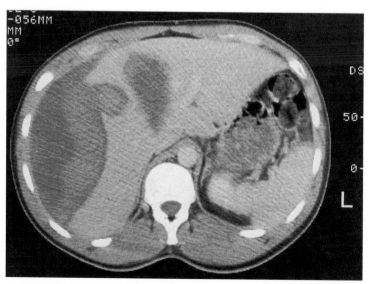

Figure 18.1 • CT image of a 25-year-old male who sustained a blunt injury to the right chest wall but was admitted to hospital haemodynamically stable. The scan shows a substantial subcapsular haematoma associated with an intraparenchymal laceration. This patient was managed successfully without operation.

Some authors recommend performing a whole-body CT (head, C-spine, chest, abdomen, pelvis) as the standard diagnostic tool during the early phase for patients with polytrauma, advocating that this will alter treatment in up to 34% of patients with blunt trauma.[26] A 30% reduction in mortality using this approach has also been reported.[27] Other arguments in favour of an imaging survey are the reduction in time from admission to intervention and consistency in managing haemodynamically unstable patients.[28]

In the UK, with the advent of the Major Trauma Network, most patients with significant HPB trauma will be managed in a Major Trauma Centre (MTC). The protocols described above mean that such patients will either proceed rapidly to theatre for laparotomy, or to CT for full 'head, neck, spine, thorax, abdomen, and pelvis' assessment. In this way early and highly detailed visceral imaging can be used to inform management decisions.

Other diagnostic/therapeutic modalities for the assessment and treatment of liver injury

Non-invasive imaging techniques such as magnetic resonance imaging (MRI) have the advantage of being free of ionising radiation, but increased cost aside, the time taken to produce a scan means that this technique is not yet widely used in the trauma setting.

Angiography plays a vital role in the non-operative management of liver injuries. Extravasation of contrast seen on CT requires emergency angiography and therapeutic angiographic embolisation for ongoing blood loss.[29] Angioembolisation is also reported following damage control surgery prior to removal of packs if re-bleeding is suspected.[30,31]

CT is the gold standard to define the extent of injury in a stable patient and can be applied rapidly in the context of UK Major Trauma Centres.

Management of liver injury: selection of patients for non-operative management

The feasibility of non-operative management of patients with intra-abdominal solid organ injury was first established in paediatric surgery but was subsequently extended to adult practice. Richie and Fonkalsrud described successful conservative management of four patients with liver injury in an era before the availability of CT.[32] Further indirect evidence for the feasibility of a non-operative approach came from a report published by White and Cleveland[33] in the same year. They reported a consecutive series of 126 patients with liver trauma, all of whom underwent laparotomy. Interestingly, 67 patients in this series (53%) had placement of a drain to the subhepatic space as their only liver-related surgical intervention at laparotomy. Subsequent studies have recognised that 50–80% of liver injuries stop bleeding spontaneously and this has led to a non-operative approach for blunt liver trauma in selected patients.

Non-operative management of liver trauma is now a well-established treatment option. Trunkey's group in Portland, Oregon, first defined in 1985 the following criteria for the selection of patients for non-operative management:

- haemodynamic stability;
- absence of peritoneal signs;
- availability of good-quality CT;
- an experienced radiologist;
- ability to monitor patients in an intensive care setting;
- facility for immediate surgery (and by implication, availability of an experienced liver surgeon);
- simple liver injury with <125 mL of free intraperitoneal blood;
- absence of other significant intra-abdominal injuries.[34]

Farnell et al. extended the threshold of haemoperitoneum to 250 mL and described specific liver injuries suitable for non-operative management.[35] Feliciano suggested subsequently that any blunt hepatic injury, regardless of its magnitude, should be managed without operation if the patient was haemodynamically stable and had a haemoperitoneum of <500 mL.[36] The degree of liver injury amenable to successful non-operative management has gradually extended over recent years, and most authors now believe that the ultimate decisive factor in favour of non-operative management is haemodynamic stability of the patient at presentation or after initial resuscitation, irrespective of the grade of liver injury on CT or the amount of haemoperitoneum.[37,38]

A 22-month prospective study from Memphis of the initial non-operative treatment of haemodynamically stable blunt hepatic trauma patients compared outcome to a matched cohort of blunt hepatic trauma patients treated operatively.[39] The study reported that of 136 patients with blunt trauma, 24 (18%) underwent emergency surgery. Of the remaining 112 patients, 12 (11%) failed conservative management (for causes not related to the liver injury in seven) and the remaining 100 patients were treated successfully without operation. Of these, 30% had minor injuries (grades I and II) but 70% had major injuries (grades III–V). This study concluded that non-operative management was safe for haemodynamically stable patients and that this was independent of the CT-delineated grade of the liver injury. The blood transfusion requirement and the incidence of abdominal complications were lower in the non-operatively treated group.

Reporting a single institutional experience, Boone et al. stated that 46 (36%) of 128 consecutive patients with blunt liver trauma were successfully treated non-operatively, including 23 patients with grade III and IV injuries.[37] A review of 495 patients from the published literature noted a success rate for non-operative treatment of 94%.[40] This was accomplished with a mean transfusion rate of 1.9 units, a complication rate of 6% and a mean hospital stay of 13 days. There were no liver-related deaths, nor were there any missed enteric injuries.

The current consensus view is that successful selection of patients for conservative treatment after blunt abdominal trauma cannot be carried out by CT alone, but that an overall assessment of suitability for such an approach must take into account the findings of careful repeated clinical examination and the results of close monitoring of haemodynamic and haematological parameters. If non-operative management is selected, haemodynamic instability is the predominant indication for intervention early in the clinical course whilst intervention (often radiological or endoscopic) may be required later for management of bile leak or intrahepatic collections.

If a non-operative strategy is selected, it should be borne in mind that the risk of hollow organ injury increases in proportion to the number of solid organs injured[41] and that there is a small but significant risk of delayed haemorrhage. However, it appears that the natural course of liver injuries is more analogous to that of lung or kidney injuries, rather than splenic injuries, in that any deterioration is usually gradual, with a fall in haemoglobin level or an increase in fluid requirement, rather than acute haemodynamic decompensation. Therefore, with close supervision, patients who fail with an initial non-operative approach can be detected early and treated appropriately.

Although non-operative management of haemodynamically stable patients with liver trauma has become the standard of care over the past decade, the role of in-hospital follow-up CT to monitor the injury remains controversial. Demetriades et al. reported that follow-up CT at a mean of 10 days after surgical intervention showed a 49% incidence of liver-related complications, most of which required subsequent intervention.[42] However, other authors suggest there is little evidence that follow-up CT provides additional information and rarely changes management.[43]

The management policy for abdominal gunshot injuries in most centres continues to be a mandatory laparotomy, regardless of the clinical presentation;[44] however, several studies have reported successful non-operative management of selected liver gunshot injuries.[45,46] In the study by Omoshoro-Jones et al., 26.6% of patients who presented with liver gunshot injuries were managed non-operatively, with an overall success rate of 94% and a morbidity rate of 36%, of which 3% were liver-related.[45] This approach is associated with the risk of failure to detect concomitant intra-abdominal visceral injury and therefore should only be considered in specialist centres with experience in management of liver trauma and appropriate facilities to deal with any complications that arise.

✓ Non-operative management is safe for haemodynamically stable patients with CT evidence of liver injury.

Operative management of liver injury

General strategy

Primary operative intervention is indicated for liver injury if the patient is haemodynamically unstable. Important prerequisites for a successful outcome are: adequate blood, platelets, fresh-frozen plasma and cryoprecipitate; an intensive care unit; the necessary diagnostic facilities to monitor and detect potential complications; and an experienced trauma and hepatobiliary surgeon. Although this is the ideal, in the recent past patients with liver trauma would routinely present to surgeons without specialist hepatobiliary experience and without the facilities available in liver surgery units. With the introduction of MTCs, this situation is now much less likely. However every operating general surgeon should have a basic understanding of the principles of HPB haemorrhage control. Once haemostatic control is achieved, specialist advice may be sought. Unfortunately the nature of HPB trauma has repeatedly demonstrated that anatomically misjudged initial surgical manoeuvres can lead to irretrievable situations. Therefore, the non-specialist should seek early assistance from an HPB surgeon.

Theatre set-up, patient positioning and choice of incision

The patient should be positioned in the crucifix position (both arms out on boards) with skin preparation applied from knees to neck. Following draping, access for both laparotomy and thoracotomy should be possible. The patient should be warmed. The theatre team should open general and liver instrument trays with additional vascular clamps. An autotransfusion (cell salvage) device should be available.

A long midline incision is the only appropriate incision for an emergency laparotomy. It has the advantages that it can be made rapidly, and extended proximally (to enter the chest after median sternotomy) or distally as required. Access to the liver can be improved by converting the incision into a 'T' by adding a right transverse component or to a 'Y' by adding a right lateral thoracotomy, although extension of the incision into the chest is exceptional. In situations where a delayed operation is being carried out after initial conservative management, for example to treat bile leakage or perform delayed resectional debridement, a subcostal incision with fixed costal margin retraction affords excellent access to the liver.

The authors advocate routine early use of a table-mounted retractor. Access is vitally important in high-grade injury and many HPB trauma scenarios will definitely require this level of access for a successful outcome.

> ✔ Surgeons operating on HPB trauma patients should be intimately familiar with their local table-mounted retractor.

Initial manoeuvres and intraoperative assessment

The operation should begin in the same manner as employed for non-differentiated trauma. Once the abdomen has been entered, blood and clots should be removed and packs inserted into each quadrant of the abdomen. In high-grade liver injury it will be clear at this point that a great deal of blood is flowing from the right upper quadrant. In stressful situations such as these it can be helpful to keep some simple sequential steps in mind. In the case of a significant liver injury the author uses:

- **PUSH** – Gently compress the liver closing any significant wounds and restore the anatomical shape. If bleeding stops, continue with PACKING the liver as definitive management.
- **PACK** – Bleeding stops = portovenous injury (packing only sufficient).
  Bleeding continues …
- **PRINGLE** – Bleeding stops = arterial injury (definitive procedure required).
  Bleeding continues …

Perihepatic packing

In many surgical texts 'four quadrant packing' constitutes the sum total of the instruction offered.

However, in the case of the right upper quadrant and HPB trauma, pack insertion requires a little more thought and technique. Perihepatic packing of the liver is aimed at restoring the anatomical conformation of the organ. As mentioned above, the most common injuries associated with major haemorrhage are distracted lacerations occurring near fixed ligamentous attachments. In order to 'reduce' the liver, these ligaments must be mobilised sufficiently to allow packs to compress lacerations within the liver parenchyma. Consider the example of a right/left laceration; blind direct packing over the dome of the liver results in the right lobe of the liver being pushed away from the left (which is fixed by the falciform ligament). The distraction is aggravated and the injury extended, potentially into major intra-parenchymal vessels. Such manoeuvres worsen hepatic injury and cause harm.

Such issues are easily avoided by dividing the falciform and right triangular ligaments prior to pack insertion. It is the authors' practice to rapidly divide the falciform ligament (using hand-held diathermy) until air is seen to rush into the coronary ligament. The left hand is then moved smoothly over the dome of the liver until the apex of the right triangular ligament is located. This can be isolated between fingers and divided, thus allowing medial rotation of the right lobe until the exposed raw surface of the right lobe contacts the corresponding left lobe surface (much like closing a book). The pressure achieved by packing should not be too aggressive – no degree of packing will overcome hepatic arterial bleeding; the aim is to overcome portovenous pressures. If this is greatly exceeded, necrosis will occur. Ongoing haemorrhage despite correct packing should lead to a Pringle manoeuvre (see below) and further assessment/intervention. It is not an indication for more aggressive and tighter packing.

A typical example of a well-reduced liver will have packs placed 'under' the right lobe between the posterior abdominal wall and the capsule, as well as over the anterior laceration (**Fig. 18.2**).

In most cases simple packing will induce haemostasis. At this point, further evaluation of the extent of liver injury should be delayed until the anaesthetist has replenished adequately the intravascular volume and stabilised the blood pressure. Attempts to evaluate the liver injury before adequate resuscitation may result in further blood loss, with worsening hypotension and acidosis.

The packs can subsequently be gently removed to allow a detailed evaluation of the type and extent of the liver injury. It should be borne in mind that a subcapsular haematoma may cover an area of ischaemic tissue and that parenchymal lacerations may be associated with damage to segmental bile ducts. If bleeding is arrested satisfactorily with

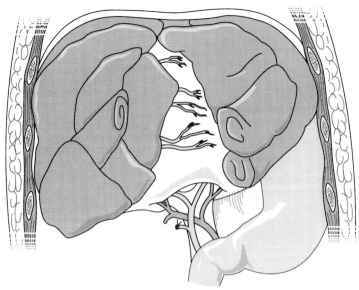

Figure 18.2 • Placement of gauze packs around the liver to compress the fracture.
Reproduced from Berne TV, Donovan AJ. Section 10. Injury and haemorrhage. In: Blumgart LH, Fong Y, editors. Surgery of the liver and biliary tract, 3rd edition. Vol. 2. Edinburgh: Churchill Livingstone; 1994. With permission from Elsevier.

low pressure packing, the appropriate decision is to reapply and plan to relook in 48 hours. In the vast majority of cases, haemostasis will occur and on delayed removal no further bleeding is seen. Occasionally the specialist HPB surgeon may directly repair a venous injury. The benefit of achieving immediate definitive repair is balanced against the increased risk of a packing strategy and should not be routinely undertaken.

In other situations where it is thought that definitive control of haemorrhage cannot be obtained, or patients are deemed critically unstable, coagulopathic or acidotic, perihepatic packing should be employed. Such an approach follows the principles of damage control surgery – rapid perihepatic packing, temporary closure of the abdomen with a negative-pressure device (Abthera™) and transfer to the intensive care unit (ICU) as soon as possible for continued resuscitation and rewarming. When the metabolic derangements have been corrected or improved, the patient can be taken back to theatre or transferred to a specialist centre for re-exploration and definitive treatment.[47]

The principal complications and limitations of perihepatic packing can be considered as 'early' or 'late'. Early complications include failure to control haemorrhage. However, this is relatively uncommon. Excessive packing will compromise caval blood flow, although this can be avoided by using an appropriate technique. The principal late complications of packing are infection and multiple organ dysfunction. The risk of septic complications led to a recommendation that liver packs should

be removed as soon as possible. However, Nicol et al. reported in a series of 93 patients requiring liver packing that an early re-look laparotomy at 24 hours rather than at 48 hours or later was associated with a higher incidence of re-bleeding necessitating re-packing, without any difference in the incidence of liver-related complications or intra-abdominal collections.[48]

> ✔ The first re-look laparotomy following packing for a liver injury should ideally be performed after 36–48 hours, only when hypotension, hypothermia, coagulopathy and acidosis have been corrected and appropriate personnel and equipment are available.

The Pringle manoeuvre

This is defined as temporary digital compression of the free edge of the lesser omentum (Pringle manoeuvre; **Fig. 18.3**). If there is active bleeding despite packing, a Pringle manoeuvre can be used diagnostically and compression can be maintained with an atraumatic vascular clamp (**Fig. 18.4**). If haemorrhage is arrested upon clamping, an arterial injury is diagnosed. The options for definitive management at this point are angiographic embolisation or the surgical options detailed below. If packing or a Pringle manoeuvre does not control bleeding, a hepatic vein or retrohepatic caval injury is suspected. Strategies to deal with these are described below. The clamp should be occluded only to the degree necessary to compress the blood

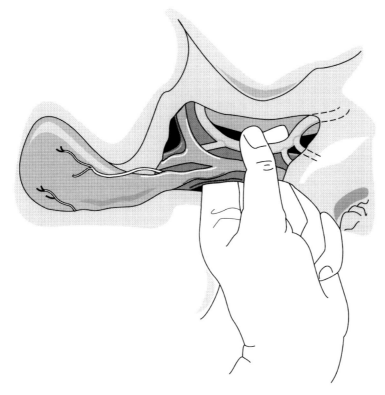

Figure 18.3 • Manual occlusion of the structures of the portal triad – the Pringle manoeuvre.

vessels and not to injure the common bile duct. A normal liver can tolerate inflow occlusion for up to 1 hour; however, the ability of a damaged liver to tolerate ischaemia may be impaired. Where a Pringle manoeuvre is concerned, the adage 'as long as is required, as short as possible' is best applied.

If there is significant hepatic venous bleeding, hepatic outflow control may also be required. Access to the suprahepatic cava is difficult even for the experienced liver surgeon, and in patients with an injured liver, such attempts can prove fatal. Consideration should be made of accessing and clamping the inferior vena cava within the pericardium either through opening the chest or splitting the diaphragm. Total vascular occlusion of the liver requires control of the inferior vena cava below the liver in addition to the suprahepatic cava but is poorly tolerated by an injured liver.

Techniques for hepatic surgical haemostasis

Exposed bleeding vessels can be suture-ligated, clipped or repaired to achieve haemostasis. The ultrasonic dissector is useful in removing damaged and non-viable hepatic parenchyma whilst exposing blood vessels. Diathermy coagulation can also be used.

Liver sutures are absorbable sutures on a large curved blunt-tipped needle, often used in conjunction with a bolster of haemostatic material. They can be used to approximate a fissured parenchymal injury and thus control haemorrhage as an alternative to exploration of the depths of the injury. The disadvantages of this technique are that vessels may continue to bleed, resulting in a cavitating haematoma, bile duct injuries may not be detected and the suture itself may cause further bleeding, ischaemia or intrahepatic bile duct injury (**Fig. 18.5**) and therefore this technique is not advocated.

Haemostatic adjuncts are a valuable part of the arsenal for liver injury. Fibrin glue has been used as an adjunctive measure; however, there are concerns regarding the use of fibrin glue in humans. Fatal hypotension following application of fibrin glue into a deep hepatic laceration has been reported.[49] There are a number of absorbable haemostatic patches available that have the advantage of allowing pressure to be applied and a number of them are impregnated with thrombin and fibrin to augment local coagulation.[50]

Resectional debridement

This technique involves removal of devitalised liver tissue down to normal parenchyma using the lines of the injury, rather than anatomical planes, as the

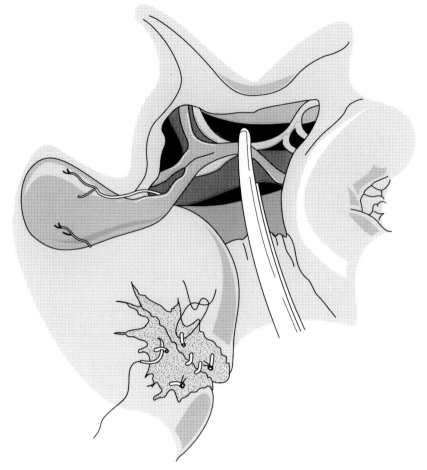

Figure 18.4 • Occlusion of the structures in the portal triad using a soft non-crushing clamp.

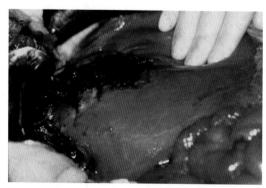

Figure 18.5 • Operative photograph demonstrating a liver injury with necrosis at the site of previously inserted liver sutures that had been applied in an attempt to arrest haemorrhage.

boundaries of the resection.[51] The optimum timing may be to combine debridement with pack removal, as necrotic tissue will be well demarcated at 48 hours post-injury. Resectional debridement is by definition 'non-anatomical' and may expose segmental bile ducts (**Fig. 18.6**). Disrupted bile ducts exposed in the periphery of the liver should be sutured or ligated in order to prevent postoperative bile leaks, as this troublesome complication will not necessarily be treatable by endoscopic transampullary biliary stenting. It is better to anticipate and avoid this complication.

Anatomical liver resection

The practical difficulties of undertaking formal anatomical liver resection in a patient with a significant liver injury, who will frequently have associated shock, coagulopathy and concomitant injury, are

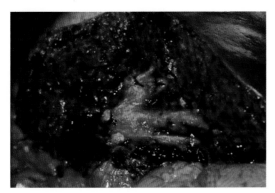

Figure 18.6 • Debridement of a liver injury managed 3 days before by packing has left the branches of the right portal pedicle exposed.

such that this type of treatment is not used widely. It is generally accepted that anatomical resections should be reserved for situations in which no other procedure adequately achieves haemostasis, such as with deep liver lacerations involving major vessels and/or bile ducts, where there is extensive devascularisation, or if there is major hepatic venous bleeding.

Strong et al. reported a single-centre series of 37 patients that underwent anatomical resection for liver trauma from an institutional experience of 287 patients with liver injury treated over a 13-year period.[52] Twenty-seven of these patients underwent right hemihepatectomy and overall there were three postoperative deaths (8% mortality rate). However, these excellent results achieved by a technically skilled liver surgeon and his unit may not be reproduced if the technique were more widely used.

Management of hepatic venous and retrohepatic caval injury

Suspicion that one of these serious injuries is present should be raised if the Pringle manoeuvre fails to arrest haemorrhage. In this situation, it is vital that a systematic approach be adopted. Injudicious mobilisation of the liver can cause exsanguination or embolisation of air or detached fragments of liver parenchyma. Therefore it is important to exclude anatomical vascular variants as a source of persistent bleeding. For example, there may be bleeding from the left liver due to the presence of a left hepatic artery arising from the left gastric artery or there may be bleeding from the right liver due to an aberrant right hepatic artery. These anatomical variants should be considered.

Persistent bleeding may then indicate the presence of hepatic venous or retrohepatic caval injury. These injuries account for about 10% of liver trauma cases, and there is no clear consensus on an optimal management strategy. Total vascular exclusion (clamping of the inferior vena cava and suprahepatic cava in addition to the Pringle manoeuvre) may be used. However, clamping the vena cava will seriously compromise venous return in a situation of major trauma and may be unwise. Veno-venous bypass (shunt from common femoral vein to left internal jugular or axillary vein) has the advantage of preserving venous return but is unlikely to be available. Atriocaval shunting has also been described and, combined with a Pringle manoeuvre, allows total vascular isolation of the liver; however, the reported mortality is such that the technique is no longer applied. Chen et al. reported on a series of 19 patients with blunt juxtahepatic venous injury from a group of 92 patients with blunt liver trauma over a 2-year period.[53] Ten of the 20 patients with isolated right hepatic vein injury were treated using an atriocaval shunt but the mortality in these 20 patients was 18 (80%), with one survivor in both the shunted and non-shunted groups. Of four patients with combined right and left hepatic vein injury, one was treated by liver transplantation but all four patients in this group died. The overall mortality rate in patients with juxtahepatic vein injury was 63%. The opportunity to optimise the outcome in patients with these serious injuries probably lies in packing followed by transfer to a specialist liver surgery unit.

Ex vivo surgery and liver transplantation

Ringe and Pichlmayr[54] reported a consecutive series of eight patients with severe liver trauma treated by total hepatectomy followed by liver transplantation. These patients had all undergone prior surgery for trauma, which had been followed by severe complications – uncontrollable bleeding in four and massive necrosis in four. Where a donor liver was not immediately available a temporary portocaval shunt was used as a bridging procedure. There was a high mortality in this group, with six out of eight patients dying from multiple organ failure or sepsis. The authors concluded that total hepatectomy can be a potentially life-saving procedure in exceptional emergencies in patients with major liver injuries. Heparinised coated tubes such as the Gott shunt can be used to bridge caval defects if total hepatectomy and excision of a caval segment is required in order to obtain haemostasis.[55] The shunt acts as a temporary bridge during the anhepatic phase and has been reported to remain patent over an 18-hour period. Whilst experience of this sort of surgery is extremely infrequent, awareness of the therapeutic potential is useful and small series continue to report encouraging results.[56]

Complications of liver trauma

Complications of non-operative management

Complications of non-operative management of liver trauma can be considered in three main categories. First, it should be borne in mind that complications can arise as a result of inappropriate selection of a patient for conservative management. If a patient has continued bleeding this may present as episodes of hypotension requiring fluid and blood replacement, impaired renal function and there may be evidence of coagulopathy. These features represent not so much a 'complication' as the natural progression of a patient with continued active intra-abdominal bleeding, and in such a case the policy of non-operative intervention will require reappraisal.

The second group of complications are those relating to coexisting injuries that have not been recognised at the time of initial presentation or become apparent after initial delay. Bile leaks may manifest as biliary peritonitis or as a localised bile collection. Endoscopic retrograde cholangiopancreatography (ERCP) is useful in diagnosing the source of a bile leak in patients with liver trauma treated non-operatively and also in postoperative patients. Perforations of the intestine are also at risk of being missed as the signs of abdominal tenderness may be attributed to intra-abdominal blood from the liver injury. The risk of missing this type of injury can be minimised by regular careful clinical observation. Intestinal perforation may become apparent on CT by the presence of free intraperitoneal fluid or gas. In Sherman et al.'s series of patients with liver trauma treated non-operatively, 4 of 30 (13%) patients initially treated without operation required subsequent laparotomy.[39] These were due to splenic injury in three patients and renal injury in one patient. Although the grade of injury to these organs is not specified, in all cases the injuries became apparent after a period of clinical observation. However, the authors concluded that this risk of missed solid organ injury does not obviate the benefits of initial non-operative management.

The third category of complication relates to the late complications of liver injury. Liver injury may give rise to a transient increase in liver transaminase enzymes. Their persistent elevation suggests significant liver injury. Septic complications such as intra-abdominal abscess and bile leak are recognised late complications and may require radiological, endoscopic or surgical intervention.

Postoperative complications after surgery for liver trauma

The complications after liver surgery for trauma are similar to those encountered after any form of hepatic surgery. Haemorrhage in the immediate postoperative period may be due to coagulopathy related to large-volume transfusion and may require correction with fresh-frozen plasma and platelet concentrates. If there is no evidence of a significant coagulopathy and bleeding continues, CT angiography may provide diagnostic information. Selective mesenteric angiography may permit therapeutic embolisation, but if this is unsuccessful, re-laparotomy will be indicated to assess and control the source of bleeding and to remove retained blood and clot. Bleeding in the later postoperative period may be due to haemobilia or bleeding from the biliary tree into the gut. It has been reported to occur in 1.2% of patients with liver trauma.[57]

Postoperative sepsis may be due to infected collections of bile or blood, or related to devitalised segments of liver parenchyma. CT is of value in diagnosis and may be used to guide placement of drains. Bile leakage from a drain site is not uncommon and usually ceases spontaneously; however, if it persists, ERCP may be all that is required to define the site of the leak and allow temporary stent placement. Arteriovenous fistula is not an uncommon complication after liver injury and can manifest as an arterioportal fistula resulting in portal hypertension.

Outcome after liver injury

The outcome after liver trauma is related not only to the severity of the injury but also to the severity of any associated injury. Most series report mortality rates of approximately 10–15%; however, the large variation in case mix between different centres makes comparison difficult. In a large series of 1000 cases of liver trauma from Houston, an overall mortality of 10.5% was reported.[8] White and Cleveland documented a similar mortality rate, with eight deaths occurring in a consecutive series of 126 patients (6.3%).[33] The results in the series reported by Schweizer et al. recorded an overall mortality rate of 12% (21 deaths in 175 patients), with a progressively higher mortality rate associated with an increasing grade of liver injury.[58] In a series of 337 patients, Kozar et al. reported 37 hepatic-related complications in 25 patients; 63% (5 of 8) of patients with grade V injuries developed complications, 21% (19 of 92) of patients had grade IV injuries, but only 1% (1 of 130) of patients had grade III injuries.[59] The mechanism of injury has an important bearing on the mortality rate, with blunt trauma carrying a higher mortality rate (10–30%) than penetrating liver trauma (0–10%). While most early deaths seem to be due to uncontrolled haemorrhage and associated injuries, most late deaths result from head injuries and sepsis with multiple organ failure.

Extrahepatic biliary tract trauma

Non-iatrogenic injury to the extrahepatic biliary tract is uncommon and encountered only rarely by surgeons outside specialist hepatobiliary centres. Most injuries are due to penetrating rather than blunt abdominal trauma. Biliary tract injury is diagnosed infrequently before operation and is often only recognised incidentally at laparotomy. Extrahepatic bile duct injury due to blunt trauma is only rarely associated with injury to the portal vein or hepatic artery. This may be explained by the increased length, tortuosity and elasticity of the vascular structures. Furthermore, a vascular injury, especially portal vein rupture, is likely to be associated with a high immediate mortality.

Incidence of biliary injury

The reported incidence of injury to the extrahepatic biliary system varies between 1% and 5% of patients who sustain abdominal trauma.[60] In a review of 5070 patients who sustained blunt and penetrating abdominal trauma, Penn reported a 1.9% incidence of gallbladder injury.[61] Soderstrom et al. identified 31 patients (2.1%) with gallbladder injury in a group of 1449 patients who sustained blunt abdominal trauma and underwent exploratory laparotomy.[62] In a further review of 949 patients undergoing laparotomy for acute trauma, there were 32 injuries to the gallbladder (3.4%) and five to the common bile duct (0.5%).[63] Burgess and Fulton reported that, over a 5-year period, 24 of 184 patients with abdominal trauma had extrahepatic bile duct or gallbladder injury as well as liver injury.[64] They reported that this injury was often seen with severe hepatic trauma and in association with multiple organ injury. Dawson et al. reviewed the results of treatment of all patients with porta hepatis injuries presenting to a level I trauma centre in Seattle over an 11-year period.[65] A total of 21 patients (0.21% of 10 500 admissions) had injuries to the portal triad, of whom 11 (52%) died. Isolated extrahepatic bile duct injury occurred in four of these patients. Injuries to the portal vein or hepatic artery, either in isolation or in association with extrahepatic bile duct injury, were associated with the worst prognosis. Of note is the fact that in none of the 21 cases was the diagnosis of the injury made preoperatively.[66] Most series report a median age of approximately 30 years and there are many reports in children.

Classification of biliary injury

The gallbladder is the most frequently injured part of the extrahepatic biliary tract. The largest reported series of extrahepatic biliary tract injuries consists of 53 patients, of whom 45 (85%) sustained injury to the gallbladder and eight (15%) had an injury to the bile duct.[66] Kitahama et al. reported the gallbladder to be involved in 32 (80%) of 40 patients, while ductal injury occurred in 12 (30%), some patients having multiple injuries.[67]

Injury to the gallbladder resulting from blunt trauma can be classified as contusion, avulsion or perforation. In addition to these three main types of injury, Penn added traumatic cholecystitis as a pathological entity.[68] The most common type of gallbladder injury is perforation. Avulsion of the gallbladder may refer to the organ being partially or completely torn from the liver bed while still attached to the bile duct, or it may signify complete separation from all attachments with the organ lying free in the abdomen. Contusion is probably under-reported, as it will be recognised only if laparotomy is performed. The natural course of an untreated gallbladder contusion is not known, although it is likely that the majority resolve without further complication. It has been speculated that an intramural haematoma might result in necrosis of the gallbladder wall and result in a subsequent perforation. There have been a number of reports of delayed rupture of the gallbladder, and it is plausible that unrecognised contusion of the gallbladder might lead to such a delayed presentation.

Bile duct injury is classified according to the site of injury and according to whether the transection is partial or complete. Partial duct injuries are often referred to as 'tangential' wounds. Penetrating injuries can affect any part of the extrahepatic biliary system; however, the commonest sites of injury due to blunt trauma are at the point where the common bile duct enters the pancreas and where the biliary confluence exits from the liver. These sites are at points of maximum fixation, which accounts for their propensity to injury.

Isolated injury to the extrahepatic biliary tract is very uncommon. The liver is the organ most commonly injured in association with biliary tract trauma (approximately 80% of cases), with the duodenum, stomach, colon and pancreas being the next most frequently reported. Associated vascular injuries are relatively rare; however, inferior vena cava and portal vein injuries are more commonly reported than those to the hepatic artery, renal vessels or aorta.

Presentation and diagnosis of biliary injury

Clinical presentation of the vast majority of bile duct injuries can be divided into two broad categories. The first contains patients in whom clinical signs or associated injury lead to laparotomy with early diagnosis and surgical management (early presentation); these patients generally present with hypovolaemic shock or signs of an acute abdomen. The second category of patient has a delay (>24 hours) in diagnosis and definitive therapy (delayed presentation). These patients comprised over half the cases (53.2%) in a review of combined series.[68] In addition, a third category of patient, representing a very small proportion of those who sustain a bile duct injury, may present with obstructive jaundice months or even years after the initial trauma (late presentation). In these patients, the bile duct injury is always isolated. Compromise of the blood supply to the duct may occur either at the time of the primary injury or at operation during the Pringle manoeuvre, and this may contribute to the development of a late biliary stricture. Bourque et al. reported that the delay between clinical presentation and surgical intervention for isolated bile duct injury averaged 18 days, with a range from several hours to 60 days.[69] Michelassi and Ranson reported that biliary injury was not recognised at initial operation in 11 (12%) of 91 patients with extrahepatic biliary tract trauma,[68] whereas Dawson and Jurkovich reported that 41% of bile duct injuries were missed at initial laparotomy.[70]

If a non-operative course of management for abdominal trauma is adopted, suspicion of an extrahepatic bile duct injury may be raised by CT evidence of a central liver injury involving the porta hepatis or the head of the pancreas, the presence of fluid collections in the subhepatic space, or evidence of periportal tracking of haematoma.[23] The diagnostic procedure of choice is ERCP, and if a duct injury is identified this may be treated by endoscopic stenting.[71]

Intraoperative recognition of biliary tract injury requires a high index of suspicion. The presence of free bile in the peritoneal cavity, or the presence of bile staining in the hepatoduodenal ligament or retroperitoneum, is a sign of injury to the extrahepatic biliary tract. Biliary tract injury must also be suspected if there is profuse bleeding from the hepatic artery or portal vein, particularly following blunt trauma, as the bile duct is also likely to be injured. Penetrating wounds near the porta hepatis require careful examination. If routine dissection does not reveal the location of the injury, fine-needle intraoperative cholangiography via the gallbladder or common bile duct may identify the site. Cystic duct cholangiography should be considered after cholecystectomy for traumatic gallbladder injury to avoid missing an associated bile duct injury.

It is possible for a patient who has sustained blunt abdominal trauma to be discharged from hospital only to return days or weeks later with a combination of symptoms and signs, including jaundice, abdominal distension, nausea, vomiting, anorexia, abdominal pain, low-grade fever or weight loss – a clinical picture similar to that seen in patients with intraperitoneal bile leakage following cholecystectomy. When jaundice develops after abdominal trauma, missed extrahepatic biliary injury must be considered.

Operative management of biliary injury

Many patients with extrahepatic biliary tract injury present in shock due to associated haemorrhage, and the priority at laparotomy is to identify and control haemorrhage. The report of Dawson et al. demonstrates that these patients are at risk of exsanguinating on the operating table.[65] Injuries to the gallbladder are best treated by cholecystectomy.[72] Primary repair of a clean and simple partial or complete transection of the common duct using absorbable sutures such as 4/0 polydioxanone over a T-tube inserted through a separate choledochotomy has been described. However, this type of repair is not appropriate if there is any evidence of duct contusion, loss of ductal tissue or possible injury to the hepatic artery as this may increase the risk of late development of an ischaemic stricture. In general, it is therefore safer to recommend that most injuries should be managed by fashioning a Roux-en-Y hepatico-jejunostomy as in the management of iatrogenic bile duct injuries. Such a repair should be undertaken by a surgeon experienced in these anastomoses, as the best outcomes are achieved at the first repair.

Outcome after biliary injury

Injuries of this nature are associated with a mortality rate of 10% from concomitant injuries.[67] Septic complications and bile leakage account for most of the early morbidity and may require operative intervention. Late morbidity after repair of a traumatic biliary tract injury is unusual; however, jaundice or episodes of ascending cholangitis suggest a stricture of the ductal system.

Pancreatic trauma

Injuries to the pancreas are uncommon, accounting for 1–4% of severe abdominal injuries, and usually occur in young men. In a report of 51 425 patients from the Trauma Register of the German Society of Trauma Surgery, 9268 (18%) had documented abdominal injuries and 284 (3.1%) had a pancreatic injury.[73]

Mechanisms of pancreatic injury

Deceleration injury and direct blunt trauma are major mechanisms of pancreatic trauma, with the neck of the gland being at risk of transection across the vertebral column. In children, the classic injury arises from bicycle handlebars. The deep location of the pancreas means that considerable force is needed to cause an injury and this level of force will often be sufficient to damage other organs.

Diagnosis of pancreatic injury

Pancreatic injury should be suspected in any patient with penetrating trauma to the trunk, particularly if the entry site is between the nipples and the iliac crest, and in any patient with blunt compression trauma of the upper abdomen.

In an early study, Moretz et al. found that there was no reliable correlation between initial serum amylase and pancreatic injury.[74] In a later report, Takishima et al. retrospectively studied admission serum amylase values in a series of 73 patients with blunt pancreatic trauma treated in a single institution over a 16-year period.[75] Sixty-one (84%) of these patients had a raised serum amylase level. Of interest, the serum amylase level was found to be abnormal in all patients admitted more than 3 hours after trauma. Recent studies suggest that lipase may be a more sensitive marker of pancreatic injury than amylase.[76]

For those patients not requiring immediate laparotomy for haemodynamic instability, contrast-enhanced CT is the investigation of choice (**Fig. 18.7**) for pancreatic injury and to exclude concomitant intra-abdominal visceral injury. Reported CT features of pancreatic injury include free intraperitoneal fluid, localised fluid in the lesser sac, retroperitoneal fluid, pancreatic oedema or swelling and changes in the peripancreatic fat. The presence of fluid in the lesser sac between the pancreas and the splenic vein is reported by Lane et al. to be a reliable sign in blunt pancreatic injury.[77] However, Sivit and Eichelberger reported that this radiological sign was rarely the only abnormal CT finding in pancreatic injury.[78] It should be borne in mind that many of these CT features are also seen in acute pancreatitis (and furthermore that acute pancreatitis may occur as a result of blunt abdominal trauma). There is also evidence from older studies that CT tends to underdiagnose pancreatic injury. Akhrass et al.

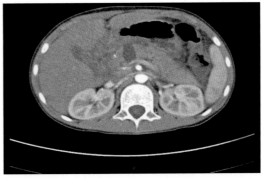

Figure 18.7 • CT showing a complete transection of the neck of the pancreas in an 8-year-old boy who had fallen out of a tree.

evaluated the clinical course of 72 patients with pancreatic injury admitted over a 10-year period.[79] Seventeen of these patients underwent CT as part of their initial assessment and this was reported as normal in nine. Eight of these patients underwent laparotomy (principally for suspected associated splenic injury) and three were found to have pancreatic injury requiring distal pancreatectomy. Newer, non-invasive imaging modalities such as magnetic resonance cholangiopancreatography (MRCP) have been reported in the assessment of patients with suspected pancreatic trauma.[80] Increased sophistication with the use of this technique may allow for accurate assessment of pancreatic ductal integrity; however, this is not indicated in the acute situation with a hypotensive patient and is best reserved for delayed imaging when ductal injury is suspected.

Classification of pancreatic injury

Of the various proposed classification schemes, Lucas suggested in an early report that appropriate treatment be formulated according to the type of injury.[81] This classification system divides pancreatic injuries into three groups:

- grade I – superficial contusion with minimal damage;
- grade II – deep laceration or transection of the left portion of the pancreas;
- grade III – injury of the pancreatic head (**Fig. 18.8**).

The American Association for the Surgery of Trauma (AAST) Organ Injury Scale is widely used to classify pancreatic trauma (Table 18.2). The most common site of injury is the neck of the pancreas. The relative frequency of pancreatic injuries reported in collected reviews is represented in **Fig. 18.9**. The AAST organ injury scale is the

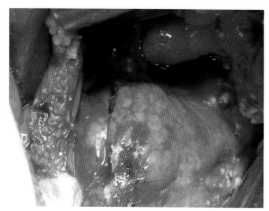

Figure 18.8 • Operative photograph of a transection injury along the neck of the pancreas resulting from a direct blow to the abdomen. This injury was managed by distal pancreatectomy and splenectomy.

most widely used and can be used to determine the management.

Initial management of pancreatic injury

In a major retrospective clinical casenote review of pancreatic trauma from six hospitals, Bradley et al. demonstrated a significant association between pancreas-related morbidity and injury to the main pancreatic duct.[83] Delayed intervention (due to delay in recognition of main pancreatic duct injury) was associated with high morbidity. In this study, CT was unreliable for the assessment of main pancreatic ductal integrity and an accurate assessment required ERCP; however, MRCP with contrast could be used.

✅ Assessment of the integrity of the main pancreatic duct is critical to the treatment of pancreatic injury.

Operative management of pancreatic injury

The mainstay of treatment remains operative as pancreatic injuries are usually diagnosed at laparotomy undertaken because of injury to surrounding structures. The region of the head of the pancreas should be thoroughly inspected and retroperitoneal blood, gas or bile around the duodenum or head of pancreas are markers of an injury that requires further thorough evaluation. Equally in blunt trauma laparotomy, the body of the pancreas should always be inspected for injury.

The important principles at operation are to gain good access to allow thorough inspection of the gland. Access to the lesser sac is best done by creating a window in the gastrocolic omentum outside the gastroepiploic arcade to allow examination of the body of the pancreas. A Kocher manoeuvre is necessary to permit palpation of the head of the pancreas between the thumb and fingers. A thorough inspection of the base of the transverse mesocolon is also undertaken. Injury to the pancreas is suspected if retroperitoneal haemorrhage can be seen through the base of the mesocolon or the lesser omentum. Absence of any sign of haemorrhage over the pancreas and duodenum makes injury unlikely.

Experience of patients with pancreatic injury from Durban led to the recommendation for operative treatment in patients with penetrating or gunshot injury and signs of peritoneal irritation.[84] In this large series of 152 patients with pancreatic trauma presenting over a 5-year period, 63 patients had been shot, 66 stabbed and 23 had blunt trauma. The mainstay of treatment was exploratory laparotomy followed by drainage of the pancreatic injury site. Large-bore soft Silastic drains were used to minimise the risk of drain erosion into a major vessel. The mortality rates were 8% after gunshot injury, 2% after stab wounds and 10% after blunt trauma. The majority of these deaths were attributed to damage of other organs. The proportions of patients that

Table 18.2 • Classification of pancreatic from the American Association for the Surgery of Trauma (AAST)

Grade*	Type of injury	Description of injury
I	Haematoma	Minor contusion without duct injury
II	Laceration	Superficial laceration without duct injury
III	Haematoma	Major contusion without duct injury or tissue loss
IV	Laceration	Major laceration without duct injury or tissue loss
V	Laceration	Distal transection or parenchymal injury with duct injury
	Laceration	Proximal† transection or parenchymal injury involving ampulla
	Laceration	Massive disruption of pancreatic head

*Advance one grade for multiple injuries up to grade III.
†Proximal pancreas is to the patient's right of the superior mesenteric vein.

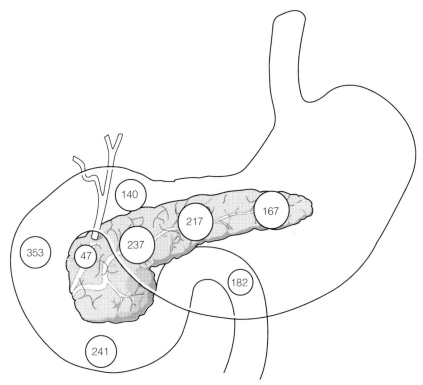

Figure 18.9 • Distribution of pancreatic injuries in the world literature. Note the preponderance of injuries in the junctional area of the neck of the gland.
Reproduced from Frey CF, Wardell JW. Section 9. Injuries to the pancreas. In: Trede M, Carter DC, editors. Surgery of the pancreas. Edinburgh: Churchill Livingstone; 1993. With permission from Elsevier.

developed pancreatic fistulas in the three groups were 14%, 9% and 13%, respectively. The authors concluded that 'conservative' surgical drainage (avoiding pancreatic resection) was justified after pancreatic injury.

The management of pancreatic injuries of the body/tail depends on the integrity of the pancreatic duct. For AAST grade I and II injuries where there is only a haematoma or laceration of the duct but no duct injury, closed system drainage is all that is required.

Grade III injuries involve the pancreatic duct and are to the left of the superior mesenteric vein (SMV). These are managed by distal pancreatectomy, with closure of the duct by suture or staples and placement of a closed drain system.

Spleen-preserving distal pancreatectomy is occasionally performed in the elective setting; rarely it is possible in pancreatic trauma, and only when the patient is haemodynamically stable and the injury is limited to the pancreas. Grade IV injuries are to the right of the SMV and involve the parenchyma and duct but not the ampulla; drainage is advocated.

Simplified management guidelines based on the treatment protocols developed during the treatment of 124 pancreatic injuries at the University of Tennessee[85] also advocate simple drainage alone for proximal pancreatic injuries. Of 37 (30%) patients with proximal injuries, the 'pancreas-related' morbidity was 11% – principally the sequelae of pancreatic fistulas. Of 87 distal pancreatic injuries, the integrity of the main pancreatic duct was not established in 54 (62%). Patients thought to have a high probability of duct transection were treated by distal pancreatectomy. A concern with simple drainage for injuries in the head of the pancreas is persistent pancreatic fistula, and thus a surgical alternative is to drain the head of the pancreas into a Roux-en-Y limb of jejunum.

Moncure and Goins described their experience over a 6-year period with a consecutive series of 44 patients with pancreatic injury,[86] of which penetrating abdominal trauma accounted for the majority of cases. Coexistent duodenal injuries were treated by primary closure in 21% and more complex duodenal exclusion techniques were used in 20%. The most frequent complications were intra-abdominal abscesses (31%) and pancreatic fistulas (16%).

Krige et al. reported on a series of 110 patients with pancreatic injuries after blunt trauma.[87] One hundred and one patients underwent a total of 123 operations, including drainage of the pancreatic injury ($n = 73$), distal pancreatectomy ($n = 39$) and Whipple resection ($n = 5$). The overall complication rate was 74.5% and the mortality rate was 16.4%. Only two of the 18 deaths were attributable to the pancreatic injury. Mortality increased exponentially as the number of associated injuries increased.

Finally, in grade V injuries where there is devitalisation of the head of the pancreas with massive disruption, damage control techniques should be applied as the initial part of a staged Whipple procedure. These are a major challenge, but fortunately are relatively rare, occurring in approximately 5% of all pancreatico-duodenal injuries.[88] However, where indicated it is the only option for survival and can be performed successfully. Where trauma pancreatico-duodenectomy is required, a staged approach is essential. Removal of the resection specimen should represent the end of the first stage. The stomach and jejunum may be left stapled, and the bile duct tied off (to allow dilatation and an easier hepatico-jejunostomy) or drained. The cut surface of the pancreatic neck should also be drained. The surgeon may also consider total pancreatectomy at this point, especially if it is judged that the patient would not survive a later pancreatico-jejunostomy leak. The second stage would follow temporary abdominal closure (using an Abthera device) and a period of resuscitation on ICU (24–48 hours). Ideally the reconstruction would then be performed with a physiologically well patient, free of inotropic or pressor organ support. The principles of treatment are to ensure that haemorrhage from concomitant injuries is dealt with first, as this is likely to be the major source of mortality. Similarly, a prolonged operative procedure should be avoided in a potentially unstable patient and the involvement of an experienced pancreatic surgeon is desirable.

Duodenal injuries can be closed primarily or drained into a Roux loop. Bile duct injuries may be repaired primarily over a T-tube or drained into a Roux limb of jejunum.

> ✅ Trauma pancreatico-duodenectomy is indicated in rare cases of severe pancreatico-duodenal complex disruption.

Complications of pancreatic injury

The most common post-traumatic complications include necrotising pancreatitis, pseudocyst formation, pancreatic abscesses and pancreatic fistula. Cerwenka et al. reported the incidence of these complications to be 15%, 9%, 6% and 4%, respectively.[89] The principles regarding management are similar to those for treating these complications when they arise as a result of pancreatitis or pancreatic surgery. Inflammation of the pancreas after trauma behaves in much the same way as acute biliary or acute alcohol-induced pancreatitis, with the possible exception that there is a higher incidence of development of local complications such as pseudocyst – possibly relating to the nature of duct disruption in trauma. The Cape Town group reported that, of a series of 64 patients with pancreatic trauma, pseudocysts developed in 15 patients (23%), of whom eight had a duct injury demonstrated by endoscopic retrograde pancreatography.[90] Patients with pseudocysts related to distal duct injury were treated successfully by percutaneous aspiration. Three patients with duct injuries in the neck/body region underwent distal pancreatectomy. Pseudocysts related to ductal injury in the head of the pancreas were drained internally by Roux-en-Y cyst-jejunostomy. The authors concluded that traumatic pancreatic pseudocysts associated with a peripheral duct injury may resolve spontaneously, whereas those associated with injuries to the proximal duct would more likely require surgical intervention. Alternative treatment strategies include endoscopic transpapillary or transmural drainage of the pseudocyst.

The incidence of pancreatic fistula after surgery for trauma is dependent on the type of procedure, with some evidence that the fistula rate is higher after drainage procedures than after resection. Successful insertion of pancreatic duct stents has been reported for management of major pancreatic duct disruption; however, the incidence of long-term ductal stricture is high and therefore the role of pancreatic duct stenting needs to be further defined.[91]

> ✅ Management of post-traumatic pseudocysts and fistulas will depend on the time from injury, presence of ongoing ductal leak, site of leak and presence of debris within a pseudocyst cavity. The optimal treatment strategy should involve a multidisciplinary approach in a specialist unit employing similar principles to those of managing these complications following an attack of acute pancreatitis.

Conclusion

The contemporary management of patients with suspected liver, biliary or pancreatic injury involves simultaneous clinical assessment and haemostatic resuscitation followed, in haemodynamically stable patients, by CT. If surgical intervention is required, the mainstay of treatment is to control haemorrhage. In European healthcare systems, the optimum care of the patient may consist of packing followed by transfer to a regional hepato-pancreato-biliary unit. A paper by Hoyt et al. examining preventable causes of death in 72 151 admissions with abdominal trauma to North American level I trauma centres identified abdominal injury as the cause of death in 287, with liver injury being responsible for 92 deaths.[92] Delays in packing were highlighted as a preventable cause of death, as was a need for better understanding of the endpoints to be achieved by packing. The conclusion of this large survey was that the management of liver injury remains a major technical challenge.

Acknowledgement

The authors wish to thank John-Joe Reilly.

Key points

- Management of patients with suspected liver, biliary or pancreatic injury involves simultaneous clinical assessment and haemostatic resuscitation.
- Haemodynamic instability resistant to blood resuscitation associated with clinical signs of peritonism is an indication for immediate laparotomy.
- Patients who are haemodynamically stable or who respond to initial fluid resuscitation should undergo immediate CT.
- Laparotomy is generally required for patients with an abdominal gunshot wound.

Liver trauma

- Non-operative management of liver trauma is now a well-established treatment option and should be augmented with angiographic techniques where a contrast blush is detected on CT.
- Significant liver haemorrhage can initially be controlled at operation by manual compression of the liver parenchyma, appropriate liver packing, or application of the Pringle manoeuvre.
- Perihepatic packing is a highly effective technique to control venous bleeding from the liver.
- Resectional debridement of non-viable hepatic parenchyma may be undertaken successfully where inflow/outflow vessels are injured.
- Other techniques to control haemorrhage include hepatotomy and suture ligation of vessels within the laceration, although this technique should only be employed by surgeons experienced in both trauma and liver surgery.
- Postoperative complications include bile leakage or sepsis, and may require radiological, endoscopic or surgical intervention.

Extrahepatic biliary tract trauma

- This uncommon injury is more likely to be due to penetrating rather than blunt abdominal trauma.
- It is rarely diagnosed before operation and is usually recognised incidentally at laparotomy.
- Concomitant vascular injury of the portal vein or hepatic artery is rare.
- ERCP may demonstrate bile leakage and allow therapeutic insertion of a biliary stent.
- Definitive operative intervention for gallbladder trauma is cholecystectomy.
- Roux-en-Y hepatico-jejunostomy is the operation of choice for most injuries to the bile duct.

Pancreatic trauma

- This is most commonly diagnosed by CT; however, in the non-acute setting, contrast MRCP may be undertaken to assess pancreatic duct integrity and may allow therapeutic stenting if leakage of contrast is identified.
- Exploratory laparotomy and drainage of the pancreas is recommended for pancreatic parenchyma injuries.
- Main pancreatic duct injuries in the neck, body and tail may be managed by distal pancreatectomy.
- Pancreatico-duodenectomy is indicated in rare cases of severe pancreatico-duodenal complex disruption.

Key references

39. Croce MA, Fabian TC, Menke PG, et al. Nonoperative management of blunt hepatic trauma is the treatment of choice for hemodynamically stable patients: results of a prospective trial. Ann Surg 1995;221(6):744–53; discussion 53–5. PMID: 7794078.

This study concluded that non-operative management was safe and the procedure of choice for haemodynamically stable patients and that this was independent of the CT grade of the liver injury.

87. Krige JE, Kotze UK, Hameed M, et al. Pancreatic injuries after blunt abdominal trauma: an analysis of 110 patients treated at a level 1 trauma centre. S Afr J Surg 2011;49(2):58, 60, 2–4 passim. PMID: 21614975.

This study reported on a series of 110 patients with pancreatic injuries after blunt trauma. Excellent results were achieved applying drainage, or distal pancreatectomy depending on the location of the injury and integrity of the pancreatic duct.

92. Hoyt DB, Bulger EM, Knudson MM, et al. Death in the operating room: an analysis of a multi-center experience. J Trauma 1994;37(3):426–32. PMID: 8083904.

This study reported on the preventable causes of death in 72151 admissions with abdominal trauma to North American level I trauma centres. Abdominal injury was identified as the cause of death in 287, with liver injury responsible for 92 deaths. The importance of early application of liver packing as the predominant surgical technique in the management of liver trauma was highlighted.

Index

NB: Page numbers followed by *f* indicate figures, *t* indicate tables and *b* indicate boxes.

Index